Type 1 Diabetes: Diagnosis and Management

Type 1 Diabetes: Diagnosis and Management

Editor: Solomon Fleming

AMERICAN
MEDICAL PUBLISHERS
www.americanmedicalpublishers.com

AMERICAN
MEDICAL PUBLISHERS
www.americanmedicalpublishers.com

Cataloging-in-Publication Data

Type 1 diabetes : diagnosis and management / edited by Solomon Fleming.
p. cm.
Includes bibliographical references and index.
ISBN 978-1-63927-128-3
1. Diabetes. 2. Diabetes--Diagnosis. 3. Diabetes--Treatment. 4. Diabetes--Complications.
5. Endocrine glands--Diseases. 6. Carbohydrate intolerance. I. Fleming, Solomon.
RC660 .T97 2022
616.462--dc23

American Medical Publishers,
41 Flatbush Avenue,
1st Floor, New York,
NY 11217, USA

ISBN 978-1-63927-128-3 (Hardback)

Contents

Preface

The world is advancing at a fast pace like never before. Therefore, the need is to keep up with the latest developments. This book was an idea that came to fruition when the specialists in the area realized the need to coordinate together and document essential themes in the subject. That's when I was requested to be the editor. Editing this book has been an honour as it brings together diverse authors researching on different streams of the field. The book collates essential materials contributed by veterans in the area which can be utilized by students and researchers alike.

Type 1 diabetes is a form of diabetes in which very little or no amount of insulin is produced by the pancreas. It is also known as juvenile diabetes. The major symptoms of type 1 diabetes include frequent urination, increased hunger and thirst, weight loss, blurry vision, tiredness and poor wound healing. It is caused by genetic or environmental factors. Insulin therapy is given to the patients of type 1 diabetes. It is done by giving insulin injection just under the skin or it is delivered by an insulin pump. It is necessary to maintain proper diabetic diet and regular exercise for the management of type 1 diabetes. Various other complications are further developed by this type of diabetes such as heart disease, stroke, kidney failure and eye damage. This book covers in detail some existent theories and innovative concepts revolving around type 1 diabetes. It consists of contributions made by international experts. Researchers and students will be assisted by this book.

Each chapter is a sole-standing publication that reflects each author´s interpretation. Thus, the book displays a multi-facetted picture of our current understanding of application, resources and aspects of the field. I would like to thank the contributors of this book and my family for their endless support.

Editor

Effects of Pravastatin on Type 1 Diabetic Rat Heart with or without Blood Glycemic Control

Jeong Jin Min,[1,2] Byung-Seop Shin,[1] Jong-Hwan Lee,[1] Yunseok Jeon,[2] Dae Kyun Ryu,[1] Sojin Kim,[1] and Young Hee Shin[1]

[1] *Department of Anesthesiology and Pain Medicine, Samsung Medical Center, Sungkyunkwan University School of Medicine, Seoul, Republic of Korea*
[2] *Department of Anesthesiology and Pain Medicine, Seoul National University Hospital, Seoul National University College of Medicine, Seoul, Republic of Korea*

Correspondence should be addressed to Jong-Hwan Lee; jonghwanlee75@gmail.com

Academic Editor: Mark Yorek

Although statins have been suggested to attenuate the progression of diabetic cardiomyopathy, its effect without glycemic control remains unclear. Therefore, we evaluated the effect of pravastatin on diabetic rat hearts according to glycemic control. Rats were randomly divided into five groups: control (C), diabetes (D), diabetes with insulin (I), diabetes with pravastatin (P), and diabetes with insulin and pravastatin (IP). Eight weeks after allocated treatments, the heart was extracted and analyzed following echocardiography. Cardiac fibrosis was measured using Masson's trichrome stain. Cardiac expression of collagen I/III, matrix metalloproteinase (MMP)-2, MMP-9, and angiotensin-converting enzyme (ACE)/ACE2 was evaluated by immunohistochemistry and/or Western blot. Enzyme-linked immunosorbent assay was used for measuring reactive oxygen species (ROS). Diabetic groups without glycemic control (D and P) showed significantly impaired diastolic function and increased levels of cardiac fibrosis, collagen I/III, MMP-2, MMP-9, and ROS production. However, there were little significant differences in the outcomes among the control and two glucose-controlled diabetic groups (I and IP). Groups C and IP showed more preserved ACE2 and lower ACE expressions than the other groups did (D, I, and P). Our study suggested glycemic control would be more important to attenuate the progression of diabetic cardiomyopathy than pravastatin medication.

1. Introduction

Statin therapy is generally recommended in diabetic patients with cardiovascular risk factors or overt cardiovascular disease [1]. Many previous studies have shown that statins are effective to prevent major cardiac and cerebrovascular events [2, 3], which are related to the so-called "pleotropic" actions of statins including anti-inflammation, antithrombotic, antiatherosclerosis, antiproliferation, and reducing oxidative stress [4].

Statin treatment has also been suggested to reduce the progression of diabetic cardiomyopathy. Diabetic cardiomyopathy, which was first identified in 1972, is a separate disease from other well-established diabetic cardiovascular complications (e.g., coronary artery disease and cardiac autonomic neuropathy) and increases the risk of heart failure and cardiac mortality [5, 6]. Protective effects of statins on diabetic cardiomyopathy have been reported to improve cardiovascular remodeling by suppression of arterial wall thickening and myocardial fibrosis, restoration of left ventricular diastolic function, preservation of angiotensin-converting enzyme-2 (ACE2), and reduction of oxidative stress [7–10].

However, when using lipophilic statins (i.e., atorvastatin, simvastatin, or rosuvastatin) in diabetic patients, concerns regarding the progression of glucose intolerance [11] through alteration of insulin sensitivity or glucose uptake by adipocytes remain [12–16]. In contrast to those lipophilic statins, hydrophilic statins such as pravastatin and fluvastatin do not deteriorate glycemic control [7, 11, 14–16] because of the pharmacokinetic differences including hydrophilicity [4, 17].

In a previous study, we suggested that a combination of fluvastatin and insulin appears to be more effective than insulin alone in the diabetic heart [8]. However, considering that glucose control by insulin is the main therapy for diabetes, whether a clinical dose of statin would be protective in cases where blood glucose is not controlled remains unclear. In addition, the protective effects of statins on the diabetic heart may differ among statins. Therefore, in the present study, we evaluated the effect of pravastatin on cardiac function, myocardial fibrosis, oxidative stress, and ACE2 expression according to the presence of glycemic control in diabetic rat hearts. We hypothesized that early cotreatment of pravastatin and insulin would have more beneficial effects on cardiac protection than insulin-alone treatment.

2. Materials and Methods

This study was reviewed and approved by the Animal Care and Use Committee at Samsung Medical Center (IACUC number 20140203003), and the animal experiments were conducted in accordance with the Samsung Biomedical Research Institute guidelines for animal experiments.

2.1. Experimental Animal Modeling and Care. Seven-week-old male Lewis (inbred Wistar) rats ($n = 87$) were used in this study. All rats were housed at $22 \pm 3^{\circ}C$ with 40–60% humidity in a 12/12-hour light/dark cycle. All animal experiments were performed in a semipathogen-free barrier zone at the Samsung Laboratory Animal Research Center. Rats were randomly allocated into one of 5 groups according to the insulin or pravastatin treatment after diabetic modeling: (i) group C (control rats, $n = 16$), (ii) group D (untreated diabetic rats, $n = 18$), (iii) group I (diabetic rats receiving insulin treatment, $n = 18$), (iv) group P (diabetic rats receiving pravastatin treatment, $n = 17$), and (v) group IP (diabetic rats receiving cotreatment of insulin and pravastatin, $n = 18$). Diabetes was induced by an intravenous injection of 65 mg/kg streptozotocin (STZ); in group C, the same volume of citrate buffer (pH 4.5) was administered. Three days after STZ injection, blood glucose levels were measured using a OneTouch Ultra® Blood Glucose Meter (LifeScan Inc., Milpitas, CA), and a glucose level higher than 300 mg/dl was considered as a successful diabetic induction. In the groups treated with insulin (group I and group IP), the blood glucose level of each rat was measured twice daily (at 7 a.m. and 7 p.m.) and Lantus® (insulin glargine, Sanofi-Aventis, France) was administered at 2–10 U/kg to achieve a normal blood glucose range for eight weeks from the day of diagnosis. In the statin treatment group (group P and group IP), a calculated dose of pravastatin (20–25 mg/kg/day) was dissolved in water and orally administered once every evening by an oral gavage using a feeding catheter for eight weeks from the day of diagnosis. Standard rat chow and tap water were provided *ad libitum* throughout the study period.

2.2. Echocardiography. Eight weeks after treatment, each group of rats was anesthetized with isoflurane/oxygen, and transthoracic echocardiographic images were acquired using a Vevo® 2100 high-resolution imaging system (VisualSonics Inc., Toronto, Canada). Two-dimensional parasternal short-axis images were measured at the level of the midpapillary muscle, and M-mode tracings were recorded. Left ventricular end-diastolic area, left ventricular end-systolic area, left ventricular internal dimension in diastole, and left ventricular internal dimension in systole were measured, and left ventricular fractional area change (LV-FAC) and left ventricular fractional shortening (LV-FS) were calculated as previously described [8]. Mitral peak flow velocities at early diastole and atrial contraction were recorded using a pulsed Doppler technique in parasternal long-axis view, and the ratio of the early (E) to late (A) ventricular filling velocities (E/A ratio) was calculated. All measurements were performed by an experienced technician who was blinded to animal group allocation. Three representative cardiac cycles were analyzed and averaged for each measurement.

2.3. Biochemical Measurements. After echocardiography, blood glucose levels and body weights were measured. Blood samples were also collected from the abdominal aorta and then immediately centrifuged to measure total cholesterol, low-density lipoprotein, high-density lipoprotein, and triglycerides. Euthanasia was performed by cervical dislocation under deep anesthesia, and the heart was extracted and weighed.

2.4. Histology and Immunohistochemistry. Hearts extracted from 9–11 rats were formalin fixed, paraffin embedded, and sliced into 4 μm sections. Sections were deparaffinized in xylene, rehydrated in graded alcohol, and transferred to 0.01 M phosphate-buffered saline (PBS, pH 7.4). Myocardial collagen depositions were stained by Masson's trichrome and measured. Conventional immunohistochemistry for collagen I/III, angiotensin-converting enzyme (ACE), and ACE2 expressions was performed by the same method as previously described [8]. For analyses, slides were scanned using a ScanScope AT digital slide scanner (Aperio, Vista, CA), and images were analyzed using the Aperio ImageScope Positive Pixel Count algorithm. To quantify immunohistochemical expression, 7 to 10 fields in each slide (at a magnification of 20 times) were randomly chosen and color positivity of pixels within the fields was automatically detected after setting the appropriate input parameters. Color positivity was presented as three different levels, strong positive, moderate positive, and weak positive, according to the strength of the color expression. For further analyses, we defined positivity as follows:

$$\text{Positivity} = \frac{\text{number of (strong positive + moderate positive) pixels}}{\text{total number of pixels in the selected fields}}. \quad (1)$$

2.5. Western Blot Analysis. Proteins were extracted from heart tissue obtained from 9–11 rats for each experimental group. Cardiac myocytes were placed on ice for 15 minutes and then sonicated for 30 s; whole-cell protein lysates were recovered by centrifugation. The protein concentration of the supernatant was determined using a Bradford reagent method (Bio-Rad, Hercules, CA, USA). Proteins

Table 1: Demographic, laboratory, and echocardiographic data after eight weeks of treatment.

	Group C	Group D	Group I	Group P	Group IP	*P* value
BWt (g)	387 (375.8–401)$^{†, ‡, \S, ‖}$	226 (215–293)	352 (320–370)$^{†, \S}$	246.5 (236–255)	352 (329.5–366)$^{†, \S}$	<0.001
HWt (g)	1.18 (1.15–1.27)$^{†, ‡, \S}$	0.81 (0.77–0.85)$^{*, ‡, ‖}$	1.07 (0.98–1.11)$^{*, †, \S}$	0.87 (0.80–0.92)$^{*, ‡, ‖}$	1.09 (1.02–1.17)$^{†, \S}$	<0.001
HWt/BWt (%)	0.31 (0.3–0.33)$^{†, \S}$	0.39 (0.36–0.41)$^{*, ‡, ‖}$	0.31 (0.3–0.34)$^{†, \S}$	0.35 (0.33–0.39)$^{*, ‡}$	0.32 (0.31–0.37)†	0.002
Blood glucose (mg/dl)	142 (133–153)$^{†, \S}$	443 (403–470)$^{*, ‡, ‖}$	141 (89–149)$^{†, \S}$	438 (417–505)$^{*, ‡, ‖}$	119 (83–151)$^{†, \S}$	<0.001
Lipid profile (mg/dl)						
Total cholesterol	82.5 (77–91.5)	93 (85.25–103)	81.5 (72–86)	79.5 (71–81)	88 (84–90)	0.01
Triglyceride	65 (41–77.5)†	145 (138–325.5)*	124 (86–140)*†	92.5 (74–137)*†	106 (65–145.5)*†	<0.001
HDL	74 (71.5–76.5)$^{†, ‡}$	60 (58–74)$^{*, ‖}$	68 (60–72)$^{*, ‖}$	69 (65–75)$^{‖}$	79 (74–81)$^{†, ‡, ‖}$	0.004
LDL	11.5 (11-12.5)	15 (10–17.25)	11 (10–13.25)	10 (10-11)	12 (10.25–13)	0.118
Echocardiographic variables						
FAC (%)	61 (58–68)$^{†, \S}$	38 (29–43)$^{*, ‡, \S, ‖}$	60 (53–62)†	52 (45–56)$^{*, †, ‖}$	63 (60–72)$^{†, \S}$	<0.001
FS (%)	53 (49–54)$^{†, ‡, \S}$	39 (37–43)$^{*, ‖}$	45 (41–48)*	41 (34–45)$^{*, ‖}$	53 (41–63)$^{†, \S}$	0.0014
E/A ratio	1.8 (1.5–2.5)$^{†, \S}$	0.9 (0.8–0.9)$^{*, ‡, ‖}$	1.8 (1.2–1.9)$^{†, \S}$	0.8 (0.7–0.8)$^{*, ‡, ‖}$	1.7 (1.5–2.3)$^{†, \S}$	<0.001

Data are presented as the median (IQR). *P* values were calculated using a Kruskal-Wallis one-way analysis of variance on ranks. The Tukey test was used for multiple comparisons. BWt: body weight; HWt: heart weight; HDL: high-density lipoprotein; LDL: low-density lipoprotein; FAC: fractional area change; FS: fractional shortening; E/A: the ratio of the early (E) to late (A) ventricular filling velocities. $^{*}P < 0.05$ versus group C, $^{†}P < 0.05$ versus group D, $^{‡}P < 0.05$ versus group I, $^{\S}P < 0.05$ versus group P, and $^{‖}P < 0.05$ versus group IP.

were resolved by electrophoresis by sodium dodecyl sulfate-polyacrylamide gel electrophoresis (SDS-PAGE) or native PAGE as appropriate under denaturing conditions. The proteins were transferred to nitrocellulose membranes (BioTrace™ NT, Pall Corp., USA). After blocking in Tris-buffered saline with Tween 20 (TBS-T, 10 mM Tris, 150 mM NaCl, 0.1% Tween 20) containing 5% bovine serum albumin (BSA) for one hour, the membranes were incubated overnight with primary antibody in 3% BSA in TBS-T at 4°C. Membranes were then washed with TBS-T and incubated in 3% BSA in HRP-conjugated IgG secondary antibodies for 1 hour. Membranes were washed again with TBS-T, and the immunocomplexes were detected using a chemiluminescence reagent kit (Amersham Corp., Arlington Heights, IL, USA). The primary antibodies used for immunoblotting studies were collagen I antibody (ab6308, Abcam Inc.), collagen III antibody (ab7778, Abcam Inc.), matrix metalloproteinase- (MMP-) 2 antibody (ab79271, Abcam Inc.), MMP-9 antibody (ab137867, Abcam Inc.), ACE antibody (ab11734, Abcam Inc.), or ACE2 antibody (ab87436, Abcam Inc.). Immunoblotting for β-actin was performed to verify equivalent protein loading.

2.6. Enzyme-Linked Immunosorbent Assay (ELISA). The concentration of reactive oxygen species (ROS) in the rat myocardium was measured using a commercial rat ROS ELISA kit (CSB-E15037r, CUSABIO®, Wuhan, Hubei, China). In brief, rat heart tissue was mechanically homogenized in PBS and stored overnight at −20°C. After two freeze-thaw cycles to break the cell membranes, the homogenized samples were centrifuged for 5 min at 5000 rpm and 4°C. Each supernatant was then transferred into a fresh test-tube and stored at −80°C, and the level of ROS was determined by ELISA kit following the manufacturer's recommended procedures.

2.7. Statistical Analysis. All statistical analyses were performed using SPSS for Windows (version 21.0, SPSS Inc., Chicago, IL, USA). Data are presented as median (interquartile range, IQR). Normality of the data distribution was determined with a Shapiro-Wilk test. Differences among groups were tested using a one-way analysis of variance or a Kruskal-Wallis one-way analysis of variance on ranks as appropriate, followed by Tukey's test using ranks for multiple comparisons. In Western blot analysis, the protein expression result in group C was used as a reference (with a reference value of "1"), and a one-sample signed rank test with Bonferroni correction was used when comparing group C with other groups (groups D, I, P, and IP). A *P* value less than 0.05 was considered statistically significant.

3. Results

3.1. Demographic and Laboratory Characteristics (Lipid Profile). Diabetes was successfully induced in all rats. Of the 87 rats used in the experiment, 3 rats expired (2 died during diabetic modeling, and 1 from group D died after the echocardiographic exam), and thus 84 rats were included in the final analysis. Table 1 shows the demographic and laboratory data of the rats after 8 weeks of each treatment. Diabetic rats without glycemic control (group D and group P) showed significantly lower body and heart weights compared with the other groups. For the lipid profile, group D showed the highest blood triglyceride level. However, group P, which was the diabetic group receiving pravastatin single treatment, showed a comparable lipid profile results to groups I and IP. The insulin-treated diabetic group without statin therapy

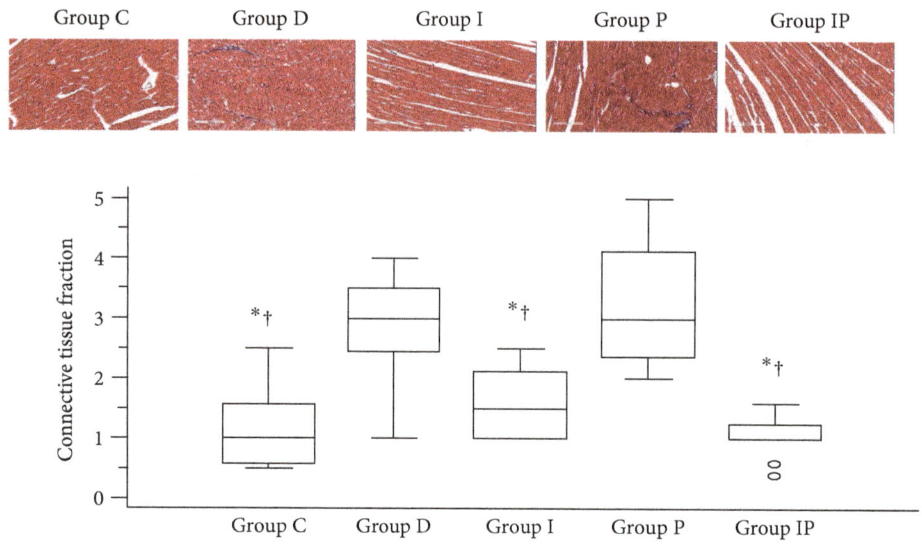

FIGURE 1: Masson's trichrome stain of the myocardium with the connective tissues stained blue. Boxes and lines represent medians and interquartile ranges, respectively. Dots represent the outliers. The upper part represents the images (with 20 times magnification) and the lower part shows the quantitative analysis. $^{*}P < 0.05$ versus group D, $^{\dagger}P < 0.05$ versus group P.

(group I) showed comparable levels of triglycerides and low-density lipoproteins with rats on statin therapy (group P and group IP).

3.2. Echocardiography (Cardiac Function). The echocardiographic data after 8 weeks of treatment are shown in Table 1. The median values of LV-FAC in diabetic rats without glycemic control (group D and group P) were significantly reduced compared with those in the other groups. The values of LV-FS were also lower in group D and group P compared with those in group C and group IP. The E/A ratio, which indicates left ventricular diastolic function, was significantly lower in group D and group P than in the other groups (Table 1).

3.3. Histology. Masson's trichrome was used to stain the cardiac connective tissue blue. There were significant differences in the median cardiac connective tissue fraction among the five groups ($P < 0.0001$). The cardiac connective tissue fraction was significantly higher in the diabetic rats with poor glycemic control (group D and group P) than other groups (Figure 1). However, there were no significant differences in the cardiac connective tissue fraction among groups C, I, and IP (Figure 1).

3.4. Collagen and MMP-2, MMP-9 Protein Cardiac Expression. Immunohistochemistry and Western blot analyses demonstrated that cardiac expression of collagen I and III was significantly increased in group D and group P compared with those in the other groups (Figures 2 and 3). Group I showed higher expression of collagen I by immunohistochemistry analysis compared with group C and group IP (Figure 2(a)). However, expression of collagen III shown by immunohistochemistry (Figure 3(a)) and collagens I and III shown by Western blot analyses results (Figures 2(b) and 3(b)) was comparable among group C, group I, and group IP.

Cardiac expression of MMP-2 and MMP-9 was significantly increased in the high blood glucose groups (group D and group P) as compared with those in other groups as shown by Western blot analyses (Figure 4). The MMP-2 expression in group I was higher than group C, which was comparable to the expression level of group IP (Figure 4(a)). Group C and group IP showed comparable results in both MMP-2 and MMP-9 expression levels (Figures 4(a) and 4(b)).

3.5. ROS Production. The ELISA demonstrated that the median reactivity of ROS in heart tissue homogenate was significantly increased in group D and group P compared with the other groups (Figure 5). Group C showed the lowest value of ROS reactivity. No significant differences in ROS reactivity were observed between group I and group IP (Figure 5).

3.6. Cardiac ACE and ACE2 Protein Expression. In immunohistochemistry analysis, the ACE expression level was significantly lower in group C compared to groups D, I, and P, while ACE expression in group IP showed no significant difference from that of the group C (Figure 6(a)). For ACE2, higher expressions were observed in groups C and IP compared to the other groups (Figure 6(b)). In Western blot analyses, ACE protein expression was significantly lower in groups C and IP than in the other groups (Figure 6(c)). In contrast, ACE2 cardiac protein expression was significantly preserved in groups C and IP compared to those in the other groups (Figure 6(d)).

4. Discussion

4.1. Major Findings. In this experimental study, we observed the cardiac effects of pravastatin under two different conditions of blood glucose control in the STZ-induced diabetic rat model. Under poor glycemic control, diabetic rats showed

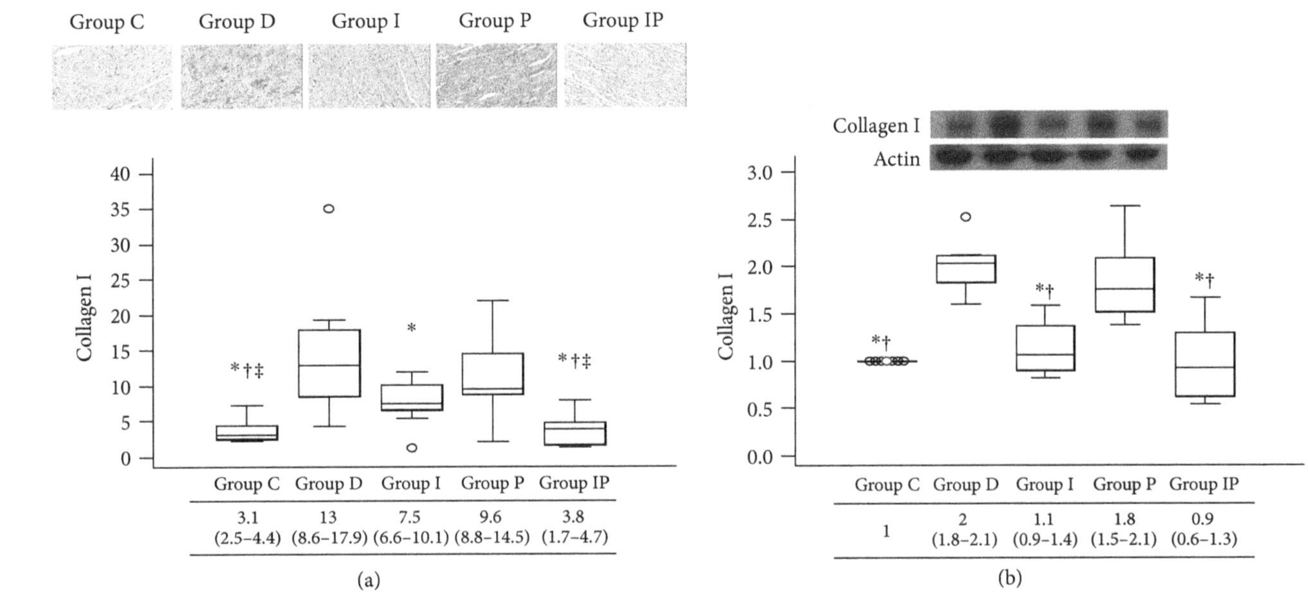

FIGURE 2: Representative micrograph of immunohistochemistry (a) and Western blot photograph for cardiac protein expression (b) of collagen I. Boxes and lines represent medians and interquartile ranges, respectively. Dots represent the outliers. The upper part represents the images (with 20 times magnification in immunohistochemistry) and the lower part shows the quantitative analysis. $^{*}P < 0.05$ versus group D, $^{\dagger}P < 0.05$ versus group P, and $^{\ddagger}P < 0.05$ versus group I.

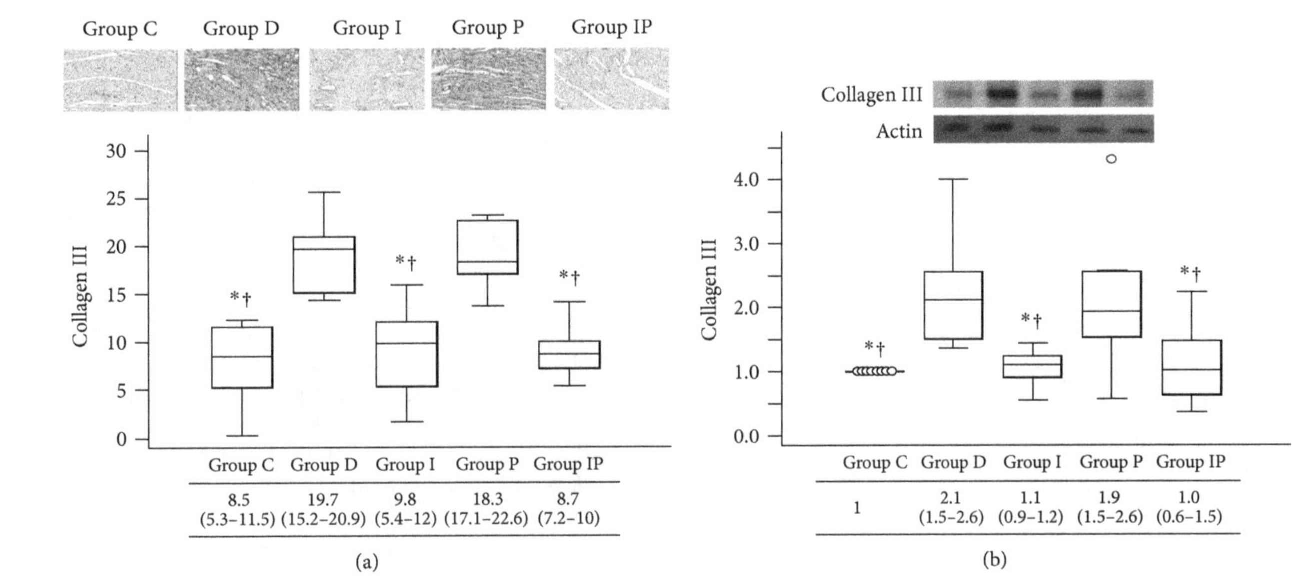

FIGURE 3: Representative micrograph of immunohistochemistry (a) and Western blot photograph for cardiac protein expression (b) of collagen III. Boxes and lines represent medians and interquartile ranges, respectively. Dots represent the outliers. The upper part represents the images (with 20 times magnification in immunohistochemistry) and the lower part shows the quantitative analysis. $^{*}P < 0.05$ versus group D, $^{\dagger}P < 0.05$ versus group P.

significantly impaired cardiac function and increased levels of cardiac fibrosis and ROS production regardless of pravastatin treatment. When blood glucose levels were well controlled from the early stage of diabetes with insulin, diabetic rats showed comparable results with nondiabetic rats in cardiac function, fibrosis, MMP expression, and ROS production, regardless of additional treatment with oral pravastatin. Although cardiac ACE2 expression seemed to be more preserved in the combination treatment group receiving pravastatin and insulin than in the insulin-alone group, this did not lead to meaningful differences in other outcomes in our study.

4.2. Pathophysiology of Diabetic Cardiomyopathy and Statin. Diabetic cardiomyopathy is defined as left ventricular dysfunction in diabetic patients without coronary artery

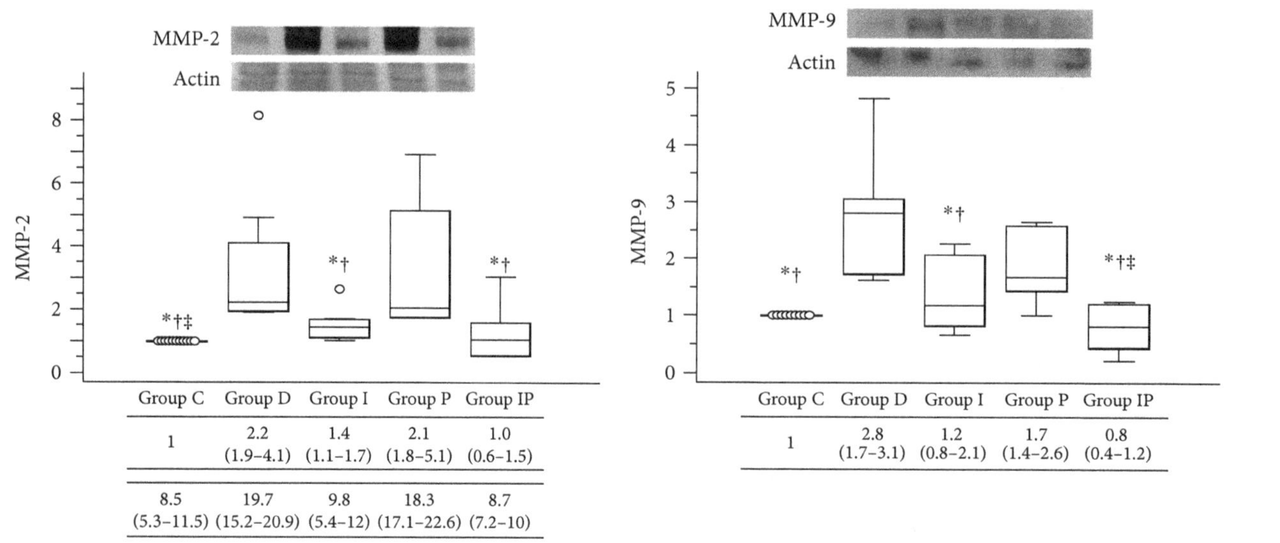

FIGURE 4: Representative Western blot photographs for cardiac protein expression of MMP-2 (a) and MMP-9 (b). Boxes and lines represent medians and interquartile ranges, respectively. Dots represent the outliers. $^*P < 0.05$ versus group D, $^\dagger P < 0.05$ versus group P, and $^\ddagger P < 0.05$ versus group I. MMP: matrix metalloproteinase.

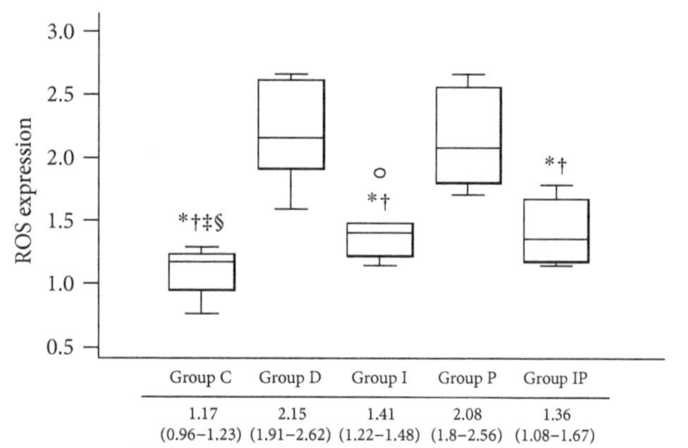

FIGURE 5: Cardiac expressions of reactive oxygen species measured by enzyme-linked immunosorbent assay. Boxes and lines represent medians and interquartile ranges, respectively. Dots represent the outliers. $^*P < 0.05$ versus group D, $^\dagger P < 0.05$ versus group P, $^\ddagger P < 0.05$ versus group I, and $^\S P < 0.05$ versus group IP.

disease or other potential etiological conditions [18] and, morphologically, is mainly characterized by cardiac hypertrophy and adverse remodeling associated with myocardial fibrosis. The pathogenesis of diabetic cardiomyopathy has a multifactorial basis. Several suggested mechanisms include metabolic disturbances, insulin resistance, microvascular disease, renin-angiotensin system activation, and excessive oxidative stress [5]. Among the various mechanisms, the role of oxidative stress has been strongly suggested in many studies [19–22], and therefore beneficial effects of statins and antioxidant treatments on the management of diabetic complications have been extensively investigated and reported.

4.3. Results of Our Study. Previously, we suggested that a combination of fluvastatin and insulin may be more effective than insulin-alone treatment in diabetic hearts with regard to reducing myocardial fibrosis and preserving cardiac function and ACE2 expression [8]. However, in that study, the sole effect of fluvastatin on diabetic cardiomyopathy could not be explained because of the absence of an experimental group receiving a single fluvastatin treatment. In the present study, we included experimental groups observing both the sole effect of each treatment (group I or group P) and the effect in combination (group IP) on diabetic rat hearts. Our results suggest that glycemic control is the primary factor involved in reducing the progression of diabetic cardiomyopathy. Contrary to our expectations, once blood glucose was well controlled with insulin, the addition of pravastatin treatment did not make a significant difference in most of the study outcomes. Two insulin-treated groups with good glycemic control (group I versus group IP) showed comparable results regardless of the use of pravastatin in cardiac function, fibrosis, collagen expression, MMP activation, or ROS production.

Moreover, between the two diabetic groups without glycemic control (group D versus group P), pravastatin treatment did not bring any beneficial effects compared to the untreated group showing comparable progression of diabetic cardiomyopathy. These results are inconsistent with previous findings that statin treatment itself was effective in reducing myocardial fibrosis and cardiac dysfunction in the diabetic condition without specific comments for glycemic control [7].

There are several explanations for the results of our study. First, because we started and maintained good glycemic control from a very early stage of diabetes, diabetic complications may have been prevented or delayed in the insulin-treated rats during our study period. In clinical practice, a chronic hyperglycemic period generally exists until the initial diagnosis of diabetes, and in this situation, increased levels of inflammatory proteins and oxidative stress are

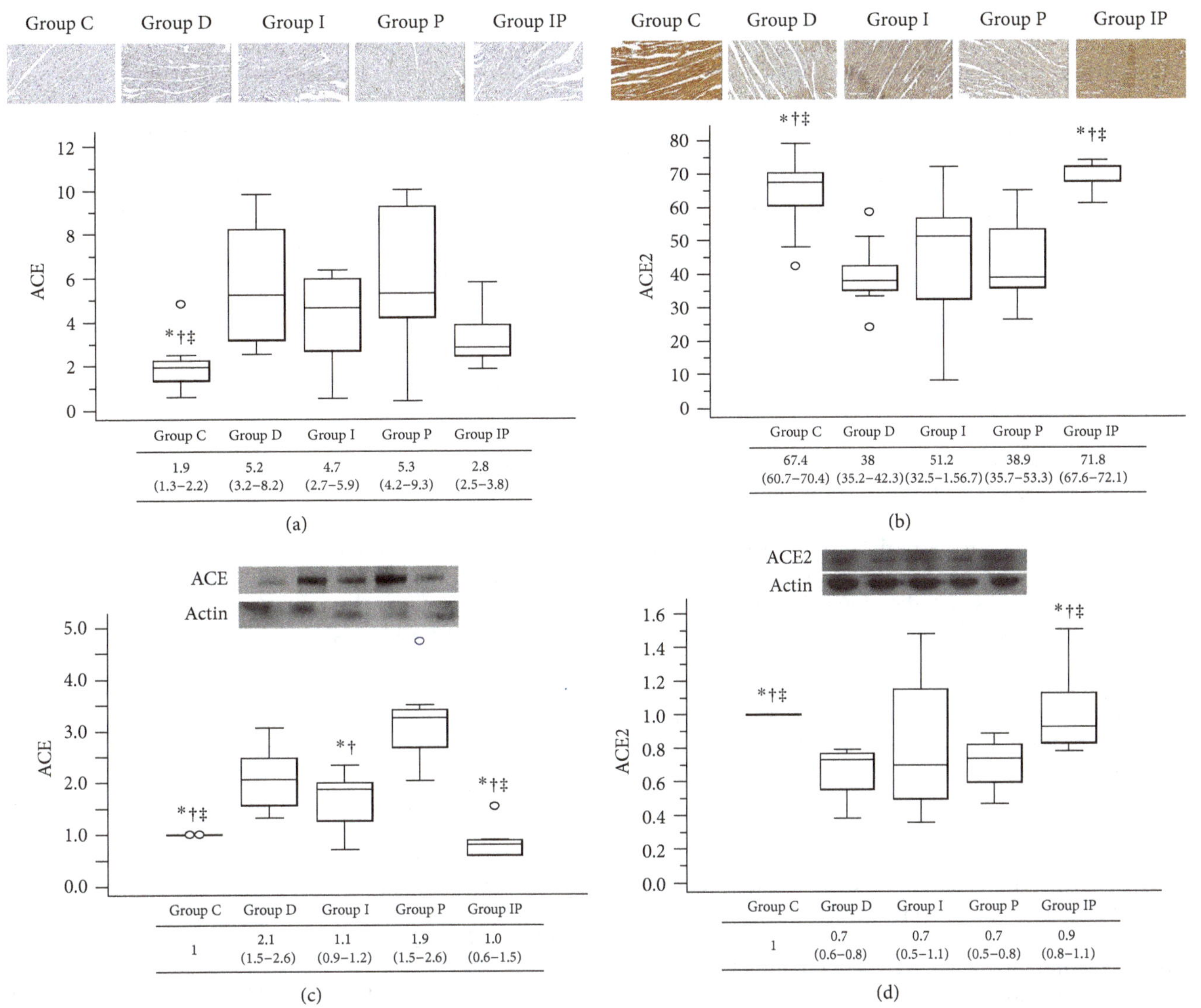

Figure 6: Representative micrographs of immunohistochemistry for ACE (a) and ACE2 (b) and Western blot photographs for cardiac protein expression for ACE (c) and ACE2 (d). Boxes and lines represent medians and interquartile ranges, respectively. Dots represent the outliers. The upper part represents the images (with 20 times magnification in immunohistochemistry) and the lower part shows the quantitative analysis. $^*P < 0.05$ versus group D, $^\dagger P < 0.05$ versus group P, and $^\ddagger P < 0.05$ versus group I. ACE: angiotensin-converting enzyme.

not completely restored even with the later normalization of blood glucose [23]. This phenomenon results from "glycemic memory," in that once ROS production is increased in the early hyperglycemic environment, ROS-induced cellular dysfunction and mitochondrial DNA damage may occur and persist independently with later glycemic control. Secondly, the different dosage of pravastatin used for treatment in our study (20–25 mg/kg/day) may have affected our results. In previous experimental studies, much higher doses of pravastatin (100 mg/kg/day) effectively reduced cardiac fibrosis and MMP activity [24]. Another pravastatin study, which showed the preventive effect of cardiovascular remodeling in a type II diabetic model, also used higher dose of pravastatin (100 mg/kg/day) [7]. However, considering that the recommended dosage of pravastatin is 40 mg/day in human clinical practice, the pravastatin dosage we used was not an underdose for rats of much smaller size than human. Third, the results may be due to the unique pharmacokinetic characteristics of pravastatin such as lower plasma protein binding, hydrophilic nature, different primary metabolic pathways, and dual routes of elimination [17, 25, 26]. Pravastatin has shown different effects on the progression of glucose intolerance [11, 12] and side effects compared with other statins [27]. Moreover, in a previous study, which observed the effects of various statins for MMP activity and vascular smooth muscle proliferation, only pravastatin showed different results from other statins (fluvastatin, simvastatin, lovastatin, and atorvastatin) [28].

4.4. Statin and ACE2. Interestingly, cardiac ACE2 expression was more preserved in the pravastatin-treated group among glucose-controlled rats in our study. However, this did not lead to a meaningful difference in the levels of cardiac fibrosis or ROS production. The effects of pravastatin might not have been high enough to sufficiently reduce the MMP upregulation or cardiac collagen deposition. In our previous study, additive treatment with fluvastatin in glucose-controlled diabetic rats led to more preserved cardiac ACE2 expression as well as in the cardiac fibrosis and diastolic cardiac function than did the insulin-only treated group. Although fluvastatin is less potent than pravastatin with regard to lipid-lowering effects, the differences in pleiotropic effects among statins remain unclear because there are insufficient data.

4.5. Potential Benefits of Hydrophilic Statins in Diabetic Patients. When making a therapeutic selection between statin agents in diabetic patients for primary prevention purpose, there are some factors that must be considered. Although all statins are generally well tolerated, some side effects such as drug interactions, muscle toxicity, insomnia, and cognitive dysfunction have been related to statin use. These side effects are more likely to occur with the use of lipophilic statins. In this regard, hydrophilic statins have some advantages compared to lipophilic statins especially in diabetic or elderly patients taking multiple medications. Among hydrophilic statins, pravastatin has not deteriorated glycemic control and is less likely to displace albumin-bound drugs such as warfarin because of its lower plasma protein binding [26]. Moreover, in clinical situations where patients must receive multiple medications, pravastatin may have the fewest drug interactions because it is not metabolized by CYP450 [17]. In patients with impaired renal function, fluvastatin is preferred because fluvastatin is the drug that is least affected by renal elimination [17]. However, further evaluation is needed to identify appropriate agents and adequate doses to provide optimal therapeutic efficacy including the pleiotropic effect of statins for each individual patient's condition.

4.6. Study Limitations. There were several limitations in our study. First, since we started glycemic control immediately after the confirmation of diabetic induction, there was no experimental group with a chronic hyperglycemic period before starting insulin treatment, and we did not observe the effect of statin under such condition with glycemic memory, which is common in the real-life clinical situation. Second, we did not observe the long-term effects of pravastatin after 8 weeks. Although 8 weeks is sufficient to develop diabetic cardiomyopathy in the groups without glycemic control, a longer follow-up might be needed in groups with controlled-blood glucose because the onset and progression of diabetic cardiomyopathy may be delayed under good glycemic control. Moreover, lipid profiles were normalized in the pravastatin-treated groups, and therefore long-standing use of statins may make a difference even between the groups with poor glucose control because dyslipidemia may also play a role in the development of microvascular complications [5, 29, 30]. Third, we used semiquantitative methods to analyze the study outcomes (immunostaining, Western blotting, and ELISA), although they are popular techniques used in biomedical research. Fourth, our experimental model was type I diabetes induced by STZ injection. Although the STZ-induced diabetic rat model is an established experimental model for research of diabetic cardiomyopathy [8, 9, 31, 32] and models of type 1 and type 2 diabetes have been used interchangeably to understand pathophysiological mechanisms of diabetic cardiomyopathy [32], it is difficult to extend our study results to all diabetic conditions. Finally, the lipid-lowering effect of statin would be different in rodents; therefore, rat models might not be perfect to evaluate the effects of statin. However, in this experimental study, we aimed to evaluate the pleiotropic effects of statin independent from its lipid-lowering effects. Moreover, many previous studies have used rats or mice to evaluate the protective effects of statin on the cardiovascular system.

5. Conclusions

In conclusion, this experimental study with type 1 diabetic rat models revealed that glycemic control is the primary condition attenuating the progression of diabetic cardiomyopathy even with pravastatin treatment. Further studies may be needed to identify a regimen for optimal pleiotropic effects of pravastatin on the heart in different types of diabetes.

Conflicts of Interest

The authors have no commercial, proprietary, or financial interests in the products or companies described in this article.

Authors' Contributions

Jeong Jin Min and Byung-Seop Shin contributed equally to this work.

Acknowledgments

This study was supported by Faculty Research Fund, Sungkyunkwan University, 2014 (SMX1132231) and 2015 (SMX1150511). The authors thank the Basic Research Support Center of Samsung Biomedical Research Institute for their help in analyzing the immunohistochemistry images, and the authors also thank Hee-Jong Kim and Eo-Jin Lee for their contributions in animal care and Western blot analysis.

References

[1] American Diabetes Association, "8. Cardiovascular disease and risk management," *Diabetes Care*, vol. 38, Supplement 1, pp. S49–S57, 2016.

[2] Y. H. Chen, B. Feng, and Z. W. Chen, "Statins for primary prevention of cardiovascular and cerebrovascular events in diabetic patients without established cardiovascular diseases: a meta-analysis," *Experimental and Clinical Endocrinology & Diabetes*, vol. 120, no. 2, pp. 116–120, 2012.

[3] P. M. Kearney, L. Blackwell, R. Collins et al., "Efficacy of cholesterol-lowering therapy in 18,686 people with diabetes in 14 randomised trials of statins: a meta-analysis," *The Lancet*, vol. 371, no. 9607, pp. 117–125, 2008.

[4] P. Gazzerro, M. C. Proto, G. Gangemi et al., "Pharmacological actions of statins: a critical appraisal in the management of

cancer," *Pharmacological Reviews*, vol. 64, no. 1, pp. 102–146, 2012.

[5] J. M. Pappachan, G. I. Varughese, R. Sriraman, and G. Arunagirinathan, "Diabetic cardiomyopathy: pathophysiology, diagnostic evaluation and management," *World Journal of Diabetes*, vol. 4, no. 5, pp. 177–189, 2013.

[6] I. Falcao-Pires and A. F. Leite-Moreira, "Diabetic cardiomyopathy: understanding the molecular and cellular basis to progress in diagnosis and treatment," *Heart Failure Reviews*, vol. 17, no. 3, pp. 325–344, 2012.

[7] Y. Yu, K. Ohmori, Y. Chen et al., "Effects of pravastatin on progression of glucose intolerance and cardiovascular remodeling in a type II diabetes model," *Journal of the American College of Cardiology*, vol. 44, no. 4, pp. 904–913, 2004.

[8] Y. H. Shin, J. J. Min, J. H. Lee et al., "The effect of fluvastatin on cardiac fibrosis and angiotensin-converting enzyme-2 expression in glucose-controlled diabetic rat hearts," *Heart and Vessels*, vol. 32, no. 5, pp. 618–627, 2016.

[9] T. Shida, T. Nozawa, M. Sobajima, H. Ihori, A. Matsuki, and H. Inoue, "Fluvastatin-induced reduction of oxidative stress ameliorates diabetic cardiomyopathy in association with improving coronary microvasculature," *Heart and Vessels*, vol. 29, no. 4, pp. 532–541, 2014.

[10] Q. M. Dai, J. Lu, and N. F. Liu, "Fluvastatin attenuates myocardial interstitial fibrosis and cardiac dysfunction in diabetic rats by inhibiting over-expression of connective tissue growth factor," *Chinese Medical Journal*, vol. 124, no. 1, pp. 89–94, 2011.

[11] M. Kanda, K. Satoh, and K. Ichihara, "Effects of atorvastatin and pravastatin on glucose tolerance in diabetic rats mildly induced by streptozotocin," *Biological and Pharmaceutical Bulletin*, vol. 26, no. 12, pp. 1681–1684, 2003.

[12] G. Muscogiuri, G. Sarno, A. Gastaldelli et al., "The good and bad effects of statins on insulin sensitivity and secretion," *Endocrine Research*, vol. 39, no. 4, pp. 137–143, 2014.

[13] M. Ishikawa, A. Namiki, T. Kubota et al., "Effect of pravastatin and atorvastatin on glucose metabolism in nondiabetic patients with hypercholesterolemia," *Internal Medicine*, vol. 45, no. 2, pp. 51–55, 2006.

[14] M. Ishikawa, F. Okajima, N. Inoue et al., "Distinct effects of pravastatin, atorvastatin, and simvastatin on insulin secretion from a β-cell line, MIN6 cells," *Journal of Atherosclerosis and Thrombosis*, vol. 13, no. 6, pp. 329–335, 2006.

[15] A. Takaguri, K. Satoh, M. Itagaki, Y. Tokumitsu, and K. Ichihara, "Effects of atorvastatin and pravastatin on signal transduction related to glucose uptake in 3T3L1 adipocytes," *Journal of Pharmacological Sciences*, vol. 107, no. 1, pp. 80–89, 2008.

[16] K. K. Koh, M. J. Quon, S. H. Han et al., "Differential metabolic effects of pravastatin and simvastatin in hypercholesterolemic patients," *Atherosclerosis*, vol. 204, no. 2, pp. 483–490, 2009.

[17] P. H. Chong, J. D. Seeger, and C. Franklin, "Clinically relevant differences between the statins: implications for therapeutic selection," *The American Journal of Medicine*, vol. 111, no. 5, pp. 390–400, 2001.

[18] L. Ernande and G. Derumeaux, "Diabetic cardiomyopathy: myth or reality?," *Archives of Cardiovascular Diseases*, vol. 105, no. 4, pp. 218–225, 2012.

[19] M. Seddon, Y. H. Looi, and A. M. Shah, "Oxidative stress and redox signalling in cardiac hypertrophy and heart failure," *Heart*, vol. 93, no. 8, pp. 903–907, 2007.

[20] F. Giacco and M. Brownlee, "Oxidative stress and diabetic complications," *Circulation Research*, vol. 107, no. 9, pp. 1058–1070, 2010.

[21] S. Uemura, H. Matsushita, W. Li et al., "Diabetes mellitus enhances vascular matrix metalloproteinase activity: role of oxidative stress," *Circulation Research*, vol. 88, no. 12, pp. 1291–1298, 2001.

[22] K. Huynh, B. C. Bernardo, J. R. McMullen, and R. H. Ritchie, "Diabetic cardiomyopathy: mechanisms and new treatment strategies targeting antioxidant signaling pathways," *Pharmacology & Therapeutics*, vol. 142, no. 3, pp. 375–415, 2014.

[23] T. Nishikawa, D. Edelstein, and M. Brownlee, "The missing link: a single unifying mechanism for diabetic complications," *Kidney International*, vol. 58, Supplement 77, pp. S26–S30, 2000.

[24] S. Ichihara, A. Noda, K. Nagata et al., "Pravastatin increases survival and suppresses an increase in myocardial matrix metalloproteinase activity in a rat model of heart failure," *Cardiovascular Research*, vol. 69, no. 3, pp. 726–735, 2006.

[25] T. Hatanaka, "Clinical pharmacokinetics of pravastatin: mechanisms of pharmacokinetic events," *Clinical Pharmacokinetics*, vol. 39, no. 6, pp. 397–412, 2000.

[26] M. Schachter, "Chemical, pharmacokinetic and pharmacodynamic properties of statins: an update," *Fundamental & Clinical Pharmacology*, vol. 19, no. 1, pp. 117–125, 2005.

[27] R. Bitzur, H. Cohen, Y. Kamari, and D. Harats, "Intolerance to statins: mechanisms and management," *Diabetes Care*, vol. 36, Supplement 2, pp. S325–S330, 2013.

[28] S. Bellosta, N. Ferri, L. Arnaboldi, F. Bernini, R. Paoletti, and A. Corsini, "Pleiotropic effects of statins in atherosclerosis and diabetes," *Diabetes Care*, vol. 23, Supplement 2, pp. B72–B78, 2000.

[29] L. A. Leiter, "The prevention of diabetic microvascular complications of diabetes: is there a role for lipid lowering?," *Diabetes Research and Clinical Practice*, vol. 68, Supplement 2, pp. S3–S14, 2005.

[30] J. Stamler, O. Vaccaro, J. D. Neaton, and D. Wentworth, "Diabetes, other risk factors, and 12-yr cardiovascular mortality for men screened in the multiple risk factor intervention trial," *Diabetes Care*, vol. 16, no. 2, pp. 434–444, 1993.

[31] W. Hsueh, E. D. Abel, J. L. Breslow et al., "Recipes for creating animal models of diabetic cardiovascular disease," *Circulation Research*, vol. 100, no. 10, pp. 1415–1427, 2007.

[32] H. Bugger and E. D. Abel, "Rodent models of diabetic cardiomyopathy," *Disease Models & Mechanisms*, vol. 2, no. 9-10, pp. 454–466, 2009.

2

Integration of Routine Parameters of Glycemic Variability in a Simple Screening Method for Partial Remission in Children with Type 1 Diabetes

Nina Nielens,[1] Olivier Pollé,[1] Annie Robert,[2] and Philippe A. Lysy[1]

[1]*Pediatric Endocrinology Unit, Cliniques Universitaires Saint Luc, Av. Hippocrate 10, 1200 Brussels, Belgium*
[2]*Pôle Epidémiologie et Biostatistique, Institut de Recherche Expérimentale et Clinique, Université Catholique de Louvain, Av. Hippocrate 10, 1200 Brussels, Belgium*

Correspondence should be addressed to Philippe A. Lysy; philippe.lysy@uclouvain.be

Academic Editor: Georgia Fousteri

Although different criteria were used to define partial remission in type 1 diabetes, the IDAA1C formula has prevailed as it correlates with stimulated C-peptide levels. Our retrospective study evaluated clinical variables associated with the occurrence of IDAA1C-defined partial remission in a series of 239 pediatric patients. Diabetic ketoacidosis and age at diagnosis, but no other clinical feature, influenced the occurrence of remission. We then evaluated whether parameters of glycemic variability used in clinical routine may reliably define partial remission, as these would alleviate confounding factors related to insulin treatment. Using multiple linear regression, we observed that HbA_{1C} levels and percentage of normoglycemia were efficient and sufficient to predict partial remission. These parameters were entered into a formula, called glycemic target-adjusted HbA_{1C} ($GTAA_{1C}$), that corresponded to $HbA_{1C(\%)} - (3 \times \%$ of normoglycemic $\text{values}_{(70-180\ \text{mg/dL})})$. With a threshold of 4.5, this alternative formula predicted partial remission with a sensitivity and a specificity of 72.3% and 92%, respectively, and yielded strong correlation with IDAA1C levels and BETA-2 score, which is a correlate of β-cell function after islet transplantation. We propose $GTAA_{1C}$, based on routine and objective markers of glycemic variability, as a valid alternative for definition of partial remission in type 1 diabetes.

1. Introduction

In type 1 diabetes (T1D), there is a longstanding autoimmune attack of pancreatic β-cells [1] recognizable by seroconversion of specific antibodies [2] that develops on genetic susceptibility grounds [3] and leads to symptomatic insulinopenia when β-cell mass is drastically reduced [4]. Since the fall of insulin stores is abrupt, it is thought that dysregulation of glucose homeostasis is contemporaneous to overt onset (i.e., polyuria and polydipsia) of the disease. Alleviation of hyperglycemia by administration of exogenous insulin is accompanied in about 60% of patients by a rapid reduction of daily insulin requirements (DIR) for maintenance of normal glycemia and HbA_{1C} levels [5]. This defines a transitory state of partial remission (PR) (or "honeymoon period") with residual β-cell function, improved insulin sensitivity [6], and reduced risk of severe hypoglycemia (SH) [7, 8]. As such, PR represents a key period—between 7 and 9 months [9, 10]—in the early management of diabetes: PR seems to be optimal to introduce new diets, immunotherapies, and strategies to preserve and/or expand β-cell mass [4, 11].

The definition of PR, being of particular clinical importance, has been variously addressed and remains a matter of debate [12]. The Hvidoere study group on childhood diabetes proposed the identification of remitters using the insulin dose-adjusted hemoglobin A_{1C} (IDAA1C) formula [13], which strongly correlated with residual β-cell function estimated by stimulated C-peptide levels during mixed-meal tolerance test, when being lower or equal to 9. To validate the IDAA1C definition, the Hvidoere cohort was further compared to a Danish cohort of patients, which had different age and C-peptide secretion profiles, such that the sensitivity and specificity of IDAA1C to predict C-peptide levels were lower than expected [14]. Similarly, Hao et al. described good correlations between IDAA1C and peak C-peptide (>0.2 pmol/mL) levels during the first three years after diagnosis, but rather low sensitivity of IDAA1C itself (≈50% in children and ≈67% in adults) [15]. Yet the IDAA1C threshold (i.e., ≤9) was successfully used elsewhere to identify remitters [10, 16, 17] and level out other parameters, such as daily insulin dose per kilogram of body weight [12].

A common feature of clinically meaningful PR is that patients harbor low levels of glycemic variability (GV) (e.g., standard deviation, coefficient of variability, and percentage of normoglycemia), which is a recognized feature of residual β-cell function since more than three decades [18]. As opposed to daily insulin dose, parameters of GV might per se represent a better assessment of PR since it only refers to objective measures, whereas for patients without electronic logs of insulin doses, correction units may not always be recorded [19]. In this study, we analyzed a retrospective cohort of patients with the aim to develop a definition of PR using parameters independent of DIR and which significantly correlates with hallmarks of β-cell function.

2. Patients and Methods

The study was designed as an observational study with a retrospective cohort of 239 children and adolescents with T1D-attending outpatient clinic in a tertiary health care center (Cliniques Universitaires Saint Luc) and followed in our pediatric diabetes clinic from diagnosis (from 1998 to 2013) to adulthood (18–20 years of age). The local ethical committee approved the study protocol. The study was conducted in accordance to the Declaration of Helsinki. T1D was diagnosed according to International Society for Pediatric and Adolescent Diabetes (ISPAD) guidelines [20] and based on symptoms of insulinopenia, elevated blood glucose (expressed in mg/dL) and HbA_{1C}, positive anti-islet antibodies (GAD65, IA2, and insulin), and lack of family history of genetic diabetes. Biometrics (age, height z-score, and BMI z-score) and biological features (blood glucose, HbA_{1C}) were collected at diagnosis and at each consultation (postdiagnosis consultations occurred at 15 days, 1 month and then every 3 months; only fully adherent patients were recorded). At diagnosis, measures included screening of DKA (defined as pH < 7.3 and/or bicarbonate < 16 mM) and postprandial C-peptide levels (AutoDELFIA C-peptide, PerkinElmer Life and Analytical Sciences), which were assayed every year. Z-scores for height and BMI were assessed using Belgian Flemish reference charts [21]. HbA_{1C} was determined by high-capacity liquid chromatography with iron-resin exchange.

Insulin doses were adjusted for pre- and postprandial glycemic targets according to ISPAD guidelines [20], when available, or to our institution's guidelines. SH was defined as loss of consciousness, coma with or without convulsions, or alteration of consciousness impeding the capacity for oral sugar ingestion (need of a tier for IM glucagon administration). Occurrence of SH was monitored at each consultation (as per our institution's guidelines). Only patients that performed at least five measurements of capillary BG were included in the study. Self-monitoring data were recorded during each consultation. PR was defined as IDAA1C ≤ 9, according to definition by Mortensen et al. [13]: A1C (%) + [4 × insulin dose (U/kg/day)].

Data were analyzed using the GraphPad and Sigmaplot software. Categorical variables were analyzed using chi-square test or Fisher's exact test for small samples. Continuous variables were analyzed using unpaired *t*-test or Mann–Whitney rank sum test, according to the statistical distribution. ANOVA with or without R tests was used, according to the statistical distribution, when there were more than two groups. Normality of distribution was verified through Shapiro-Wilk testing. For continuous variables, data were expressed as mean ± standard deviation when normally distributed, and as median and interquartiles (q25%–q75%) when not. Correlation analysis was used to evaluate relationship between variables. When building logistic regression models, all significant variables in univariate analyses were entered into a multivariate logistic regression. Results are expressed as odds ratio (OR) with 95% confidence intervals. Logistic regression analyses were performed using IBM SPSS Statistics 21.0 software. $P < 0.05$ was considered significant.

3. Results

3.1. Determinants of Partial Remission. In the 239 newly diagnosed patients with T1D, remission occurred in 71.1% ($n = 170$, all being partial) with similar rates of remission in girls (46.9%) and boys (53.1%), although girls were significantly older than boys at diagnosis (Table 1). While age at diagnosis did not influence PR occurrence globally, children less than 5 years of age were significantly less likely than children aged 5–10 years to enter PR (resp., 59% and 77.3%, $P = 0.035$). When children were grouped according to gender, a striking age stratification of PR risk was found for girls only: no more than 19.2% of girls diagnosed before the age of 5 entered PR as compared to 78% and 91% in the groups aged 5–10 and ≥10 years old, respectively ($P < 0.001$). Mean duration of PR was 8.9 ± 8.6 months (range 1.8–44.3), without influence of gender or age.

Characteristics of DKA at diagnosis and of HbA_{1C} and C-peptide evolution are described in Table S1 and Figure 1. Data were similar to what we described earlier [10], with few exceptions. At baseline, mean HbA_{1C} levels were 10.8 ± 2.7% and positively correlated with age, but not with gender, in the PR group (HbA_{1C} of 9.7 ± 1.9%, 10.4 ± 2.2%, and 11.4 ± 3.1% for the <5 years, 5–10 years, and ≥10 years, resp.; $P = 0.002$) (Figures 1(a) and 1(b)). Median basal C-peptide levels at diagnosis and after one and two years were 0.19 (0.1–0.33) pmol/mL, 0.16 (0.05–0.35) pmol/mL, and 0.08 (0–0.22) pmol/mL, respectively ($P < 0.001$) (Figures 1(c) and 1(d)). At baseline and during follow-up, children >10 years of age had significantly higher C-peptide levels than other age groups, as described elsewhere [10, 14]. Also, C-peptide values at baseline were higher in girls (0.21 [0.12–0.39] pmol/mL) than in boys (0.16 [0.07–0.30] pmol/mL) ($P < 0.01$) but this difference was not observed

Table 1: Characteristics of the clinical series at diagnosis.

		Total ($n = 239$)	PR ($n = 170$)	No PR ($n = 69$)	P^a
Gender n (%)					0.6
Girls		112 (46.9)	78 (69.6)	34 (30.4)	0.3
	<5 yrs n (%)	9 (8)	5 (55.6)	4 (44.4)	
	5–10 yrs n (%)	41 (36.6)	32 (78)	9 (22)	
	≥10 yrs n (%)	62 (55.4)	41 (66.1)	21 (33.9)	
Boys		127 (53.1)	92 (72.4)	35 (27.6)	0.2
	<5 yrs n (%)	30 (23.6)	18 (60)	12 (40)	
	5–10 yrs n (%)	47 (37)	36 (76.6)	11 (23.4)	
	≥10 yrs n (%)	50 (39.4)	38 (76)	12 (24)	
Age at Δ					0.1
	<5 yrs n (%)	39 (16.3)	23 (59)	16 (41)	
	5–10 yrs n (%)	88 (36.8)	68 (77.3)	20 (22.7)	
	≥10 yrs n (%)	112 (46.9)	79 (70.5)	33 (29.5)	
	Mean (yrs[b])	9.1 ± 3.8	9.2 ± 3.6	8.8 ± 4.34	
	Median (yrs[c])	9.7 (6.3–11.9)	9.67 (6.6–11.8)	9.67 (5.3–12.2)	0.7
	Range (yrs)	0.8–16.4	1.8–16.4	0.8–16.2	
	Girls (yrs)[c]	10.3 (7.2–12.3)	10 (7.2–12.2)	11.3 (7.7–12.2)	0.03
	Boys (yrs)[c]	8.9 (5–11.6)	9.4 (5.7–11.5)	7.5 (3.5–11.5)	

[a]Categorical variables were analyzed using chi-square test; ages at diagnosis were analyzed using Mann–Whitney rank sum test (PR-no PR). [b]Mean ± SD; [c]median and interquartile range (q25%–q75%); Δ: diagnosis; yrs: years.

later on during follow-up. In our cohort, the presence of PR according to the IDAA1C definition was predictive of a C-peptide value higher than 0.3 pmol/mL, with a 51% sensitivity and 80.2% specificity. The best correlation was observed among children <5 years at diagnosis, with a sensitivity of 57.7% and a specificity of 84.8%. In multivariate logistic regression, DKA ($P = 0.04$) and an age of 5–10 years ($P = 0.01$) were the only variables at diagnosis that were associated with a higher chance of experiencing PR.

We found 87.5% and 71.7% of patients positive at diagnosis for anti-IA2 and anti-GAD65 antibodies, respectively. Girls were more likely to be positive for anti-GAD65 than boys (84% versus 60.7%, resp.; $P = 0.002$). When comparing patient subgroups, no significant difference was found for islet antibody titers (i.e., anti-IA2, anti-GAD65, and anti-insulin) and no association could be found between these titers and PR occurrence. Positive (i.e., ≥20 U/mL) anti-transglutaminase antibodies were found in 4.6% of patients at diagnosis, without correlation with the onset of PR. Also, during the three-year follow-up after diagnosis, only a trend toward lower risk of SH episodes in the PR group could be observed (23.5% in PR versus 34.8% in no PR group, resp.; $P = 0.075$) (Table S2). However, this difference was significant when we considered only patients aged <10 years (29.7% in PR versus 55.6% in no PR group; $P = 0.006$). Finally, we found no seasonal influence on the probability of PR.

3.2. Prediction of PR Based on Routine Parameters of GV. We aimed to predict PR with indexes of glucose homeostasis used in clinical routine, that is, HbA_{1C}, percentage of normoglycemia (% normoglycemia), mean blood glucose, standard deviation to the mean (SD), and coefficient of variation (CV, equal to DS divided by mean blood glucose). When these parameters were run in multivariate analysis, we observed that only HbA_{1C} levels and percentage of normoglycemia significantly (with a significant P value or with a significant correlation coefficient) influenced PR prediction as defined by the IDAA1C criterion (Table S3). These were integrated into a new formula for PR prediction, as follows: glycemic target-adjusted HbA_{1C} or $GTAA_{1C}$, being equal to $HbA_{1C(\%)} - (3 \times [\%\ \text{normoglycemia}_{(70\text{–}180\ \text{mg/dL})}])$, predicted PR when scored ≤4.5. As expected, $GTAA_{1C}$ strongly correlated with IDAA1C ($r^2 = 0.71$, $P < 0.001$) and predicted IDAA1C-defined PR with 73.2% sensitivity and 92% specificity. When $GTAA_{1C}$ was evaluated for its capacity to predict PR in patients from different age groups, it showed high specificity for patients <5 years (99.3%, with 64.4% sensitivity, $r^2 = 0.79$) and high sensitivity for patients >10 years (80.9%, with 86.5% specificity, $r^2 = 0.73$), whereas for patients aged 5–10 years, sensitivity and specificity 67.7% and 95.4%, respectively, ($r^2 = 0.75$). No effect of gender was found on sensitivity and specificity of $GTAA_{1C}$.

With $GTAA_{1C}$, PR rates were slightly lower than with IDAA1C: 66.1% of patients entered PR, among those 70.5% of girls and 62.2% of boys were included ($P = 0.17$). Interestingly, there was a significant age-dependent distribution of PR rate with the $GTAA_{1C}$ definition, as PR occurred in 43.6%, 60.2%, and 78.6%, respectively, in children aged <5 years, 5–10 years, and ≥10 years at diagnosis ($P < 0.001$). Also, $GTAA_{1C}$-defined PR were slightly shorter than its

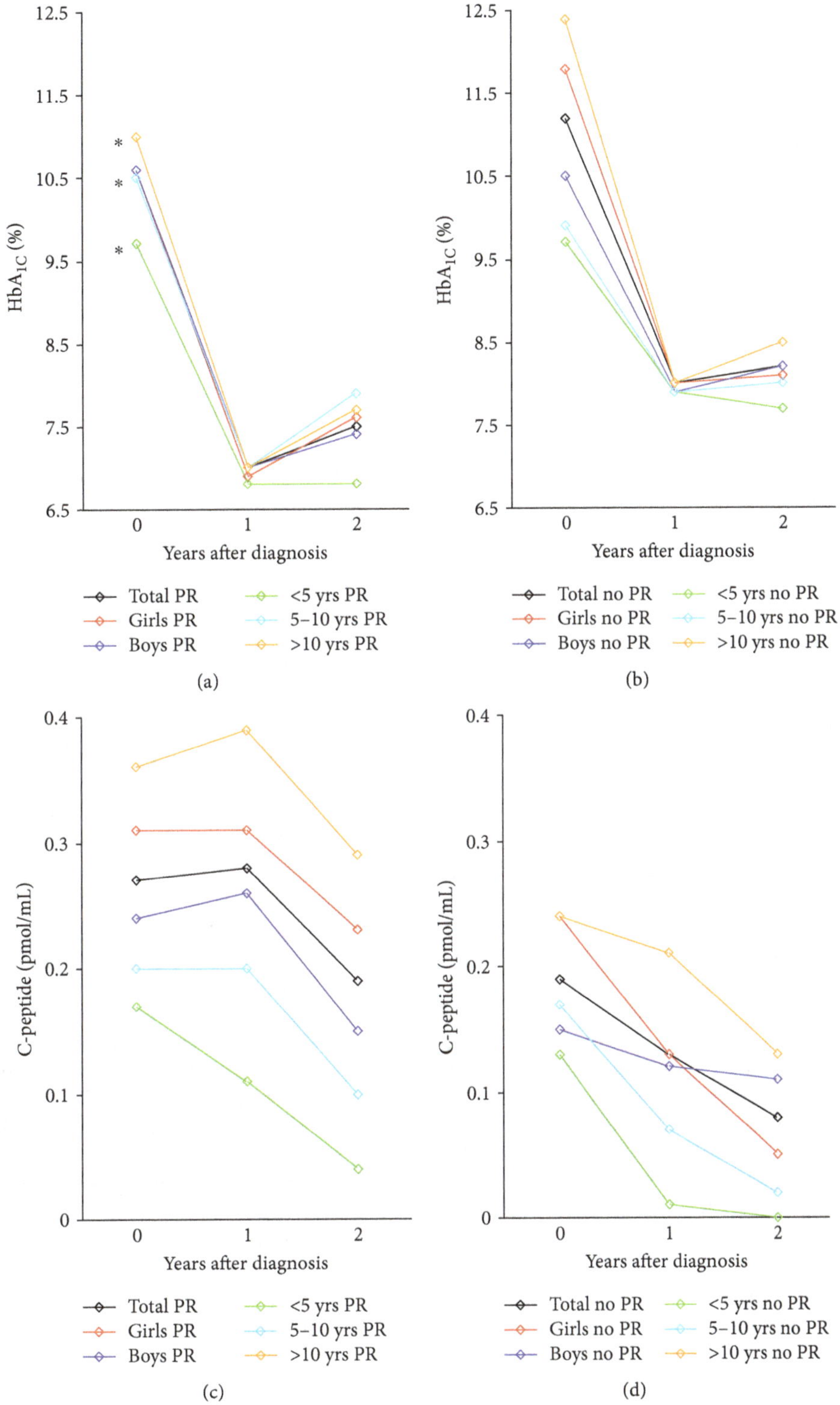

FIGURE 1: Evolution of HbA_{1C} and C-peptide values at diagnosis and during follow-up. Graphs represent mean HbA_{1C} levels (in %) in PR (a) and no PR (b) groups, mean C-peptide values (in pmol/mL) in PR (c) and no PR (d) groups at diagnosis, and one and two years postdiagnosis. Mean HbA_{1C} levels were at 10.6 ± 2.6% in PR and 11.2 ± 3% in no PR group ($P = 0.33$). Those levels were, respectively, at 6.9% (6.2–7.5) and 7.7% (6.9–8.6) at one year ($P < 0.001$) and at 7.5% (6.7–8.1) and 7.7% (6.9–8.5) at two years ($P = 0.023$), in patients with PR and without PR. For the remitter group, median C-peptide levels were, respectively, at 0.21 pmol/mL (0.11–0.35), 0.22 pmol/mL (0.1–0.41), and 0.11 pmol/mL (0–0.28) at diagnosis, one year and two years postdiagnosis. For the nonremitter group, median C-peptide levels were, respectively, at 0.15 pmol/mL (0.1–0.23), 0.05 pmol/mL (0–0.17), and 0 pmol/mL (0–0.09) at diagnosis, one year and two years postdiagnosis. *Compared HbA_{1C} levels at diagnosis among age subgroups (i.e., 9.7 ± 1.9%, 10.4 ± 2.2%, and 11.4 ± 3.1% for the <5 years, 5–10 years, and ≥10 years, resp.; $P = 0.0017$).

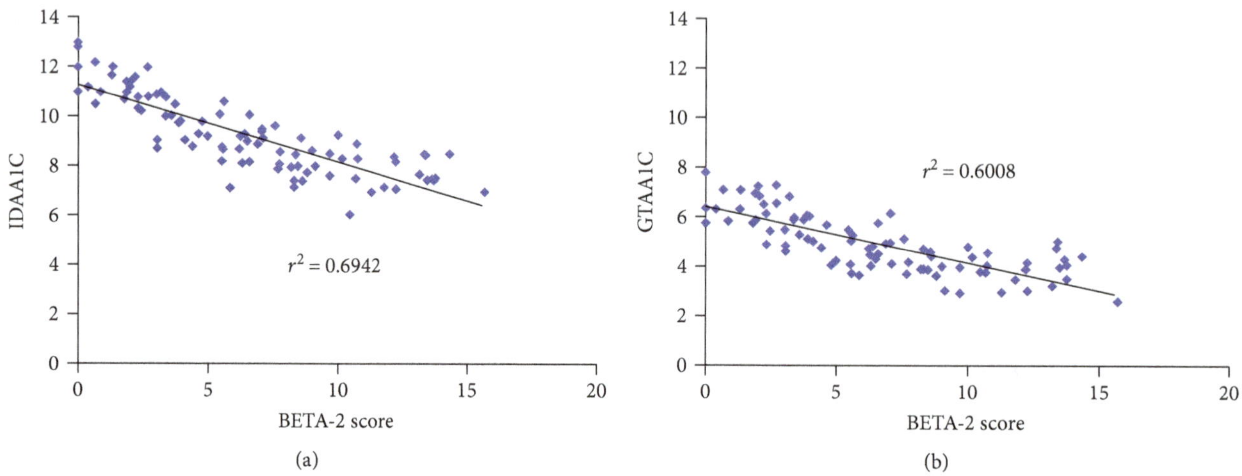

FIGURE 2: Correlation of BETA-2 score with IDAA1C and $GTAA_{1C}$ definitions of PR. Graphs show correlation between BETA-2 score and IDAA1C-based ((a) $P < 0.001$) or $GTAA_{1C}$-based ((b) $P < 0.001$) criteria for PR in a subgroup of 90 patients from our cohort. These correlations (BETA-2 and IDAA1C versus BETA-2 and $GTAA_{1C}$) were not statistically different in multivariate analysis. Related r^2 were noted in the corresponding graphs.

IDAA1C counterpart and averaged 8.3 ± 8.04 months without differences for gender or age.

Levels of $GTAA_{1C}$ at 3 months postdiagnosis were inversely correlated with PR duration ($r^2 = 0.26$, $P < 0.001$) and, when calculated to be ≤ 3.5, between 3.5 and 4 and between 4 and 4.5, these levels predicted a PR duration >300 days in 47.9%, 29.3%, and 5.9% of patients ($P < 0.001$) (Figure S1). Among children with $GTAA_{1C}$ values at 3 months postdiagnosis >4.5, only 22% experienced PR, whereas when it levelled above 5, only 11.7% of patients had characteristics of PR. These predictions were not significantly different when PR was characterized according to the IDAA1C criterion (Figure S1).

Because the $GTAA_{1C}$ definition only refers to parameters of GV, we confronted its levels calculated in our series of patients with a score reflecting β-cell function. We chose the BETA-2 score [22], which integrates biomarkers extracted from a morning fasted blood sample (i.e., C-peptide [nM], plasma glucose [mM], HbA_{1C} [%]) and DIR (total units/kg body weight) and which was validated in the setting of islet transplantation in patients with T1D. Because we wanted to limit our investigations in patients with a regular follow-up, by excluding all samplings performed in a clinical trial setting, we restricted our analysis to patients with blood samples drawn during the consultation, that is, in postprandial state. Comparison of BETA-2 score with both IDAA1C and $GTAA_{1C}$ yielded robust correlation criteria ($r^2 = 0.69$ and 0.60, resp.) (Figure 2). This confirmed, at least indirectly, the potential of $GTAA_{1C}$ to reflect residual β-cell function in patients with T1D.

4. Discussion

Although several groups studied characteristics of PR in patients with T1D [9, 13, 23, 24], since 2009, most common prediction studies relied on the IDAA1C formula, which is a valid predictor of PR and stimulated C-peptide values above 0.3 pmol/mL [13]. Despite being validated by different authors [10, 14, 15, 25] and widely used [10, 11, 26, 27], IDAAC1 has two main limitations. First, the correlation of IDAA1C with C-peptide loses specificity and sensitivity with age [13, 14, 17] and tends to underestimate C-peptide levels in children presenting a score above 9 [14–16]. This is especially true in the ">10-year" group where this formula does not discriminate between residual insulin secretion and increased insulin resistance [13, 14]. Second, this score depends on two variables: HbA_{1C} and DIR, which may depend on multiple confounding factors such as hospital guidelines, clinicians' habits, and patient/parents own management of insulin injections. Moreover, DIR estimation does not take into account insulin correction doses [15, 17]. PR might thus be better defined by objective parameters of GV, as those correlate with glucose control [28].

Hirsch et al. [29] define GV as the degree to which a patient's blood glucose level fluctuates between high (hyperglycemia) and low (hypoglycemia) levels, which are known inducers of oxidative stress [30–33], increased comorbidities, and lower residual C-peptide secretion [4, 28, 34]. GV is per se associated with increased cardiovascular risk, as shown in nondiabetic subjects and in diabetic patients stratified for GV parameters but having similar HbA_{1C} levels [35–37]. Among multiple GV parameters [38], clinicians only use in routine the percentage of normoglycemia, the mean glucose level and related standard deviation, and the coefficient of variation of glucose. In 2015, Buckingham and coworkers [16] showed that the percentage of normoglycemia, although not directly integrating peak and nadir glycemic values, is a good predictor of stimulated C-peptide levels above 0.2 pmol/mL if 60% of glucose measurements lie between 3.9 and 7.8 mM, although a clear-cut threshold value was not met. This study suggests the potential of simple GV parameters to serve as variables in the definition of PR.

In our study, we first investigated prevalence and key indicators of remission in a cohort of children with new-onset T1D and then proposed an alternative formula to IDAA1C to predict PR independently of DIR. Using the IDAA1C formula, we found a prevalence of remission of 71% with a mean PR duration of 8.9 months and a peak prevalence 3 months after onset, as described elsewhere [10, 13, 14, 17, 25] even with different PR definition [39]. Also in agreement with previous studies [9, 10, 27, 40, 41] were the findings that T1D onset in patients between 5–10 years and higher C-peptide levels at diagnosis were more frequent in remitters, that younger onset (<5 years) of T1D was associated with a lower rate of PR and that presence of DKA ($pH < 7.3$) at diagnosis was negatively correlated with PR. Also, while other studies [10, 17, 42] described a negative correlation between anti-islet antibodies and PR, we found no such correlation within our cohort, which may partly be explained by the retrospective design of our study. We also did not find correlation between gender, HbA_{1C} levels, and season at diagnosis with PR. A negative association between the risk of SH in the two first years postdiagnosis and age at diagnosis was observed, in accordance with other studies [43–46] and might be explained by difficulties to recognize and react to symptoms of hypoglycemia, and to the lack of consistent meals in the youngest group of patients. We also found a significant reduction of SH rates in patients <10 years that entered PR (23.5% versus 34.8%).

After validating IDAA1C in our cohort, we aimed to generate a new formula integrating GV parameters (as suggested elsewhere [16]) that can be easily measured in routine clinical practice. We therefore ran multiple linear regression to compare IDAA1C with different GV variables and isolated two parameters correlating with IDAA1C: HbA_{1C} and percentage of normoglycemia. A new alternative PR definition, independent of DIR and integrating GV parameters, was generated and corresponded to $GTAA_{1C}$ (being equal to $HbA_{1C(\%)} - [3 \times \%\ \text{normoglycemia}_{(70-180\ \text{mg/dL})}]$), predictive of PR when ≤4.5. Since $GTAA_{1C}$ was generated by reference to IDAA1C, the correlation between both formula was strong ($r^2 = 0.71$). $GTAA_{1C}$ yielded high sensitivity (72.3%) and specificity (92%) in predicting IDAA1C-defined PR. In our patients, prevalence of PR and mean PR duration was slightly lower with $GTAA_{1C}$ (66.1% and 8.3 months) than with IDAAC (71.1% and 8.9 months). Using $GTAA_{1C}$, PR prediction was more specific (99.3%) in younger children and more sensible (80.9%) in older children groups but maintained good correlation scores with IDAA1C throughout every age subgroups. $GTAA_{1C}$ tended to underestimate PR in young children (41% versus 59%) due to lower sensitivity (64.4%) in the young children group (<5 years) and to overestimate PR in older children (>10 years) (75% versus 70.5%) due to lower specificity (86.5%).

Episodes of SH were previously shown to be reduced in patients with T1D and residual-stimulated C-peptide levels >0.04 pmol/mL [8, 34] and in patients with late-onset diabetes [43–46]. In a study reanalyzing DCCT data, Kilpatrick and colleagues [47] demonstrated independent correlation between SH and each three of these parameters, HbA_{1C}, mean blood glucose and GV (each of those three being more stable during PR). Therefore, PR should be considered as a protective factor against SH, as we observed in our study for children <10 years ($P = 0.006$). Paradoxically, we found no significant differences in the risk of presenting SH between remitter and nonremitters in the >10-year group, which might be explained by the insufficient discrimination of patients with reduced insulin sensitivity by IDAA1C in the postpubertal group.

C-peptide secretion is considered as the gold standard measure for residual insulin secretion in diabetic patients [48]. Pioneer studies [49, 50] have shown increased C-peptide secretion three months after initiation of insulin therapy, linking stimulated C-peptide with PR occurrence [49]. One limitation of our study comes from C-peptide measurements performed randomly rather than after fasting or stimulation tests. However, our investigations were aimed at characterizing PR and developing new PR definition by using routine clinical parameters. Stimulated C-peptide tests might represent a better reflect of β-cell function [51] but lacked prediction value for description of PR [14, 16] or to assess clinically significant endogenous insulin secretion in immunoprevention studies [52] or in longitudinal studies of patients with longstanding T1D [53]. Moreover, our data converged with previous studies that characterized C-peptide values at diagnosis of T1D and during follow-up [13, 15, 16].

β-Score [54], revised as BETA-2 score [22], was developed to determine graft function after islet transplantation in patients with complicated T1D. *BETA*-2 score is calculated on biological markers measured in a single blood sampling (i.e., fasting C-peptide, fasting glucose, DIR, and HbA_{1C} levels) and negatively correlates with stimulated glucose values. Parameters of GV are other valuable tools to evaluate outcomes of islet grafts. The team of Vantyghem et al. [55] found that mean glucose was a valid determinant of islet graft function with negative ($R = -0.65$ with β-score) correlation with continuous glucose-monitoring values. Furthermore, Barton et al. [56] showed that GV and SH were competitive parameters, as compared to insulin doses, to predict islet secretion function. Recent study showed that GV evaluated by SD glucose and CONGA4 score was more reliable than HbA_{1C} to assess islet function and risk of clinical events such as SH [57]. We therefore compared $GTAA_{1C}$ with BETA-2 score in our cohort of patients and found a strong correlation of $r^2 = 0.60$ between those parameters, indirectly confirming $GTAA_{1C}$ ability to reflect residual β-cell function.

In this study, we describe characteristics of PR in a Belgian cohort of pediatric patients with T1D and underline the paucity of clinical determinants, besides DKA, for prediction of PR occurrence. Moreover, we propose the $GTAA_{1C}$ criterion as a new definition of PR, based on routine clinical parameters of GV and independent from insulin treatment management, which showed strong correlation with parameters of β-cell function. Longitudinal studies are now mandatory for external validation of the potential of $GTAA_{1C}$ to identify PR patients with new-onset T1D.

Conflicts of Interest

The authors declare that they have no conflicts of interest.

Authors' Contributions

Nina Nielens and Olivier Pollé contributed equally to this work, and they are thus sharing the first authorship.

References

[1] T. L. van Belle, K. T. Coppieters, and M. G. von Herrath, "Type 1 diabetes: etiology, immunology, and therapeutic strategies," *Physiological Reviews*, vol. 91, no. 1, pp. 79–118, 2011.

[2] R. A. Watkins, C. Evans-Molina, J. S. Blum, and L. A. DiMeglio, "Established and emerging biomarkers for the prediction of type 1 diabetes: a systematic review," *Translational Research*, vol. 164, no. 2, pp. 110–121, 2014.

[3] P. A. Lysy, "Update on genetic determinants of type1 diabetes," *Journal of Molecular and Genetic Medicine*, vol. 08, no. 03, pp. 126–133, 2014.

[4] E. Akirav, J. A. Kushner, and K. C. Herold, "β-cell mass and type 1 diabetes: going, going, gone?," *Diabetes*, vol. 57, no. 11, pp. 2883–2888, 2008.

[5] I. M. Hramiak, J. Dupre, and D. T. Finegood, "Determinants of clinical remission in recent-onset IDDM," *Diabetes Care*, vol. 16, no. 1, pp. 125–132, 1993.

[6] H. Yki-Järvinen, R. A. DeFronzo, and V. A. Koivisto, "Normalization of insulin sensitivity in type I diabetic subjects by physical training during insulin pump therapy," *Diabetes Care*, vol. 7, no. 6, pp. 520–527, 1984.

[7] The Diabetes Control and Complications Trial group, "Hypoglycemia in the diabetes control and complications trial," *Diabetes*, vol. 46, no. 2, pp. 271–286, 1997.

[8] J. S. Sørensen, J. Johannesen, F. Pociot et al., "Residual β-cell function 3–6 years after onset of type 1 diabetes reduces risk of severe hypoglycemia in children and adolescents," *Diabetes Care*, vol. 36, no. 11, pp. 3454–3459, 2013.

[9] M. Abdul-Rasoul, H. Habib, and M. Al-Khouly, ""The honeymoon phase" in children with type 1 diabetes mellitus: frequency, duration, and influential factors," *Pediatric Diabetes*, vol. 7, no. 2, pp. 101–107, 2006.

[10] A. Pecheur, T. Barrea, V. Vandooren, V. Beauloye, A. Robert, and P. A. Lysy, "Characteristics and determinants of partial remission in children with type 1 diabetes using the insulin-dose-adjusted A1C definition," *Journal of diabetes research*, vol. 2014, Article ID 851378, 7 pages, 2014.

[11] M. Fonolleda, M. Murillo, and F. Vázquez, "Remission phase in paediatric type 1 diabetes: new understanding and emerging biomarkers," *Hormone Research in Paediatrics*, vol. 88, no. 5, pp. 307–315, 2017.

[12] R. L. Lundberg, K. R. Marino, A. Jasrotia et al., "Partial clinical remission in type 1 diabetes: a comparison of the accuracy of total daily dose of insulin of <0.3 units/kg/day to the gold standard insulin-dose adjusted hemoglobin A_{1c} of ≤9 for the detection of partial clinical remission," *Journal of Pediatric Endocrinology and Metabolism*, vol. 30, no. 8, pp. 823–830, 2017.

[13] H. B. Mortensen, P. Hougaard, P. Swift et al., "New definition for the partial remission period in children and adolescents with type 1 diabetes," *Diabetes Care*, vol. 32, no. 8, pp. 1384–1390, 2009.

[14] M. L. Max Andersen, P. Hougaard, S. Pörksen et al., "Partial remission definition: validation based on the insulin dose-adjusted HbA1c (IDAA1C) in 129 Danish children with new-onset type 1 diabetes," *Pediatric Diabetes*, vol. 15, no. 7, pp. 469–476, 2014.

[15] W. Hao, S. Gitelman, L. A. DiMeglio, D. Boulware, C. J. Greenbaum, and Type 1 Diabetes TrialNet Study Group, "Fall in C-peptide during first 4 years from diagnosis of type 1 diabetes: variable relation to age, HbA_{1c}, and insulin dose," *Diabetes Care*, vol. 39, no. 10, pp. 1664-1670, 2016.

[16] B. Buckingham, P. Cheng, R. W. Beck et al., "CGM-measured glucose values have a strong correlation with C-peptide, HbA_{1c} and IDAAC, but do poorly in predicting C-peptide levels in the two years following onset of diabetes," *Diabetologia*, vol. 58, no. 6, pp. 1167–1174, 2015.

[17] K. Nagl, J. M. Hermann, M. Plamper et al., "Factors contributing to partial remission in type 1 diabetes: analysis based on the insulin dose-adjusted HbA1c in 3657 children and adolescents from Germany and Austria," *Pediatric Diabetes*, vol. 18, no. 6, pp. 428–434, 2017.

[18] M. Fukuda, A. Tanaka, Y. Tahara et al., "Correlation between minimal secretory capacity of pancreatic β-cells and stability of diabetic control," *Diabetes*, vol. 37, no. 1, pp. 81–88, 1988.

[19] G. Kramer, N. Kuniss, C. Kloos et al., "Principles and frequency of self-adjustment of insulin dose in people with diabetes mellitus type 1 and correlation with markers of metabolic control," *Diabetes Research and Clinical Practice*, vol. 116, pp. 299–305, 2016.

[20] M. E. Craig, C. Jefferies, D. Dabelea, N. Balde, A. Seth, and K. C. Donaghue, "Definition, epidemiology, and classification of diabetes in children and adolescents," *Pediatric Diabetes*, vol. 15, Supplement S20, pp. 4–17, 2014.

[21] M. Roelants, R. Hauspie, and K. Hoppenbrouwers, "References for growth and pubertal development from birth to 21 years in Flanders, Belgium," *Annals of Human Biology*, vol. 36, no. 6, pp. 680–694, 2009.

[22] S. Forbes, R. A. Oram, A. Smith et al., "Validation of the BETA-2 score: an improved tool to estimate beta cell function after clinical islet transplantation using a single fasting blood sample," *American Journal of Transplantation*, vol. 16, no. 9, pp. 2704–2713, 2016.

[23] A. Dost, A. Herbst, K. Kintzel et al., "Shorter remission period in young versus older children with diabetes mellitus type 1," *Experimental and Clinical Endocrinology & Diabetes*, vol. 115, no. 01, pp. 33–37, 2007.

[24] H. P. Chase, T. A. MacKenzie, J. Burdick et al., "Redefining the clinical remission period in children with type 1 diabetes," *Pediatric Diabetes*, vol. 5, no. 1, pp. 16–19, 2004.

[25] O. M. Neylon, M. White, M. A. O´Connell, and F. J. Cameron, "Insulin-dose-adjusted HbA_{1c}-defined partial remission phase in a paediatric population-when is the honeymoon over?," *Diabetic Medicine*, vol. 30, no. 5, pp. 627-628, 2013.

[26] J. J. Couper, M. J. Haller, A. G. Ziegler, M. Knip, J. Ludvigsson, and M. E. Craig, "Phases of type 1 diabetes in children and adolescents," *Pediatric Diabetes*, vol. 15, Supplement S20, pp. 18–25, 2014.

[27] İ. Esen, F. Demirel, D. Tepe, and Ö. Kara, "Frequency of partial remission and related factors in children and adolescents diagnosed with type 1 diabetes mellitus," *International Journal of Diabetes in Developing Countries*, vol. 35, no. 3, pp. 230–235, 2015.

[28] J. M. Lachin, I. Bebu, R. M. Bergenstal et al., "Association of glycemic variability in type 1 diabetes with progression of microvascular outcomes in the diabetes control and complications trial," *Diabetes Care*, vol. 40, no. 6, pp. 777–783, 2017.

[29] I. B. Hirsch, "Glycemic variability and diabetes complications: does it matter? Of course it does!," *Diabetes care*, vol. 38, no. 8, pp. 1610–1614, 2015.

[30] L. Quagliaro, L. Piconi, and R. Assaloni, "Intermittent high glucose enhances apoptosis related to oxidative stress in human umbilical vein endothelial cells: the role of protein kinase C and NAD(P)H-oxidase activation," *Diabetes*, vol. 52, no. 11, pp. 2795–2804, 2003.

[31] L. Monnier, E. Mas, C. Ginet et al., "Activation of oxidative stress by acute glucose fluctuations compared with sustained chronic hyperglycemia in patients with type 2 diabetes," *JAMA*, vol. 295, no. 14, pp. 1681–1687, 2006.

[32] A. Ceriello, K. Esposito, L. Piconi et al., "Oscillating glucose is more deleterious to endothelial function and oxidative stress than mean glucose in normal and type 2 diabetic patients," *Diabetes*, vol. 57, no. 5, pp. 1349–1354, 2008.

[33] E. M. Horváth, R. Benkő, L. Kiss et al., "Rapid 'glycaemic swings' induce nitrosative stress, activate poly(ADP-ribose) polymerase and impair endothelial function in a rat model of diabetes mellitus," *Diabetologia*, vol. 52, no. 5, pp. 952–961, 2009.

[34] M. W. Steffes, S. Sibley, M. Jackson, and W. Thomas, "β-cell function and the development of diabetes-related complications in the diabetes control and complications trial," *Diabetes Care*, vol. 26, no. 3, pp. 832–836, 2003.

[35] M. Lind, A. M. Svensson, M. Kosiborod et al., "Glycemic control and excess mortality in type 1 diabetes," *New England Journal of Medicine*, vol. 371, no. 21, pp. 1972–1982, 2014.

[36] E. B. Levitan, Y. Song, E. S. Ford, and S. Liu, "Is nondiabetic hyperglycemia a risk factor for cardiovascular disease?: a meta-analysis of prospective studies," *Archives of Internal Medicine*, vol. 164, no. 19, pp. 2147–2155, 2004.

[37] J. Sherr, V. W. Tamborlane, and D. Xing, "Achievement of target A1C levels with negligible hypoglycemia and low glucose variability in youth with short-term type 1 diabetes and residual β-cell function," *Diabetes Care*, vol. 35, no. 4, pp. 817–820, 2012.

[38] Y. Saisho, "Glycemic variability and oxidative stress: a link between diabetes and cardiovascular disease?," *International Journal of Molecular Sciences*, vol. 15, no. 10, pp. 18381–18406, 2014.

[39] P. Pozzilli, S. Manfrini, R. Buzzetti et al., "Glucose evaluation trial for remission (GETREM) in type 1 diabetes: a European multicentre study," *Diabetes Research and Clinical Practice*, vol. 68, no. 3, pp. 258–264, 2005.

[40] S. A. Bowden, M. M. Duck, and R. P. Hoffman, "Young children (<5 yr) and adolescents (>12 yr) with type 1 diabetes mellitus have low rate of partial remission: diabetic ketoacidosis is an important risk factor," *Pediatric Diabetes*, vol. 9, no. 3, Part 1, pp. 197–201, 2008.

[41] E. Böber, B. Dündar, and A. Büyükgebiz, "Partial remission phase and metabolic control in type 1 diabetes mellitus in children and adolescents," *Journal of Pediatric Endocrinology and Metabolism*, vol. 14, no. 4, pp. 435–441, 2001.

[42] K. R. Marino, R. L. Lundberg, A. Jasrotia et al., "A predictive model for lack of partial clinical remission in new-onset pediatric type 1 diabetes," *PLoS One*, vol. 12, no. 5, article e0176860, 2017.

[43] V. M. Wagner, M. Grabert, and R. W. Holl, "Severe hypoglycaemia, metabolic control and diabetes management in children with type 1 diabetes in the decade after the diabetes control and complications trial – a large-scale multicentre study," *European Journal of Pediatrics*, vol. 164, no. 2, pp. 73–79, 2005.

[44] W. Clarke, T. Jones, A. Rewers, D. Dunger, and G. J. Klingensmith, "Assessment and management of hypoglycemia in children and adolescents with diabetes," *Pediatric Diabetes*, vol. 10, Supplement 12, pp. 134–145, 2009.

[45] A. Johansen, B. Kanijo, S. Fredheim et al., "Prevalence and predictors of severe hypoglycemia in Danish children and adolescents with diabetes," *Pediatric Diabetes*, vol. 16, no. 5, pp. 354–360, 2015.

[46] E. Cengiz, D. Xing, J. C. Wong et al., "Severe hypoglycemia and diabetic ketoacidosis among youth with type 1 diabetes in the T1D exchange clinic registry," *Pediatric Diabetes*, vol. 14, no. 6, pp. 447–454, 2013.

[47] E. S. Kilpatrick, A. S. Rigby, K. Goode, and S. L. Atkin, "Relating mean blood glucose and glucose variability to the risk of multiple episodes of hypoglycaemia in type 1 diabetes," *Diabetologia*, vol. 50, no. 12, pp. 2553–2561, 2007.

[48] J. P. Palmer, G. A. Fleming, C. J. Greenbaum et al., "C-Peptide is the appropriate outcome measure for type 1 diabetes clinical trials to preserve β-cell function: report of an ADA workshop, 21–22 October 2001," *Diabetes*, vol. 53, no. 1, pp. 250–264, 2004.

[49] E. B. Sochett, D. Daneman, C. Clarson, and R. M. Ehrlich, "Factors affecting and patterns of residual insulin secretion during the first year of type 1 (insulin-dependent) diabetes mellitus in children," *Diabetologia*, vol. 30, no. 7, pp. 453–459, 1987.

[50] J. J. Couper, I. Hudson, G. A. Werther, G. L. Warne, J. M. Court, and L. C. Harrison, "Factors predicting residual β-cell function in the first year after diagnosis of childhood type 1 diabetes," *Diabetes Research and Clinical Practice*, vol. 11, no. 1, pp. 9–16, 1991.

[51] A. G. Jones and A. T. Hattersley, "The clinical utility of C-peptide measurement in the care of patients with diabetes," *Diabetic Medicine*, vol. 30, no. 7, pp. 803–817, 2013.

[52] N. Sherry, W. Hagopian, J. Ludvigsson et al., "Teplizumab for treatment of type 1 diabetes (protégé study): 1-year results from a randomised, placebo-controlled trial," *The Lancet*, vol. 378, no. 9790, pp. 487–497, 2011.

[53] H. A. Keenan, J. K. Sun, J. Levine et al., "Residual insulin production and pancreatic β-cell turnover after 50 years of diabetes: Joslin medalist study," *Diabetes*, vol. 59, no. 11, pp. 2846–2853, 2010.

[54] E. A. Ryan, B. W. Paty, and P. A. Senior, "β-Score: an assessment of β-cell function after islet transplantation," *Diabetes Care*, vol. 28, no. 2, pp. 343–347, 2005.

[55] M. C. Vantyghem, V. Raverdy, and A. S. Balavoine, "Continuous glucose monitoring after islet transplantation in type 1 diabetes: an excellent graft function (β-score greater than 7) is required to abrogate hyperglycemia, whereas a minimal function is necessary to suppress severe hypoglycemia (β-score greater than 3)," *The Journal of Clinical Endocrinology & Metabolism*, vol. 97, no. 11, pp. E2078–E2083, 2012.

[56] F. B. Barton, M. R. Rickels, R. Alejandro et al., "Improvement in outcomes of clinical islet transplantation: 1999-2010," *Diabetes Care*, vol. 35, no. 7, pp. 1436–1445, 2012.

[57] D. J. Holmes-Walker, J. E. Gunton, W. Hawthorne et al., "Islet transplantation provides superior glycemic control with less hypoglycemia compared with continuous subcutaneous insulin infusion or multiple daily insulin injections," *Transplantation*, vol. 101, no. 6, pp. 1268–1275, 2017.

3

Variables to Be Monitored via Biomedical Sensors for Complete Type 1 Diabetes Mellitus Management: An Extension of the "On-Board" Concept

Ignacio Rodríguez-Rodríguez,[1] **José-Víctor Rodríguez**,[2] **and Miguel-Ángel Zamora-Izquierdo**[1]

[1]*Universidad de Murcia, Spain*
[2]*Universidad Politécnica de Cartagena, Spain*

Correspondence should be addressed to Ignacio Rodríguez-Rodríguez; ignacio.rodriguez1@um.es

Academic Editor: Michaelangela Barbieri

Type 1 diabetes mellitus (DM1) is a growing disease, and a deep understanding of the patient is required to prescribe the most appropriate treatment, adjusted to the patient's habits and characteristics. Before now, knowledge regarding each patient has been incomplete, discontinuous, and partial. However, the recent development of continuous glucose monitoring (CGM) and new biomedical sensors/gadgets, based on automatic continuous monitoring, offers a new perspective on DM1 management, since these innovative devices allow the collection of 24-hour biomedical data in addition to blood glucose levels. With this, it is possible to deeply characterize a diabetic person, offering a better understanding of his or her illness evolution, and, going further, develop new strategies to manage DM1. This new and global monitoring makes it possible to extend the "on-board" concept to other features. This well-known approach to the processing of variable "insulin" describes some inertias and aggregated/remaining effects. In this work, such analysis is carried out along with a thorough study of the significant variables to be taken into account/monitored—and how to arrange them—for a deep characterization of diabetic patients. Lastly, we present a case study evaluating the experience of the continuous and comprehensive monitoring of a diabetic patient, concluding that the huge potential of this new perspective could provide an acute insight into the patient's status and extract the maximum amount of knowledge, thus improving the DM1 management system in order to be fully functional.

1. Introduction

Diabetes is a metabolic disease, characterized by chronic hyperglycemia resulting from the body's inability to produce and/or use insulin. In a nondiabetic human, glucose homeostasis is a closed-loop system which is able to regulate blood glucose (BG) levels. Unfortunately, this regulation is not possible in patients suffering from type 1 diabetes mellitus (DM1), who do not produce any insulin (a strong hormone able to reduce hyperglycemia), and, therefore, they must exogenously inject this hormone (or wear an insulin pump) in order to reduce their BG levels. Hence, diabetic people must check their BG levels manually (typically through glucose meters which analyze patients' capillary blood samples obtained via finger pricking) several times a day and, based on these data, as well as other factors like meals and exercise, decide when and how much insulin is required to avoid hyperglycemia.

However, a great many new technological advances achieved in recent years offer a new perspective for diabetes management and can constitute a real revolution within this field. An artificial pancreas (AP) is presumed to comprise a continuous glucose monitoring (CGM) device, which is aimed at checking the patient's glucose levels in real time, and a pump which should inject into his or her body the amount of insulin (and glucagon, if applicable) stipulated by a control system based on a closed loop [1-2]. Therefore, CGM has become a cornerstone in diabetes care and future

AP prototypes [3], since it can provide the magnitude, tendency, frequency, and duration of glucose level fluctuations almost every minute.

However, some situations cannot be explained solely by the provided CGM data. Sometimes, medical staff may need to question patients about their daily routine or about other specific circumstances for some particular moment, so that they can have a comprehensive understanding. Unfortunately, people remember the context in a subjective way, so doctors and patients cannot analyze the background properly.

Fortunately, beyond CGM, other devices in the field of biometrics allow maintaining a 24-hour monitoring of the patient, recording important information about the person's health, and could also be of relevance in an AP context. In this way, variables like temperature, exercise, heart rate, and perspiration (among others) can be monitored continuously. Advances in biomedical science allow easy and mobile data collection [4-5].

As there is no global monitoring of a diabetic patient, going beyond BG levels alone, there is a necessity to describe the physiological aspects of patients' evolution and current conditions more exhaustively and in much more detail than before. In the present paper, a thorough analysis of the significant variables to be taken into account and monitored in diabetic patients for a fully functional and meaningful DM1 management system will be presented.

In addition, the concept of being "on-board" was widely treated in diabetes research related to the insulin effect. With this, the remaining effect of fast insulin of previous bolus can be taken into account since it should be noted that it can be acting with low intensity for several hours. This idea has been recurrently studied in literature and introduced in a practical way in bolus calculators [6], also taking into account other variables such as the carbohydrate to insulin ratio [7] or the influence of circadian variability in this insulin on-board (IOB) [8]. This interpretation will be extended and justified—as a novelty—to other continuously measured features indicated in this paper.

This paper is organized as follows: Section 2 presents CGM as a cornerstone, with a brief review of the currently offered possibilities. Some other necessary devices for a complete DM1 management system are described in Section 3. Then, as a result of the different possibilities of monitoring, an almost complete characterization of a diabetic patient (the significant variables to be taken into account) is proposed in Section 4. Section 5 presents a case study and then Section 6 analyzes some challenges to be faced by this idea. The conclusions and possibilities offered by this novel global outlook are given in Section 7.

2. Continuous Glucose Monitoring (CGM)

Currently, it is not possible to think of an approach to an artificial pancreas without a CGM device. This mechanism constitutes a revolution in diabetes care, since it can provide for the magnitude, tendency, frequency, and duration of the fluctuations of the glucose levels in diabetic patients [9]. Compared with conventional glucose monitoring (fingerstick, capillary blood glucose monitoring), which provides between three to ten measurements of glucose level per day, CGM can deliver up to one measurement per minute (i.e., 1440 data points per day). Therefore, this sampling frequency is sufficient to be the input of a control system, although Kovatchev et al. indicate [10] that CGM still suffers from some limitations, such as random noise and a transient loss of sensitivity. So, in order to get a complete monitoring of a diabetic person, the first decision is to choose a proper CGM.

A frequent complaint is the time lag between the data provided by the CGM and the real glucose level in the bloodstream of the patient. This is due to the fact that the CGM is not measured directly from the blood: the value that the CGM device offers is an estimate based on the interstitial fluid glucose which exists under the skin, whose level is delayed some minutes with respect to the actual value present in the bloodstream. This fact can be perceived as being a disadvantage. However, recent research has found that this time lag is not more than 5 to 10 minutes [11]. Moreover, mathematical methods can suitably compensate for the lack of accuracy due to this delay. In fact, some tests deployed by Basu et al. confirmed a delay of just 6 minutes [12].

The accuracy of these devices can be evaluated by means of two standards: the mean absolute relative difference (MARD) and the Clarke error grid [13]. The MARD is defined as the result of a mathematical calculation that measures the average disparity between the CGM sensor and the reference measurement. The lower the MARD, the smaller the average error and the more accurate the device can be considered to be. The most accurate CGM devices reach maximum values of the MARD of between 6% and 8%. The main commercialized CGM devices are presented in Table 1.

Dexcom is probably the most accurate CGM system available. In its most recent version (Dexcom G5), a MARD of 9% is reached thanks to the new 505 software, which features the same advanced algorithm as that used in artificial pancreas research. The life of the sensor is seven days, according to the manufacturer's specifications, but users can usually restart it when this expires. The G5 model has several features, such as the possibility of displaying the glucose levels on a smartphone, without the necessity of carrying the Dexcom receiver. The previous version (Dexcom G4 PLATINUM) cannot transmit to a smartphone (just to a Dexcom receiver), but both are able to be connected to an Animas Vibe insulin pump. Other combinations can also be found, like the integration of a t:slim insulin pump with the Dexcom G4 and G5.

Medtronic also offers CGM sensors: Medtronic Enlite, together with their insulin pumps, although it is also possible to use the sensor separately. Its MARD (13.60%) is a little bit higher than that of the Dexcom devices, and the approved life of the sensor is 6 days, although it can be reactivated for up to twelve days. By adding a specific Bluetooth device, it is possible to show the results on a smartphone.

At this moment, the US Food and Drug Administration (FDA) has approved a device with a CGM gadget and an insulin pump, capable of stopping the insulin infusion in case of hypoglycemia (Medtronic 530G) and, recently, the FDA has also approved the Medtronic 670G, which is also able

Table 1: Current commercialized CGM sensor systems.

Company	Model	Features		MARD
Abbott	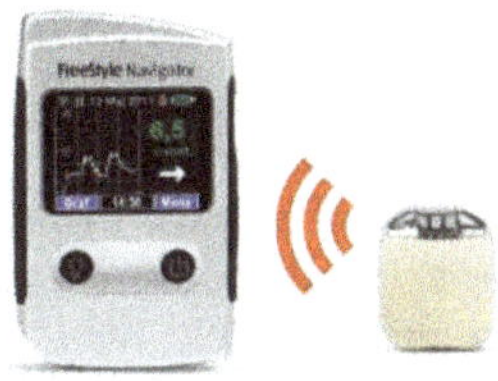 Navigator II	Trend marks Rate-of-change alerts Alarms (hyper/hypo) 5-day lifetime	Calibration recommended up to 72 h	14.5% [26]
	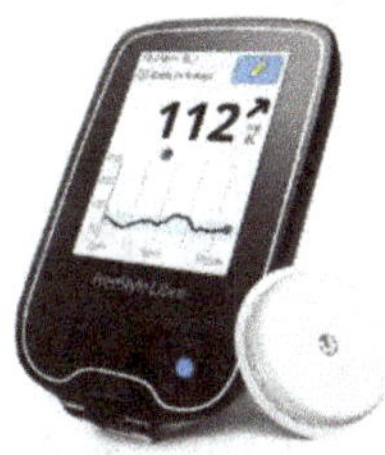 FreeStyle Libre	Trend marks No alerts or alarms 14-day lifetime NFC communication with smartphone	Read approaching meter to sensor (NFC technology) No calibration needed	11.4% [27]
Dexcom	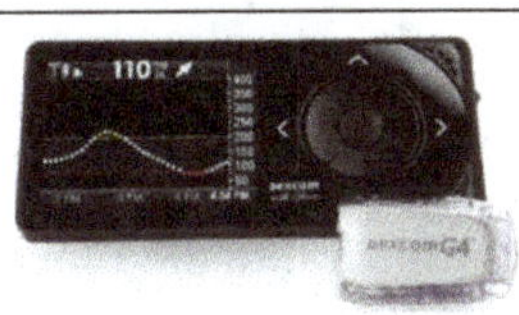 G4 Platinum	Trend marks Rate-of-change alerts Alarms (hyper/hypo) 7-day lifetime	Remote monitoring Calibration every 12 h	13% [28] (Original algorithm)
	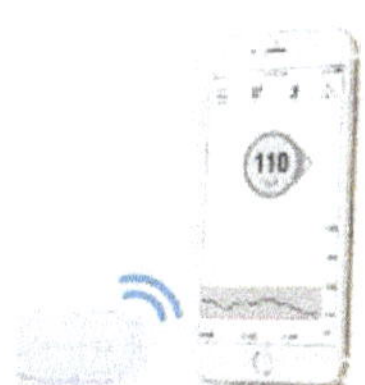 G5 Mobile	Trend marks Rate-of-change alerts Alarms (hyper/hypo) 7-day lifetime	Remote monitoring Wireless communication with smartphone Calibration every 12 h	9% [29]
Medtronic	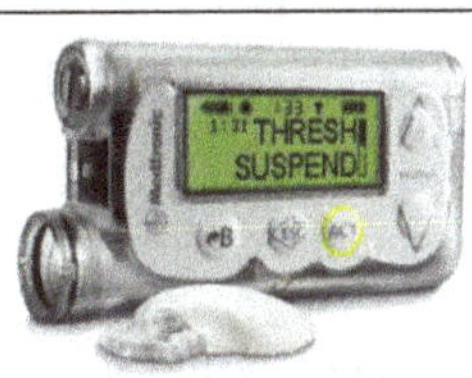 Enlite Sensor	Trend marks Rate-of-change alerts Alarms (hyper/hypo) 6-day lifetime	Integration with Medtronic 530G insulin pumps Calibration every 12 h	13.6% [30]
	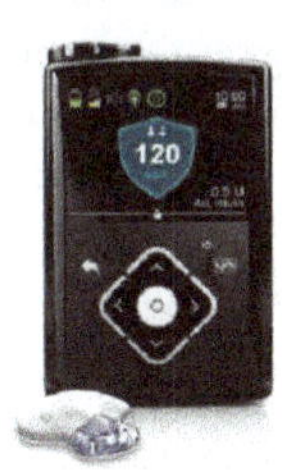 Guardian Sensor 3	Trend arrows Rate-of-change alerts Alarms (hyper/hypo) 7-day lifetime	Integration with Medtronic 670G insulin pumps Calibration every 12 h	9.1% [31]
Senseonics	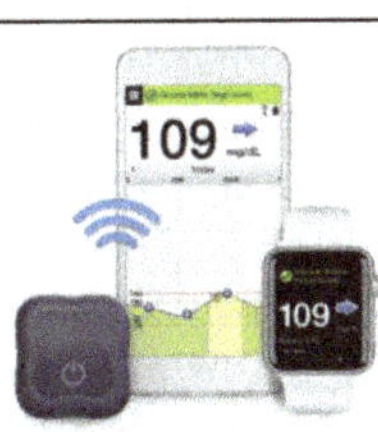 Eversense	Trend arrows Rate-of-change alerts Alarms (hyper/hypo) 90-day lifetime	Communication with smartphone Sensor inserted under the skin	11.6% [32]

to minimize hyperglycemia thanks to its connection to the CGM gadget.

Abbott now has two products available. The first one is the FreeStyle Navigator II, which was the most accurate CGM device until the new Dexcom algorithm 505 appeared. It presents a MARD of 11%, but, unfortunately, it is only available in certain countries, such as the United Kingdom, the Netherlands, and Israel. It provides a new glucose value every minute, in contrast to the Dexcom G5, where it is necessary to wait 5 minutes for a new value to be offered. The official life of the sensor is 5 days but it may last longer. One disadvantage is that an initial calibration by finger prick glucose monitoring is necessary and, from time to time, a new calibration is required. This is also true for the Dexcom and Medtronic devices.

Abbott has also offered the FreeStyle Libre from the end of 2014 [14]. Strictly speaking, it is not a real CGM device since the glucose information is not transmitted continuously (although it is stored and can be read by scanning the sensor with the receiver), so it is not possible to set alarms for low or high values of glucose. The sensor is placed on the arm and the information can then be transmitted via NFC, known as the "Flash System." It achieves a MARD of 11.4% and the sensors have a longer life (14 days), but they cannot be restarted. One of its perks is that it does not need to be calibrated.

All of the CGM devices use different algorithms to minimize the delay between the glucose levels present in the bloodstream and those measured under the skin (interstitial fluid) when trying to predict the next value. This delay, mainly when glucose levels are changing fast, results in inaccuracy, the predicted values not being reliable under those circumstances. To avoid this, many improvements have been implemented in CGM. Denoising, enhancement of raw data accuracy, and minimizing error due to the delay introducing a correction are the three main key challenges [15].

The denoising algorithm could be based on an adaptive self-tunable Bayesian smoother [16] able to automatically estimate in real time the signal-to-noise ratio present on the CGM. The other denoising algorithms that can be used here are, e.g., those presented by Palerm and Bequette [17] and Mahmoudi et al. [18].

The enhancement module is proposed in [19] grounded in a stochastic deconvolution-based recalibration algorithm, which rescales the CGM data using a simple linear regressor whose parameters are recalculated every time a new SMBG value is available. The other enhancement/recalibration algorithms that can be exploited in this step are, e.g., those presented by Barcelo-Rico et al. [20] (adaptive calibration) and Kirchsteiger et al. [21] (LMI-based approach).

In the prediction stage, a simple but effective predictor based on an autoregressive model of order one can be used [22], whose key feature is the real-time estimation of the predictor's parameters using a recursive least squares implementation, exploiting a forgetting factor to smartly weigh previously acquired data. Other sophisticated prediction algorithms can be used, including other signals like IOB or physical activity: Zecchin et al. [23] (neural network), Zarkogianni et al. [24] (taking into account physical activity), and Georga et al. [25] (regression models).

3. Additional Commercial Smart Devices to Be Included in a Full DM1 Monitoring System

Some new technological advances have brought innovative developments in this area. In the commercial market, it is possible to find new devices which have revolutionized monitoring possibilities.

At the moment, smartphones present a level of adaptability that is unachievable by any other device. They allow us to

(1) keep the software responsible to model the dynamics of the system, make a glucose prediction, optimize a solution, and control the process

(2) gather information between CGM devices and an insulin pump. The possibilities of connectivity are enormous. Today, a mobile phone is able to communicate not only via 4G but also through Bluetooth, Wi-Fi, NFC, Ant+, etc., which offers a plethora of different choices

(3) send data and information to the Cloud, to be either stored or computed (Cloud computing)

(4) forward emergency calls in case the patient is at risk

(5) update its software when required

Furthermore, smartphones provide a wide range of possibilities in the field of monitoring. Nowadays, the inclusion of accelerometer sensors, gyroscopes, and pedometers allows physical activity to be quantified. Other uses could be to measure physiological features such as heart rate, using camera flash (admittedly with a large uncertainty), and some are able to register the environmental temperature. In any case, these attributes are often used recreationally. In the following paragraphs, some other more specific and more accurate sensors will be described.

These possibilities have been tested in experiments performed by Place et al. [33]; in real time, patients' evolution has been followed from different locations. Other publications have studied the use of a smartphone as a device capable of sending an emergency call, providing the location via GPS in case the patient is at risk [34].

However, there are some doubts as to whether smartphones will be approved as medical devices (class III, high risk). The controller application installed in the phone has to be reliable, so as to avoid conflicts with other applications running on the device. Other circumstances, such as a discharge of the battery or lost connectivity, would have to be prevented. These pros and cons are exposited in Rigla [35].

In another vein, groundbreaking advances in electronics have introduced miniaturization and more powerful innovations in biometrics, the field in which measurable biological characteristics are studied. It is now possible to measure certain variables, most of them being vital signs (such as the heart rate and exercise), in a continuous mode. All of these measurements play a part in the complex balance of blood glucose and must be taken into account. Some years ago, it was difficult to obtain a full-day's data, but, nowadays, devices such as smartbands, smartwatches, and other fitness and medical wearables make this objective easily attainable, offering a lot of useful information [36]. These innovations have potential in the health field due to their ability to collect different types of data and presenting them in a user-friendly way. In addition, they have potential due to their connectivity; they are usually provided with a Bluetooth connection. However, they are restricted by their size, length of battery life, and the fact that these devices are sometimes conceived for non-health care, professional uses. These factors cast some doubts on their accuracy [37], but, in any case, they can provide data of an appropriate order of magnitude. A compilation of the most popular and affordable fitness smartbands is presented in Table 2, along with a summary of their main features. As we can see, these devices can provide a wide range of physiological features and, therefore, can provide a good characterization of the patient. To complete the monitoring, some other medical devices could be worn by the patient in order to measure temperature, blood pressure, etc.

Therefore, although the use of novel devices (accelerometers, electrocardiograms, thermistors, etc.) has been tested, they have only been studied in isolated trials and not included in DM1 management systems. Some of them (but not all) have been used together with CGM devices, sometimes with the sole aim of studying the relationship between BG and other features and sometimes to predict glycemia levels. It should be said that a 24-hour simultaneous monitoring of all the features has not been carried out nor has a study of the types of variables, the correlations between them, ranks of influence on the BG, and a valuable set of features used for modeling the evolution of glycemia.

4. Significant Variables to Be Monitored for Complete Diabetes Management

4.1. Types of Variables: The Idea of Something On-Board. According to the nature of the feature under study and how it changes through time, it is possible to distinguish three different types of variables, each one requiring specific handling.

4.1.1. Pulse Variables. These features interact with the system at one point and then stop. However, this impulse, with a given strength, has the capability to unbalance the system, creating a disruption. In this sense, insulin boluses and meals, and just indicating the exact time when they take place, are pulse variables, and it is known that these features are zero most of the time [38]. They are considered to be discrete events, regardless of the time that it takes to end their influence.

4.1.2. Trending Variables. In this case, it is not only necessary to know the value in the current moment, but, furthermore, a corresponding trend is critical in order to know previous states and then extrapolate (or predict) future values. Examples of this are glycemia, exercise, and heart rate. However, in the scientific literature, it is not possible to find a discussion about how many past values are necessary to take into account in these kinds of variables.

4.1.3. "On-Board" Variables. This is a well-known concept that has been introduced in several previously published works, in order to explain the remaining influence of previous insulin doses (IOB). In this case, the maximum effect has already ceased but the remaining tails of the insulin curve still have a remarkable influence, especially when there were several punctual injections throughout the experiment. In this way, an insulin dose presents its maximum effect at 90 minutes but the mentioned tails could have an influence, even throughout the 6 hours after injection. As these action times can oscillate because of external causes such as exercise, this remaining effect will be the subject of discussion in the next sections. The idea of IOB has been introduced in several previous works, as in [39], where the possibility of a prediction of glucose levels in a 20-minute horizon using proportional integral derivative (PID) controllers is studied. The integral component of the algorithm could cause hypoglycemia, and this is, in essence, the IOB contribution. This paper also presents the concept of "exercise on-board." After physical activity, the glucose demand from the muscles is still particularly high, in order for them to recover after the effort. This has a permanent and sustained effect in both glycemic demand and insulin sensibility, as previously explained. Therefore, this idea will be modeled with an accumulated amount of exercise in the previous hours. Following the same philosophy, meals not only disturb the system equilibrium in a single moment (ingestion) but they also have a critical influence in a range of several hours. So, meal furthers more of the disruption in glycemia created at the time of eating (which should be better understood as an "announcement"); later, after digestion, the glucose resulting from the metabolic processes is dumped into the blood or, among other destinations, stored as glycogen in muscles and the liver. This glycogen can be directly correlated with the amount of food (mainly carbohydrates) ingested in the hours preceding the measurement, and it can affect the amount of glycemia dumped as glucose into the bloodstream. Hence, the innovative concept of "meal on-board," as accumulated food, makes sense in explaining this circumstance. The amount of hours needed to consider this fact will need to be discussed deeply. On the other hand, rest level is also an influential variable in glycemia control. A low amount of sleeping time tends to result in rising blood glucose levels because of a higher necessity for stress hormones, which have a hyperglycemic effect. Therefore, it seems reasonable to take account of lack of sleep (sleep deprivation on-board) as well. Even with this idea, it is possible to discuss the influence of the daily routine. Some kind of "schedule on-board" could make sense, and this concept will be developed later. The limit of this sum will be also the object of discussion in future works.

Taking these ideas into account, we can list and describe a complete set of features that can be monitored in order to produce a global description of the patient, capturing his or her physiological history as well as their present condition.

Table 2: Main currently commercialized smartbands.

Company	Model	Sleep	Distance	Steps	Calories	Waterproof	Heart rate	Interface	Battery
Fitbit	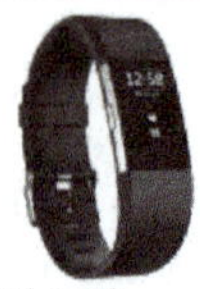 Fitbit Charge 2	✓ High accuracy	✓	✓ High accuracy	✓	Small	✓	iPhone Android	4–7 days
	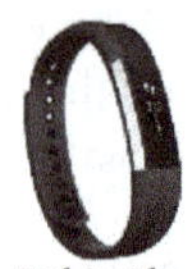 Fitbit Alta	✓	✓	✓	✓	Small	✖	iPhone Android	4–7 days
	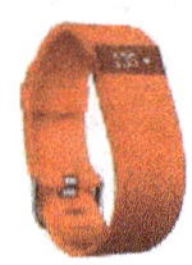 Fitbit Charge HR	✓	✓	✓	✓	1–2 m	✓	Web iPhone Android	1–2 weeks
	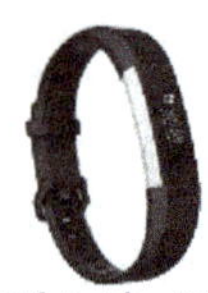 Fitbit Alta HR	✓	✓	✓	✓	Small	✓	Web Android	1–2 weeks
Polar	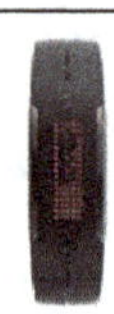 Loop	✓	✓	✓	✖	Small	✖	iPhone Android	1–2 weeks
Garmin	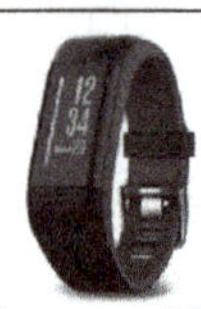 Vivosmart HR +	✓ High accuracy	✓	✓ High accuracy	✓	5 m	✓	iPhone Android	4–7 days
	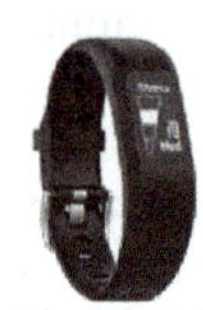 Vívosmart 3	✓	✓	✓	✓	Small	✓	iPhone Android	4–7 days
Jawbone	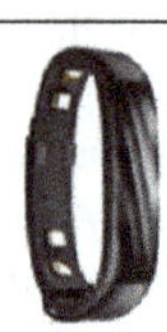 Up 3	✓ High accuracy	✓	✓ High accuracy	✓	Small	✓	iPhone Android	1–2 weeks
Xiaomi	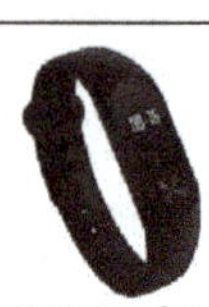 Mi Band 2	✓ High accuracy	✓	✓ High accuracy	✓	Small	✓	iPhone Android	2–3 weeks

4.2. Identified Variables. At present, most of the previous literature on diabetes management systems has only taken into account glycemia and insulin levels, and sometimes an estimation of meals, but it seems reasonable to incorporate additional variables that could also influence glucose levels as far as it is possible to measure or estimate them. It seems that there is a general agreement in using glycemia, insulin, and meal as remarkable variables [40, 41], and the studies with this set of variables are a majority, but it is also possible to find works involving just previous glycemia data as the only variable in use (like those that can be found in autoregressive model approaches [22]) or in [42], just adding insulin to glycemia and using an autoregressive with exogenous term model. There is also a lot of studies in the last years taking into account other variables, mainly exercise, both in silico and in vivo [43], and also considering the possibility of heart rate, temperature, etc. These ideas will be presented in the following lines. In any case, to the best of the authors' knowledge, there is no previous work using a comprehensive characterization of the diabetic patient, examining a global and integral overview.

In this section, a comprehensive list of the significant variables for a complete DM1 control system is analyzed. Some of them have been previously discussed in the scientific literature, but others are presented in this paper for the first time.

4.2.1. Current and Previous Glucose Bloodstream Levels. This is one of the principal variables. In addition to traditional capillary blood monitoring, which consists of discrete glucose values, new CGM devices offer enough accuracy and a good sample frequency [44] to be one of the inputs to a continuous control algorithm.

4.2.2. Insulin. This hormone has an exogenous origin in a diabetic patient, who has to make a decision about the dose to be injected. As it is the variable which primarily governs how much glucose level will decrease due to hypoglycemic response, this could be the main variable requiring optimization. It is necessary to differentiate three ways of taking insulin into account.

Instantaneous Insulin Input. It refers to recent doses, especially fast-acting insulin (boluses). This type of insulin usually has an effect for two and a half hours, with a maximum peak effect at 90 minutes.

Basal Insulin. It covers 24 hours, compensating for the normal and slow dump of glucose into the blood (due to the action of glucagon) from the glycogen stored mainly within the liver.

Accumulated Insulin (IOB). This concept has been taken into account in some of the scientific literature and means the insulin amount that is currently in the body (and which is, therefore, active). It involves basal insulin and remaining fast insulin, which can be acting with low intensity (but still noticeable) for several hours. It is assumed to have a remarkable effect for the previous eight hours [45], although another research points to an active range of the previous five to eight hours [46].

4.2.3. Exercise. Physical activity increases the muscles' demand for glucose; it is necessary to a normal workout. It also raises blood circulation, so insulin is used up faster and its effectiveness is increased because exercise temporarily makes the cellular walls more permeable, which lets glucose enter the cells more effectively [47]. This could lead to the risk of hypoglycemia and a lower requirement of insulin (however, it should be noted that exercise could cause hyperglycemia in the absence of insulin). Exercise also leads to a reduction of our reservoir of glycogen, which is slowly dumped into the bloodstream throughout the day and relatively faster when hypoglycemia is taking place. Thus, it is possible to make a distinction between three aspects regarding exercise.

Recent Exercise. Physical effort has an immediate consequence in glycemia. Thus, it would be reasonable to continuously measure this variable.

Intensity of Exercise. The duration can define not only the type of exercise but also the intensity since, for example, the more power or strength are involved, the more there is influence on the insulin's action.

Accumulated Exercise (Exercise On-Board (EOB)). Although the increased effect of exercise on both blood glucose and insulin requirements starts to decrease at the same time the physical activity is being performed, a remaining effect can act for up to 48 hours afterwards [48-49]. Moreover, it is proven that regular activity increases the sugar bloodstream equilibrium and reduces the need for insulin [50]. Therefore, the concept of EOB appears to be very necessary if a rigorous glucose prediction method is to be obtained. For this reason, this variable is one of the innovative proposals of this paper.

4.2.4. Meals. What we eat and when we do it have a great influence on blood glucose levels. Food is mainly transformed and absorbed as glucose, which is dumped into the blood, raising glycemia almost instantly. This interaction has been described and modeled by using processing software [51]. Three aspects should be noted regarding meals.

Notification of Ingestion. As meals have a fast impact on blood glucose levels, an agile response in an artificial pancreas would be necessary. Unfortunately, the system cannot act as quickly as desired, so any preparation regarding the glucose level increase derived from food intake would be welcome.

Meal (Carbohydrate Counting). How fast and how much the blood glucose level increases depend mainly on the amount of carbohydrates that is present, and so, such information should be registered. It is generally difficult and inefficient to measure the exact amounts that are consumed (patients are sometimes confused when evaluating this parameter because it is a subjective assessment), but, usually, diabetic people have been trained in how to measure meals and carbohydrate counting, based on standardized tables. The speed with which some meals are absorbed and reflected in glycemia has been studied by Bell et al. [52]. In that study, the absorption of fats is estimated at five hours (due to CGM); on the other hand, protein generates a peak at three hours but is less marked and carbohydrate levels peak in about two hours. Of course, meals are a mix of these three components, and the time of the highest total contribution will be very diverse.

Accumulated Intakes (Meal On-Board (MOB)). In the long term, food intake increases glycogen reservoirs, and so, on the one hand, the eventual hypoglycemic reaction will be fast, but, on the other, glucose levels will normally be higher due to the slow and continuous dumping of glucagon and consequent liberation of glucose (mainly from the glycogen stored within the liver). Moreover, it should be noted that there can be interactions between the main types of macronutrients when it comes to their absorption, since one can be delayed by the effect of another. For example, the ingestion of fat can slow down the absorption of carbohydrates [53]. In fact, an excessive ingestion of fat can lower the sensitivity of the body to insulin [54]), but, on the other hand, the intake of fiber can slow down the absorption of carbohydrates [55]. Regarding the above statement, the idea of a "meal on-board" concept has arisen and seems reasonable. Unfortunately, to the best of the authors' knowledge, there is no research which takes this idea into account. In this sense, this variable is first presented in the present paper.

4.2.5. Stress. Stress hormones also have a hyperglycemic influence [56]. Adrenaline and cortisol are secreted for several reasons. In this case, two important aspects should be noted.

Sleep Quality at Night. Poor quality of rest at night or too few hours of sleep can lead to an altered glucose metabolism and to an insulin resistance (i.e., hyperglycemic effects) [57]. Therefore, another novel variable is proposed: sleep deprivation on-board (SDOB), since the hyperglycemic response derived from sleep deprivation can last for several hours. Thus, an estimation of the number of hours slept should be considered.

Heart Rate. An increase of this parameter can be due to several causes. Evidently, this value increases when exercising. However, if such an increase is not related to physical activity, it could also be generated by stressful situations [58]. Moreover, the heart rate can also be indicative of a hypoglycemia episode [59]; the relationship with hyperglycemia has also been studied [60].

4.2.6. Temperature. This parameter can be a symptom of hypoglycemia, becoming lower under these circumstances [61]. However, long-term patients with frequent drops of glucose levels often present a lack of symptoms, not realizing their low-glucose state until the situation is risky. On the other hand, hyperthermia (which is normally the signal of a concurrent illness) usually has hyperglycemic effects [62]. Completing this view, correlation between a hypothermic state could lead to subsequent hyperglycemia [63].

4.2.7. Perspiration. This is another expression of hypoglycemia. As with temperature, this symptom can go unnoticed in long-term patients [64].

4.2.8. Blood Pressure. Arterial hypertension is commonly associated with type 2 diabetes because of the so-called *metabolic syndrome* (which involves insulin resistance) and also with type 1 long-term diabetes patients, generally due to kidney malfunction. Therefore, high blood pressure could point to a poor control of glycemia [65] and lead to complications involving the heart, eyes, kidneys, and blood vessels.

4.2.9. Schedule (Time). As we are always involved in a set of customs and habits, patients' schedules tend to be similar from one day to the next. It is usually possible to identify a weekly pattern, especially in the case of diabetic patients, since this is generally helpful in controlling their diabetes. Several tasks are usually carried out routinely at the same hour, such as working, eating, practicing sports, or injecting insulin. Thus, by identifying both the hour and the day of the week, it should be possible to anticipate and predict the evolution of the system. Another advantage of recording the schedule is the identification of the basal insulin evolution. New types of slow-acting insulin [66] have an almost flat profile, but it should be noted that it is not 100% flat. Therefore, the hourly absorption and its alterations should be taken into account. In fact, going further, another innovative variable can be considered: schedule on-board (ScOB), which can be seen as the persistence in time of a daily routine, in terms of its impact on glucose levels, when a routine is changed or modified.

4.2.10. Others. Other features that could be considered in the system, in order to reach personalized solutions, could be

(i) age

(ii) sex

(iii) height

(iv) weight

(v) body-mass index

There are also some other patient's features, situations, and concurrent (chronic or temporary) illnesses that could affect glucose levels. This issue results in a wide discussion and varies from a patient to another. For instance, special attention has also been developed in some particular diabetic women's circumstances, like pregnancy [67], where the deployment of a specific planning has resulted in an improvement in gestation and childbirth. Continuing with special situations in the life of diabetic women, it is necessary to pay attention to menstruation, menopause [68], or the progression of osteoporosis [69].

In another vein, influence of psychiatric illness has been discussed in [70], concluding the importance of taking into account this coexisting disease. Other concurrent illnesses, especially those derived from diabetes, are also mandatory to bear in mind and be considered as a "variable" to characterize a diabetes patient. In this area, it is possible to name cardiovascular and renal impairment [71] and others like diabetic foot and retinopathy [72], where the importance of considering these simultaneous circumstances and implementing a combined approach has been successfully probed. Although the casuistry of these concurrent situations is so extensive and needs to be studied case by case by specialized

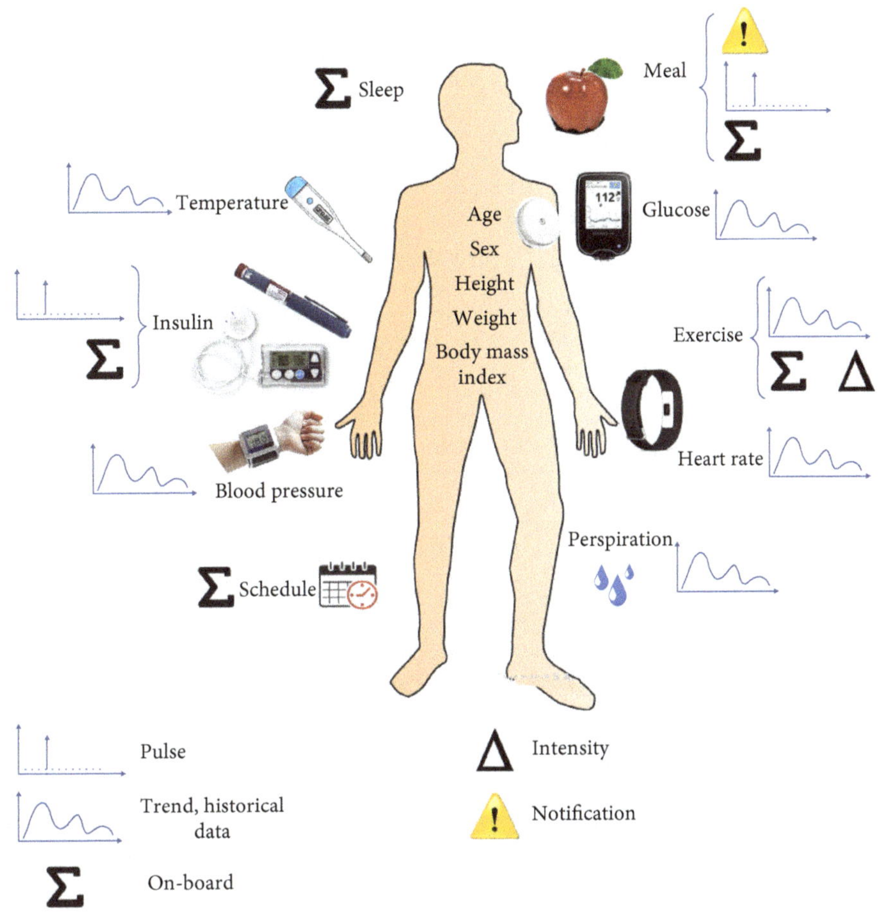

FIGURE 1: How to characterize a diabetic person using continuous monitoring devices.

medical staff, a deep characterization like that exposed in the present work could provide more exact information and tune exactly a personal diabetes care.

So, although it would be reasonable to add other variables if they have any significance, only the ones that can easily be measured with noninvasive devices are listed above.

Figure 1 summarizes all of the points analyzed in this section.

5. Case Study: Results of a Comprehensive Monitoring System

In order to explore the possibilities of the monitoring described above, a case study was carried out. For that, the following devices were used:

(1) *Abbott Freestyle Libre*: this groundbreaking device allows accurate and affordable 24-hour glucose monitoring. It also makes it possible to register meals as carbohydrate portions (CP) (one CP is equal to 10 g of carbohydrate) and the insulin dosage (units)

(2) *Fitbit Charge HR*: this is an advanced tracking wristband that gives an automatic, continuous heart rate and activity tracking during workouts and throughout the day. It records number of steps, distance, floors climbed, and sleep time. It stays connected wirelessly and can be synchronized with a smartphone and computer to monitor trends. With this smartband the following features were recorded: steps, heart rate, and sleep.

Patients also recorded their meal intake and schedule, indicating periods of work time or playing sports.

Although we listed other features (temperature, blood pressure, and perspiration), they were not monitored due to limitations in the chosen devices, and the additional devices would not have been able to be acquired easily and/or were not affordable. As this was a preliminary study, we considered the measured features with the available tools to be relevant enough to make a first evaluation of the monitoring experience.

The patient studied was a healthy man, 25 years old, DM1 for 12 years, and with diabetes under control. We considered this individual to be a good example for a preliminary study. He was under continuous monitoring for 14 days. In this period, he continued with his daily routine, including work, sports, dietary habits, and insulin dosages. The monitoring was carried out in a passive way, so there was no intervention in his diabetes treatment. A physician checked his medical condition daily, with the aim of assuring the safety of the process.

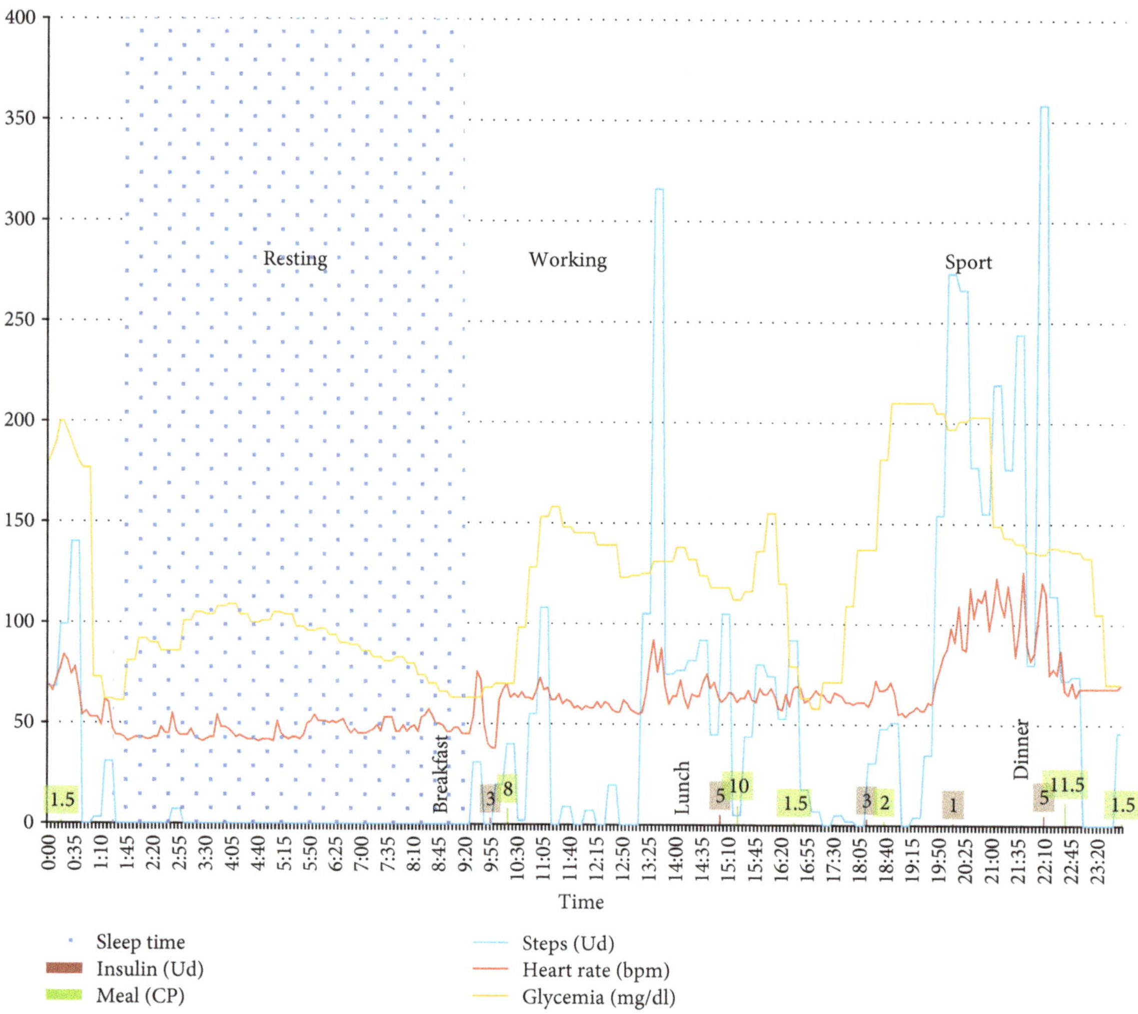

Figure 2: A complete 24-hour monitoring of a diabetic person.

Data were collected every 5 minutes, although it could have been recorded with a higher frequency. At this rate, the datasheet comprises more than 24,000 measurements; the level of detail achieved is really high. However, in terms of data storage, it is easily affordable.

Figure 2 shows the results from a few days and represents an example of the results that can be achieved.

As can be observed, the data provides more information than a simple glucose graph, and, therefore, caregivers can better understand the phenomena that influence the patient's status. With just a glance, it is now possible to understand glycemia evolution just by looking at the relationship with physical activity, for example.

Furthermore, all of the data can easily be transmitted to a smartphone or to the Cloud because of the connections of the CGM and smartbands, or other medical devices, mainly via Bluetooth. With all of these values, the possibilities that arise using machine learning techniques are boundless. It is in this context that the derived "on-board" variables are especially meaningful and have sense to be generated, that this idea encloses aggregative significance, and it is in this situation where the power of this perspective can be completely exploited.

6. Challenges to Be Overcome

However, beyond the promising view given above, some challenges still need to be solved. If we want wearable devices to play a crucial role in diabetes monitoring and management, one aspect that has to be ensured is energy supply. Batteries are now able to cover several hours (a few days at best), but we cannot rely on devices which lose power in a short period of time. On the other hand, another challenge is to get the prices of these devices lower, since today some of these devices are unaffordable for some parts of the population. Of course, another issue is to ensure their security and privacy [73]. Finally, it is necessary to deal with the acceptance level of telemedicine. A continuous monitoring that records personal data and provides a complete characterization of the patient could be considered to be interference in their private life. This could lead to an attitude of rejection from the user. These issues are compiled in [74], where it is explained that variables such as age, gender, and previous experiences with telemedicine can modulate its level of acceptance.

As can be seen, some areas need to be improved on, but, on the other hand, new horizons now seem to be opening up.

Modeling techniques based on artificial intelligence methods open up the possibility of predicting glycemia and anticipating actuation. This will help us follow the different stages of the so-called "Kowalski Path" [75] which needs to be followed in order to obtain an artificial pancreas. Unfortunately, such methods have not been studied taking into account the preceding considerations. In this sense, the fields of work that have been opened up are immense and promising. Implementing a predictive model in order to forecast the evolution of the patient is something highly desirable. It could anticipate risky situations or even provide decision support. Unfortunately, the development and validation of models using machine learning techniques are far from complete, laying aside in all the studies some features that could improve the model.

A complete monitoring leads to an enormous amount of data that needs to be transformed into knowledge. In this regard, it is necessary to study complete technological platforms that allow proper diabetes management, taking advantage of improvements in information and communication technologies (ICT); however, this is outside the scope of this paper. These architectures make no sense if they are partial and consider only some features of the patient's status. In this sense, this paper is a good beginning to lay down the basis for such a purpose, in order for future research to develop a complete ICT framework for efficient DM1 management.

Developing a fully operational ICT-based platform could help in information exchange between caregivers and medical staff, provide a better way to manage emergency situations, allow pattern identification, and optimize solutions to deal with DM1.

In addition to these advantages, the clearer and more complete explanation of the patient's evolution is a good benefit, as far as it results in a physician's better understanding of the context of their illness and thus improves the chosen treatment.

This idea of using ICT and developing a telemedicine framework has been studied and put into practice many times, for instance, as early as 2008, the INCA (Intelligent Control Assistant for Diabetes) system [76] or the DIAdvisor [77] in 2010, with excellent results. The possibilities of a remote blood glucose monitoring have also been exposed more recently in [78]. All of these issues have been specifically analyzed in a previous work of the authors [79], with an extended evaluation of the historical development of theses ICT-based platforms, their pros and cons, and a proposal of a complete diabetes telemedicine system in an ICT environment.

7. Conclusions

Our world is changing in a very remarkable way and continuously being updated due to advances in technology. All of these improvements have become revolutionary in many fields, making life easier in a lot of respects. In the struggle to obtain a definitive way to monitor and control diabetes, some improvements have occurred due to the development of new devices like those with CGM.

However, this monitoring is not enough to fully define the evolution of a diabetic person. There is a wide set of subjective features that need to be taken into account in the patient's mind. This also implies that caregivers cannot analyze all of the influences on a patient's condition and this can lead to a wrong interpretation.

As we have shown, it is now possible to find wearable monitoring systems that provide a lot of information about the human body. Smartbands, new medical devices, and CGM harvest thousands of measurements per day, which was something unthinkable some years ago. Moreover, as presented in this paper, a wide and definitely complete range of novel variables needs to be monitored for a full diabetes control system, and, furthermore, the idea of "on-board" has been extended to other features. This compilation had not been proposed so completely before and allows the description of patients in a global, comprehensive way. As an example of the possibilities of this monitoring, a case study has been discussed.

In future work, we will take advantage of these new perspectives. The content of this paper could contribute to the development of new information and communication technology (ICT) platforms for a global management system of DM1, as well as the development of a complete and totally operational artificial pancreas.

Conflicts of Interest

The authors declare no conflict of interest.

Authors' Contributions

Ignacio Rodríguez-Rodríguez searched for previous literature approaches and prepared a proposal. José-Víctor Rodríguez and Miguel-Ángel Zamora-Izquierdo completed the manuscript and outlined the issues.

Acknowledgments

This work has been sponsored by the Spanish Ministry of Economy and Entrepreneurship through the PERSEIDES (ref. TIN2017-86885-R) and CHIST-ERA (ref. PCIN-2016-010) projects and by the European Commission through the H2020-ENTROPY-649849 EU project.

References

[1] T. Peyser, E. Dassau, M. Breton, and J. S. Skyler, "The artificial pancreas: current status and future prospects in the management of diabetes," *Annals of the New York Academy of Sciences*, vol. 1311, no. 1, pp. 102–123, 2014.

[2] C. Cobelli, E. Renard, and B. Kovatchev, "Artificial pancreas: past, present, future," *Diabetes*, vol. 60, no. 11, pp. 2672–2682, 2011.

[3] B. Kovatchev, "The artificial pancreas in 2017: the year of transition from research to clinical practice," *Nature Reviews Endocrinology*, vol. 14, no. 2, pp. 74–76, 2018.

[4] T. A. Elwi, H. M. Al-Rizzo, D. G. Rucker, and H. R. Khaleel, "Effects of twisting and bending on the performance of a miniaturized truncated sinusoidal printed circuit antenna for

wearable biomedical telemetry devices," *AEU-International Journal of Electronics and Communications*, vol. 65, no. 3, pp. 217–225, 2011.

[5] S. A. Kumar and T. Shanmuganantham, "Design and analysis of implantable CPW fed bowtie antenna for ISM band applications," *AEU-International Journal of Electronics and Communications*, vol. 68, no. 2, pp. 158–165, 2014.

[6] P. Herrero, J. Bondia, O. Adewuyi et al., "Enhancing automatic closed-loop glucose control in type 1 diabetes with an adaptive meal bolus calculator–*in silico* evaluation under intra-day variability," *Computer Methods and Programs in Biomedicine*, vol. 146, pp. 125–131, 2017.

[7] D. Rodbard, "Optimizing the estimation of carbohydrate-to-insulin ratio and correction factor," *Diabetes Technology & Therapeutics*, vol. 20, no. 2, pp. 94–97, 2018.

[8] R. Visentin, C. Dalla Man, Y. C. Kudva, A. Basu, and C. Cobelli, "Circadian variability of insulin sensitivity: physiological input for in silico artificial pancreas," *Diabetes Technology & Therapeutics*, vol. 17, no. 1, pp. 1–7, 2015.

[9] G. Cappon, G. Acciaroli, M. Vettoretti, A. Facchinetti, and G. Sparacino, "Wearable continuous glucose monitoring sensors: a revolution in diabetes treatment," *Electronics*, vol. 6, no. 3, p. 65, 2017.

[10] B. P. Kovatchev, E. Renard, C. Cobelli et al., "Feasibility of outpatient fully integrated closed-loop control first studies of wearable artificial pancreas," *Diabetes Care*, vol. 36, no. 7, pp. 1851–1858, 2013.

[11] K. J. C. Wientjes and A. J. M. Schoonen, "Determination of time delay between blood and interstitial adipose tissue glucose concentration change by microdialysis in healthy volunteers," *The International Journal of Artificial Organs*, vol. 24, no. 12, pp. 884–889, 2001.

[12] A. Basu, S. Dube, S. Veettil et al., "Time lag of glucose from intravascular to interstitial compartment in type 1 diabetes," *Journal of Diabetes Science and Technology*, vol. 9, no. 1, pp. 63–68, 2015.

[13] D. J. Cox, W. L. Clarke, L. Gonder-Frederick et al., "Accuracy of perceiving blood glucose in IDDM," *Diabetes Care*, vol. 8, no. 6, pp. 529–536, 1985.

[14] L. Leelarathna and E. G. Wilmot, "Flash forward: a review of flash glucose monitoring," *Diabetic Medicine*, vol. 35, no. 4, pp. 472–482, 2018.

[15] A. Facchinetti, "Continuous glucose monitoring sensors: past, present and future algorithmic challenges," *Sensors*, vol. 16, no. 12, p. 2093, 2016.

[16] A. Facchinetti, G. Sparacino, and C. Cobelli, "Online denoising method to handle intraindividual variability of signal-to-noise ratio in continuous glucose monitoring," *IEEE Transactions on Biomedical Engineering*, vol. 58, no. 9, pp. 2664–2671, 2011.

[17] C. C. Palerm and B. W. Bequette, "Hypoglycemia detection and prediction using continuous glucose monitoring—a study on hypoglycemic clamp data," *Journal of Diabetes Science and Technology*, vol. 1, no. 5, pp. 624–629, 2007.

[18] Z. Mahmoudi, M. Dencker Johansen, J. S. Christiansen, and O. K. Hejlesen, "A multistep algorithm for processing and calibration of microdialysis continuous glucose monitoring data," *Diabetes Technology & Therapeutics*, vol. 15, no. 10, pp. 825–835, 2013.

[19] S. Guerra, A. Facchinetti, G. Sparacino, G. De Nicolao, and C. Cobelli, "Enhancing the accuracy of subcutaneous glucose sensors: a real-time deconvolution-based approach," *IEEE Transactions on Biomedical Engineering*, vol. 59, no. 6, pp. 1658–1669, 2012.

[20] F. Barcelo-Rico, J. L. Diez, P. Rossetti, J. Vehi, and J. Bondia, "Adaptive calibration algorithm for plasma glucose estimation in continuous glucose monitoring," *IEEE Journal of Biomedical and Health Informatics*, vol. 17, no. 3, pp. 530–538, 2013.

[21] H. Kirchsteiger, L. Zaccarian, E. Renard, and L. del Re, "LMI-based approaches for the calibration of continuous glucose measurement sensors," *IEEE Journal of Biomedical and Health Informatics*, vol. 19, no. 5, pp. 1697–1706, 2015.

[22] G. Sparacino, F. Zanderigo, S. Corazza, A. Maran, A. Facchinetti, and C. Cobelli, "Glucose concentration can be predicted ahead in time from continuous glucose monitoring sensor time-series," *IEEE Transactions on Biomedical Engineering*, vol. 54, no. 5, pp. 931–937, 2007.

[23] C. Zecchin, A. Facchinetti, G. Sparacino, and C. Cobelli, "Jump neural network for online short-time prediction of blood glucose from continuous monitoring sensors and meal information," *Computer Methods and Programs in Biomedicine*, vol. 113, no. 1, pp. 144–152, 2014.

[24] K. Zarkogianni, K. Mitsis, E. Litsa et al., "Comparative assessment of glucose prediction models for patients with type 1 diabetes mellitus applying sensors for glucose and physical activity monitoring," *Medical & Biological Engineering & Computing*, vol. 53, no. 12, pp. 1333–1343, 2015.

[25] E. I. Georga, V. C. Protopappas, D. Polyzos, and D. I. Fotiadis, "Evaluation of short-term predictors of glucose concentration in type 1 diabetes combining feature ranking with regression models," *Medical & Biological Engineering & Computing*, vol. 53, no. 12, pp. 1305–1318, 2015.

[26] D. Rodbard, "Continuous glucose monitoring: a review of recent studies demonstrating improved glycemic outcomes," *Diabetes Technology & Therapeutics*, vol. 19, Supplement 3, pp. S-25–S-37, (2017).

[27] T. Bailey, B. W. Bode, M. P. Christiansen, L. J. Klaff, and S. Alva, "The performance and usability of a factory-calibrated flash glucose monitoring system," *Diabetes Technology & Therapeutics*, vol. 17, no. 11, pp. 787–794, 2015.

[28] V. Matuleviciene, J. I. Joseph, M. Andelin et al., "A clinical trial of the accuracy and treatment experience of the Dexcom G4 sensor (Dexcom G4 system) and Enlite sensor (Guardian REAL-time system) tested simultaneously in ambulatory patients with type 1 diabetes," *Diabetes Technology & Therapeutics*, vol. 16, no. 11, pp. 759–767, 2014.

[29] FDA Advisory Panel, "FDA advisory panel votes to recommend non-adjunctive use of Dexcom G5 mobile CGM," *Diabetes Technology & Therapeutics*, vol. 18, no. 8, pp. 512–516, 2016.

[30] T. S. Bailey, A. Ahmann, R. Brazg et al., "Accuracy and acceptability of the 6-day Enlite continuous subcutaneous glucose sensor," *Diabetes Technology & Therapeutics*, vol. 16, no. 5, pp. 277–283, 2014.

[31] M. P. Christiansen, S. K. Garg, R. Brazg et al., "Accuracy of a fourth-generation subcutaneous continuous glucose sensor," *Diabetes Technology & Therapeutics*, vol. 19, no. 8, pp. 446–456, 2017.

[32] M. P. Christiansen, L. J. Klaff, R. Brazg et al., "A prospective multicenter evaluation of the accuracy of a novel implanted continuous glucose sensor: PRECISE II," *Diabetes Technology & Therapeutics*, vol. 20, no. 3, pp. 197–206, 2018.

[33] J. Place, A. Robert, N. Ben Brahim et al., "DiAs web monitoring: a real-time remote monitoring system designed for artificial pancreas outpatient trials," *Journal of Diabetes Science and Technology*, vol. 7, no. 6, pp. 1427–1435, 2013.

[34] E. Dassau, L. Jovanovic, F. J. Doyle III, and H. C. Zisser, "Enhanced 911/global position system wizard: a telemedicine application for the prevention of severe hypoglycemia—-monitor, alert, and locate," *Journal of Diabetes Science and Technology*, vol. 3, no. 6, pp. 1501–1506, 2009.

[35] M. Rigla, "Smart telemedicine support for continuous glucose monitoring: the embryo of a future global agent for diabetes care," *Journal of Diabetes Science and Technology*, vol. 5, no. 1, pp. 63–67, 2011.

[36] S. Ding and M. Schumacher, "Sensor monitoring of physical activity to improve glucose management in diabetic patients: a review," *Sensors*, vol. 16, no. 4, p. 589, 2016.

[37] M. A. Case, H. A. Burwick, K. G. Volpp, and M. S. Patel, "Accuracy of smartphone applications and wearable devices for tracking physical activity data," *JAMA*, vol. 313, no. 6, pp. 625-626, 2015.

[38] H. Kirchsteiger, H. Efendic, F. Reiterer, and L. del Re, "Alternative frameworks for personalized insulin–glucose models," in *Prediction Methods for Blood Glucose Concentration. Lecture Notes in Bioengineering*, H. Kirchsteiger, J. Jørgensen, E. Renard, and L. Re, Eds., pp. 1–29, Springer, Cham, 2016.

[39] G. M. Steil, K. Rebrin, C. Darwin, F. Hariri, and M. F. Saad, "Feasibility of automating insulin delivery for the treatment of type 1 diabetes," *Diabetes*, vol. 55, no. 12, pp. 3344–3350, 2006.

[40] H. Kirchsteiger, R. Johansson, E. Renard, and L. D. Re, "Continuous-time interval model identification of blood glucose dynamics for type 1 diabetes," *International Journal of Control*, vol. 87, no. 7, pp. 1454–1466, 2014.

[41] J. Bondia and J. Vehi, "Physiology-based interval models: a framework for glucose prediction under intra-patient variability," in *Prediction Methods for Blood Glucose Concentration. Lecture Notes in Bioengineering*, H. Kirchsteiger, J. Jørgensen, E. Renard, and L. Re, Eds., Springer, Cham, 2016.

[42] G. C. Estrada, L. del Re, and E. Renard, "Nonlinear gain in online prediction of blood glucose profile in type 1 diabetic patients," in *2010 49th IEEE Conference on Decision and Control (CDC)*, pp. 1668–1673, Atlanta, GA, USA, December 2010.

[43] S. K. Garg, S. A. Weinzimer, W. V. Tamborlane et al., "Glucose outcomes with the in-home use of a hybrid closed-loop insulin delivery system in adolescents and adults with type 1 diabetes," *Diabetes Technology & Therapeutics*, vol. 19, no. 3, pp. 155–163, 2017.

[44] D. Rodbard, "Continuous glucose monitoring: a review of successes, challenges, and opportunities," *Diabetes Technology & Therapeutics*, vol. 18, Supplement 2, pp. S2-3–S2-13, 2016.

[45] S. D. Patek, L. Magni, E. Dassau et al., "Modular closed-loop control of diabetes," *IEEE Transactions on Biomedical Engineering*, vol. 59, no. 11, pp. 2986–2999, 2012.

[46] C. Ellingsen, E. Dassau, H. Zisser et al., "Safety constraints in an artificial pancreatic β cell: an implementation of model predictive control with insulin on board," *Journal of Diabetes Science and Technology*, vol. 3, no. 3, pp. 536–544, 2009.

[47] L. B. Borghouts and H. A. Keizer, "Exercise and insulin sensitivity: a review," *International Journal of Sports Medicine*, vol. 21, no. 1, pp. 1–12, 2000.

[48] J. T. Devlin, M. Hirshman, E. D. Horton, and E. S. Horton, "Enhanced peripheral and splanchnic insulin sensitivity in NIDDM men after single bout of exercise," *Diabetes*, vol. 36, no. 4, pp. 434–439, 1987.

[49] D. S. King, P. J. Baldus, R. L. Sharp, L. D. Kesl, T. L. Feltmeyer, and M. S. Riddle, "Time course for exercise-induced alterations in insulin action and glucose tolerance in middle-aged people," *Journal of Applied Physiology*, vol. 78, no. 1, pp. 17–22, 1995.

[50] C. Zecchin, A. Facchinetti, G. Sparacino et al., "Physical activity measured by physical activity monitoring system correlates with glucose trends reconstructed from continuous glucose monitoring," *Diabetes Technology & Therapeutics*, vol. 15, no. 10, pp. 836–844, 2013.

[51] C. Dalla Man, R. A. Rizza, and C. Cobelli, "Meal simulation model of the glucose-insulin system," *IEEE Transactions on Biomedical Engineering*, vol. 54, no. 10, pp. 1740–1749, 2007.

[52] K. J. Bell, C. E. Smart, G. M. Steil, J. C. Brand-Miller, B. King, and H. A. Wolpert, "Impact of fat, protein, and glycemic index on postprandial glucose control in type 1 diabetes: implications for intensive diabetes management in the continuous glucose monitoring era," *Diabetes Care*, vol. 38, no. 6, pp. 1008–1015, 2015.

[53] T. Hung, J. L. Sievenpiper, A. Marchie, C. W. C. Kendall, and D. J. A. Jenkins, "Fat versus carbohydrate in insulin resistance, obesity, diabetes and cardiovascular disease," *Current Opinion in Clinical Nutrition and Metabolic Care*, vol. 6, no. 2, pp. 165–176, 2003.

[54] J. C. Lovejoy, "The influence of dietary fat on insulin resistance," *Current Diabetes Reports*, vol. 2, no. 5, pp. 435–440, 2002.

[55] T. G. Kiehm, J. W. Anderson, and K. Ward, "Beneficial effects of a high carbohydrate, high fiber diet on hyperglycemic diabetic men," *The American Journal of Clinical Nutrition*, vol. 29, no. 8, pp. 895–899, 1976.

[56] M. Housiaux, H. Dorchy, and O. Luminet, "Influence of an emotional level of conscience on the glycemic equilibrium in type 1 diabetic children and adolescents," *Diabetes & Metabolism*, vol. 34, article A33, 2008.

[57] K. L. Knutson, K. Spiegel, P. Penev, and E. Van Cauter, "The metabolic consequences of sleep deprivation," *Sleep Medicine Reviews*, vol. 11, no. 3, pp. 163–178, 2007.

[58] J. Taelman, S. Vandeput, A. Spaepen, and S. Van Huffel, "Influence of mental stress on heart rate and heart rate variability," *4th European Conference of the International Federation for Medical and Biological Engineering. IFMBE Proceedings, vol. 22*, J. Vander Sloten, P. Verdonck, M. Nyssen, and J. Haueisen, Eds., , pp. 1366–1369, Springer, Berlin, 2009.

[59] C. Alexakis, H. O. Nyongesa, R. Saatchi et al., "Feature extraction and classification of electrocardiogram (ECG) signals related to hypoglycaemia," in *Computers in Cardiology, 2003*, pp. 537–540, Thessaloniki Chalkidiki, Greece, September 2003.

[60] R. D. Buñag, T. Tomita, and S. Sasaki, "Chronic sucrose ingestion induces mild hypertension and tachycardia in rats," *Hypertension*, vol. 5, no. 2, pp. 218–225, 1983.

[61] K. Johansen, S. Ellegaard, and S. Wex, "Detection of nocturnal hypoglycemia in insulin-treated diabetics by a skin temperature-skin conductance meter," *Acta Medica Scandinavica*, vol. 220, no. 3, pp. 213–217, 1986.

[62] J. Feldman and E. Gellhorn, "The influence of fever on the vago-insulin and sympathetico-adrenal systems," *Endocrinology*, vol. 29, no. 1, pp. 141–143, 1941.

[63] T. Melhuish, "Linking hypothermia and hyperglycemia," *Nursing Management*, vol. 40, no. 12, pp. 42–45, 2009.

[64] V. McAulay, I. J. Deary, and B. M. Frier, "Symptoms of hypoglycaemia in people with diabetes," *Diabetic Medicine*, vol. 18, no. 9, pp. 690–705, 2001.

[65] A. Lurbe, J. Redon, J. M. Pascual, J. Tacons, V. Alvarez, and D. C. Batlle, "Altered blood pressure during sleep in normotensive subjects with type I diabetes," *Hypertension*, vol. 21, no. 2, pp. 227–235, 1993.

[66] Novo Nordisk, *Novo Nordisk Receives Complete Response Letter in the US for Tresiba® and Ryzodeg®*, 2013, https://www.novonordisk.com/bin/getPDF.1676900.pdf.

[67] P. Kekäläinen, M. Juuti, T. Walle, and T. Laatikainen, "Pregnancy planning in type 1 diabetic women improves glycemic control and pregnancy outcomes," *The Journal of Maternal-Fetal & Neonatal Medicine*, vol. 29, no. 14, pp. 2252–2258, 2016.

[68] C. A. Stuenkel, S. R. Davis, A. Gompel et al., "Treatment of symptoms of the menopause: an endocrine society clinical practice guideline," *The Journal of Clinical Endocrinology & Metabolism*, vol. 100, no. 11, pp. 3975–4011, 2015.

[69] P. R. Siddapur, A. B. Patil, and V. S. Borde, "Comparison of bone mineral density, T-scores and serum zinc between diabetic and non diabetic postmenopausal women with osteoporosis," *Journal of Laboratory Physicians*, vol. 7, no. 1, pp. 43–48, 2015.

[70] J. R. Larsen, V. D. Siersma, A. S. Davidsen, F. B. Waldorff, S. Reventlow, and N. de Fine Olivarius, "The excess mortality of patients with diabetes and concurrent psychiatric illness is markedly reduced by structured personal diabetes care: a 19-year follow up of the randomized controlled study Diabetes Care in General Practice (DCGP)," *General Hospital Psychiatry*, vol. 38, pp. 42–52, 2016.

[71] L. Tong and S. Adler, "Glycemic control of type 2 diabetes mellitus across stages of renal impairment: information for primary care providers," *Postgraduate Medicine*, vol. 130, no. 4, pp. 381–393, 2018.

[72] E. Y. Chew, "There is level 1 evidence for intensive glycemic control for reducing the progression of diabetic retinopathy in persons with type 2 diabetes," *Endocrine*, vol. 49, no. 1, pp. 1–3, 2015.

[73] E. Vayena, J. Dzenowagis, J. S. Brownstein, and A. Sheikh, "Policy implications of big data in the health sector," *Bulletin of the World Health Organization*, vol. 96, no. 1, pp. 66–68, 2018.

[74] M. J. Rho, H. S. Kim, K. Chung, and I. Y. Choi, "Factors influencing the acceptance of telemedicine for diabetes management," *Cluster Computing*, vol. 18, no. 1, pp. 321–331, 2015.

[75] A. Kowalski, "Pathway to artificial pancreas systems revisited: moving downstream," *Diabetes Care*, vol. 38, no. 6, pp. 1036–1043, 2015.

[76] E. J. GÓmez, M. E. H. PÉrez, T. Vering et al., "The INCA system: a further step towards a telemedical artificial pancreas," *IEEE Transactions on Information Technology in Biomedicine*, vol. 12, no. 4, pp. 470–479, 2008.

[77] J. U. Poulsen, A. Avogaro, F. Chauchard et al., "A diabetes management system empowering patients to reach optimised glucose control: from monitor to advisor," in *2010 Annual International Conference of the IEEE Engineering in Medicine and Biology*, pp. 5270-5271, Buenos Aires, Argentina, August 2010.

[78] G. Lanzola, E. Losiouk, S. del Favero et al., "Remote blood glucose monitoring in mHealth scenarios: a review," *Sensors*, vol. 16, no. 12, p. 1983, 2016.

[79] I. Rodríguez-Rodríguez, M. Á. Zamora-Izquierdo, and J. V. Rodríguez, "Towards an ICT-based platform for type 1 diabetes mellitus management," *Applied Sciences*, vol. 8, no. 4, p. 511, 2018.

4

DPP-4 Inhibitors as Treatments for Type 1 Diabetes Mellitus

Qixian Wang, Min Long, Hua Qu, Rufei Shen, Rui Zhang, Jing Xu, Xin Xiong, Hui Wang, and Hongting Zheng

Department of Endocrinology, Xinqiao Hospital, Third Military Medical University, Chongqing 400037, China

Correspondence should be addressed to Hongting Zheng; fnf7703@hotmail.com

Academic Editor: Raffaele Marfella

Objective. Several clinical studies have reported the application of dipeptidyl peptidase-4 (DPP-4) inhibitors as treatments for type 1 diabetes mellitus (T1DM). This study aims to review the outcomes of these existing studies and to discuss the therapeutic effects of DPP-4 inhibitors on T1DM. *Methods.* We thoroughly searched the Medline, Embase, PubMed, and Cochrane Library databases and ClinicalTrials.gov for studies concerning the use of DPP-4 inhibitors in patients with T1DM. *Results.* In preclinical trials, DPP-4 inhibitors improved the pathogenesis of T1DM. However, only a portion of the studies showed potential efficacy regarding clinical glycemic control and other clinical parameters. From this meta-analysis, pooled data from 5 randomized controlled trials revealed that the additional use of DPP-4 inhibitors resulted in a greater decrease in glycated hemoglobin A1c (HbA1c) levels (0.07%, 95% CI (−0.37%–0.23%)) than insulin monotherapy, although the decrease was not significant. A small decrease in postprandial glucose or insulin consumption was confirmed. *Conclusion.* Although DPP-4 inhibitors may be beneficial for T1DM, existing studies do not strongly support these positive effects in clinical practice. Further optimized clinical trials are needed.

1. Introduction

Type 1 diabetes mellitus (T1DM) is considered a chronic immune-mediated disease that is characterized by the selective destruction of β-cells in genetically susceptible individuals. The proportion of diabetes mellitus patients diagnosed with T1DM is estimated to be 5%–10% [1] with an annual increase of 3.8–5.6% [2–4], but this proportion may be underestimated [5]. Insulin replacement has been the mainstay of therapy for T1DM [6]. New therapies, including immunotherapy, islet transplantation, and stem cell/precursor cell transplantation, have been utilized in attempts to conquer T1DM. However, numerous defects, such as the absence of durable effectiveness, severe adverse effects (e.g., cytokine-release syndrome and transient Epstein-Barr viral infection), immunosuppression, and the scarcity of donors, limit their extended applications in patients with T1DM [7]. Only a small percentage of patients with T1DM achieve the goal of glycemic control. Moreover, treatments that address the underlying disease process are not available. Therefore, explorations of new and efficient therapies for T1DM are urgently needed [8].

Dipeptidyl peptidase-4 (DPP-4) inhibitors, which have been widely used as outstanding blood glucose-dependent antidiabetic agents for patients with type 2 diabetes mellitus (T2DM), show promise. These inhibitors prevent the degradation of incretin (glucagon-like peptide-1 (GLP-1) and glucose-dependent insulinotropic polypeptide (GIP)) by dipeptidyl peptidase-4 enzymes and therefore elevate endogenous GLP-1 levels. GLP-1 stimulates insulin secretion from β-cells in a glucose-dependent manner, suppresses glucagon secretion from α-cells, and inhibits hepatic glucose production, eventually contributing to the antihyperglycemic effect. In addition, DPP-4 inhibitors preserve the β-cell mass [9].

Recently, an increasing number of studies on the topic of DPP-4 inhibitors and T1DM have discovered their mutual characteristics of immune destruction. Insulitis was alleviated in a T1DM animal model treated with DPP-4 inhibitors [10], and the numbers of regulatory T cells, including $CD4^+CD25^+FoxP3^+$cells, which were reduced in patients with T1DM [11], increased [10]. Glucagon levels have been shown to be decreased during hyperglycemia [12–15] in several clinical trials of T1DM. However, controlled clinical trials have reported controversial effects on postprandial glycemic control, as well as the levels of glycated hemoglobin A1c (HbA1c) and other indicators. Is DPP-4 inhibitor monotherapy or its combination with insulin appropriate for patients with T1DM? Here, we performed a systematic review and meta-analysis to evaluate the roles of DPP-4 inhibitors in T1DM with the aim of directing future clinical trials.

2. Methods

2.1. Ethical Review. Our research was a study-level systematic review and meta-analysis of clinical trials. Therefore, ethical approval was not necessary for this study.

2.2. Search Strategy. This systematic review was performed according to PRISMA guidelines [16]. Two investigators (QX Wang and M Long) thoroughly searched the bibliographic databases Medline, PubMed, Embase, and the Cochrane Library for published articles describing DPP-4 inhibitors and T1DM up to March 10, 2017. In addition, we explored relevant unpublished data at ClinicalTrials.gov. The search strategy used for PubMed (http://www.ncbi.nlm.nih.gov/pubmed/) and the Cochrane Library (http://www.cochranelibrary.com/) was ("dipeptidyl peptidase-4 inhibitors" OR "dpp-4 inhibitor" OR dutogliptin OR alogliptin OR linagliptin OR saxagliptin OR sitagliptin OR vildagliptin) AND ("type 1 diabetes" OR t1dm). Publications were searched in Medline and Embase using the same strategy on one website (http://www.embase.com/). Additionally, all references of the articles downloaded from these databases were rapidly checked, and we manually searched 360 relevant articles. We did not employ any restrictions on publication year, specimen, or language.

2.3. Eligibility Criteria. We used the following selection criteria to ensure the inclusion of all relevant studies: (1) controlled clinical studies on the topic of DPP-4 inhibitors; (2) studies in which subjects were restricted to a diagnosis of type 1 diabetes, including patients with latent autoimmune diabetes in adults (LADA); and (3) studies reporting changes in control and experimental groups after treatment with respect to at least one indicator (HbA1c, insulin dosage, or blood glucose).

The exclusion criteria were as follows: (1) studies that did not meet any of the above inclusion criteria; (2) comments, reviews, abstracts, and articles other than original papers; and (3) duplicated data from the same laboratory.

Two investigators (QX Wang and M Long) independently searched the titles and abstracts as well as the full text, if necessary. All ambiguities were clarified by discussion with a third investigator (HT Zheng).

2.4. Data Extraction. The outcomes were recorded in detail. The primary outcome parameters studied here were classified as variations in β-cell function (detectable C-peptide levels) and glycemic control (the HbA1c, fasting blood glucose, and 2-hour postprandial blood glucose levels, as well as the area under the curve (AUC) for the blood glucose levels during a specific period). Insulin dosage, cholesterol, triglycerides, and adverse events were classified as secondary outcomes. We extracted the following data: treatment option, length of study, sample size, average age, duration of T1DM, body mass index (BMI), study design, and number of research centers. Briefly, all relevant data available that might impact the results were extracted and input into a predesigned table.

2.5. Quality Assessment. We used the Cochrane Risk of Bias Tool for Randomized Controlled Trials to assess the quality of the literature and the risk of bias.

2.6. Data Synthesis. We used the change in the value of the outcome to evaluate the therapeutic effect and emphasize the benefits of the combination of DPP-4 inhibitors with insulin versus insulin monotherapy. Because some articles reported the sample sizes (N), means (M), and standard deviations (SD) for females and males, we adopted the formula from chapter 7.7.3 of the Cochrane Handbook to synthesize M_{1+2} and SD_{1+2} data for systematic review. The formulas were

$$M_{1+2} = \frac{N_1 M_1 + N_2 M_2}{N_1 + N_2},$$
$$\mathrm{SD}_{1+2} = \sqrt{\frac{(N_1 - 1)\mathrm{SD}_1^2 + (N_2 - 1)\mathrm{SD}_2^2 + (N_1 N_2/(N_1 + N_2))\left(M_1^2 + M_2^2 - 2M_1 M_2\right)}{N_1 + N_2 - 1}}. \quad (1)$$

We adopted the following formula to assess continuous variation in parameters, such as the HbA1c levels:

$$\mathrm{SD}_{\mathrm{E,change}} = \sqrt{\mathrm{SD}_{\mathrm{E,baseline}}^2 + \mathrm{SD}_{\mathrm{E,final}}^2 - 2 \times \mathrm{Corr} \times \mathrm{SD}_{\mathrm{E,baseline}}^2 \times \mathrm{SD}_{\mathrm{E,final}}^2}. \quad (2)$$

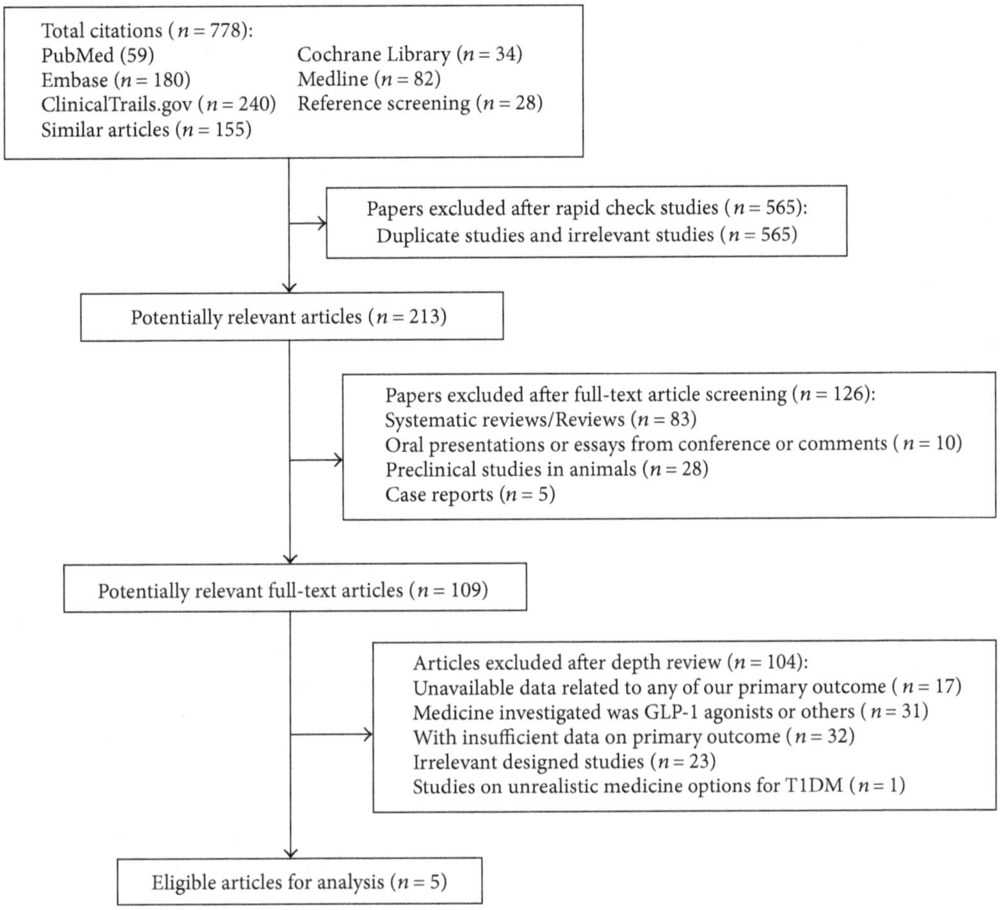

FIGURE 1: Flowchart illustrating the article screening process.

2.7. Data Analysis. The analysis software Manager Review Version 5.2 (Cochrane Collaboration, Software Update, Oxford, UK) was used to synthesize the data, and 95% confidence intervals (95% CI) were calculated. We reported the mean difference (MD) for indicators of efficacy, including the HbA1c, fasting blood glucose, and 2-hour postprandial blood glucose levels and other continuous variables. The relative risk ratio (RR) was used for dichotomous variables, such as indicators evaluating safety. If the indicators were reported in fewer than 3 studies, we summarized the result of each study individually. Statistical significance was set to an α of 0.05. Heterogeneity between trials was estimated using the I^2 statistic [17]. If significant heterogeneity was observed between studies, the results were reported using a random-effects model, and a sensitivity analysis was performed using the "leave one out" approach to explore the source of the heterogeneity. Then, a subgroup analysis was conducted, if applicable.

3. Results

3.1. Literature Retrieval. The literature retrieval process is shown in Figure 1. Two investigators searched the databases, and all relevant lists of studies were retrieved. Together with the reference lists from similar studies, a total of 778 titles and their keywords were identified. After a rapid check, we excluded 565 articles that were either duplicated or obviously irrelevant. Then, we screened the potential relevant full texts among the remaining 213 articles. By excluding inappropriate types of articles or studies researching undesired populations after an in-depth screen of the full texts, we obtained 109 potential articles. After we repeatedly studied these chosen articles and discussed their inclusion with Hongting Zheng, 5 randomized controlled trials (RCTs) were eventually considered eligible for this meta-analysis and systematic review.

Two hundred fifty-three participants, including 120 C-peptide-positive patients, from 5 RCTs were included in this meta-analysis and systematic review. Regarding medicine options, four studies [8, 18–20] examined the effects of combination therapy comprising sitagliptin and insulin compared with insulin monotherapy on T1DM, and the other study [13] investigated vildagliptin. Insulin injections were described in detail for both the experimental and control groups. Twelve patients from the study by Hari et al. [19] used an insulin analogue; conversely, patients from the other four studies used human insulin or an analogue. Only a few patients from the study by Garg et al. [20] received a continuous subcutaneous insulin infusion (CSII). Among the included studies, one study [18] was conducted on LADA patients. This study was designed to determine whether sitagliptin protected islet β-cells in patients with LADA.

Regarding indicators, the earliest initiated study was an 8-week crossover study from Sweden [13] that focused on the modulation of glucagon levels by vildagliptin. Two studies [18, 19] focused on changes in the levels of hormones regulating glycemia after DPP-4 inhibitor treatment of patients with new-onset T1DM to explore the advantages of a sitagliptin and insulin combination compared with insulin monotherapy. A multicenter, randomized, placebo-controlled clinical trial from the United States [8] aimed to test the efficacy of the combination of lansoprazole with sitagliptin on T1DM. A randomized, double-blind, placebo-controlled trial with the largest sample size (125 subjects) conducted in the United States [20] aimed to explore the effect of sitagliptin on the postprandial glucagon and GLP-1 levels. Table 1 shows the characteristics of the included studies. We also examined the inclusion and exclusion criteria for the participants enrolled in each study.

3.2. Assessment of Study Quality. We evaluated the risk of bias using Review Manager version 5.2. Figure 2 illustrates the summarized risk of bias. Three studies had a risk of selection bias attributed to random sequence generation. None of the studies had a high risk of selection bias (allocation concealment), reporting bias, performance bias, detection bias, or attrition bias. The results were unclear regarding whether other biases were present.

3.3. Results of the Meta-Analysis and Systematic Review

3.3.1. Primary Outcomes

(1) β-Cell Function: C-Peptide. The additional effects of DPP-4 inhibitors on the C-peptide level remain controversial. One study [18] reported a positive effect and concluded that sitagliptin at least attenuated the progressive decrease in the C-peptide levels. Three studies [8, 19, 20] did not observe a notable effect, and one study [13] did not address this subject. The study by Zhao et al. [18] selected patients with recent-onset LADA who presented with a fasting C-peptide level (FCP) ≥ 200 or a 2-hour postprandial C-peptide (2 h CP) level ≥ 400 pmol/L. After 1 year of treatment, the participants who were administered sitagliptin and insulin had no evident decrease in their fasting C-peptide levels, 2-hour postprandial C-peptide levels, or ΔCP (ΔCP = 2hCP–FCP), whereas the patients administered insulin monotherapy displayed significantly decreased FCP, 2hCP, and ΔCP values. As shown in the study by Hari et al. [19], among patients with new-onset T1DM who presented with stimulated C-peptide levels ≥ 0.1 ng/mL, C-peptide was elevated by 0.0067 ± 0.19 ng/mL or -0.05 ± 0.28 ng/mL in the groups treated with sitagliptin alone or the combination of sitagliptin and insulin, respectively. However, neither the changes in the C-peptide levels in the groups nor between the groups were significant ($P > 0.05$). In the study by Griffin et al. [8], the AUCs for the 2 hour C-peptide levels at 6 and 12 months declined significantly in the groups that received one year of combination therapy with sitagliptin and lansoprazole or the placebo control, but the difference between the treatment groups was insignificant. In contrast, only 8 (13%) patients in the experimental group and 12 (19%) patients in the control group had detectable C-peptide levels (above 16 pmol/L) among the participants enrolled in the study by Garg et al. [20], and the C-peptide-positive patients who were randomly allocated to receive sitagliptin had a nonsignificant trend toward decreased HbA1c levels, mean glucose levels, and duration of hyperglycemia. The data were not available for the C-peptide-negative patients. All 28 participants with T1DM enrolled in the study by Farngren et al. [13] were initially C-peptide-negative and antibody-positive, but the researchers did not evaluate whether the C-peptide levels increased. In conclusion, 120 patients with T1DM included in this systematic review were C-peptide-positive, and the increase in the fasting C-peptide level, which was measured as an indicator of β-cell function, could not be confirmed in the group treated with DPP-4 inhibitors. Therefore, whether patients with a higher baseline C-peptide level, a shorter duration, and differential insulin usage will benefit more from combination therapy with any DPP-4 inhibitor remains unknown.

(2) Glycemic Control: HbA1c. As a main outcome indicator, specific data on the HbA1c levels were available in four RCTs. Individually, three RCTs did not observe a significant improvement in the HbA1c levels when the patients were treated with sitagliptin [19, 20] or vildagliptin [13] in addition to insulin therapy. The authors in the other RCT [18] did not estimate the difference themselves, although the forest plot (shown in Figure 3(a)) showed an advantage for the HbA1c levels in the group that received combination treatment including sitagliptin over insulin monotherapy. Overall, a meta-analysis of these four studies (shown in Figure 3(a)) suggested that the addition of DPP-4 inhibitor treatment resulted in a greater decrease (0.07%) in the HbA1c level in patients with T1DM (95% CI: −0.37%–0.23%), albeit with significant heterogeneity. A sensitivity analysis was conducted to explore the sources of heterogeneity, and the heterogeneity became acceptable after the study by Farngren et al. [13] was removed. Thus, we hypothesize that the heterogeneity may be caused by different clinical characteristics, such as the study design (a single-center crossover study), negative baseline C-peptide status, and the use of different medicines (vildagliptin was used in Farngren et al.'s study, while the other studies used sitagliptin). Then, we performed a subgroup analysis. The vildagliptin subgroup showed advantages over insulin monotherapy in reducing HbA1c levels (0.32% (95% CI: −0.38%–0.26%)) in the study by Farngren et al. [13]. However, the subgroup of the other three studies on sitagliptin suggested that it was no better than insulin monotherapy. As shown in Figure 3(b), the change in the HbA1c levels in the experimental group was 0.22% (95% CI: −0.24%–0.68%) higher than the change in the control group, but the difference was not significant ($P = 0.23$, >0.05).

(3) Glycemic Control: Glycemic Fluctuation. Amazingly, after 16 weeks of treatment, the group receiving DPP-4 inhibitors had lower postprandial blood glucose levels and lower glucagon levels in the study by Garg et al., although the 4-hour AUCs for glycemia were not different between groups [20]. However, other studies did not provide evidence confirming

Table 1: Characteristics of the included studies.

Studies	Hari et al. (NCT01235819)	Griffin et al. (NCT01155284)	Garg et al. (NCT01227460)	Zhao et al. (NCT01159847)	Farngren et al. (NCT01147276)
Experimental treatment	Sitagliptin (100 mg, qd) + insulin[a] (premix insulin)	Sitagliptin (100/50 mg, qd) + lansoprazole (60/30 mg, qd) + insulin (unspecified)	Sitagliptin (100 mg, qd) + insulin[b] (premixed insulin excluded)	Sitagliptin (100 mg, qd) + insulin (unspecified)	Vildagliptin (50 mg, bid) + insulin[c] (long-acting and short-acting insulin)
Control treatment[d]	Insulin (bid-tid)	Placebo + insulin	Placebo + insulin	Insulin	Placebo + insulin
Treatment period (weeks)	52	52	16	52	8
Experimental samples	6	40	63	15	14
Control samples	6	18	62	15	14
Average age (years)	27.15 ± 4.20	16.18 ± 5.78	37.99 ± 14.01	47.45 ± 3.27	U
Mean duration of T1DM	33.25 ± 9.37 d	103.41 ± 51.74 d	21.01 ± 11.00 y	1.4 ± 0.20 y	11.0 ± 4.30 y
Average BMI (kg/m^2)	21.50 ± 3.39	21.51 ± 3.95	27.45 ± 4.54	23.35 ± 0.85	24.8 ± 3.30
Design	RCT	RCT	RCT	RCT	RCT
Number of centers	1	3	3	1	1
HbA1c at baseline (%)	9.75 ± 0.83	7.18 ± 1.09	8.55 ± 0.70	6.45 ± 0.20	7.49 ± 0.55
Cholesterol at baseline (mmol/L)	U	U	U	4.65 ± 0.16	U
C-peptide at baseline (pmol/L)	0.395 ± 0.15[e]	685.44 ± 412.36	≥16 pmol/L[f]	401.75 ± 52.27[g]	U
LDL-C at baseline (mmol/L)	U	U	U	2.75 ± 0.13	U
Triglyceride at baseline (mmol/L)	U	U	U	1.2 ± 0.1	U
Inclusion criteria	Recent T1DM < 3 m, GAD^+ or stimulated CP < 0.5 ng/mL, age < 30 y	Aged 11–36 y, <6 m	Aged 18–80 y, after diagnosed for 1 y, BMI < 35 kg/m^2	Aged 25–70 y, FCP ≥ 200/2 hCP ≥ 400 pmol/L, duration < 3 y, LADA	Age > 18 y, duration of 2–20 y, HbA1c of 6.5–8.5%
Exclusion criteria	C-peptide < 0.1 ng/mL, age > 30 y, pancreatic disease	Risk of pancreatitis, pregnant	BMI ≥ 35 kg/m^2	Other autoimmune diseases, insulin > 0.8 U/kg/d, renal disease	Pregnant or lactating, acute infection, liver disease, blood donor, using GH or oral steroid

d: days; m: months; y: years. Data are presented as the mean ± SD or as numbers (percentages). U: unknown; NG: not given; GH: growth hormone; BMI: body mass index; RCT: randomized controlled trial. [a]Patients initially were started on a twice daily premixed insulin regime (25% insulin Lispro and 75% insulin Lispro protamine) and later shifted to a three-times-daily premixed regime depending on their glycemic profiles. [b]Patients may be using insulin via a continuous subcutaneous insulin infusion (CSII) or multiple daily injections (MDI) containing bolus and basal insulin. [c]Twenty-six patients were treated with daily basal-bolus injections; their mean insulin dose was 30 U/d (long-acting insulin; 0.37 ± 0.07 U/kg) and 31 U/d (short-acting insulin; 0.37 ± 0.09 U/kg). Two patients were treated with a continuous sc insulin infusion [daily dose 60 and 36 U (0.67 and 0.52 U/kg), resp.]. [d]The insulin dosages used were consistent with the experimental group. [e]ng/mL; [f]only 20 patients were reported to be C-peptide-positive; [g]fasting C-peptide level.

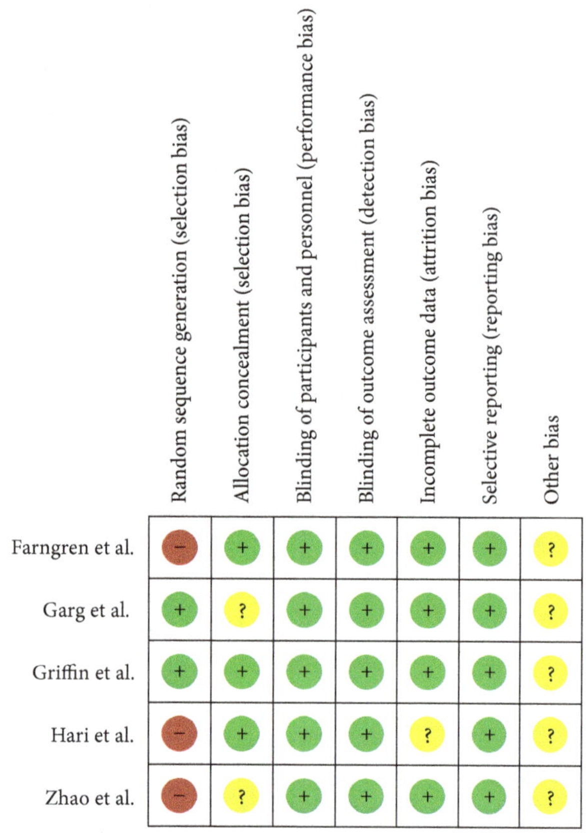

Figure 2: Risk of bias summary of included studies.

the ability of DPP-4 inhibitors to improve the blood glucose levels. As shown in the study by Griffin et al., the AUCs for the 2-hour blood glucose levels increased by 2.04 mmol/L (95% CI: 1.09–2.99) in the group receiving sitagliptin and lansoprazole combined with insulin and by 3.05 mmol/L (95% CI: 1.17–4.92) in the insulin monotherapy group, but the difference between the groups was not significant [8]. Zhao et al. did not observe a significant difference in the fasting blood glucose or postprandial blood glucose levels between the two groups [18]. The remaining two studies [13, 19] did not report data on glycemic control.

3.3.2. *Secondary Outcomes*

(1) Other Relevant Indicators. Regarding the insulin dosage, two studies [19, 20] provided raw data. The study by Hari et al. [19] revealed a significantly greater decrease in daily insulin consumption in the sitagliptin group (23.7 ± 13.9 U) than in the control group (15.2 ± 9.5 U) at the end of one year. According to the results from the other study [20], the changes in the total daily insulin dosage were −2.04 ± 11.45 U and 0.22 ± 9.17 U; however, the authors concluded that the change in the daily insulin dose (total units, units per kg/day, and basal and bolus units) did not change. Zhao et al. [18] reported a lack of difference in the insulin dosage at baseline and after treatment between groups. Farngren et al. [13] showed that the change in the insulin dosage was not significantly altered after treatment. Conversely, in the study by Griffin et al. [8], the insulin dosage increased over time in both groups and was significantly increased for the experimental group over time.

According to Garg et al. [20], the GLP-1 levels measured after 30 and 60 minutes in the sitagliptin group were significantly elevated after 16 weeks of treatment, whereas the GIP level measured at the 1-hour time point in the meal challenge test decreased. No differences in other relevant indicators, including the BMI, body weight, and lipid profiles, were observed between the experimental groups that received an additional DPP-4 inhibitor treatment and the control groups. Zhao et al. [18] did not observe significant differences in the BMI, weight, or lipid profiles (including low-density lipoprotein cholesterol, high-density lipoprotein cholesterol, triglycerides, and total cholesterol) between the treatment groups after treatment with sitagliptin for 12 months. In the study by Hari et al. [19], the BMI was significantly increased ($1.5 \pm 2.15\,kg/m^2$, $P < 0.05$) in the insulin monotherapy group, and the body weight was also increased but did not significantly differ between groups. Garg et al. [20] consistently reported a lack of significant differences in the body weight or BMI between groups.

(2) Overall Adverse Events and Side Effects. We believe that hypoglycemia is one vital adverse event that deserves more attention when antidiabetic agents are added to insulin therapy. The study by Hari et al. [19] observed a high incidence of hypoglycemia, including severe hypoglycemia (4/6 versus 3/6 in the sitagliptin group compared with the insulin monotherapy group). Griffin et al. [8] reported adverse events of severe hypoglycemia (<2.06 mmol/L) in 11 (24%) and 7 (32%) of the patients in the experimental and control groups, respectively. Additionally, hypoglycemia (<3.33 mmol/L) occurred in 44 (96%) and 19 (86%) patients in these two groups, respectively. Only one patient in the control group experienced severe hypoglycemia and required an insulin dosage adjustment after a period of 16 weeks in Garg et al.'s study [20]. In the study by Zhao et al. [18], a low incidence of hypoglycemia (<3.9 mmol/L) occurred, and no severe hypoglycemia was reported. Finally, none of these studies observed a significant difference in the incidence of hypoglycemia. We tried to obtain information regarding the time spent in hypoglycemia, but the studies included in the present meta-analysis did not report this information. In another study [13], hypoglycemia was designed to be induced by a hyperinsulinemic hypoglycemic clamp and therefore was not valued as an adverse event. These authors revealed that the most common adverse event was a common cold, and no serious adverse events occurred. Because DPP-4 inhibitors elevate the endogenous GLP-1 levels, we also examined the incidence of pancreatitis. Three studies [8, 19, 20] emphasized the exclusion of patients with a history of pancreatitis or an increased risk of pancreatitis. Importantly, no pancreatitis events were reported throughout the periods of any of the included studies. Overall side effects that seemed to occur at a greater frequency in the experimental group included gastrointestinal disorders; infections and infestations; injury; poisoning; procedural complications; nervous system disorders; respiratory, thoracic, and mediastinal disorders; and skin and subcutaneous tissue disorders, but the frequencies

Study of subgroup	Experimental group Mean	SD	Total	Control group Mean	SD	Total	Weight	Mean difference IV, Random, 95% CI
Farngren et al.	−0.34	0.1	14	−0.02	0.07	14	31.1%	−0.32 [−0.38, −0.26]
Garg et al.	−0.07	0.7	63	−0.12	0.75	62	25.8%	0.05 [−0.20, 0.30]
Hari et al.	−2.1	0.54	6	−2	0.63	6	12.5%	−0.10 [−0.76, 0.56]
Zhao et al.	−0.2	0.13	15	−0.3	0.13	15	30.6%	0.10 [0.01, 0.19]
Total (95% CI)			**98**			**97**	**100.0%**	**−0.07 [−0.37, 0.23]**

Heterogeneity: $\tau^2 = 0.08$; $\chi^2 = 56.37$, $df = 3$ ($P < 0.00001$); $I^2 = 95\%$

Test for overall effect: $Z = 0.44$ ($P = 0.66$)

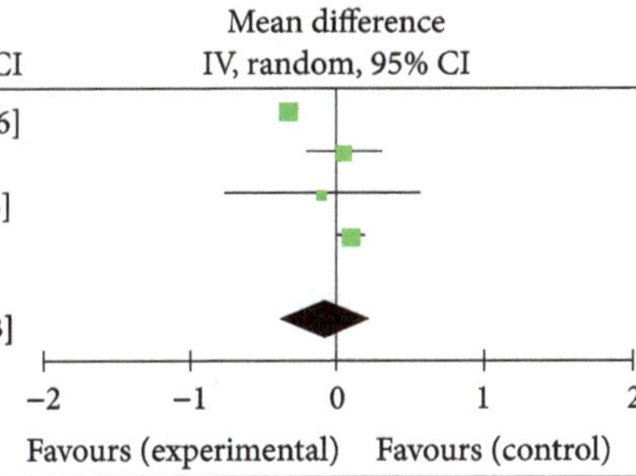

(a)

Study of subgroup	Experimental group Mean	SD	Total	Control group Mean	SD	Total	Weight	Mean difference IV, Random, 95% CI
1.6.1 Sitagliptin versus control								
Garg et al.	−0.07	0.7	63	−0.12	0.75	62	59.4%	0.07 [−0.28, 0.42]
Hari et al.	−2.1	0.54	6	−2	0.63	6	13.8%	−0.16 [−1.29, 0.98]
Zhao et al.	−0.2	0.13	15	−0.3	0.13	15	26.8%	0.75 [0.00, 1.49]
Subtotal (95% CI)			**84**			**83**	**100.0%**	**0.22 [−0.24, 0.68]**

Heterogeneity: $\tau^2 = 0.06$; $\chi^2 = 2.96$, $df = 2$ ($P = 0.23$); $I^2 = 33\%$

Test for overall effect: $Z = 0.94$ ($P = 0.35$)

Test for subgroup differences: not applicable

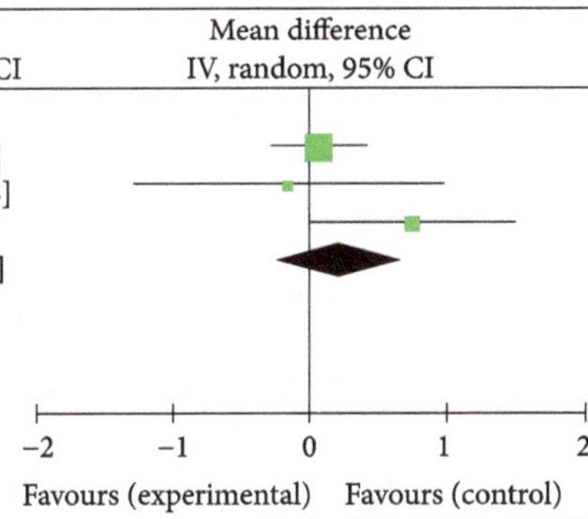

(b)

Figure 3: Forest plot of HbA1c.

were not statistically significant [8]. Records of adverse effects from Garg et al. [20] included a skin rash and a need for esophageal cancer surgery that finally led to treatment interruption. For most of the studies included in the present review, significant differences in the incidences of various adverse events were not observed between the two groups. All authors concluded that no serious side effects were confirmed to be clearly related to the DPP-4 inhibitors, including hypoglycemia, and other causes led to discontinuation from further participation; in addition, ketoacidosis and pancreatitis were not reported.

4. Discussion

Due to their recommended use as first-line antidiabetic agents by the American Association of Clinical Endocrinologists (AACE), DPP-4 inhibitors are currently widely used as outstanding monotherapeutic or combination therapeutic agents for T2DM. However, no DPP-4 inhibitor for T1DM has received authorization for application. No currently available treatment has shown lasting disease remission, although insulin is life-saving. Meanwhile, the life expectancy of patients with T1DM has substantially improved in recent decades. Therefore, additional management strategies are needed. Any novel treatment option (newer) in addition to insulin may produce a qualitative leap. Emerging studies have reported evidence that an elevation of serum DPP-4 activity is related to the pancreatic autoimmune process, intestinal proinflammatory alterations, and hepatobiliary injury [21–23] (i.e., DPP-4 may contribute to T1DM pathology). Additionally, inhibition of DPP-4 activity has shown a potential therapeutic effect in patients with T1DM. In fundamental studies, inhibition of DPP-4 activity alleviated insulitis and stimulated β-cell proliferation [10], markedly increased the β-cell mass and number of proliferating β-cells [24], elevated the glucose-stimulated insulin and C-peptide concentrations [25], and increased the total insulin levels [26], eventually delaying the diabetogenic autoimmune response [27, 28]. DPP-4 inhibitors (P32/98, DA1229, and MK0431) substantially decreased the blood glucose levels in animal models of T1DM [29–31] and even resulted in normoglycemia in some cases [32]. Moreover, DPP-4 inhibition increased the survival of islet grafts [33] and improved diabetic retinopathy [34]. According to clinical studies, patients with T1DM displayed higher DPP-4 levels [35, 36]. Consequently, we believe that treatment with DPP-4 inhibitors is a practical therapeutic strategy for T1DM, and thus, we sought to identify evidence from clinical practice. Numerous studies have provided evidence for the therapeutic effect of DPP-4 inhibitors in patients with T1DM. In clinical studies, DPP-4 inhibitors reduced the prandial insulin dose and its daily dosage [13, 37], inhibited glucagon secretion [13, 15], and decreased the blood glucose levels in patients with T1DM (2-hour postprandial and 24-hour AUCs) [37]. However, some clinical studies did not show any obvious improvement in the blood glucose levels, AUCs of the C-peptide levels, or HbA1c levels [18, 20]. Therefore, the therapeutic effects of DPP-4 inhibitors on T1DM remain controversial, and a comprehensive conclusion must be drawn after summarizing the currently available evidence.

Here, we systematically reviewed all relevant publications and performed a meta-analysis of five randomized controlled clinical trials on the effects of DPP-4 inhibitors on T1DM. We were also interested in another clinical trial (NCT00622284), which was originally intended to investigate the efficacy of linagliptin compared to glimepiride administration for 104 weeks as an add-on therapy to preferably >1500 mg of metformin in patients with T2DM with insufficient glycemic control. Some of the participants were reclassified as LADA depending on the tested autoantibodies during the trial. Further investigation found that these LADA patients demonstrated progressively increasing C-peptide levels and slightly decreasing HbA1c levels after linagliptin-metformin treatment compared to the baseline levels [38], hinting at a possible therapeutic effect of DPP-4 inhibitors on T1DM. Considering the heterogeneity, we excluded this study from our meta-analysis. Based on the pooled data in our meta-analysis, treatment with DPP-4 inhibitors neither resulted in a significantly greater decrease in the HbA1c levels nor further reduced the insulin dosage or affected the weight or BMI in patients with T1DM. Unfortunately, we were unable to perform a pooled analysis of the data on the fasting blood glucose or prandial blood glucose levels because the raw data or changes were not available for some studies. Although benefits, including declining fasting blood glucose levels [39], prandial blood glucose levels [13, 20, 37], AUCs of 24-hour blood glucose levels [37], and HbA1c levels, as well as reductions in the insulin dosages [37], have been reported by individual studies, these effects failed to be revealed in other similar studies. The discrepancy may be caused by different baseline characteristics (such as C-peptide levels) of the enrolled populations, different lengths of follow up [39], and other variables. DPP-4 inhibitors significantly increased the GLP-1 and GIP levels [13, 14, 40], reduced the glucagon levels during hyperglycemia, and sustained glucagon counterregulation during hypoglycemia in patients with T1DM [13, 14]. Fortunately, the absence of relevant severe side effects promises more studies regarding security to validate the therapeutic effects.

The limitations of this review include the small number of RCTs and the absence of some data. More desirable studies and raw data will enable us to perform a stratified analysis and further explore the roles of DPP-4 inhibitors as treatments for T1DM. Another limitation is that immunological indicators have not been reported in any studies, although conclusive evidence has been established for the immunoregulatory effects of DPP-4 inhibitors. In addition, almost none of the studies included in this review reported the full-scale adverse effects that were reported during the treatment of T2DM, such as cardiovascular events and tumors, which were the most common, severe, and vital adverse effects [41]. Pharmacotherapy for T1DM is required throughout the patient's lifetime; therefore, the application of any novel medicine requires a very thorough long-term cost/benefit analysis (i.e., for cancer and other relevant endpoints). Therefore, we believe that a lack of a cost/benefit analysis is one limitation.

As discussed above, more studies should be recruited to elucidate the roles of DPP-4 inhibitors in appropriately selected patients with T1DM. A larger sample size, a longer follow-up, unified characteristics of participants (such as diabetes duration and C-peptide levels), the comprehensive monitoring of glycemia and relevant hormone levels, the use of immunological indicators (such as $CD4^+$ and $CD8^+$ T cells), and a report of full-scale adverse effects should be the focus of future studies.

Conflicts of Interest

None of the authors have conflicts of interest to declare.

Authors' Contributions

Qixian Wang and Min Long contributed equally to this work.

Acknowledgments

This review article was funded by grants from the National Key R&D Program of China (no. 2016YFC1101100 to Hongting Zheng) and the National Natural Science Foundation of China (nos. 81471039, 81270893, and 81228023 to Hongting Zheng).

References

[1] American Diabetes Association, "Standards of medical care in diabetes–2010," *Diabetes Care*, vol. 33, Supplement 1, pp. S11–S61, 2010.

[2] J. H. Kim, C. G. Lee, Y. A. Lee, S. W. Yang, and C. H. Shin, "Increasing incidence of type 1 diabetes among Korean children and adolescents: analysis of data from a nationwide registry in Korea," *Pediatric Diabetes*, vol. 17, no. 7, pp. 519–524, 2016.

[3] C. Gong, X. Meng, Y. Jiang, X. Wang, H. Cui, and X. Chen, "Trends in childhood type 1 diabetes mellitus incidence in Beijing from 1995 to 2010: a retrospective multicenter study based on hospitalization data," *Diabetes Technology & Therapeutics*, vol. 17, no. 3, pp. 159–165, 2015.

[4] F. S. Fazeli, P. C. Souverein, M. M. van der Vorst et al., "Increasing trends in the incidence and prevalence rates of type 1 diabetes among children and adolescents in the Netherlands," *Pediatric Diabetes*, vol. 17, no. 1, pp. 44–52, 2016.

[5] T. H. Lipman, K. L. Levitt, S. J. Ratcliffe et al., "Increasing incidence of type 1 diabetes in youth: twenty years of the Philadelphia Pediatric Diabetes Registry," *Diabetes Care*, vol. 36, no. 6, pp. 1597–1603, 2013.

[6] K. M. Munir and S. N. Davis, "The treatment of type 1 diabetes mellitus with agents approved for type 2 diabetes mellitus," *Expert Opinion on Pharmacotherapy*, vol. 16, no. 15, pp. 2331–2341, 2015.

[7] P. Pozzilli, E. Maddaloni, and R. Buzzetti, "Combination immunotherapies for type 1 diabetes mellitus," *Nature Reviews Endocrinology*, vol. 11, no. 5, pp. 289–297, 2015.

[8] K. J. Griffin, P. A. Thompson, M. Gottschalk, J. H. Kyllo, and A. Rabinovitch, "Combination therapy with sitagliptin and lansoprazole in patients with recent-onset type 1 diabetes

(REPAIR-T1D): 12-month results of a multicentre, randomised, placebo-controlled, phase 2 trial," *The Lancet Diabetes & Endocrinology*, vol. 2, no. 9, pp. 710–718, 2014.

[9] J. J. Holst, "The physiology of glucagon-like peptide 1," *Physiological Reviews*, vol. 87, no. 4, pp. 1409–1439, 2007.

[10] L. Tian, J. Gao, J. Hao et al., "Reversal of new-onset diabetes through modulating inflammation and stimulating beta-cell replication in nonobese diabetic mice by a dipeptidyl peptidase IV inhibitor," *Endocrinology*, vol. 151, no. 7, pp. 3049–3060, 2010.

[11] A. Zoka, G. Barna, A. Somogyi et al., "Extension of the $CD4^{+}Foxp3^{+}CD25^{-/low}$ regulatory T-cell subpopulation in type 1 diabetes mellitus," *Autoimmunity*, vol. 48, no. 5, pp. 289–297, 2015.

[12] E. Kutoh, "Sitagliptin is effective and safe as add-on to insulin in patients with absolute insulin deficiency: a case series," *Journal of Medical Case Reports*, vol. 5, no. 1, p. 117, 2011.

[13] J. Farngren, M. Persson, A. Schweizer, J. E. Foley, and B. Ahren, "Vildagliptin reduces glucagon during hyperglycemia and sustains glucagon counterregulation during hypoglycemia in type 1 diabetes," *The Journal of Clinical Endocrinology & Metabolism*, vol. 97, no. 10, pp. 3799–3806, 2012.

[14] J. E. Schopman, J. B. Hoekstra, B. M. Frier et al., "Effects of sitagliptin on counter-regulatory and incretin hormones during acute hypoglycaemia in patients with type 1 diabetes: a randomized double-blind placebo-controlled crossover study," *Diabetes, Obesity and Metabolism*, vol. 17, no. 6, pp. 546–553, 2015.

[15] J. E. Foley, M. Ligueros-Saylan, Y. L. He et al., "Effect of vildagliptin on glucagon concentration during meals in patients with type 1 diabetes," *Hormone and Metabolic Research*, vol. 40, no. 10, pp. 727–730, 2008.

[16] D. Moher, A. Liberati, J. Tetzlaff, and D. G. Altman, "Preferred reporting items for systematic reviews and meta-analyses: the PRISMA statement," *BMJ*, vol. 62, no. 10, article b2535, pp. 1006–1012, 2009.

[17] J. P. Higgins, S. G. Thompson, J. J. Deeks, and D. G. Altman, "Measuring inconsistency in meta-analyses," *BMJ*, vol. 327, no. 7414, pp. 557–560, 2003.

[18] Y. Zhao, L. Yang, Y. Xiang et al., "Dipeptidyl peptidase 4 inhibitor sitagliptin maintains β-cell function in patients with recent-onset latent autoimmune diabetes in adults: one year prospective study," *The Journal of Clinical Endocrinology & Metabolism*, vol. 99, no. 5, pp. E876–E880, 2014.

[19] K. K. Hari, A. Shaikh, and P. Prusty, "Addition of exenatide or sitagliptin to insulin in new onset type 1 diabetes: a randomized, open label study," *Diabetes Research and Clinical Practice*, vol. 100, no. 2, pp. e55–e58, 2013.

[20] S. K. Garg, E. G. Moser, B. W. Bode et al., "Effect of sitagliptin on post-prandial glucagon and GLP-1 levels in patients with type 1 diabetes: investigator-initiated, double-blind, randomized, placebo-controlled trial," *Endocrine Practice*, vol. 19, no. 1, pp. 19–28, 2013.

[21] T. Varga, G. Firneisz, G. Nagy, and A. Somogyi, "Elevated serum dipeptidyl peptidase-4 activity in type 1 diabetes mellitus: a direct comparison," *Orvosi Hetilap*, vol. 151, no. 22, pp. 899–902, 2010.

[22] K. Blaslov, T. Bulum, and L. Duvnjak, "Circulating dipeptidyl peptidase-4 activity is associated with insulin resistance in type 1 diabetic patients," *Journal of Diabetes and Its Complications*, vol. 29, no. 3, pp. 390–394, 2015.

[23] G. Firneisz and A. Zoka, "Elevation of serum dipeptidyl peptidase-4 activity in type 1 diabetes: potential explanations and implications," *Diabetes Research and Clinical Practice*, vol. 127, pp. 291-292, 2017.

[24] D. H. Kim, J. C. Lee, M. K. Lee, K. W. Kim, and M. S. Lee, "Treatment of autoimmune diabetes in NOD mice by Toll-like receptor 2 tolerance in conjunction with dipeptidyl peptidase 4 inhibition," *Diabetologia*, vol. 55, no. 12, pp. 3308–3317, 2012.

[25] L. Ding, C. A. Gysemans, G. Stange et al., "Combining MK626, a novel DPP-4 inhibitor, and low-dose monoclonal CD3 antibody for stable remission of new-onset diabetes in mice," *PLoS One*, vol. 9, no. 9, article e107935, 2014.

[26] M. P. de Amorim, O. M. Monteiro, J. J. Rossoni, M. E. Silva, W. G. de Lima, and D. C. Costa, "Vildagliptin induces β-cell neogenesis and improves the lipid profile in a later phase of type 1 diabetes," *Current Pharmaceutical Biotechnology*, vol. 16, no. 1, pp. 60–65, 2015.

[27] M. T. Julian, N. Alonso, R. Colobran et al., "CD26/DPPIV inhibition alters the expression of immune response-related genes in the thymi of NOD mice," *Molecular and Cellular Endocrinology*, vol. 426, pp. 101–112, 2016.

[28] J. Jelsing, N. Vrang, S. B. van Witteloostuijn, M. Mark, and T. Klein, "The DPP4 inhibitor linagliptin delays the onset of diabetes and preserves β-cell mass in non-obese diabetic mice," *Journal of Endocrinology*, vol. 214, no. 3, pp. 381–387, 2012.

[29] J. A. Pospisilik, J. Martin, T. Doty et al., "Dipeptidyl peptidase IV inhibitor treatment stimulates β-cell survival and islet neogenesis in streptozotocin-induced diabetic rats," *Diabetes*, vol. 52, no. 3, pp. 741–750, 2003.

[30] J. M. Cho, H. W. Jang, H. Cheon et al., "A novel dipeptidyl peptidase IV inhibitor DA-1229 ameliorates streptozotocin-induced diabetes by increasing β-cell replication and neogenesis," *Diabetes Research and Clinical Practice*, vol. 91, no. 1, pp. 72–79, 2011.

[31] S. F. A. Da, M. A. Dias, V. B. Leme et al., "Dipeptidyl peptidase IV inhibitor improves the salivary gland histology of spontaneously diabetic mice," *Archives of Oral Biology*, vol. 58, no. 7, pp. 755–761, 2013.

[32] W. L. Suarez-Pinzon, G. S. Cembrowski, and A. Rabinovitch, "Combination therapy with a dipeptidyl peptidase-4 inhibitor and a proton pump inhibitor restores normoglycaemia in non-obese diabetic mice," *Diabetologia*, vol. 52, no. 8, pp. 1680–1682, 2009.

[33] S. J. Kim, C. Nian, D. J. Doudet, and C. H. McIntosh, "Inhibition of dipeptidyl peptidase IV with sitagliptin (MK0431) prolongs islet graft survival in streptozotocin-induced diabetic mice," *Diabetes*, vol. 57, no. 5, pp. 1331–1339, 2008.

[34] A. Goncalves, C. Marques, E. Leal et al., "Dipeptidyl peptidase-IV inhibition prevents blood-retinal barrier breakdown, inflammation and neuronal cell death in the retina of type 1 diabetic rats," *Biochimica et Biophysica Acta (BBA) - Molecular Basis of Disease*, vol. 1842, no. 9, pp. 1454–1463, 2014.

[35] T. Varga, A. Somogyi, G. Barna et al., "Higher serum DPP-4 enzyme activity and decreased lymphocyte CD26 expression in type 1 diabetes," *Pathology Oncology Research*, vol. 17, no. 4, pp. 925–930, 2011.

[36] S. Osawa, D. Kawamori, N. Katakami et al., "Significant elevation of serum dipeptidyl peptidase-4 activity in young-adult type 1 diabetes," *Diabetes Research and Clinical Practice*, vol. 113, pp. 135–142, 2016.

[37] S. L. Ellis, E. G. Moser, J. K. Snell-Bergeon, A. S. Rodionova, R. M. Hazenfield, and S. K. Garg, "Effect of sitagliptin on glucose control in adult patients with type 1 diabetes: a pilot, double-blind, randomized, crossover trial," *Diabetic Medicine*, vol. 28, no. 10, pp. 1176–1181, 2011.

[38] O. E. Johansen, B. O. Boehm, V. Grill et al., "C-peptide levels in latent autoimmune diabetes in adults treated with linagliptin versus glimepiride: exploratory results from a 2-year double-blind, randomized, controlled study," *Diabetes Care*, vol. 37, no. 1, pp. e11–e12, 2014.

[39] O. Giampietro, C. Giampietro, L. D. Bartola, M. C. Masoni, and E. Matteucci, "Sitagliptin as add-on therapy in insulin deficiency: biomarkers of therapeutic efficacy respond differently in type 1 and type 2 diabetes," *Drug Design, Development and Therapy*, vol. 7, pp. 99–104, 2013.

[40] J. E. Foley, M. C. Bunck, D. L. Moller-Goede et al., "Beta cell function following 1 year vildagliptin or placebo treatment and after 12 week washout in drug-naive patients with type 2 diabetes and mild hyperglycaemia: a randomised controlled trial," *Diabetologia*, vol. 54, no. 8, pp. 1985–1991, 2011.

[41] A. C. Tricco, J. Antony, P. A. Khan et al., "Safety and effectiveness of dipeptidyl peptidase-4 inhibitors versus intermediate-acting insulin or placebo for patients with type 2 diabetes failing two oral antihyperglycaemic agents: a systematic review and network meta-analysis," *BMJ Open*, vol. 4, no. 12, article e005752, 2014.

5

Not Only Glycaemic But Also Other Metabolic Factors Affect T Regulatory Cell Counts and Proinflammatory Cytokine Levels in Women with Type 1 Diabetes

Katerina Stechova,[1] Jana Sklenarova-Labikova,[2] Tereza Kratzerova,[3] Pavlina Pithova,[1] and Dominik Filipp[4]

[1]*Department of Internal Medicine, 2nd Medical Faculty, Charles University and University Hospital Motol, Prague, Czech Republic*
[2]*Department of Paediatrics, 2nd Medical Faculty, Charles University and University Hospital Motol, Prague, Czech Republic*
[3]*Department of Physiology, 2nd Medical Faculty, Charles University, Prague, Czech Republic*
[4]*Laboratory of Immunobiology, Institute of Molecular Genetics of the ASCR, Prague, Czech Republic*

Correspondence should be addressed to Katerina Stechova; katerina.stechova@lfmotol.cuni.cz

Academic Editor: Ruben Varela-Calvino

Type 1 diabetic (T1D) patients suffer from insulinopenia and hyperglycaemia. Studies have shown that if a patient's hyperglycaemic environment is not compensated, it leads to complex immune dysfunctions. Similarly, T1D mothers with poor glycaemic control exert a negative impact on the immune responses of their newborns. However, questions concerning the impact of other metabolic disturbances on the immune system of T1D mothers (and their newborns) have been raised. To address these questions, we examined 28 T1D women in reproductive age for the relationship between various metabolic, clinical, and immune parameters. Our study revealed several unexpected correlations which are indicative of a much more complex relationship between glucose and lipid factors (namely, glycosylated haemoglobin Hb1Ac, the presence of one but not multiple chronic diabetic complications, and atherogenic indexes) and proinflammatory cytokines (IL-1alpha and TNF-alpha). Regulatory T cell counts correlated with HbA1c, diabetic neuropathy, lipid spectra parameters, and IL-6 levels. Total T-helper cell count was interconnected with BMI and glycaemia variability correlated with lipid spectra parameters, insulin dose, and vitamin D levels. These and other correlations revealed in this study provide broader insight into the association of various metabolic abnormalities with immune parameters that may impact T1D mothers or their developing child.

1. Introduction

Type 1 diabetes (T1D) is a T-helper 1- (Th1-) mediated autoimmune disease that is characterized by a lack of insulin due to autoimmune destruction of pancreatic beta cells [1]. T1D develops more often in young individuals and, at the time of diagnosis, is typically associated with an acute complex metabolic disturbance in the absence of microvascular or macrovascular chronic diabetic complications. In this sense, if diabetes compensation gauged through the levels of glycosylated haemoglobin (HbA1c) is appropriate, T1D patients are relatively healthy people with normal body weight. However, after several years of disease progression, their health gradually worsens and chronic diabetic complications may occur. In fact, they gradually become biologically older, with more apparent health impairment than what is typical for their age-related peers [2]. Overweight and obesity also continue to be more prevalent among individuals with T1D. These conditions are related to worsened insulin sensitivity which further increases the risks of comorbidities, such as metabolic syndrome, and leads to further development and deterioration of T1D-associated microvascular and macrovascular diseases [3]. T1D patients may also suffer from additional autoimmune diseases (the most common is thyroid gland autoimmunity) due to the inclination of their immune system to autoreactivity [4]. Taken together, T1D in a long term represents a multifactorial pathogenic continuum rather than a single-disease entity of autoimmune origin.

In our previous study, we analyzed the impact of maternal diabetes on the immune responses of newborns. Notably, we evaluated the effect of maternal glycaemic control on the cytokine profile of newborn cord blood mononuclear cells (CBMCs). The result of this study demonstrated that nonstimulated or diabetogenic autoantigen-stimulated newborn CBMCs of T1D mothers with poor glycaemic control exhibited lower cytokine and chemokine production compared to those of mothers with well-stabilized glycaemic control [5]. Consistent with this conclusion was the demonstration that high glucose concentration in culture media that mimicked "hyperglycaemia" also dampened the production of cytokines and chemokines [5]. This study not only contributed to our increasing knowledge on foetal cell reprogramming and the importance of an intrauterine environment for the future health status of the child [6], but it also raised important questions concerning the impact of other metabolic disturbances on the immune system. Specifically, we asked whether, on top of glucose metabolites, other metabolic and clinical parameters, such as lipid spectra, atherogenic indexes, vitamin D levels, and hypertension, can exert their impact on critical humoral and cellular components of the immune systems, such as proinflammatory cytokines and Treg counts, respectively. This impact could also potentially involve the interplay between the production of advanced glycation end products (AGE) and the development of chronic diabetic complications.

To provide an initial insight into these inquiries, we selected a group of T1D women in reproductive age who eventually planned to become pregnant in the future. Our study revealed several unexpected correlations which are indicative of a much more complex relationship between glucose and lipid metabolites with elements of the immune system. These results thus provide a more complex view on the interplay between the metabolic state of T1D female patients and the immune parameters that may affect a developing child.

2. Material and Methods

2.1. Study Subjects and Ethics. We examined 28 nonpregnant T1D women. Their characteristics are summarized in Table 1. Metabolic characteristics of the group studied are described in Supplementary Table 1 available online at https://doi.org/10.1155/2017/5463273. Ethical approval for this study was obtained from the local ethics committee and written informed consent was obtained from all study participants.

2.2. Cell Isolation and Flow Cytometry. Peripheral blood mononuclear cells (PBMCs) were isolated from 20 to 25 ml of peripheral blood samples via Ficoll density gradient centrifugation (Amersham Biosciences, Uppsala, Sweden). According to the recommendation of the international working group of the experts in flow cytometry [7], CD3, CD4, CD25, CD127, and FoxP3 markers were used to analyze human Treg cells using a gating strategy illustrated in Supplementary Figure 1. Specifically, CD3-FITC, CD45-PerCP, CD127-APC (Miltenyi Biotec, Bergisch Gladbach, Germany), CD4-Alexa Fluor® 700, (EXBIO a.s., Prague, Czech Republic), Foxp3-PE, and CD25-Brilliant Violet (BioLegend, San Diego, USA) antibodies (Abs) were used. For intracellular staining, we used Foxp3-Fix/Perm and Foxp3-Perm Buffers (BioLegend, San Diego, USA). The flow cytometric data were collected on a LSR II flow cytometer (BD Biosciences, Franklin Lakes, NJ, USA) and analyzed using Summit 4.3 software (Dako, Glostrup, Denmark).

Table 1: Clinical characteristics of the study population.

	Median	Range
Age (years)	35	22–42
Diabetes duration (years)	12	6–27
BMI	23.1	18.5–35
Insulin units per kg	0.7	0.4–1.4
	Present	
Autoimmune thyroiditis	21/28	
Other autoimmune disease	2/28	
Hypertension	8/28	
Dyslipidaemia	9/28 But only 1 treated	
Diabetic retinopathy	12/28	
Diabetic neuropathy	11/28	
Diabetic nephropathy	8/28	
Diabetic foot syndrome	1/28	
Multiple chronic complications (2 and more)	11/28	

2.3. Measurements of Cytokine, AGE, and Protein Levels. Serum levels of cytokines and advanced glycation end products (AGE) were measured using the Instant ELISA kit for IL-1alpha, TNF-alpha, and IL-6 (eBioscience, San Diego, USA) and OxiSelect AGE ELISA kit (Cell Biolabs, San Diego, USA). Protein concentrations were determined with a Pierce™ BCA Protein Assay Kit (Bio-Rad, California, USA).

2.4. Routine Biochemical Laboratory and Calculated Metabolic Parameters. To express insulin resistance, the whole-body estimated glucose disposal rate (eGDR) was calculated using the formula

$$\text{eGDR}\left(\text{mg}\cdot\text{kg}^{-1}\cdot\text{min}^{-1}\right) = 24.31 - (12.22 \times \text{WHR}) - (3.29 \times \text{HTN}) - (0.57 \times \text{HbA1c}), \quad (1)$$

where WHR indicates the waist-hip ratio and HTN is the presence or absence of hypertension (expressed as 1/0 in the calculation) [8]. The glycosylated haemoglobin HbA1c, native lipid laboratory parameters, and vitamin D levels were determined using routine methods of the hospital biochemical laboratory. We calculated the risk indexes, that is, the plasma atherogenic index (PAI) as log(triglycerides/HDL cholesterol) which is recommended to be below 0.1 in women, the atherogenic index (AI) as the total cholesterol/HDL cholesterol where AI < 0.1 means the lowest cardiovascular risk, AI $\geq 0.1 \leq 0.21$ as the intermediate risk, and AI > 0.21 as the highest cardiovascular risk for the patients. Remnant cholesterol was calculated as the total cholesterol

Table 2: Definitions of the grouping variables.

Grouping variable	Groups	Group definition
HbA1c	1 (perfect or acceptable T1D stabilization)	HbA1c < 7.5% DCCT
	2 (not very well stabilized)	HbA1c according to DCCT in the range of 7.5 to 9.0%
	3 (badly compensated)	HbA1c > 9.0% DCCT
Glycaemic variability	1 (acceptable glycaemia variability)	Glycaemia SD ≤ 1/3 of mean glycaemia
	2 (high glycaemia variability)	Glycaemia SD > 1/3 of mean glycaemia
eGDR	RG	eGDR < 7.5
	NRG	eGDR ≥ 7.5
The presence of chronic diabetic complications	0 (no complication)	
	1 (one chronic diabetic complication present)	
	2 (two or more chronic diabetic complications present)	
LDL cholesterol	0 (low and normal values)	LDL < 2.5 mmol/l
	1 (increased levels)	LDL ≥ 2.5 mmol/l
Hypertension	0 (low and normal values)	
	1 (increased blood pressure values or treatment with antihypertensive drugs)	Blood pressure < 130/80

minus HDL cholesterol minus LDL cholesterol [9]. Glycaemic variability was calculated from patient glycaemia which was measured by the patients glucometer or by CGM (continuous glucose monitoring) during one month before blood sampling.

2.5. Statistics. The statistical analyses were performed using SPSS 22.0 for Windows (SPSS Inc., Chicago, IL, USA). The data was examined for normality and nonparametric tests, including nonparametric correlations (Spearmann's coefficient R was calculated) that were applied. We used several grouping variables (Table 2) to test the importance of different metabolic factors. For comparisons across groups, we used the Mann-Whitney U test for 2 samples and the Kruskal-Wallis 1-way ANOVA for k samples. Significance was defined at $p < 0.05$.

3. Results

3.1. Inflammatory Cytokines. Evaluating relationships between various clinical and biochemical parameters, we found significant correlations between the production of inflammatory cytokines and the level of HbA1c, presence of chronic diabetic complications, and calculated lipid risk indexes.

Towards this end, T1D patients were split into three groups according to HbA1c values. Group 1 consisted of eight patients who exhibited perfect or acceptable T1D stabilization with HbA1c below 7.5% DCCT. Twelve patients who were classified as not well stabilized represented group 2 with HbA1c in the range of 7.5 to 9% DCCT. Finally, eight patients with HbA1c values over 9% DCCT, indicating a very bad compensation, represented group 3. When we correlated cytokine levels within these three groups (Figure 1), unexpectedly, the lowest TNF-alpha production was found in group 3 which significantly differed from that in group 1 ($p = 0.001$) and even showed tangible but not significant difference with that in group 2. No correlation between HbA1c and IL-1alpha nor with IL-6 was found.

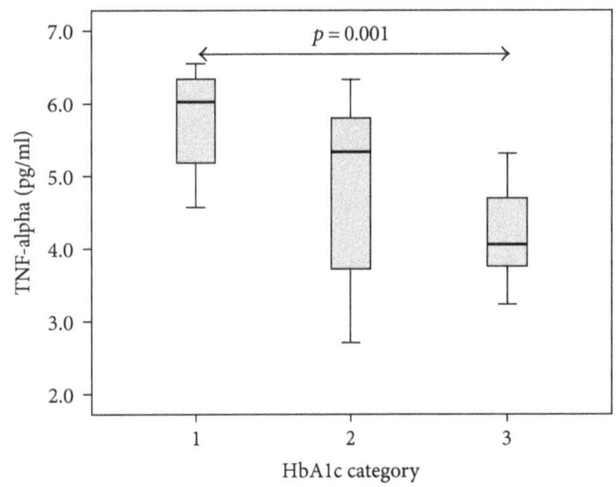

Figure 1: Inflammatory cytokines and HbA1c category. Patients with the worst diabetes stabilization (evaluated according to glycosylated haemoglobin HbA1c) had surprisingly the lowest level of proinflammatory cytokine TNF-alpha. There was a significant difference between this subgroup (marked as category 3) and the subgroup of patients with the best HbA1c (marked as category 1).

Data from our cohort of 28 patients also allowed us to correlate cytokine expression levels with the presence of chronic diabetic complications (i.e., diabetic retinopathy, nephropathy, neuropathy, and diabetic foot). In this context, 11 out of 28 patients (11/28) exhibited none of these complications at the time of sampling (marked as group 0). On the other hand, 6/28 patients suffered from only one complication (group 1) and 11/28 patients with two or more of these chronic diabetic complications comprised the final grouping (group 2). Figure 2(a) shows the comparison in IL-1alpha production between these three groups, and it was

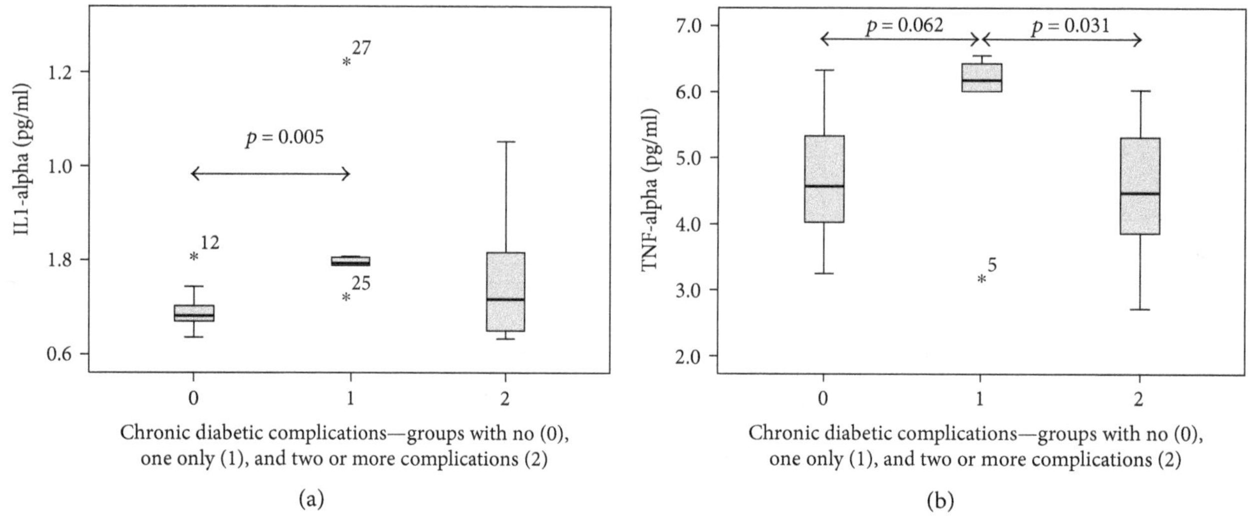

FIGURE 2: Inflammatory cytokines and chronic diabetic complications. The highest production of IL-1alpha was observed in patients with one chronic diabetic complication which significantly differed from patients without any diabetic complications. TNF-alpha expression levels were similar to those seen for IL-1alpha, but in addition, patients with multiple complications had significantly lower levels of TNF-alpha than those with only one complication. (a) IL-1alpha. (b) TNF-alpha—the highest TNF-alpha production was also observed in patients with one chronic diabetic complication.

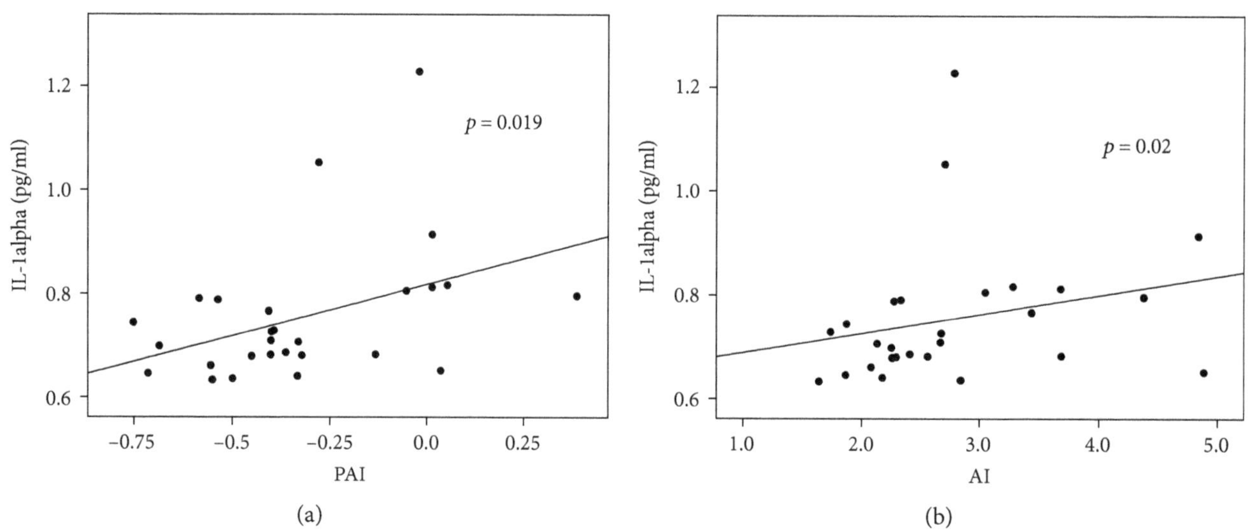

FIGURE 3: Inflammatory cytokines and calculated lipid indexes. Patients with higher calculated PAI and AI lipid indexes exhibited a significantly higher production of proinflammatory cytokine IL-1alpha ($p = 0.019$ and $R = 0.449$ for PAI and $p = 0.02$ and $R = 0.446$ for AI, resp.). (a) IL-1alpha and PAI (plasma atherogenic index). (b) IL-1alpha and AI (atherogenic index).

significantly higher in group 1 when compared to that in group 0 ($p = 0.005$). In a similar fashion, the group with only one complication (group 1) exhibited the greatest TNF-alpha production and differed significantly from both the group with multiple complications (group 2, $p = 0.031$) and the group with no complications (group 0, $p = 0.062$) (Figure 2(b)).

Next, the plasma atherogenic index (PAI) which is recommended to be below 0.1 and the atherogenic index (AI), which being below 0.1 indicates the lowest cardiovascular risk, were correlated with IL-1alpha and TNF-alpha cytokine levels. As shown in Figures 3(a) and 3(b), both PAI and AI were significantly positively correlated with IL-1alpha production ($p = 0.019$ for PAI and $p = 0.02$ for AI). There was no correlation with TNF-alpha production observed.

3.2. Treg Counts. Among many inspected relationships, we found a correlation between Treg counts and diabetes stabilization determined by HbA1c levels, the presence of diabetic neuropathy, lipid spectra, BMI, and IL-6 levels. Notably, in the group with a poor diabetes compensation (group 3, HbA1c > 9% DCCT, see above), we observed significantly lower Treg numbers in comparison to group 1 (perfect or

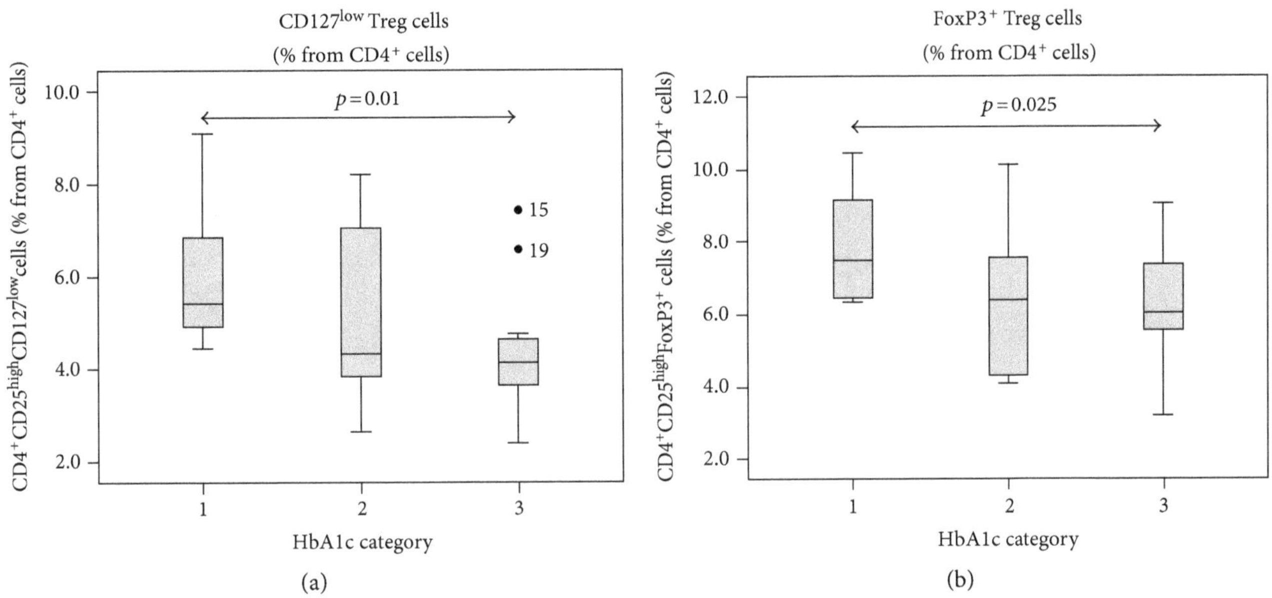

Figure 4: T regulatory cells and HbA1c category. The lowest count of Treg cells was determined in the group of patients with poor diabetes stabilization with the highest HbA1c levels (category 3) and differed significantly from that with the lowest HbA1c, independently whether Treg marker CD127^{low} or FoxP3 was used.

acceptable T1D stabilization). Importantly, this difference was irrespective of whether CD127^{low} ($p = 0.01$, Figure 4(a)) or FoxP3 positivity ($p = 0.025$, Figure 4(b)) was used as the Treg marker.

In respect to specific diabetic complications, the number of Tregs defined by the CD127 marker (CD4$^+$CD25^{high} CD127^{low}) showed a significant positive correlation with the presence of diabetic neuropathy ($p = 0.037$). Figure 5 illustrates this finding (the higher CD127^{low} Treg cell numbers in the group with neuropathy, $p = 0.04$). When Tregs were gated as FoxP3 positive cells (CD4$^+$CD25^{high}FoxP3$^+$) or as the combination of CD127^{low} and FoxP3 (CD4$^+$ CD25^{high}CD127^{low}FoxP3$^+$), positive correlations in regard to the presence of diabetic neuropathy were still apparent but failed to reach significant levels ($p = 0.369$ for CD4$^+$CD25^{high} FoxP3$^+$ and $p = 0.169$ for CD4$^+$CD25^{high}CD127^{low}FoxP3$^+$).

In contrast to diabetic neuropathy, Treg numbers as defined by CD127 (CD4$^+$CD25^{high}CD127^{low}) and/or FoxP3 markers (CD4$^+$CD25^{high}FoxP3$^+$ or CD4$^+$CD25^{high}CD127^{low} FoxP3$^+$) were inversely correlated with HDL cholesterol and ApoAI. These correlations were significant when the combination of both CD127^{low} and FoxP3$^+$ markers was used (CD4$^+$ CD25^{high}CD127^{low}FoxP3$^+$; $p = 0.005$ for HDL and $p = 0.028$ for ApoAI; Figures 6 and 7, resp.). A significant inverse correlation was observed as well as for CD4$^+$CD25^{high}CD127^{low} Treg cells and the calculated remnant cholesterol ($p = 0.03$). An apparent inverse but nonsignificant relationship for remnant cholesterol and CD4$^+$CD25^{high}FoxP3$^+$ which is CD4$^+$CD25^{high} CD127^{low}FoxP3$^+$ Treg cells was present (Figure 8).

Interestingly, the total number of CD4$^+$ T cells was also inversely correlated with the patient's body mass index (BMI, $p < 0.001$, Figure 9) whereby patients with higher BMI had a lower number of CD3$^+$CD4$^+$ T cells. In contrast, we found a positive correlation between the number of CD4$^+$CD25^{high}

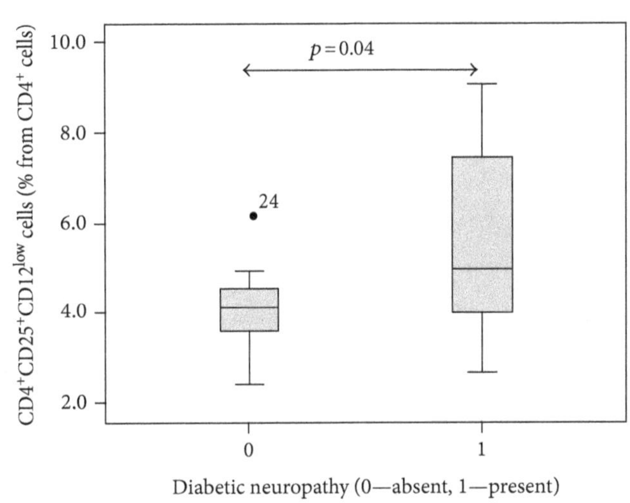

Figure 5: The presence of diabetic neuropathy and CD127^{low} Treg cells. Patients suffering from diabetic neuropathy showed a significantly higher number of CD127^{low} Treg cells than patients with no complications.

CD127^{low} Tregs and a patient's BMI, even though this correlation did not reach significance ($p = 0.087$; data not shown).

Tregs as defined by the CD127 and/or FoxP3 markers were also positively correlated with IL-6 levels with $p = 0.003$ for CD4$^+$CD25^{high}CD127^{low}, $p = 0.051$ for CD4$^+$CD25^{high}FoxP3$^+$, and $p = 0.016$ for CD4$^+$CD25^{high}CD127^{low}FoxP3$^+$ (Figure 10).

3.3. *Other Metabolic Parameters with Possible Impact to Immune Reactions*

3.3.1. Vitamin D. The group with the worst HbA1c levels had significantly lower vitamin D levels ($p = 0.009$ when

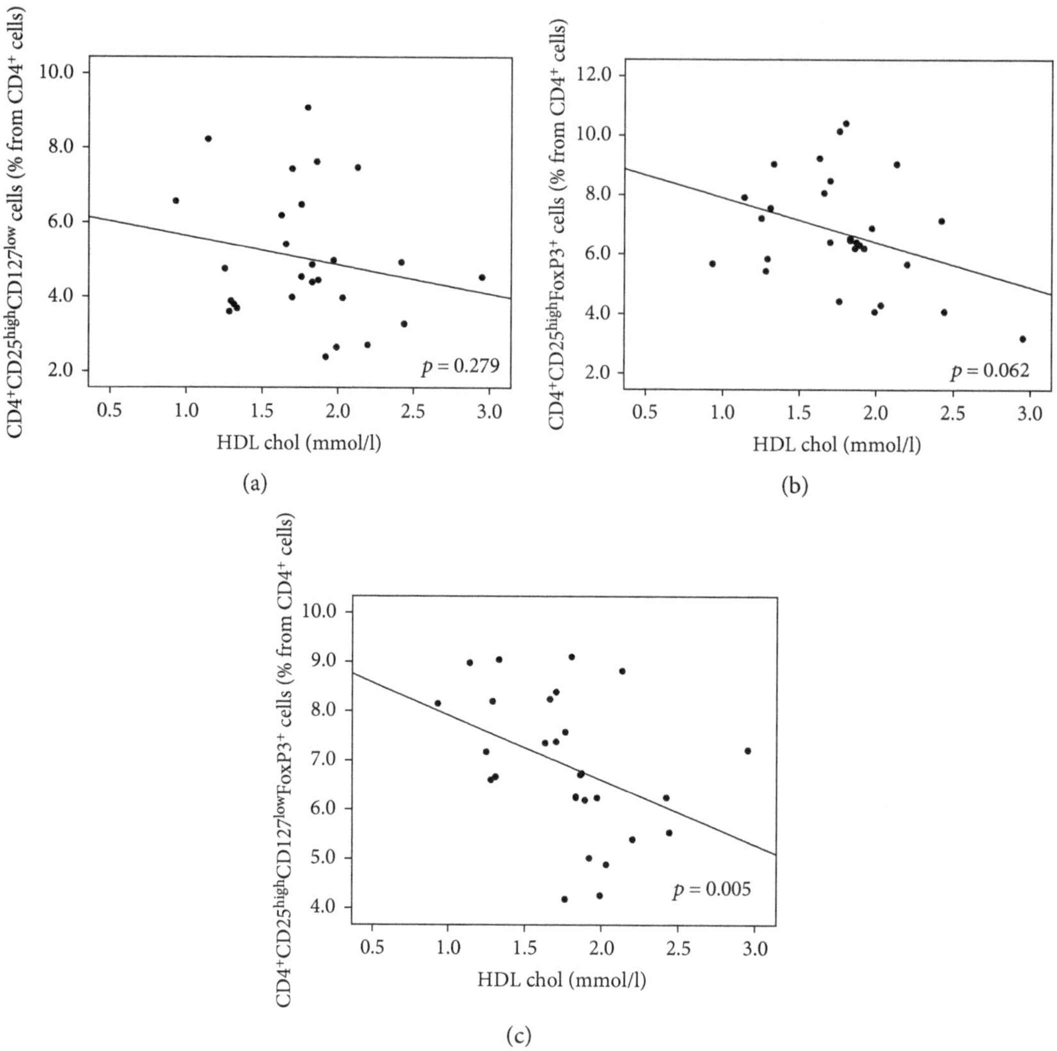

FIGURE 6: (a–c) The relationship between T regulatory cells and HDL level. Higher level of HDL cholesterol correlated with lower Treg numbers. This correlation was significant in the case of $CD127^{low}FoxP3^{+}$ cells ($p = 0.005$, $R = -0.52$). The same trend was observed for both $CD127^{low}$ and $FoxP3^{+}$ Treg cells but failed to reach significant levels ($p = 0.279$ and $R = -0.216$ for $CD127^{low}$ Treg cells and $p = 0.062$ and $R = -0.357$ for $FoxP3^{+}$ Treg cells). (a) $CD127^{low}$ Treg cells (% from $CD4^{+}$cells). (b) $FoxP3^{+}$ Treg cells (% from $CD4^{+}$cells). (c) $CD127^{low}FoxP3^{+}$ cells (% from $CD4^{+}$cells).

compared with group 1 and $p = 0.02$ when compared with group 2; Supplementary Figure 2a). Higher glycaemic variability also significantly correlated with lower vitamin D levels ($p = 0.047$, Supplementary Figure 2b). We observed that diabetic patients with LDL cholesterol levels that exceeded the recommended value (LDL cholesterol should be <2.5 mmol/l) had also significantly lower vitamin D levels ($p = 0.019$; Supplementary Figure 3).

Figure 11 summarizes the correlations between immune and metabolic parameters revealed in this study.

4. Discussion

It is well known that each diabetic patient may eventually become immunologically compromised, particularly if diabetes lasts for a long period of time and is poorly stabilized. In this context, it has been shown that the high frequency of infections among diabetic patients is caused by hyperglycaemia that leads to complex immune dysfunctions, that is, an impairment of neutrophil function, antioxidant system, and humoral immunity [10]. Many diabetes-related comorbidities along with overweight or obesity (if present) may also considerably contribute to immune dysregulation. Currently, there is an emerging consensus among diabetologists on the importance of description and understanding of other aspects of diabetes-associated cellular and genetic changes, such as metabolomics and epigenetics. We are learning how biochemical parameters can imprint our genetic information and eventually understand how these can affect the lives of our newborns via intrauterine transmission. Bidirectional interactions between the immune system and whole-body metabolism is being increasingly recognized, and consequently, a new research field of immunometabolism with a particular focus on immunoregulatory and proinflammatory mechanisms has been recently established [6, 11]. These new trends and our

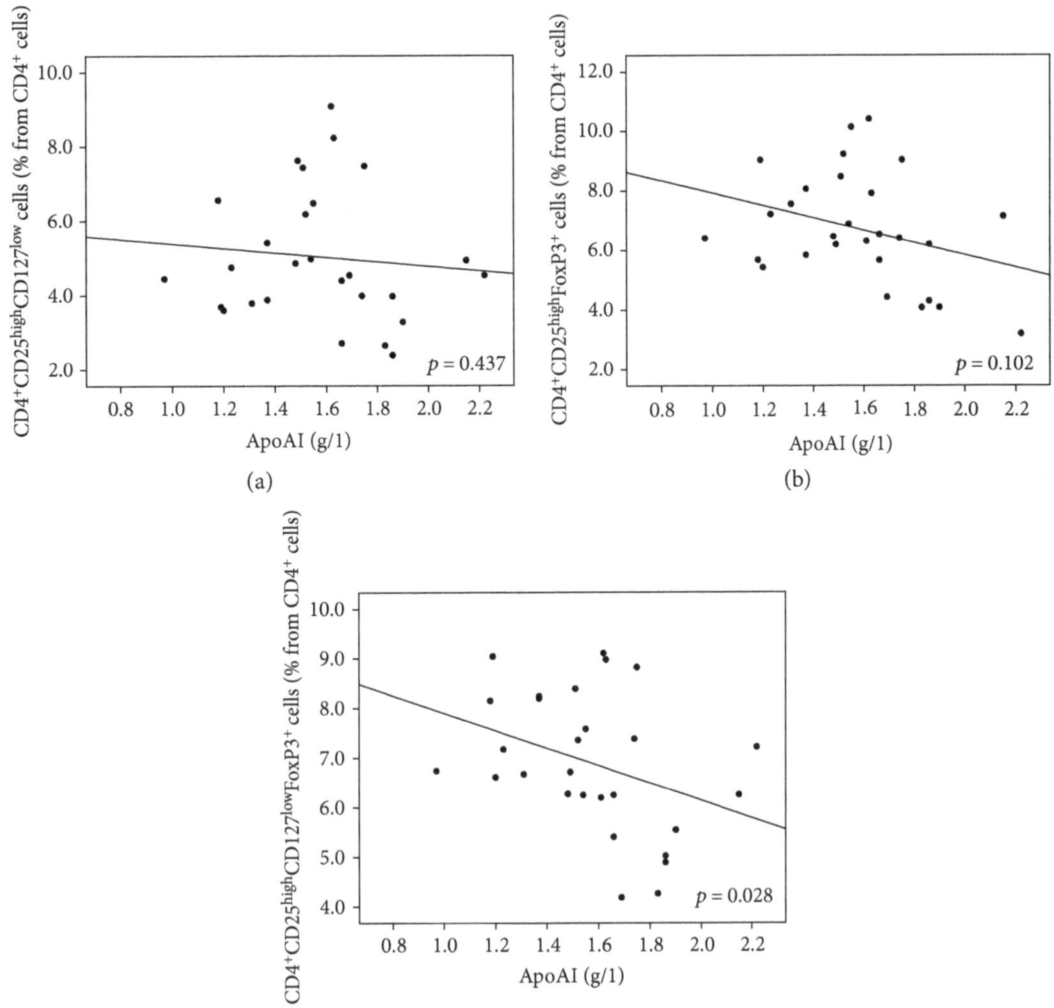

(c)

FIGURE 7: (a–c) The relationship between T regulatory cells and ApoAI. Higher level of ApoAI correlated with lower Treg numbers. This correlation was significant in the case of $CD127^{low}FoxP3^+$ cells ($p = 0.028$, $R = -0.416$). The same trend was observed for both $FoxP3^+$ and $CD127^{low}$ Treg cells but failed to reach significant levels ($p = 0.102$, $R = -0.315$ and $p = 0.437$, $R = -0.156$, resp.). (a) $CD127^{low}$ Treg cells (% from $CD4^+$cells). (b) $FoxP3^+$ Treg cells (% from $CD4^+$cells). (c) $CD127^{low}FoxP3^+$ Treg cells (% from $CD4^+$cells).

previous research related to this topic inspired us to study the complex interplay between metabolic and immune factors of T1D patients in general and, in this context, the effect of T1D mothers on their offspring, in particular.

The parameter that is widely used to monitor lasting hyperglycaemia is the level of HbA1c. It reflects the glycaemic status of an individual for approximately the last 3 months [12], and not surprisingly, this factor exerts important correlations with several immune and metabolic parameters. For example, it has been reported that hyperglycaemia itself has immunosuppressive and proinflammatory effects [10]. Consistent with a recent report [13], we also observed a lower number of Treg cells in patients with higher HbA1c levels. However, while the HbA1c level is a very useful parameter for evaluating diabetes stabilization, it does not reflect the glycaemic variability which is increasingly used as an important marker in the development of chronic diabetic complications that determines a patient's long-term prognosis [1]. We failed to correlate glycaemia standard deviation (SD), considered to be a basic parameter that represents glycaemia variability [14], with immunoregulatory functions and/or proinflammatory cytokine production in our study. On the other hand, glycaemia SD correlated with lipid spectra parameters, insulin dose (data not shown), and vitamin D which may indicate the rather indirect effect of glycaemic variability to immune parameters. Thus, our data support the view that changes in immune parameters and occurrence of chronic diabetes complications reflect the total time spent in hyperglycaemic state.

One interesting finding is that both poor HbA1c values and higher glycaemic variabilities were associated with lower vitamin D levels. In this sense, a majority of samples used in our study were collected in the spring/summer season (April–September) when vitamin D levels are not dramatically affected by the low sun exposure of our patients. Vitamin D is important for proper immune function, and there are reports that low vitamin D levels are associated with the development of autoimmune conditions

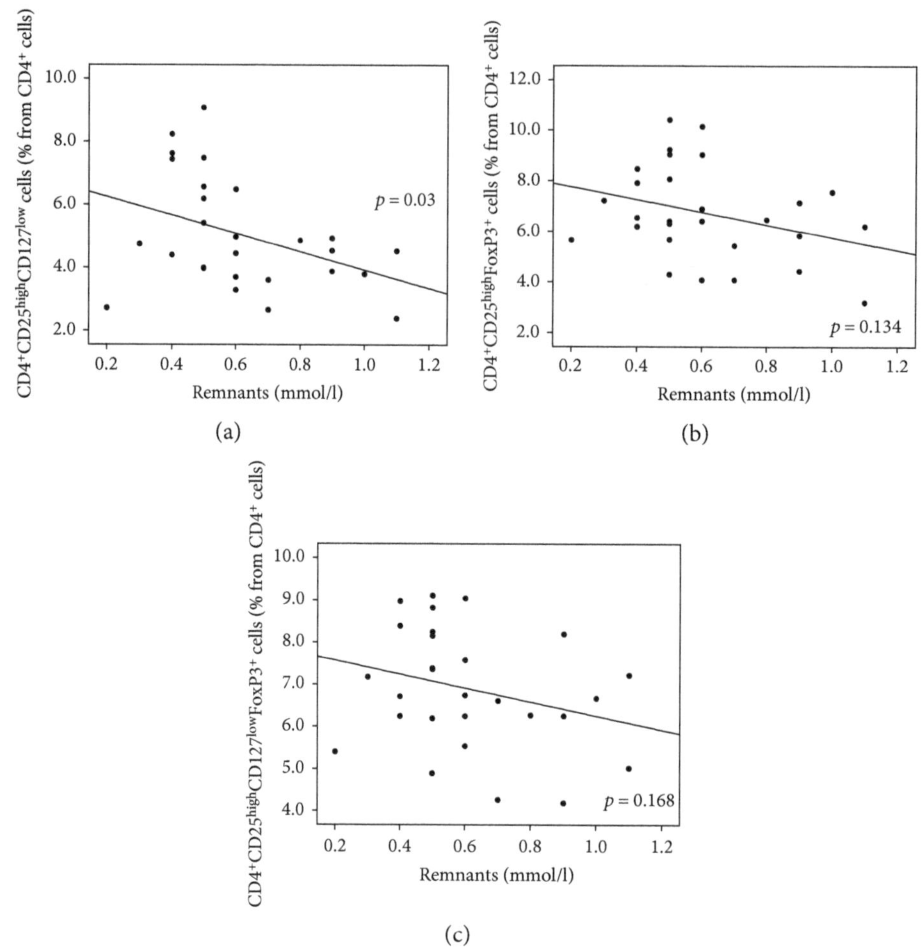

FIGURE 8: (a–c) The relationship between T regulatory cells and calculated "remnant cholesterol". Higher calculated remnant cholesterol was correlated to lower Treg numbers. This correlation was significant in the case of $CD127^{low}$ Treg cells ($p = 0.03$, $R = -0.418$). The similar trend was observed for $FoxP3^+$ as well as for $CD127^{low}FoxP3^+$ Treg cells that failed to reach statistical significance ($p = 0.134$, $R = -0.29$ and $p = 0.168$, $R = -0.268$, resp.). (a) $CD127^{low}$ Treg cells (% from $CD4^+$cells). (b) $FoxP3^+$ Treg cells (% from $CD4^+$cells). (c) $CD127^{low}FoxP3^+$ Treg cells (% from $CD4^+$cells).

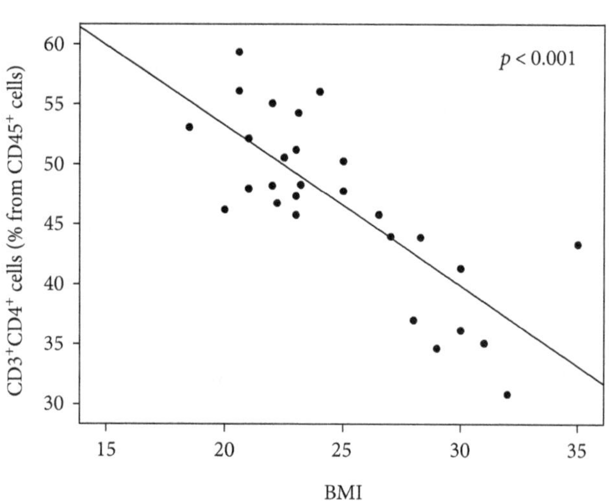

FIGURE 9: The inverse relationship between $CD3^+CD4^+$ cells (% from $CD45^+$cells) and BMI. Patients with higher BMI had significantly lower numbers of $CD3^+CD4^+$ cells (shown as % from $CD45^+$ cells). $p < 0.001$, $R = -0.65$.

including diabetes [15]. Vitamin D probably affects negative selection in the thymus, effector Th1 and Th17 pathogenesis, the responsiveness to extrinsic cell death signals, $FoxP3^+CD4^+$ Tregs and $CD4^+$ T-regulatory cell type 1 (Tr1) functions, and the Th1-Tr1 switch [15]. However, our results suggest that poorer diabetes stabilization may at least partially contribute to reduced vitamin D levels that have frequently been reported in diabetic individuals [16]. Moreover, there are reports that low vitamin D levels (which are highly prevalent worldwide) are associated with metabolic syndrome. Reciprocally, it is well known that vitamin D, via various mechanisms, can affect glycaemic control [17, 18]; therefore, the functional link between diabetes and vitamin D levels may truly be bidirectional.

Surprisingly, a poorer glycaemic control was associated with lower TNF-alpha levels, which was quite opposite to the situation that we expected. The greatest TNF-alpha production as well as IL-1alpha production was observed in patients who exhibited one chronic diabetic complication. These cytokines are mainly produced by activated macrophages, but neutrophils, epithelial cells, and endothelial

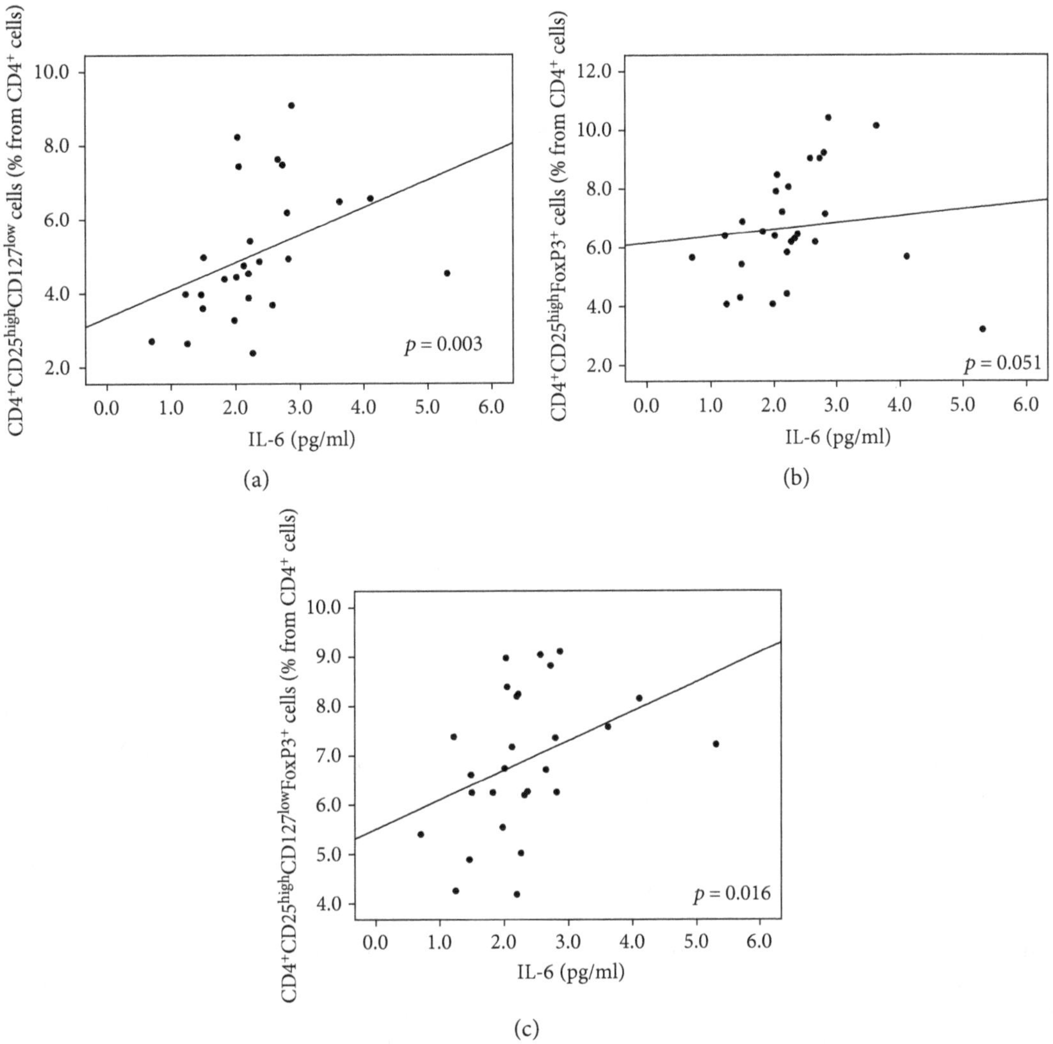

FIGURE 10: (a–c) T regulatory cells and IL-6. Higher Treg cell count correlated with higher level of proinflammatory cytokine IL-6. This relationship reached significance in the case of $CD127^{low}$ Treg cells ($p = 0.003$, $R = 0.551$) and $CD127^{low}FoxP3^{+}$ Treg cells ($p = 0.016$, $R = 0.458$). The same trend with a borderline significance was observed for $FoxP3^{+}$ Treg cells ($p = 0.051$, $R = 0.379$). (a) $CD127^{low}$ Treg cells (% from $CD4^{+}$cells). (b) $FoxP3^{+}$ Treg cells (% from $CD4^{+}$cells). (c) $CD127^{low}FoxP3^{+}$ Treg cells (% from $CD4^{+}$cells).

cells can also contribute. IL-1alpha possesses metabolic, physiological, and haematopoietic activities and plays a central role in the regulation of immune responses. For example, it affects T-helper cells causing the induction of IL-2 secretion and expression of IL-2 receptors [19]. However, there is data which suggests that IL-1alpha could be a cause of the development of chronic diabetic complications because of certain genetic variants that were shown to be positively associated with diabetic nephropathy [20]. This observation may reflect the fact that the processes underpinning the development of multiple chronic diabetic complications were still active in these participants. In contrast, in patients with multiple complications, we observed an overall exhaustion and improper activation of the innate immune mechanisms which were reflected by lower IL-1alpha levels.

We also observed a positive correlation between chronic diabetic neuropathy and Treg counts which is more difficult to explain. Such an association is likely to be indirect as defective immunoregulation by Tregs, compensated by their higher numbers, would compromise nerve protection, but we lack data to support this view [21].

Interestingly, higher IL-6 levels were associated with higher Treg numbers as defined by either of the two employed Treg markers ($CD127^{low}$ and/or FoxP3) despite the fact that the presence of IL-6 inhibits FoxP3 function by diverting Treg differentiation in favour of the Th17 phenotype [22]. These findings may indicate that imbalances between FoxP3 and retinoic acid-related orphan receptor gamma t (RORγt), the key transcription factor in Th17 cells, could be present in T1D. Such imbalances could be very important because the equilibrium between these two molecules determines CD4 T cell fate and the type of subsequently generated immune responses. The suspicion that the Treg/Th17 balance is very important for the development of T1D is also supported by our previously published study [23]. Moreover, it has been previously proposed that the development of Th1/Th17

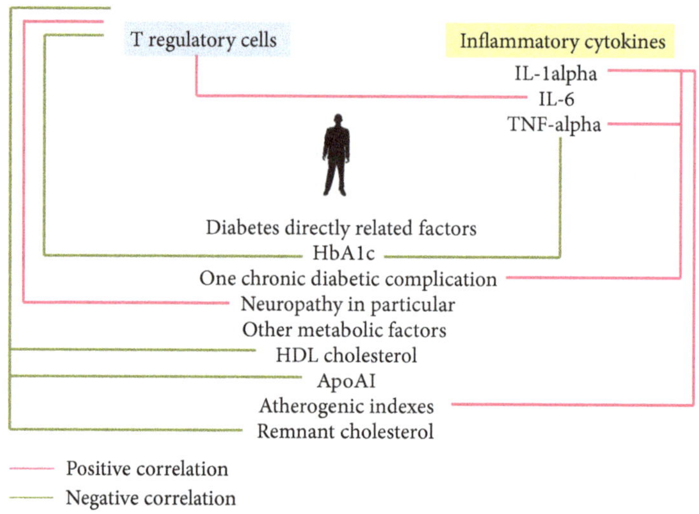

FIGURE 11: Regulatory T cell count positively correlated with the presence of neuropathy and with IL-6 level. Negative relationship was observed between regulatory T cell count and HbA1c level, HDL, ApoAI, and remnant cholesterol. IL-1alpha level was positively connected with the presence of one chronic diabetic complication (the same stands for TNF-alpha) as well as to calculated atherogenic indexes. We observed a negative relationship between TNF-alpha and HbA1c level.

plasticity may serve as a biomarker of disease progression from beta cell autoantibody positivity to clinically apparent type 1 diabetes [24].

As far as the impact of other nonimmune factors is concerned, it is known that T1D may acquire certain "T2D" (type 2 diabetes) or metabolic syndrome "features" as a patient ages, primarily when a patient's body weight increases; hence, these features may interfere with the patient's immunoreactivity. This assumption led us to concentrate on other factors related to metabolic syndrome in addition to insulin resistance. Our results also suggest that neither the presence of hypertension nor insulin resistance are linked to studied immune and metabolic parameters; one exception is being the correlation between hypertension and calculated remnant cholesterol (data not shown). In contrast, body weight was negatively correlated with the total T-helper cell count, which is consistent with recent reports which showed reductions in specific circulating lymphocyte populations in patients who are at risk of developing T2D [25].

An emerging relationship between the Treg count on one hand and HDL and ApoAI levels (ApoAI is the main protein component of HDL) on the other hand could be of clinical importance. There is an evidence of a skewed balance between anti- and proinflammatory T cell subsets in T2D patients, and it has been reported that HDL strongly affects T cell polarization [26]. Moreover, ApoAI has been found to modulate regulatory T cells in autoimmune $LDLr^{-/-}$ and $ApoAI^{-/-}$ mice [27]. Thus, our data provides additional evidence supporting direct links between these lipid factors and the number, differentiation, and function of Tregs in humans.

It is difficult to explain the level of inconsistency of our results when different Treg markers are used, that is, $CD127^{low}$ versus $FoxP3^{+}$. A group of Japanese researchers noted that $CD4^{+}CD25^{+}CD127^{low}$ T cells isolated from IPEX (Immune dysregulation, Polyendocrinopathy, Enteropathy, X-linked) patients also exhibited appreciable suppressive activity, although less than that exhibited by Treg cells from healthy controls. Their results suggest that genetically altered FoxP3 can drive the generation of functionally immature Treg cells, but intact FoxP3 is necessary for the generation of fully functional Tregs. However, T1D patients should express fully functional FoxP3. On the other hand, FoxP3 was identified as an important epigenetic modifier, and accumulating evidence suggests an intriguing functional convergence between FoxP3 and inhibitors of histone deacetylases [28, 29]. In addition, epigenetic changes may affect FoxP3 gene expression itself. Thus, due to subtle changes related to the expression of FoxP3 and CD127 in Tregs from T1D patients, discrepancies in defining Tregs using either of these markers could reveal differences. Finally, a third possibility which may explain these inconsistent results could be the fact that FACS-mediated FoxP3 analysis requires cell permeabilization, while CD127 does not. Therefore, at this point, we can only speculate if the observed discrepancy is due to the alteration of a specific Treg subset or if it is the result of Treg manipulation and staining [28, 29].

5. Conclusion

Our results show an intricate relationship between glycaemic, lipid, and immune parameters in T1D female patients. We conclude that one important factor that negatively affects immune parameters such as Treg counts, TNF-alpha production, and vitamin D levels is the total time spent in the hyperglycaemic state reflected in HbA1c values. On the other hand, glycaemia variability even though it seems not to have direct impact to studied immune parameters highly correlated with other metabolic factors including vitamin D and thus can be of potential clinical and prognostic value. Moreover at this junction, it is difficult to determine the cause and effect relationships between multiple nonimmune factors. Their associations suggest that preventing T1D patients from increasing their body weight and from developing dyslipidemia could be beneficial for a more favourable long-term prognosis from many different aspects. Our data also suggests that complementing glycaemic data with lipid clinical parameters can provide clinicians with a more comprehensive view on the immunometabolism of T1D patients and their long-term prognosis. It would be important now to extend these findings to understand if and how these complex metabolic features of T1D female patients affect the immunity and fate of their children.

Abbreviations

Apo:	Apolipoprotein
BMI:	Body mass index
Chronic diabetic complication category 0:	No complication present
Chronic diabetic complication category 1:	One chronic diabetic complication present
Chronic diabetic complication category 2:	Two or more chronic diabetic complications present
DCCT:	Diabetes Control and Complication Trial
eGDR:	Whole-body-estimated glucose disposal rate
GV:	Glucose variability
HbA1c group 1:	Perfect or acceptable T1D stabilization
HbA1c group 2:	Not well stabilized
HbA1c group 3:	Badly compensated patients
HbA1c:	Glycosylated haemoglobin
HDL:	High-density lipoproteins
IU:	Insulin units
LDL category 0:	Low and normal values
LDL category 1:	Increased levels
LDL:	Low-density lipoproteins
n.s.:	Nonsignificant
NRG:	Nonresistance group
RG:	Resistance group
SD:	Standard deviation
T1D:	Type 1 diabetes.

Conflicts of Interest

The authors declare that they have no competing interests.

Authors' Contributions

Contribution to this work by Jana Sklenarova-Labikova and Tereza Kratzerova was equal (laboratory experiments, data analysis, and manuscript writing). Pavlina Pithova and Dominik Filipp contributed equally to the analytic part of the work and the manuscript writing.

Acknowledgments

This project was supported by the project (Ministry of Health, Czech Republic) for the conceptual development of research organization 00064203 (University Hospital Motol, Prague, Czech Republic) and by Czech Diabetic Association. Dominik Filipp was supported by Grant P302/12/G101 from the Grant Agency of Czech Republic.

References

[1] M. A. Atkinson, D. L. Kaufman, L. Campbell et al., "Response of peripheral-blood mononuclear cells to glutamate decarboxylase in insulin-dependent diabetes," *Lancet*, vol. 339, no. 8791, pp. 458–459, 1992.

[2] C. F. McDaniel, "Diabetes: a model of oxidative accelerated aging," *Age (Omaha)*, vol. 22, no. 4, pp. 145–148, 1999.

[3] S. Polsky and S. L. Ellis, "Obesity, insulin resistance, and type 1 diabetes mellitus," *Current Opinion in Endocrinology, Diabetes, and Obesity*, vol. 22, no. 4, pp. 277–282, 2015.

[4] M. Kurien, K. Mollazadegan, D. S. Sanders, and J. F. Ludvigsson, "Celiac disease increases risk of thyroid disease in patients with type 1 diabetes: a nationwide cohort study," *Diabetes Care*, vol. 39, no. 3, pp. 371–375, 2016.

[5] K. Stechova, I. Spalova, M. Durilova et al., "Influence of maternal hyperglycaemia on cord blood mononuclear cells in response to diabetes-associated autoantigens," *Scandinavian Journal of Immunology*, vol. 70, no. 2, pp. 149–158, 2009.

[6] S. C. Langley-Evans, "Nutrition in early life and the programming of adult disease: a review," *Journal of Human Nutrition and Dietetics*, vol. 28, Supplement 1, pp. 1–14, 2015.

[7] S. J. Santegoets, E. M. Dijkgraaf, A. Battaglia et al., "Monitoring regulatory T cells in clinical samples: consensus on an essential marker set and gating strategy for regulatory T cell analysis by flow cytometry," *Cancer Immunology, Immunotherapy*, vol. 64, no. 10, pp. 1271–1286, 2015.

[8] C. M. Girgis, B. D. Scalley, and K. E. Park, "Utility of the estimated glucose disposal rate as a marker of microvascular complications in young adults with type 1 diabetes," *Diabetes Research and Clinical Practice*, vol. 96, no. 3, pp. e70–e72, 2012.

[9] A. Varbo, M. Benn, G. D. Smith, N. J. Timpson, A. Tybjaerg-Hansen, and B. G. Nordestgaard, "Remnant cholesterol, low-density lipoprotein cholesterol, and blood pressure as mediators from obesity to ischemic heart disease," *Circulation Research*, vol. 116, no. 4, pp. 665–673, 2015.

[10] J. Casqueiro, J. Casqueiro, and C. Alves, "Infections in patients with diabetes mellitus: a review of pathogenesis," *Indian Journal of Endocrinology and Metabolism*, vol. 16, Supplement 1, pp. S27–S36, 2012.

[11] R. Newton, B. Priyadharshini, and L. A. Turka, "Immunometabolism of regulatory T cells," *Nature Immunology*, vol. 17, no. 6, pp. 618–625, 2016.

[12] D. T. Juarez, K. M. Demaris, R. Goo, C. L. Mnatzaganian, and H. Wong Smith, "Significance of HbA1c and its measurement in the diagnosis of diabetes mellitus: US experience," *Diabetes, Metabolic Syndrome and Obesity: Targets and Therapy*, vol. 7, pp. 487–494, 2014.

[13] M. H. El-Samahy, A. A. Adly, E. A. Ismail, and N. Y. Salah, "Regulatory T cells with CD62L or TNFR2 expression in

young type 1 diabetic patients: relation to inflammation, glycemic control and micro-vascular complications," *Journal of Diabetes and Its Complications*, vol. 29, no. 1, pp. 120–126, 2015.

[14] S. Inchiostro, R. Candido, and F. Cavalot, "How can we monitor glycaemic variability in the clinical setting?" *Diabetes, Obesity & Metabolism*, vol. 15, Supplement 2, pp. 13–16, 2013.

[15] C. E. Hayes, S. L. Hubler, J. R. Moore, L. E. Barta, C. E. Praska, and F. E. Nashold, "Vitamin D actions on CD4(+) T cells in autoimmune disease," *Frontiers in Immunology*, vol. 6, p. 100, 2015.

[16] H. Al-Zubeidi, L. Leon-Chi, and R. S. Newfield, "Low vitamin D level in pediatric patients with new onset type 1 diabetes is common, especially if in ketoacidosis," *Pediatric Diabetes*, vol. 17, no. 8, pp. 592–598, 2016.

[17] R. C. Strange, K. E. Shipman, and S. Ramachandran, "Metabolic syndrome: a review of the role of vitamin D in mediating susceptibility and outcome," *World Journal of Diabetes*, vol. 6, no. 7, pp. 896–911, 2015.

[18] G. N. Thomas, R. Scragg, C. Q. Jiang et al., "Hyperglycaemia and vitamin D: a systematic overview," *Current Diabetes Reviews*, vol. 8, no. 1, pp. 18–31, 2012.

[19] C. A. Dinarello, "Immunological and inflammatory functions of the interleukin-1 family," *Annual Review of Immunology*, vol. 27, pp. 519–550, 2009.

[20] N. Nazir, K. Siddiqui, S. Al-Qasim, and D. Al-Naqeb, "Meta-analysis of diabetic nephropathy associated genetic variants in inflammation and angiogenesis involved in different biochemical pathways," *BMC Medical Genetics*, vol. 15, no. 1, p. 103, 2014.

[21] H. Bour-Jordan, H. L. Thompson, J. R. Giampaolo, D. Davini, W. Rosenthal, and J. A. Bluestone, "Distinct genetic control of autoimmune neuropathy and diabetes in the non-obese diabetic background," *Journal of Autoimmunity*, vol. 45, pp. 58–67, 2013.

[22] S. F. Ziegler and J. H. Buckner, "FOXP3 and the regulation of Treg/Th17 differentiation," *Microbes and Infection*, vol. 11, no. 5, pp. 594–598, 2009.

[23] J. Vcelakova, R. Blatny, Z. Halbhuber et al., "The effect of diabetes-associated autoantigens on cell processes in human PBMCs and their relevance to autoimmune diabetes development," *Journal of Diabetes Research*, vol. 2013, Article ID 589451, p. 10, 2013.

[24] L. Reinert-Hartwall, J. Honkanen, H. M. Salo et al., "Th1/Th17 plasticity is a marker of advanced β cell autoimmunity and impaired glucose tolerance in humans," *Journal of Immunology*, vol. 194, no. 1, pp. 68–75, 2015.

[25] H. Cucak, D. Vistisen, D. Witte, A. Philipsen, and A. Rosendahl, "Reduction of specific circulating lymphocyte populations with metabolic risk factors in patients at risk to develop type 2 diabetes," *PLoS One*, vol. 9, no. 9, article e107140, 2014.

[26] C. Zeng, X. Shi, B. Zhang et al., "The imbalance of Th17/Th1/Tregs in patients with type 2 diabetes: relationship with metabolic factors and complications," *Journal of Molecular Medicine (Berlin, Germany)*, vol. 90, no. 2, pp. 175–186, 2012.

[27] A. J. Wilhelm, M. Zabalawi, J. S. Owen et al., "Apolipoprotein A-I modulates regulatory T cells in autoimmune LDLr–/–, ApoA-I–/– mice," *The Journal of Biological Chemistry*, vol. 285, no. 46, pp. 36158–36169, 2010.

[28] H. Katoh, P. Zheng, and Y. Liu, "FOXP3: genetic and epigenetic implications for autoimmunity," *Journal of Autoimmunity*, vol. 41, pp. 72–78, 2013.

[29] K. Otsubo, H. Kanegane, Y. Kamachi et al., "Identification of FOXP3-negative regulatory T-like (CD4(+)CD25(+) CD127(low)) cells in patients with immune dysregulation, polyendocrinopathy, enteropathy, X-linked syndrome," *Clinical Immunology*, vol. 141, no. 1, pp. 111–120, 2011.

6

Association of Autoimmune Thyroid Disease with Anti-GAD Antibody ELISA Test Positivity and Risk for Insulin Deficiency in Slowly Progressive Type 1 Diabetes

Masahito Katahira,[1,2] Hidetada Ogata,[2] Takahiro Ito,[2] Tsutomu Miwata,[2] Megumi Goto,[2] Shizuka Nakamura,[2,3] and Hiromi Takashima[2]

[1]*Aichi Prefectural University School of Nursing and Health, Nagoya 463-8502, Japan*
[2]*Department of Endocrinology and Diabetes, Ichinomiya Municipal Hospital, Ichinomiya 491-8558, Japan*
[3]*Department of General Internal Medicine, Matsunami General Hospital, Gifu 501-6062, Japan*

Correspondence should be addressed to Masahito Katahira; katahira-0034@umin.net

Academic Editor: Ulrike Rothe

The presence of antiglutamic acid decarboxylase antibody (GADA) is required for the diagnosis of slowly progressive type 1 diabetes (SPT1D). We examined the factors influencing GADA determination by radioimmunoassay (GADA-RIA) and by enzyme-linked immunosorbent assay (GADA-ELISA). Sixty patients with SPT1D and 154 patients with type 2 diabetes were examined by both GADA-RIA and GADA-ELISA and for the presence of autoimmune thyroid disease (AITD). We compared the clinical characteristics of these patients based on the positivity or negativity of GADA-RIA and GADA-ELISA, and the existence or nonexistence of AITD. Thirty of 60 (50.0%) GADA-RIA-positive patients were GADA-ELISA negative, whereas none of the 154 GADA-RIA-negative patients were GADA-ELISA positive. Concomitant AITD was significantly less in patients with GADA-RIA and without GADA-ELISA and was significantly more in patients with GADA-RIA and GADA-ELISA. In GADA-RIA-positive patients, there was no significant difference in the GADA-RIA titer among the GADA-ELISA-negative patients with and without AITD, and the GADA-ELISA-positive patients without AITD; whereas the frequency of insulin deficiency was significantly higher in the patients with AITD and/or GADA-ELISA than in those without AITD and GADA-ELISA. Examination of GADA-ELISA and AITD in GADA-RIA-positive patients might be useful in predicting insulin deficiency in these patients.

1. Introduction

Type 1 diabetes (T1D) results from β-cell destruction that may ultimately lead to a clinical stage in which insulin is required for survival [1]. T1D is divided into three prevalent subtypes: fulminant, acute onset, and slowly progressive [2]. The first two subtypes are abrupt in onset when compared with type 2 diabetes (T2D) and do not necessarily require the presence of islet cell-associated autoantibodies for the diagnosis of T1D [3, 4]. However, slowly progressive T1D (SPT1D) is difficult to diagnose based on the mode of onset and requires the presence of antiglutamic acid decarboxylase antibody (GADA) and/or islet cell antibodies (ICA) [5]. The social health insurance in Japan covers the cost of a GADA test, but not an ICA test, and the presence of GADA is virtually essential for the diagnosis of SPT1D.

In Japan, since December 2015, the assay kit for measuring GADA has changed from radioimmunoassay (RIA) to enzyme-linked immunosorbent assay (ELISA). The ELISA kit was characterized by higher sensitivity and increased specificity for the detection of GADA compared with the RIA kit [6]. Oikawa et al. reported that the positive rate of GADA by ELISA (GADA-ELISA) had a tendency to be higher than that of GADA by RIA (GADA-RIA) in patients with fulminant and/or acute-onset T1D, and that the former had a tendency to be lower than the latter in patients with

SPT1D [7]. This discrepancy could have a big effect on the diagnosis of SPT1D.

It was suggested that 15% to 30% of patients with T1D have autoimmune thyroid disease (AITD) [8, 9], and the prevalence of GADA is much higher in patients with AITD than in the general population [10, 11]. The combination of T1D and AITD is called autoimmune polyendocrine syndrome type 3 [12, 13]. The reported mismatch of the results between GADA-RIA and GADA-ELISA tests showed lower GADA-RIA values [6]. Moreover, the logarithm of the GADA-RIA titer was higher in T1D patients with AITD than in those without AITD [14]. From these viewpoints, we speculated that AITD is associated with GADA-ELISA. This study aimed to clarify the differences in the clinical characteristics of patients with SPT1D or T2D based on the positivity or negativity of GADA-RIA and GADA-ELISA, and the existence or nonexistence of AITD.

2. Materials and Methods

2.1. Subjects. In this study, 60 patients with SPT1D and 154 patients with T2D who visited Ichinomiya Municipal Hospital between December 2015 and February 2016 were enrolled. All patients fulfilled the World Health Organization criteria for diabetes [1], and the patients with SPT1D fulfilled the Japan Diabetes Society criteria for SPT1D [5]. AITD was defined as the presence of Graves' disease, antithyroglobulin antibodies (TgAb), and/or anti-TPO antibodies (TPOAb). Graves' disease was diagnosed according to the guideline proposed by the Japan Thyroid Association [15]. In this study, we defined insulin deficiency based on the fulfillment of the following three criteria: (1) undergoing intensive insulin therapy, (2) not undergoing treatment with glucose-lowering agents that could accelerate insulin secretion (i.e., sulfonylureas, glinides, dipeptidyl peptidase 4 (DPP-4) inhibitors, and glucagon-like peptide 1 (GLP-1) receptor agonists), and (3) fasting C-peptide level of <0.6 ng/mL and/or two-hour postprandial C-peptide level of <1.0 ng/mL. When GADA-RIA was measured more than twice, the maximum titer of GADA-RIA was adopted. When GADA-ELISA was measured more than twice, the value of the first GADA-ELISA measurement was adopted. The study was approved by the ethics committee of the Aichi Prefectural University and Ichinomiya Municipal Hospital.

2.2. Measurements. GADA-RIA was determined at sampling using a commercially available RIA kit (GAD-Ab Cosmic, Cosmic, Tokyo, Japan), as described previously [16]. GADA-ELISA was measured using a commercially available kit (RSR Ltd., Cardiff, UK). TgAb and TPOAb were determined by electrochemiluminescence immunoassay (ECLIA) using Roche ECLusys Anti-Tg and Anti-TPO (Roche Diagnostics GmbH, Mannheim, Germany). Reference levels for these parameters were set as follows: GADA-RIA, <1.5 U/mL; GADA-ELISA, <5.0 U/mL; TgAb, <28 IU/mL; and TPOAb, <16 IU/mL. Serum C-peptide level was determined at sampling using a commercially available enzyme immunoassay kit (Kyowa Medex Co. Ltd., Tokyo, Japan). The GADA-RIA, GADA-ELISA, TgAb, TPOAb, and C-peptide tests were outsourced to Health Sciences Research Institute Inc., a commercial laboratory in Japan, and were performed according to the manufacturer's instructions.

2.3. Statistical Analysis. Results are presented as medians with interquartile ranges or as numbers. Statistical analysis was performed using PASW Statistics 24.0 (SPSS Inc., an IBM Company, Chicago, IL, USA). Group comparisons of clinical parameters were performed using the Kruskal-Wallis test, Mann–Whitney U test, or chi-square test, as appropriate. Multiple comparisons were performed using the Mann–Whitney U test with Bonferroni's correction. The correlation between GADA-RIA and GADA-ELISA was analyzed using the Spearman's rank correlation coefficient. The level of statistical significance was defined as $P < 0.05$ or the absolute value of adjusted residual > 1.96.

3. Results

3.1. Association between GADA-RIA and GADA-ELISA. In all patients, a significant correlation between GADA-RIA and GADA-ELISA was observed ($\rho = 0.730$, $P < 0.001$) (Figure 1). However, 30 of 60 (50.0%) GADA-RIA-positive patients were GADA-ELISA negative, whereas none of the 154 GADA-RIA-negative patients were GADA-ELISA positive. The positive and negative concordance rate between GADA-RIA and GADA-ELISA was 86.0%. In the GADA-RIA-positive patients ($n = 60$) and GADA-ELISA-positive patients ($n = 30$), the coefficients of correlation (ρ) between GADA-RIA and GADA-ELISA were 0.778 ($P < 0.001$) and 0.819 ($P < 0.001$), respectively.

3.2. Clinical Characteristics of the Patients Based on GADA-RIA and GADA-ELISA. We divided all patients into three groups based on the positivity or negativity of GADA-RIA and GADA-ELISA: (1) patients without GADA-RIA and GADA-ELISA (group A); (2) those with GADA-RIA and without GADA-ELISA (group B); and (3) those with GADA-RIA and GADA-ELISA (group C). Group A corresponded to patients with T2D, whereas groups B and C corresponded to patients with SPT1D. Table 1 shows the clinical characteristics of these groups.

The age of onset of diabetes was significantly younger in group C than in group A (49 (38–53) years versus 55 (47–63) years, $P = 0.028$). The titer of GADA-RIA was significantly higher in group C than in group B (36.2 (9.2–152.7) U/mL versus 4.8 (3.2–7.2) U/mL, $P < 0.001$). The interval between GADA-RIA and GADA-ELISA tests was significantly shorter in group B (2.8 (1.7–4.9) years) than in group A and group C (6.6 (2.8–8.5) and 9.0 (4.5–9.7) years, respectively, $P < 0.001$). The frequency of AITD was significantly lower in group B and higher in group C (20.0% versus 66.6%, $P < 0.001$). The frequency of insulin deficiency was significantly lower in group A and higher in group C (0.6% versus 53.3%, $P < 0.001$). The frequency of complete β-cell failure (patients with undetected C-peptide level) was significantly lower in group A and higher in group C (0.0% versus 23.3%, $P < 0.001$). The frequency of insulin use was significantly lower in group A and higher in group C (32.5% versus

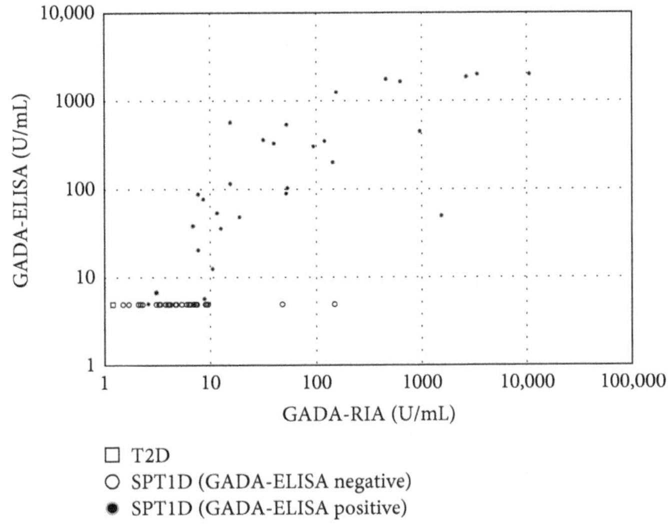

FIGURE 1: Correlation between GADA-RIA and GADA-ELISA. Dot plots show a significant correlation between GADA-RIA and GADA-ELISA titers in all patients ($\rho = 0.730$, $P < 0.001$), in GADA-RIA-positive patients with SPT1D ($\rho = 0.778$, $P < 0.001$), and in GADA-ELISA-positive patients with SPT1D ($\rho = 0.819$, $P < 0.001$).

TABLE 1: Clinical characteristics of the patients based on GADA-RIA and GADA-ELISA.

	T2D Group A ($n = 154$)	SPT1D Group B ($n = 30$)	SPT1D Group C ($n = 30$)	P value
GADA-RIA	(−)	(+)	(+)	
GADA-ELISA	(−)	(−)	(+)	
Age (years)	68 (61–75)	69 (60–75)	64 (51–69)	0.081
Gender (female/male)	70/84	8/22	17/13	0.057
BMI (kg/m^2)	23.8 (21.7–27.1)	23.1 (19.3–26.9)	23.9 (21.9–27.0)	0.440
HbA1c (%)	7.0 (6.6-7.6)	6.8 (6.5–7.6)	7.4 (6.7-8.4)	0.158
Age of onset of diabetes (years)	55 (47–63)*	54 (46–65)	49 (38–53)*	0.028
Duration of diabetes (years)	11.1 (5.5–16.6)	8.8 (5.6–16.0)	12.3 (8.9–19.8)	0.389
Interval between GADA-RIA and GADA-ELISA tests (years)	6.6 (2.8–8.5)†	2.8 (1.7–4.9)†‡	9.0 (4.5–9.7)‡	<0.001
Titer of GADA-RIA (U/mL)	—	4.8 (3.2–7.2)	36.2 (9.2–152.7)	<0.001
Titer of GADA-ELISA (U/mL)	—	—	108.8 (40.9–515.0)	—
Presence of AITD	53 (34.4)	6 (20.0)$^\$$	20 (66.7)$^\$$	<0.001
Insulin deficiency	1 (0.6)$^\$$	3 (10.0)	16 (53.3)$^\$$	<0.001
C-peptide undetected	0 (0.0)$^\$$	1 (3.3)	7 (23.3)$^\$$	<0.001
Systolic BP (mmHg)	138 (126–151)	139 (126–146)	144 (130–153)	0.670
Diastolic BP (mmHg)	76 (70–84)	80 (67–86)	76 (68–90)	0.848
Total cholesterol (mg/dL)	186 (164–210)	182 (165–215)	192 (165–216)	0.865
HDL cholesterol (mg/dL)	46 (40–55)	50 (41–59)	51 (42–61)	0.164
LDL cholesterol (mg/dL)	108 (89–128)	107 (86–126)	104 (90–127)	0.944
Non-HDL cholesterol (mg/dL)	133 (117–160)	133 (115–165)	136 (115–149)	0.870
Glucose-lowering agents				
Insulin	50 (32.5)$^\$$	12 (40.0)	23 (76.7)$^\$$	<0.001
Insulin secretagogues	120 (77.9)$^\$$	21 (70.0)	9 (30.0)$^\$$	<0.001
Others	101 (65.6)$^\$$	16 (53.3)	10 (33.3)$^\$$	<0.001

Unless noted otherwise, data are shown as median (interquartile range), or number (%). $^*P < 0.05$, group A versus group C; $^\dagger P < 0.001$, group A versus group B; $^\ddagger P < 0.001$, group B versus group C; $^\$$Absolute value of adjusted residual > 1.96. Insulin secretagogues include sulfonylureas, glinides, DPP-4 inhibitors, and GLP-1 receptor agonists. Others include biguanides, thiazolidines, α-glucosidase inhibitors, and SGLT2 inhibitors. T2D, type 2 diabetes; SPT1D, slowly progressive type 1 diabetes; GADA, anti-glutamic acid decarboxylase antibody; ELISA, enzyme-linked immunosorbent assay; BMI, body mass index; RIA, radioimmunoassay; AITD, autoimmune thyroid disease; BP, blood pressure; HDL, high-density lipoprotein; LDL, low-density lipoprotein.

73.7%, $P < 0.001$). The use of insulin secretagogues (sulfonylureas, glinides, DPP-4 inhibitors, and GLP-1 receptor agonists) and other glucose-lowering agents (biguanides, thiazolidines, α-glucosidase inhibitors, and sodium-glucose cotransporter 2 (SGLT2) inhibitors) was significantly more frequent in group A (77.9% and 65.6%, resp.) and less frequent in group C (30.0% and 33.3%, resp.) ($P < 0.001$ and $P < 0.001$, resp.). No significant difference was observed among the three groups with regard to age, gender distribution, body mass index (BMI), glycated hemoglobin (HbA1c), systolic blood pressure, diastolic blood pressure, total cholesterol, high-density lipoprotein (HDL) cholesterol, low-density lipoprotein cholesterol, and non-HDL cholesterol.

3.3. Clinical Characteristics of the Patients Based on GADA-RIA, GADA-ELISA, and AITD. We divided groups A, B, and C into two subgroups each based on the presence or absence of AITD: (1) group A without AITD (group A0), (2) group A with AITD (group A1), (3) group B without AITD (group B0), (4) group B with AITD (group B1), (5) group C without AITD (group C0), and (6) group C with AITD (group C1). Table 2 shows the clinical characteristics of these groups.

The titer of GADA-RIA was significantly higher in group C1 (74.0 (15.5–708.9) U/mL) than in groups B0, B1, and C0 (4.5 (2.3–7.7), 5.7 (4.4–6.4), and 8.3 (6.8–26.7) U/mL, respectively; $P < 0.001$). The titer of GADA-ELISA was significantly higher in group C1 than in group C0 (317.0 (71.1–1354.9) U/mL versus 38.3 (8.1–89.0) U/mL; $P = 0.005$). The frequency of insulin deficiency was significantly lower in groups A0 and A1 (1.0% and 0%, resp.), and was significantly higher in groups B1, C0, and C1 (33.3%, 70.0%, and 45.0%, respectively; $P < 0.001$). The frequency of complete β-cell failure (patients with undetected C-peptide level) was significantly lower in group A0 (0.0%) and higher in groups C0 and C1 (30.0% and 20.0%, respectively; $P < 0.001$). The frequency of insulin use was significantly lower in group A0 (32.7%) and higher in groups C0 and C1 (90.0% and 70.0%, respectively; $P = 0.001$). The use of insulin secretagogues was significantly more frequent in group A0 (83.2%) and less frequent in groups B1, C0, and C1 (33.3%, 10.0%, and 40.0%, respectively; $P < 0.001$). The use of other glucose-lowering agents was significantly more frequent in group A0 and less frequent in group C1 (70.3% versus 35.0%; $P < 0.001$). No significant difference was observed among the six groups with regard to age, gender distribution, BMI, HbA1c, age of onset of diabetes, and duration of diabetes.

4. Discussion

Although a strong correlation between GADA-RIA and GADA-ELISA was observed in this study, the coefficient of correlation between the two tests in GADA-ELISA-positive patients as well as in GADA-RIA-positive patients was lower than those previously reported in T1D ($r = 0.925, 0.979$) [7, 17]. These previous studies measured the samples by RIA and ELISA simultaneously, whereas this study measured the samples by ELISA after a long interval from the measurement by RIA. In general, GADA values in some patients with SPT1D are considered to decrease over time and finally disappear [5]. This could explain the lower coefficient of correlation between the two tests in this study than that of previous studies.

With regard to the differences in the clinical characteristics between GADA-RIA and GADA-ELISA, in patients with GADA-RIA and GADA-ELISA (group C), the age of diabetes onset was younger, the titer of GADA-RIA was higher, and insulin deficiency and insulin use were higher compared with those without GADA-RIA and GADA-ELISA (group A) and those with GADA-RIA and without GADA-ELISA (group B). These results were in accordance with the previous findings [6]. Because the interval between GADA-RIA and GADA-ELISA tests was shorter in patients with GADA-RIA and without GADA-ELISA (group B) than in those without GADA-RIA and GADA-ELISA (group A) and in those with GADA-RIA and GADA-ELISA (group C), the interval between these tests was less likely to have affected the positive and negative concordance rate between the two tests. It was speculated that the titer of GADA was originally low in group B patients (i.e., positive GADA-RIA and negative GADA-ELISA), which is in accordance with the results of a previous report [6]. On the other hand, this study demonstrated for the first time that the frequency of AITD in GADA-RIA-positive patients was high in those with GADA-ELISA and low in those without GADA-ELISA. This finding suggested that AITD might be associated with the enhancement of GADA-ELISA positivity in GADA-RIA-positive patients. Therefore, we investigated the differences in the clinical characteristics based on the presence of AITD, in addition to GADA-RIA and GADA-ELISA. In group C, the titer of GADA-ELISA was higher in patients with AITD (group C1) than in those without AITD (group C0). This finding indicated the association of AITD with the elevation of the GADA-ELISA titer in GADA-ELISA-positive patients.

In GADA-RIA-positive patients, no significant difference was observed among patients without GADA-ELISA and AITD (group B0), those with AITD and without GADA-ELISA (group B1), and those with GADA-ELISA and without AITD (group C0) with regard to the titer of GADA-RIA, which was high in those with GADA-ELISA and AITD (group C1). However, in GADA-RIA-positive patients, the frequency of insulin deficiency was higher in those with GADA-ELISA and/or AITD compared with those without GADA-ELISA and AITD. It was demonstrated that the presence of AITD contributed to the progression to β-cell failure in T1D [18, 19]. The present study suggested that the presence of AITD and/or GADA-ELISA, both of which synergistically elevate the titer of GADA-RIA, might accelerate insulin deficiency in GADA-RIA-positive patients. Moreover, in GADA-RIA-negative patients, the frequency of insulin use was low in those without AITD (group A0). Regardless of its underlying cause, diabetes mellitus is subdivided into three clinical stages: noninsulin requiring, insulin requiring for control, and insulin requiring for survival [1], the third of which corresponds to insulin deficiency. The results in the present study indicated that the percentage of patients in the stage of insulin requiring for control was low in GADA-RIA-negative patients without AITD, suggesting

Table 2: Clinical characteristics of the patients based on GADA-RIA, GADA-ELISA, and AITD.

Group	T2D		SPT1D				P value
	A0	A1	B0	B1	C0	C1	
GADA-RIA	(−)	(−)	(+)	(+)	(+)	(+)	
GADA-ELISA	(−)	(−)	(−)	(−)	(+)	(+)	
AITD	(−)	(+)	(−)	(+)	(−)	(+)	
n	101	53	24	6	10	20	
Age (years)	68 (60–75)	68 (64–75)	69 (61–75)	69 (61–72)	60 (50–68)	66 (53–69)	0.359
Gender (female/male)	41/60	29/24	6/18	2/4	4/6	13/7	0.066
BMI (kg/m^2)	23.8 (22.0–27.4)	23.8 (21.4–26.2)	23.1 (19.3–25.7)	24.4 (20.2–27.9)	23.8 (23.1–26.9)	24.0 (21.1–27.1)	0.726
HbA1c (%)	7.2 (6.7–7.6)	6.9 (6.5–7.6)	6.8 (6.4–7.5)	7.2 (6.6–9.2)	7.3 (6.8–8.2)	7.5 (6.8–8.3)	0.144
Age of onset of diabetes (years)	55 (44–61)	55 (48–65)	54 (44–66)	57 (53–63)	44 (34–53)	49 (43–54)	0.164
Duration of diabetes (years)	11.9 (6.0–17.4)	9.8 (4.9–16.0)	9.3 (5.3–17.9)	8.1 (7.0–9.3	11.4 (9.5–19.6)	12.5 (8.8–19.7)	0.677
Titer of GADA-RIA (U/mL)	—	—	4.5* (2.3–7.7)	5.7† (4.4–6.4)	8.3‡ (6.8–26.7)	74.0* †‡ (15.5–708.9)	<0.001
Titer of GADA-ELISA (U/mL)	—	—	—	—	38.3 (8.1–89.0)	317.0 (71.1–1354.9)	0.005
Insulin deficiency	1 (1.0)§	0 (0.0)§	1 (4.2)	2 (33.3)§	7 (70.0)§	9 (45.0)§	<0.001
C-peptide undetected	0 (0.0)§	0 (0.0)	1 (4.2)	0 (0.0)	3 (30.0)§	4 (20.0)§	<0.001
Glucose-lowering agents							
Insulin	33 (32.7)§	17 (32.1)	10 (41.7)	2 (33.3)	9 (90.0)§	14 (70.0)§	0.001
Insulin secretagogues	84 (83.2)§	17 (32.1)	19 (79.2)	2 (33.3)§	1 (10.0)§	8 (40.0)§	<0.001
Others (−/+)	71 (70.3)§	30 (56.6)	11 (45.8)	5 (83.3)	3 (30.0)	7 (35.0)§	0.005

Unless noted otherwise, data are shown as median (interquartile range), or number (%). $^*P < 0.01$, group B0 versus group C1; $^\dagger P < 0.001$, group B1 versus group C1; $^\ddagger P < 0.001$, group C0 versus group C1; §Absolute value of adjusted residual > 1.96. Insulin secretagogues include sulfonylureas, glinides, DPP-4 inhibitors, and GLP-1 receptor agonists. Others include biguanides, thiazolidines, α-glucosidase inhibitors, and SGLT2 inhibitors. T2D, type 2 diabetes; SPT1D, slowly progressive type 1 diabetes; GADA, anti-glutamic acid decarboxylase antibody; ELISA, enzyme-linked immunosorbent assay; BMI, body mass index; RIA, radioimmunoassay; AITD, autoimmune thyroid disease.

that the presence of AITD might accelerate insulin secretory defects in T2D. Matejková-Behanová et al. demonstrated that the frequency of AITD was high in T2D patients who had low C-peptide levels compared with those who had high C-peptide levels, although they failed to demonstrate any difference in the frequency of AITD between T2D patients treated with hypoglycemic agents and those requiring insulin [20]. Kitano et al. demonstrated in isolated rat pancreatic islets that the serum containing thyroid microsomal autoantibodies significantly suppressed glucose-induced insulin release [21]. Recently, adult-onset autoimmune diabetes with a positive T-cell response, but lacking diabetes-associated autoantibodies has been described [22, 23]. Brooks-Worrell et al. demonstrated that a significantly lower response for stimulated C-peptide was observed in T2D patients with a positive T-cell response compared with those with a negative T-cell response [23]. GADA-RIA-negative patients with AITD in the present study might include patients with a positive T-cell response.

There were several limitations in the present study. First, the small sample from a single institution may raise concerns about generalizing the data, thereby, warranting further investigation. Second, because of the nature of a cross-sectional study design, the causal relationship of the GADA-RIA and GADA-ELISA values with the future progression to an insulin-deficient state remains unknown. To clarify this point, a longitudinal prospective follow-up study will be required in the future. Third, we could not investigate other islet cell-associated autoantibodies such as autoantibodies to insulinoma-associated antigen (IA-2A), insulin (IAA), islet cells (ICA), and zinc transporter 8 (ZnT8A). In general, ICA, IAA, IA-2A, and ZnT8A were more frequent in childhood-onset than adult-onset T1D [24–26]. Sabbah et al. demonstrated that adult patients with T1D had a decreased frequency of multiple autoantibodies compared with childhood patients with T1D [24]. GADA is by far the most common autoantibody in adult-onset diabetes [27]. However, Kawasaki et al. demonstrated that the prevalence of IAA, IA-2A, and ZnT8 in diabetic patients with GADA-RIA is higher than that in T2D patients and that the determination of IAA, IA-2A, and ZnT8 improves the prediction of a future insulin insufficiency in adult-onset autoimmune diabetes [28]. In the present study, patients with insulin deficiency might have had ICA, IAA, IA-2A, or ZnT8A. Fourth, it remains unknown whether the presence of AITD can directly damage β-cells. Previous studies demonstrated that diabetic patients with GADA, especially those with a high GADA titer, had a higher frequency of thyroid-related autoantibodies compared with those without GADA [29–31]. In the present study, no significant difference was observed between GADA-RIA-positive and GADA-ELISA-negative patients without AITD (group B0) and those with AITD (group B1) with regard to complete β-cell failure. High GADA titer and/or multiple islet cell-associated autoantibodies might cause β-cell failure and the positivity of thyroid-related autoantibodies, both of which might not have a direct relationship. Otherwise, the effect of thyroid-related autoantibodies on β-cell failure might be milder compared with that of other islet cell-associated autoantibodies.

5. Conclusion

This study demonstrated for the first time that the presence of AITD in GADA-RIA-positive patients was associated with the elevation of the GADA-ELISA titer, which probably contributed to the enhancement of GADA-ELISA positivity. The presence of AITD might be associated with insulin secretory defects, not only in SPT1D, but also in T2D. We recommend that in GADA-RIA-positive patients, the presence of AITD and GADA-ELISA positivity should be examined because they might contribute to the progression to β-cell failure in these patients.

Conflicts of Interest

The authors declare that there is no conflict of interest regarding the publication of this paper.

References

[1] K. G. M. M. Alberti, P. Z. Zimmet, and WHO Consultation, "Definition, diagnosis and classification of diabetes mellitus and its complications. Part 1: diagnosis and classification of diabetes mellitus provisional report of a WHO consultation," *Diabetic Medicine*, vol. 15, no. 7, pp. 539–553, 1998.

[2] E. Kawasaki, N. Matsuura, and K. Eguchi, "Type 1 diabetes in Japan," *Diabetologia*, vol. 49, no. 5, pp. 828–836, 2006.

[3] A. Imagawa, T. Hanafusa, T. Awata et al., "Report of the Committee of the Japan Diabetes Society on the research of fulminant and acute-onset type 1 diabetes mellitus: new diagnostic criteria of fulminant type 1 diabetes mellitus (2012)," *Journal of Diabetes Investigation*, vol. 3, no. 6, pp. 536–539, 2012.

[4] E. Kawasaki, T. Maruyama, A. Imagawa et al., "Diagnostic criteria for acute-onset type 1 diabetes mellitus (2012): report of the Committee of Japan Diabetes Society on the research of fulminant and acute-onset type 1 diabetes mellitus," *Journal of Diabetes Investigation*, vol. 5, no. 1, pp. 115–118, 2014.

[5] S. Tanaka, M. Ohmori, T. Awata et al., "Diagnostic criteria for slowly progressive insulin-dependent (type 1) diabetes mellitus (SPIDDM) (2012): report by the Committee on Slowly Progressive Insulin-Dependent (Type 1) Diabetes Mellitus of the Japan Diabetes Society," *Diabetology International*, vol. 6, no. 1, pp. 1–7, 2015.

[6] Y. Oikawa, H. Tanaka, J. Uchida et al., "Slowly progressive insulin-dependent (type 1) diabetes positive for anti-GAD antibody ELISA test may be strongly associated with a future insulin-dependent state," *Endocrine Journal*, vol. 64, no. 2, pp. 163–170, 2017.

[7] Y. Oikawa, M. Tanaka, I. Horie, T. Kawamura, and A. Shiamda, "A study on the correlation between GAD antibody titers measured by ELISA kit and RIA kit (in Japanese)," *Japanese Journal of Medicine and Pharmaceutical Science*, vol. 72, no. 9, pp. 1551–1560, 2015.

[8] J. M. Barker, "Clinical review. Type 1 diabetes-associated autoimmunity: natural history, genetic associations, and screening," *Journal of Clinical Endocrinology and Metabolism*, vol. 91, no. 4, pp. 1210–1217, 2006.

[9] G. J. Kahaly and M. P. Hansen, "Type 1 diabetes associated autoimmunity," *Autoimmunity Reviews*, vol. 15, no. 7, pp. 644–648, 2016.

[10] M. E. Primo, H. Niepomniszcze, E. Poskus et al., "Frequency of pancreatic beta-cell autoimmunity markers in patients with autoimmune thyroid disease," *Medicina*, vol. 68, no. 1, pp. 37–42, 2008.

[11] M. Balakhadze, E. Giorgadze, and M. Lomidze, "The frequency of Langerhans islets β-cells autoantibodies (anti-GAD) in Georgian children and adolescents with chronic autoimmune thyroiditis," *International Journal of Endocrinology*, vol. 2016, Article ID 6597091, 4 pages, 2016.

[12] C. Betterle and R. Zanchetta, "Update on autoimmune polyendocrine syndromes (APS)," *Acta Biomed*, vol. 74, no. 1, pp. 9–33, 2003.

[13] M. P. Hansen, N. Matheis, and G. J. Kahaly, "Type 1 diabetes and polyglandular autoimmune syndrome: a review," *World Journal of Diabetes*, vol. 6, no. 1, pp. 67–79, 2015.

[14] M. Katahira, H. Maeda, T. Tosaki, and S. Segawa, "The human leukocyte antigen class II gene has different contributions to autoimmune type 1 diabetes with or without autoimmune thyroid disease in the Japanese population," *Diabetes Research and Clinical Practice*, vol. 85, no. 3, pp. 293–297, 2009.

[15] The Japan Thyroid Association, *Guideline for the Treatment of Graves' Disease in Japan (in Japanese)*, Nankodo Co., Ltd., Tokyo, 2011.

[16] M. Katahira, T. Ishiguro, S. Segawa, K. Kuzuya-Nagao, I. Hara, and T. Nishisaki, "Reevaluation of human leukocyte antigen DR-DQ haplotype and genotype in type 1 diabetes in the Japanese population," *Hormone Research*, vol. 69, no. 5, pp. 284–289, 2008.

[17] E. Kawasaki, M. Miwa, and M. Tanaka, "Basic and clinical evaluation of ELISA assay kits (Cosmic) for GADAb and IA-2Ab (in Japanese)," *Japanese Journal of Medicine and Pharmaceutical Science*, vol. 66, no. 2, pp. 345–352, 2011.

[18] S. Murao, S. Kondo, J. Ohashi et al., "Anti-thyroid peroxidase antibody, IA-2 antibody, and fasting C-peptide levels predict beta cell failure in patients with latent autoimmune diabetes in adults (LADA)—a 5-year follow-up of the Ehime study," *Diabetes Research and Clinical Practice*, vol. 80, no. 1, pp. 114–121, 2008.

[19] M. Moriguchi, S. Noso, Y. Kawabata et al., "Clinical and genetic characteristics of patients with autoimmune thyroid disease with anti-islet autoimmunity," *Metabolism*, vol. 60, no. 6, pp. 761–766, 2011.

[20] M. Matějková-Běhanová, V. Zamrazil, K. Vondra et al., "Autoimmune thyroiditis in non-obese subjects with initial diagnosis of type 2 diabetes mellitus," *Journal of Endocrinological Investigation*, vol. 25, no. 9, pp. 779–784, 2002.

[21] N. Kitano, T. Taminato, M. Seno et al., "Effect of antithyroid autoantibodies on pancreatic islet-cell function," *Acta Diabetologica Latina*, vol. 24, no. 1, pp. 9–15, 1987.

[22] E. Laugesen, J. A. Østergaard, R. D. G. Leslie, and the Danish Diabetes Academy Workshop and Workshop Speakers, "Latent autoimmune diabetes of the adult: current knowledge and uncertainty," *Diabetic Medicine*, vol. 32, no. 7, pp. 843–852, 2015.

[23] B. M. Brooks-Worrell, J. L. Reichow, A. Goel, H. Ismail, and J. P. Palmer, "Identification of autoantibody-negative autoimmune type 2 diabetic patients," *Diabetes Care*, vol. 34, no. 1, pp. 168–173, 2011.

[24] E. Sabbah, K. Savola, T. Ebeling et al., "Genetic, autoimmune, and clinical characteristics of childhood- and adult-onset type 1 diabetes," *Diabetes Care*, vol. 23, no. 9, pp. 1326–1332, 2000.

[25] V. Lampasona, A. Petrone, C. Tiberti et al., "Zinc transporter 8 antibodies complement GAD and IA-2 antibodies in the identification and characterization of adult-onset autoimmune diabetes: Non Insulin Requiring Autoimmune Diabetes (NIRAD) 4," *Diabetes Care*, vol. 33, no. 1, pp. 104–108, 2010.

[26] E. Kawasaki, K. Nakamura, G. Kuriya et al., "Differences in the humoral autoreactivity to zinc transporter 8 between childhood- and adult-onset type 1 diabetes in Japanese patients," *Clinical Immunology*, vol. 138, no. 2, pp. 146–153, 2011.

[27] M. I. Hawa, H. Kolb, N. Schloot et al., "Adult-onset autoimmune diabetes in Europe is prevalent with a broad clinical phenotype: action LADA 7," *Diabetes Care*, vol. 36, no. 4, pp. 908–913, 2013.

[28] E. Kawasaki, K. Nakamura, G. Kuriya et al., "Autoantibodies to insulin, insulinoma-associated antigen-2, and zinc transporter 8 improve the prediction of early insulin requirement in adult-onset autoimmune diabetes," *Journal of Clinical Endocrinology and Metabolism*, vol. 95, no. 2, pp. 707–713, 2010.

[29] R. Buzzetti, S. di Pietro, A. Giaccari et al., "High titer of autoantibodies to GAD identifies a specific phenotype of adult-onset autoimmune diabetes," *Diabetes Care*, vol. 30, no. 4, pp. 932–938, 2007.

[30] G. Gambelunghe, F. Forini, S. Laureti et al., "Increased risk for endocrine autoimmunity in Italian type 2 diabetic patients with GAD65 autoantibodies," *Clinical Endocrinology*, vol. 52, no. 5, pp. 565–573, 2000.

[31] S. Zampetti, M. Capizzi, M. Spoletini et al., "GADA titer-related risk for organ-specific autoimmunity in LADA subjects subdivided according to gender (NIRAD study 6)," *Journal of Clinical Endocrinology and Metabolism*, vol. 97, no. 10, pp. 3759–3765, 2012.

7

Enhancement of Adiponectin Ameliorates Nonalcoholic Fatty Liver Disease via Inhibition of FoxO1 in Type I Diabetic Rats

Xiang Xie,[1,2] Dan Yan,[1] Haobo Li,[2] Qiqi Zhu,[1] Jun Li,[1] Yong-ping Fang,[3] Chi Wai Cheung,[2] Michael G. Irwin,[2] Zhengyuan Xia,[2] and Qingquan Lian[1]

[1]*Department of Anesthesiology, The Second Affiliated Hospital and Yuying Children's Hospital, Wenzhou Medical University, Wenzhou, China*
[2]*Department of Anesthesiology, The University of Hong Kong, Pok Fu Lam, Hong Kong*
[3]*Department of General Surgery, Huizhou First Hospital, Huizhou, Guangdong, China*

Correspondence should be addressed to Zhengyuan Xia; zyxia@hku.hk and Qingquan Lian; lianqingquanmz@163.com

Academic Editor: Secundino Cigarran

Nonalcoholic fatty liver disease (NAFLD) is a common liver disease which has been previously shown to be associated with type 2 diabetes mellitus (T2DM). Recent research has indicated that type 1 diabetes mellitus (T1DM) is also involved in the development of nonalcoholic fatty liver disease, whereas the underlying mechanisms are largely unknown. Forkhead box O1 (FoxO1) and adiponectin (APN) have been proposed to play an important role in the processes in NAFLD in T1DM. We herein investigated the effects of FoxO1 and APN on the development of NAFLD and the underlying mechanism in streptozotocin-induced T1DM. Serum liver enzymes AST, ALT, and triglyceride (TG) were determined by commercially available kits. Blood glucose levels were measured by the OneTouch Ultra glucose meter. Relevant protein expression was tested by Western blot analysis. Results showed that serum AST, ALT, and TG were all significantly increased in T1DM rats, which was ameliorated by application of APN or selective inhibition of FoxO1 with AS1842856. Moreover, APN and AS1842856 both decreased the expression of liver nuclear FoxO1 which was significantly increased in diabetic rats. However, the inhibition of FoxO1 did not alter the expression of APN and its receptors. We also found that Akt1 expression was significantly declined in diabetic rat which was restored by APN and moderately and significantly increased by FoxO1 inhibition. It is concluded that APN ameliorates NAFLD via inhibition of FoxO1 through Akt1/FoxO1 signaling pathway.

1. Introduction

Nonalcoholic fatty liver disease (NAFLD), diagnosed by fat deposition in the liver without viral hepatitis or substantial alcohol consumption, is the most prevalent chronic liver disease. NAFLD represents a spectrum of liver abnormalities starting from simple hepatic steatosis to severe manifestations, such as inflammations and liver injury known as nonalcoholic steatohepatitis (NASH), which could further progress to cirrhosis, hepatocellular carcinomas, and ultimately liver failure. It is not yet entirely understood how the pathogenesis of NAFLD develops; however, the liver fat accumulation and development of inflammation and fibrosis seem to be the most important contributing factors. Previous studies have indicated that the prevalence of NAFLD in patients that suffer obesity/type II diabetes, which has been estimated to be greater than 70% [1–3], is closely linked with type 2 diabetes mellitus (T2DM) and obesity in epidemiology and pathophysiology [4]. However, recently NAFLD has been associated with type 1 diabetes mellitus (T1DM) [5], in which obesity is not considered to play a significant pathogenic role. In another study, nearly 27.7% (204/736) T1DM patients had NAFLD [6], while little research has been focused on the relationship between T1DM and NAFLD and the underlying mechanism remains unknown.

The adipose tissue has long been considered as an energy storage organ. Recently, a variety of findings illustrated its important role as an active endocrine organ that synthesizes adipokines, including adiponectin (APN), leptin, resistin, and visfatin that are involved in the progression and pathogenesis of NAFLD [7, 8]. Particularly, APN is regarded as an antidiabetic, antiatherogenic, and anti-inflammatory adipokine. It is reported that APN level was inversely related with hepatic fat accumulation [9], and plasma APN significantly decreased in patients with NAFLD, particularly in NASH patients [10]. We, therefore, supposed that increasing APN level may alleviate the pathology of NASH. Two adiponectin receptors (AdipoRs) have been identified to regulate biological effects of adiponectin, namely, AdipoR1 and AdipoR2. AdipoR1 is commonly expressed in various tissues (in relatively large amount in skeletal muscle) and selectively activating AMP-activated kinase (AMPK) in the liver, whereas AdipoR2 primarily exists in the liver [11] and mediates insulin sensitivity by activation of PPARα. Both AdipoR1 and AdipoR2 interact with globular and full-length adiponectin, mediating fatty acid oxidation and glucose uptake [12]. Recent study shows that prompting APN and inhibiting the activation and expression of forkhead box protein O1 (FoxO1) is associated with attenuation of hepatic steatosis in high-fat- and high-sugar-treated rats [13].

The transcription factor forkhead box O1 (FoxO1) is the key intracellular targets of insulin effect, contributing to the regulation of lipid and glucose metabolism [14]. After the binding of insulin to insulin receptor (IR), Akt is activated, subsequently phosphorylating and excluding FoxO1 proteins from the nucleus to the cytoplasm, thus dampening its effects to promote glucose production [15], both in isolated hepatocytes [16] and transgenic mouse models [17]. Activation of FoxO1 may lead to dysregulation of lipid and glucose metabolism whereas FoxO1 ablation improves lipogenesis and helps restore lipid metabolism homeostasis [14, 18, 19]. As a selective antagonist of FoxO1, AS1842856 reduces hepatic glucose production through inhibition of FoxO1 transactivation [20] and suppresses adipogenesis [21].

Several studies reported that FoxO1 interacts with Akt [22] and Sirtuin 1 (SIRT1) [23], affecting hepatic AdipoR1/R2 gene expression [24, 25]. Moreover, it has been indicated that FoxO1 impedes PPARγ function [26] which has been illustrated to enhance adiponectin secretion [27], while recent research also reported that adiponectin could regulate FoxO1 expression via APN-AMPK-FOXO signal pathway [28]. However, the interaction between FoxO1 and APN in NAFLD is still unclear. We hypothesize that APN ameliorates liver function by FoxO1 inhibition in NAFLD via Akt1 pathway.

2. Method and Material

2.1. Induction of Diabetes. Male Sprague-Dawley rats (250 ± 10 g, 6–8 weeks) were obtained from the Shanghai Laboratory Animal Center (Shanghai, China) and the Laboratory Animal Service Center (The University of Hong Kong). All rats were housed and given free access to standard rat chow and water. The investigation conformed to the procedures described in the Guide for the Care and Use of Laboratory Animals published by the United States National Institutes of Health (NIH Publication number 85-23, revised 1996). The experimental protocol used in this study was approved by the Wenzhou Medical University Laboratory Animal Ethics Committee and the Committee for Use of Live Animals in Teaching and Research (CULATR) of the University of Hong Kong. Diabetes was induced by a single tail vein injection of streptozotocin (STZ) at the dose of 65 mg/kg bodyweight (Sigma-Aldrich, St. Louis, MO) in 0.1 M citrate buffer (pH 4.5) or citrate buffer alone as control under anaesthesia with a combination of ketamine 67.7 mg/kg bodyweight and xylazine 6.77 mg/kg bodyweight. After 72-hour injection, blood glucose was measured using the OneTouch Ultra glucose meter (LifeScan Inc., USA), and rats with blood glucose levels over 15 mM were considered diabetic.

2.2. Treatments with APN Adenovirus and FoxO1 Inhibition with AS Treatment. Control and diabetic rats ($n = 6$ per group) were either untreated (group C, group D) or diabetic rats treated with recombinant adenovirus expressing adiponectin (group APN, $n = 6$) or luciferase injected via tail vein for 1 week prior to tissue collection [29]. The increased expression level of adiponectin was confirmed by an enzyme-linked immunosorbent assay kit (AdipoGen Inc., Incheon, South Korea). The values of APN were expressed as micrograms per milliliter in plasma. Another group of diabetic rats ($n = 6$) were treated with a selective FoxO1 inhibitor AS1842856 (AS). AS1842856 has an IC50 of 0.033 mM to inhibit FoxO1 and can potently block FoxO1 at a final concentration of 0.05–1 mM without showing cytotoxicity [20, 30]. Rats were administrated intragastrically with AS (100 mg/kg every time) or the same dose of β-cyclodextrin as solvent control 2 times a day with a 12-hour interval for a duration of 8 days before the rats were terminated. All rats were terminated at 5 weeks after induction of diabetes. Our preliminary study and/or former study showed that luciferase and β-cyclodextrin did not affect target proteins in the liver/plasma [31]; the respective groups were not shown in the result parts.

2.3. Measurements of General Characteristics. At 5 weeks after the onset of diabetes, the rats' water intake and food consumption were recorded; rats were weighed and then euthanized following anaesthesia with an intraperitoneal injection of pentobarbital sodium (65 mg/kg). Blood samples were obtained from the carotid artery after an overnight fast of 8–10 h, and plasma was extracted and stored at −80°C until analyzed. Serum total aspartate aminotransferase (AST), alanine aminotransferase (ALT), and triglyceride (TG) were determined using commercially available kits (Stanbio Laboratory, TX, USA), respectively. Liver weight was recorded for calculating the liver weight/body weight. Blood glucose levels (mM) were measured every other day by using the OneTouch Ultra glucose meter (LifeScan Inc., USA). Plasma insulin levels were analyzed using the Ultrasensitive rat Insulin ELISA Kit (Stanbio Laboratory, TX, USA).

2.4. Nucleocytoplasmic Separation. Frozen liver tissues were suspended in a buffer that contained 10 mM Tris, pH 7.5, 1.5 mM $MgCl_2$, 10 mM KCl, and 0.1% Triton X-100 and lysed by homogenization. Nuclei were recovered by microcentrifugation at 7500 rpm for 5 min. The supernatant that contained cytoplasmic and membrane protein was collected

Table 1: General characteristics.

Parameters	C	D	D + AS	D + APN
Water intake (mL/kg/day)	118.1 ± 13.7	$898.3 \pm 74.9^{**}$	$933.7 \pm 161^{**}$	$475.6 \pm 91.9^{**\#}$
Food consumption (g/kg/day)	77.5 ± 12.2	186.8 ± 13.7	$168.7 \pm 22^{**}$	$127.6 \pm 18.2^{**\#}$
Body weight (g)	455.8 ± 46.9	$294 \pm 23.6^{**}$	$276 \pm 26^{**}$	$267 \pm 24.9^{**}$
Serum insulin (ng/mL)	5.7 ± 0.9	1.2 ± 0.5	2.1 ± 0.6	$4.9 \pm 0.8^{\#}$
Plasma APN levels (mg/mL)	16.3 ± 2.5	10.2 ± 1.7	11.5 ± 2.4	$18.5 \pm 2.7^{\#}$

Data are mean ± SEM, $^{**}P < 0.01$ versus C; $^{\#}P < 0.05$ versus D.

and stored at −80°C for Western blot analysis. Nuclear proteins were extracted at 4°C by gently resuspending the nuclei pellet in a buffer that contained 20 mM Tris, pH 7.5, 20% glycerol, 1.5 mM $MgCl_2$, 420 mM NaCl, 0.2 mM EDTA, and 0.1% Triton X-100, followed by 1 h incubation at 4°C with occasional vortexing. After microcentrifugation at 13,000 revolutions/min for 15 min at 4°C, the supernatant that contained nuclear protein was collected.

2.5. Frozen Section and Staining. Fresh liver tissue was embedded in OCT compound and then stored at −80°C. After that, we cut 10 um thick sections and mounted these on gelatin-coated slides. These slides were stored at −80°C until needed. Before staining, we warmed slides at room temperature for 30–60 minutes and fix in ice-cold acetone as fixatives for 5–10 minutes, then air dry the slides for 30–60 minutes. After that, we washed the slides in PBS and proceed to standard staining procedure with hematoxylin and eosin (H&E) and Oil Red O (Sigma, USA).

2.6. Western Blotting. The protein concentration of liver lysates was quantified by bovine serum albumin and measured with the absorption of Coomassie brilliant blue in the spectrophotometer. Thereafter, the samples were frozen at −20°C for later use. Proteins were assessed by standard Western blotting as described [32]. Briefly, equal quantities of protein were separated by SDS-PAGE and transferred to polyvinylidene difluoride membranes (PVDF, Millipore, Bedford, MA, USA). The membranes were blocked in 5% nonfat dry milk diluted with Tris Buffered Saline Tween-20 (TBST) (in mmol/L: Tris-HCl 20, NaCl 150, pH 7.5, 0.1% Tween 20) at room temperature for 1 h and then probed with antibodies against FoxO1, p-FoxO1, APN, AdipoR1, Akt1, Akt2, SIRT1, acetyl-FoxO1, β-actin, GAPDH, and Histone 3 (Cell Signaling Technology, Beverly, MA, USA) at 4°C overnight. After extensive washing, the membranes were incubated with secondary horseradish peroxidase-conjugated anti-mouse or anti-rabbit antibodies (diluted 1 : 2000; Amersham Biosciences, UK). The immunoblots were visualized using an enhanced chemiluminescence detection system (Amersham Pharmacia Biotech, Uppsala, Sweden).

2.7. Statistics. All values are presented as means ± SEM. Comparisons between multiple groups were made by one-way ANOVA, followed by the Tukey test for multiple comparisons. Statistical analysis was performed by the GraphPad Prism software (GraphPad Software Inc., La Jolla, CA). P values of less than 0.05 were considered statistically significant.

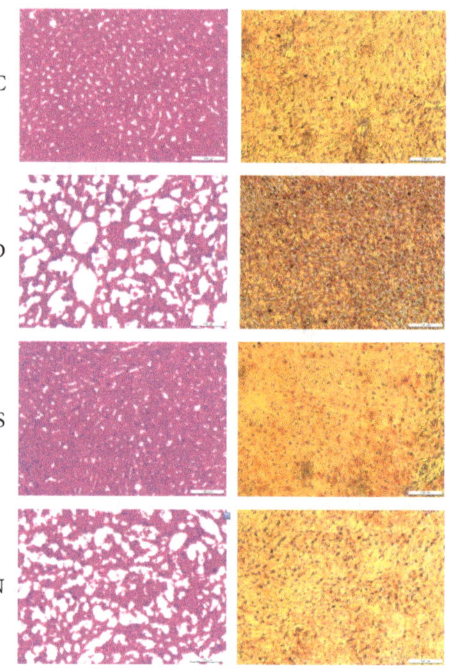

Figure 1: Representative H&E (hematoxylin and eosin) and Oil Red O staining of liver structures in different groups of rats. Images of staining under a microscope (magnification, ×20). C: control group; D: diabetic group; AS: AS-treatment group; APN: APN-treatment group.

3. Results

3.1. General Characteristics. As shown in Table 1, at five weeks of diabetes, water intake and food consumption were significantly higher while body weight was significantly lower in diabetic rats than those in nondiabetic control. And blood glucose in the diabetic rats (31.5 ± 2.6 mM) was much higher than control rats. FoxO1 inhibitor AS did not significantly affect blood glucose, nor did it have significant impact on water intake, food consumption, and body weight. APN significantly reduced water intake and food consumption but had no significant effect on body weight.

3.2. FoxO1 Inhibition and APN Supplementation Both Reduce Hepatic Fatty Infiltration in NAFLD Rats. As shown in Figure 1, under the microscope, the H&E and Oil Red O staining in the normal control group showed a clear

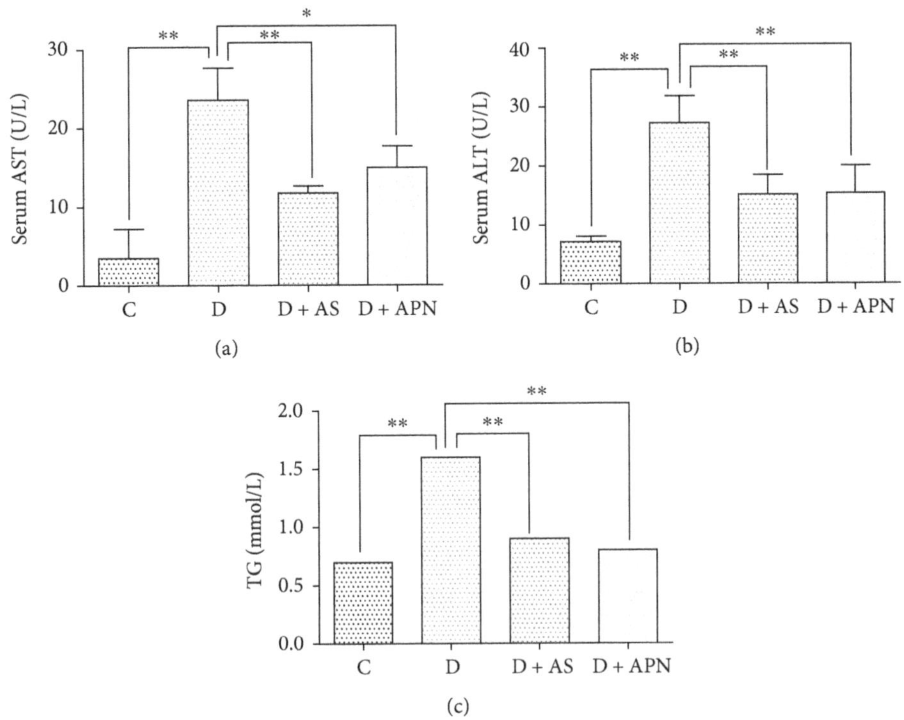

FIGURE 2: Effects of the FoxO1 inhibitor (AS) and APN on serum AST, ALT, and TG. Serum AST, ALT, and TG were determined by kits (Stanbio Laboratory, TX, USA). Values are expressed as mean ± SD, $n = 6$/group. $^*P < 0.05$, $^{**}P < 0.01$.

structure, with little fat vacuoles. While in the diabetic control group, the liver structure was not clear and filled with different sizes of fat drops. In two treatment groups (especially the AS group), the liver showed an ameliorated structure and decreased fat drops.

3.3. FoxO1 Inhibition and APN Supplementation, Respectively, Ameliorated the Liver Function in T1DM-Induced NAFLD. To investigate the effect of FoxO1 and APN on the liver function in T1DM-induced NAFLD, we first confirmed the effect of T1DM-induced NAFLD on the liver function. As shown in Figures 2(a)–2(c), serum AST, ALT, and TG were significantly increased in the diabetic group as compared with the control group. To explore the molecular mechanisms underlying the increase of serum AST, ALT, and TG, we examined the involvement of FoxO1, which is the key intracellular target of insulin effect and contributes to the regulation of lipid and glucose metabolism [14]. We found that the inhibition of FoxO1 through its selective inhibitor AS significantly decreased the serum AST, ALT, and TG compared with the solvent control, indicating the amelioration of the liver function. Also, the serum AST, ALT, and TG were apparently decreased under the treatment of APN, an antidiabetic and anti-inflammatory adipokine. Collectively, these results show that both AS and APN treatment improved the liver function in T1DM-induced NAFLD.

3.4. APN but Not the FoxO1 Inhibitor AS Reduced Blood Glucose in T1DM-Induced NAFLD Rats. We next examined the effect of AS and APN on liver weight and blood glucose in T1DM-induced NAFLD. The ratio of liver weight/body weight in the diabetic rats was about 25% higher than that in the nondiabetic rats, although the difference did not reach statistical significance. Treatment with AS or APN did not have significant influence on the ratio of liver weight/body weight (Figure 3(a)). APN but not AS significantly reduced the blood glucose level (Figure 3(b)).

3.5. FoxO1 Inhibition and APN Supplementation, Respectively, Decreased Liver Nuclear FoxO1 in T1DM-Induced NAFLD. Akt phosphorylates and excludes FoxO1 from the nucleus, retaining it to cytoplasmic compartment, thereby dampening its activity to produce glucose [33]. As shown in Figures 4(a)–4(c), the diabetic group demonstrated significant increase of nuclear FoxO1 expression. In order to further investigate how APN and AS ameliorate liver function in T1DM-induced NAFLD, we examined the effect of APN and AS on nuclear FoxO1, and the data showed that both APN and AS significantly decreased the expression of nuclear FoxO1 compared with control. AS and APN also tended to reduce nuclear p-FoxO1, but the difference did not research statistical significance.

3.6. Inhibition of FoxO1 Had No Significant Impact on the Expression of APN and AdipoR1 in T1DM-Induced NAFLD. APN is an antidiabetic adipokine which is reported to decrease after 7 weeks of T1DM induction [34], which is in accordance with our data shown in Figure 4(b). With regard to the AdipoR, we found that AdipoR1 is apparently increased in the diabetic group compared with the control group (Figure 4(a)), while application of AS did not show

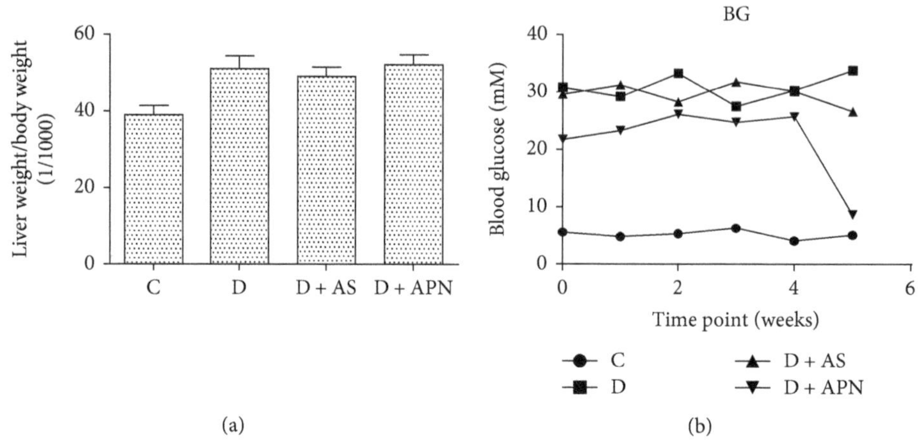

Figure 3: Effects of AS and APN on liver weight/body weight and weekly blood glucose. Blood glucose was measured by the OneTouch Ultra glucose meter. Values are expressed as mean ± SD, $n = 6$/group.

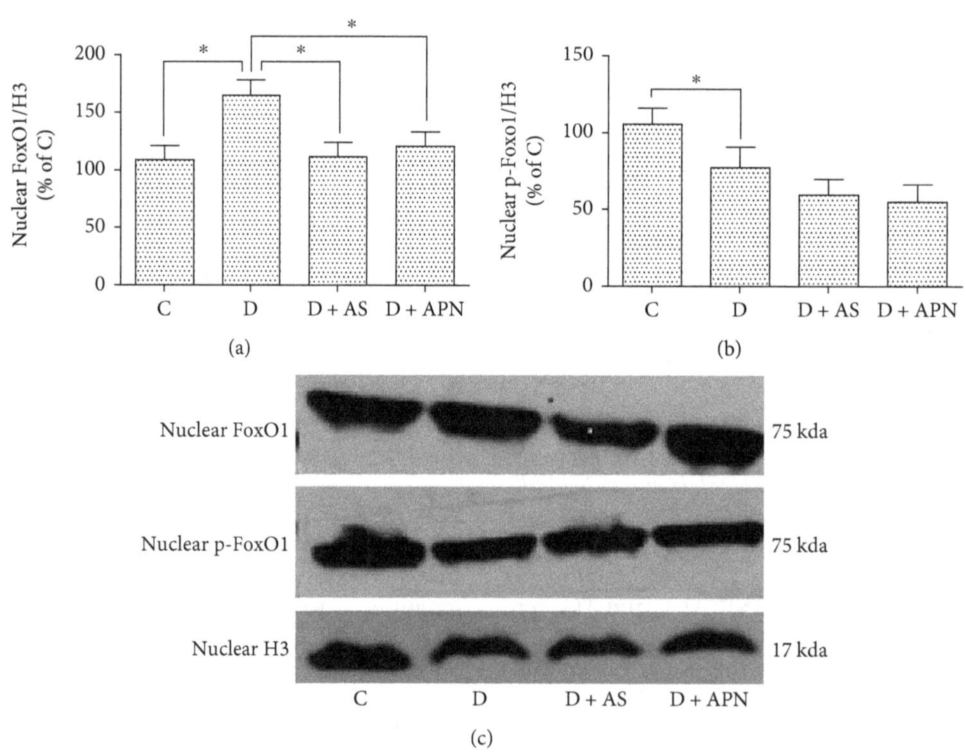

Figure 4: Effects of AS and APN on the expression of FoxO1 and p-FoxO1 in nucleus in the liver. Values are expressed as mean ± SD, $n = 6$/group. $^{*}P < 0.05$.

significant influence on the expression of APN and AdipoR1. In addition, AdipoR2 expression did not show significant difference in all groups (data not shown).

3.7. Liver Akt1 Was Significantly Reduced in Diabetic Rats and APN Restored Akt1 While AS Attenuated Reduction of Akt1 Expression. Since both APN and AS could decrease the expression of FoxO1, we further examined two subtypes of Akt, which is illustrated to function upstream of FoxO1 [35]. As shown in Figure 5, Akt1 expression was significantly reduced in the diabetic group. Application of APN restored Akt1 expression while AS moderately but significantly increased Akt1 expression. By contrast, the expression of Akt2 did not display apparent difference among all the groups.

3.8. Liver SIRT1 and Acetyl-FoxO1 Were Significantly Reduced in Diabetic Rats and Were Not Affected by Neither APN Nor AS. It has been suggested that SIRT1 was supposed to function as an upstream regulator of FoxO1 actions in the

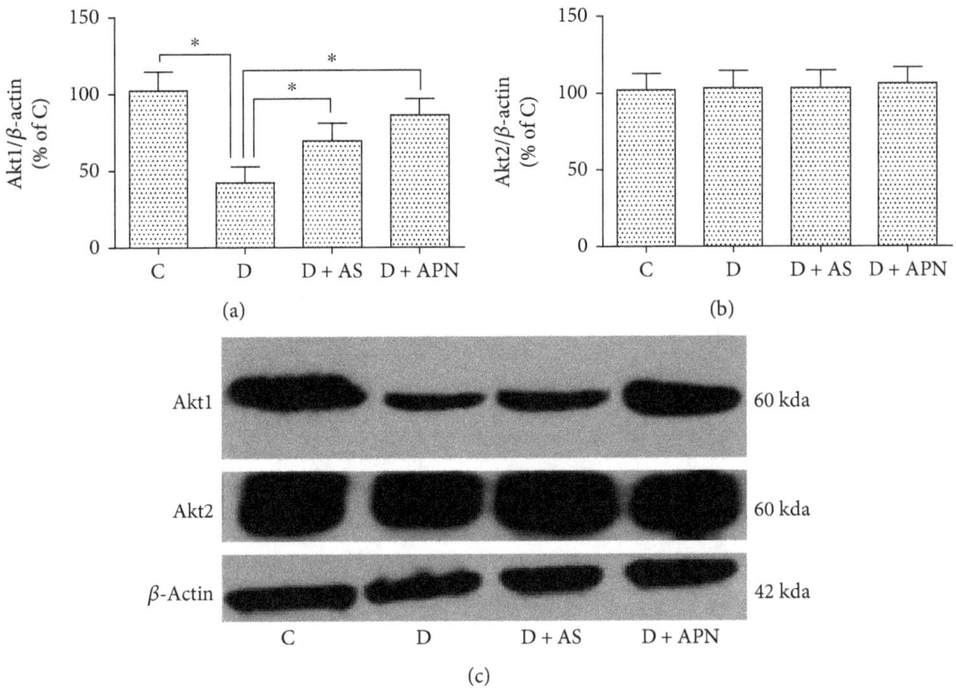

FIGURE 5: Effects of AS and APN on the expression of Akt1 and Akt2 in the liver. Values are expressed as mean ± SD, $n = 6$/group. $^*P < 0.05$.

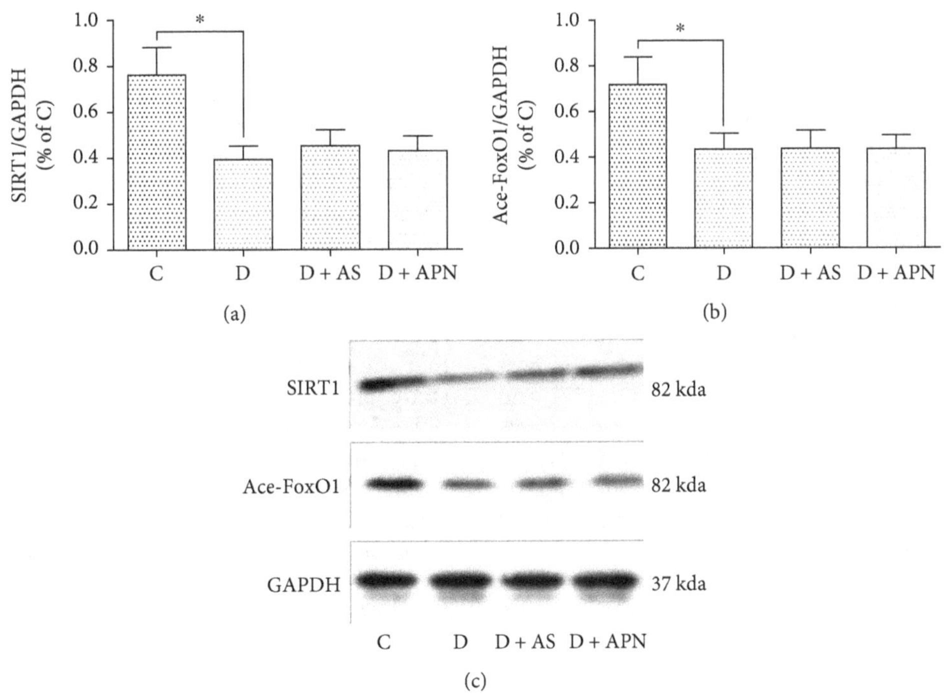

FIGURE 6: Effects of AS and APN on the expression of SIRT1 and acetyl-FoxO1 (Ace-FoxO1) in the liver. $^*P < 0.05$.

liver and other tissues and that SIRT1 usually deacetylates FoxO1 and not necessarily change the FoxO1 protein levels. We, therefore, further measured the levels of liver SIRT1 and acetyl-FoxO1. As shown in Figures 6(a)–6(c), the liver SIRT1 and acetyl-FoxO1 were significantly decreased in diabetes, while AS and APN did not have significant impact on the reductions of SIRT1 and acetyl-FoxO1 (all $P > 0.05$).

4. Discussion

As one of the worldwide metabolic diseases, NAFLD represents a disease spectrum which ranges from simple steatosis to NASH, cirrhosis to end-stage carcinoma. It has been long considered that fatty liver is closely linked with T2DM, while the association between NAFLD and T1DM lacks enough

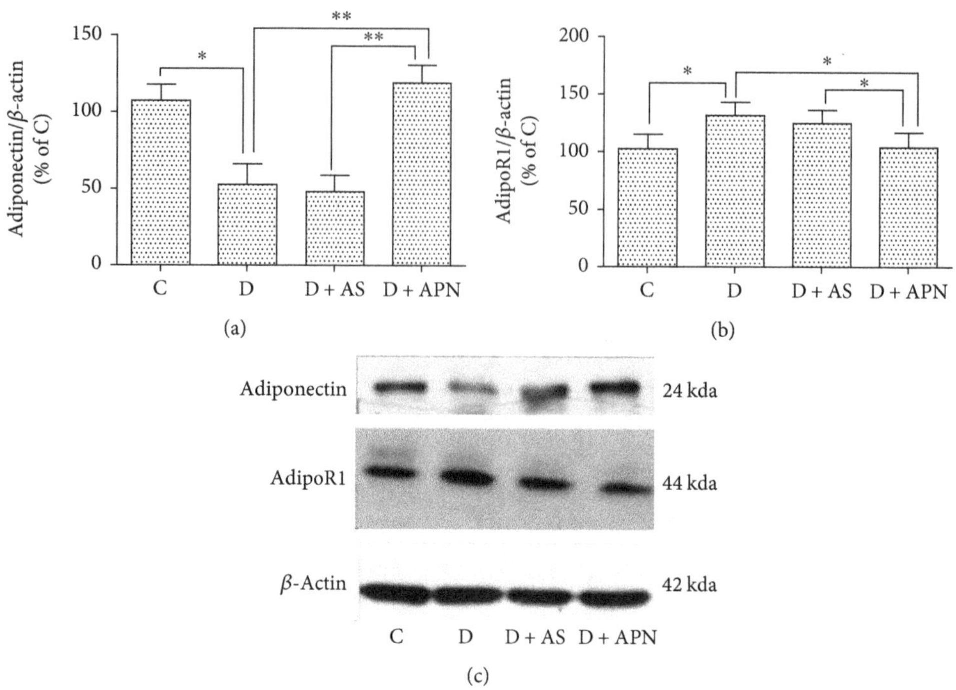

FIGURE 7: Effects of AS and APN on the expression of plasma adiponectin and liver adiponectin receptor 1 (AdipoR1) in diabetic rats. $^{*}P < 0.05$, $^{**}P < 0.01$.

attention. Although a few studies reported that the NAFLD is linked with T1DM [5, 6], the underlying mechanism is still unknown and needs further exploration.

APN is a multipurpose adipokine which is primarily secreted in adipose tissues and then released into the blood, further exerting antidiabetic and anti-inflammatory properties. In accordance with a previous study [36], we confirmed that APN significantly decreases blood glucose compared with the diabetic group, whereas AS had no obvious effect on blood glucose (Figure 3(b)). In addition, APN was reported to block cannabinoid type 1 receptor [37] and increase free fatty acid β-oxidation [38], therefore ameliorating the fat accumulation in the liver. In another study, the level of APN was found to be negatively related to the progression of NAFLD and may be a potential marker to distinguish different stages of NAFLD [9]. In this study, the serum APN level and hepatic APN expression were also significantly low in the diabetic group (Figure 7(a) and Table 1). However, the underlying molecular mechanism is still largely unknown. In the present study, we have demonstrated beneficial effects of APN on T1DM-induced NAFLD and explored its molecular mechanisms. We demonstrated that APN inhibited T1DM-induced NAFLD via reduction of the expression of FoxO1. Moreover, Akt1 signaling may represent a mechanism by which APN mediated the suppression of FoxO1 in T1DM-induced NAFLD (Figure 7).

FoxO1 is a commonly expressed member of the forkhead factor family and has long been considered to be involved in metabolic disorders, especially the lipid and glucose metabolism. On the contrary, blockade of FoxO1 increases lipogenesis and helps to restore metabolism homeostasis [14, 18, 19]. In the present study, we block the FoxO1 with selective antagonist (AS1842856) to examine its effect on T1DM-induced NAFLD. The data showed that liver function is impaired under diabetic condition, while the application of AS ameliorates liver function manifested as the reduction of ALT and AST (Figure 2). Interestingly, application of APN showed similar amelioration of liver function (Figure 2). Additionally, AS decreased the expression of nuclear FoxO1 and so did the APN (Figure 4(a)). Previous study reported that AS could change blood glucose [20]; however, in our study, blood glucose in the AS group showed no significant difference compared with the control group. We argue that this is mainly because of the different operations on the animals, since in that study mice were orally administered AS1842856 at three time points on the second day and went through fasting whereas our rats are administrated 2 times a day with a 12-hour interval for a duration of 8 days, which may have a different effect on the blood glucose. Considering that AS did not influence the level of APN (Figure 7(a)), we propose that APN is on the upstream of FoxO1 signal pathway. To confirm this hypothesis, we examined two subunits of Akt (Akt1 and Akt2). The result indicated that APN could restore the expression of Akt1 which is impaired in the diabetic group (Figure 5(a)), while Akt2 expression showed no significant difference (Figure 5(b)).

In summary, in this study, we examined the expression levels of APN and FoxO1 to explore the potential role of these two proteins in the pathology of type 1 diabetes-induced NAFLD. Findings obtained from the current study suggest that APN ameliorates NAFLD via inhibition of FoxO1 through Akt1/FoxO1 signaling pathway.

Disclosure

This paper was presented at the Experimental Biology conference in 2018 and published in part in the form of an abstract [39].

Conflicts of Interest

The authors declare that they have no conflicts of interest.

Authors' Contributions

Xiang Xie and Dan Yan contributed equally to this study.

Acknowledgments

This study was supported in part by Wenzhou City Grants (Y20160132, 2017Y0534, and 20160133) and in part by Hong Kong RGC/RGF Grant (17124614M).

References

[1] European Association for the Study of the Liver (EASL), European Association for the Study of Diabetes (EASD), and European Association for the Study of Obesity (EASO), "EASL-EASD-EASO Clinical Practice Guidelines for the management of non-alcoholic fatty liver disease," *Journal of Hepatology*, vol. 64, no. 6, pp. 1388–1402, 2016.

[2] Q. M. Anstee, G. Targher, and C. P. Day, "Progression of NAFLD to diabetes mellitus, cardiovascular disease or cirrhosis," *Nature Reviews Gastroenterology & Hepatology*, vol. 10, no. 6, pp. 330–344, 2013.

[3] N. Stefan and H. U. Haring, "The metabolically benign and malignant fatty liver," *Diabetes*, vol. 60, no. 8, pp. 2011–2017, 2011.

[4] M. G. Radaelli, F. Martucci, S. Perra et al., "NAFLD/NASH in patients with type 2 diabetes and related treatment options," *Journal of Endocrinological Investigation*, vol. 41, no. 5, pp. 509–521, 2018.

[5] S. Gancheva, A. Bierwagen, K. Kaul et al., "Variants in genes controlling oxidative metabolism contribute to lower hepatic ATP independent of liver fat content in type 1 diabetes," *Diabetes*, vol. 65, no. 7, pp. 1849–1857, 2016.

[6] R. Vendhan, A. Amutha, R. M. Anjana, R. Unnikrishnan, and V. Mohan, "Clinical profile of non alcoholic fatty liver disease among young patients with type 1 diabetes mellitus seen at a diabetes speciality centre in India," *Endocrine Practice*, vol. 20, no. 12, pp. 12494–11257, 2014.

[7] L. Abenavoli, C. Luigiano, P. H. Guzzi et al., "Serum adipokine levels in overweight patients and their relationship with non-alcoholic fatty liver disease," *Panminerva Medica*, vol. 56, no. 2, pp. 189–193, 2014.

[8] L. Abenavoli and V. Peta, "Role of adipokines and cytokines in non-alcoholic fatty liver disease," *Reviews on Recent Clinical Trials*, vol. 9, no. 3, pp. 134–140, 2014.

[9] L. Abenavoli, L. di Renzo, P. H. Guzzi, R. Pellicano, N. Milic, and A. de Lorenzo, "Non-alcoholic fatty liver disease severity, central fat mass and adinopectin: a close relationship," *Clujul Medical*, vol. 88, no. 4, pp. 489–493, 2015.

[10] S. A. Polyzos, K. A. Toulis, D. G. Goulis, C. Zavos, and J. Kountouras, "Serum total adiponectin in nonalcoholic fatty liver disease: a systematic review and meta-analysis," *Metabolism*, vol. 60, no. 3, pp. 313–326, 2011.

[11] T. Yamauchi, J. Kamon, Y. Ito et al., "Cloning of adiponectin receptors that mediate antidiabetic metabolic effects," *Nature*, vol. 423, no. 6941, pp. 762–769, 2003.

[12] T. Yamauchi, Y. Nio, T. Maki et al., "Targeted disruption of AdipoR1 and AdipoR2 causes abrogation of adiponectin binding and metabolic actions," *Nature Medicine*, vol. 13, no. 3, pp. 332–339, 2007.

[13] X. Liu, W. Tong, X. Zhao, H. Zhang, Y. Tang, and X. Deng, "Chinese herb extract improves liver steatosis by promoting the expression of high molecular weight adiponectin in NAFLD rats," *Molecular Medicine Reports*, vol. 16, no. 4, pp. 5580–5586, 2017.

[14] I. S. O-Sullivan, W. Zhang, D. H. Wasserman et al., "FoxO1 integrates direct and indirect effects of insulin on hepatic glucose production and glucose utilization," *Nature Communications*, vol. 6, no. 1, p. 7079, 2015.

[15] A. Brunet, A. Bonni, M. J. Zigmond et al., "Akt promotes cell survival by phosphorylating and inhibiting a Forkhead transcription factor," *Cell*, vol. 96, no. 6, pp. 857–868, 1999.

[16] P. Puigserver, J. Rhee, J. Donovan et al., "Insulin-regulated hepatic gluconeogenesis through FOXO1-PGC-1α interaction," *Nature*, vol. 423, no. 6939, pp. 550–555, 2003.

[17] M. Matsumoto, S. Han, T. Kitamura, and D. Accili, "Dual role of transcription factor FoxO1 in controlling hepatic insulin sensitivity and lipid metabolism," *The Journal of Clinical Investigation*, vol. 116, no. 9, pp. 2464–2472, 2006.

[18] J. R. Cook, M. Matsumoto, A. S. Banks, T. Kitamura, K. Tsuchiya, and D. Accili, "A mutant allele encoding DNA binding-deficient FoxO1 differentially regulates hepatic glucose and lipid metabolism," *Diabetes*, vol. 64, no. 6, pp. 1951–1965, 2015.

[19] P. M. Titchenell, Q. Chu, B. R. Monks, and M. J. Birnbaum, "Hepatic insulin signalling is dispensable for suppression of glucose output by insulin *in vivo*," *Nature Communications*, vol. 6, no. 1, p. 7078, 2015.

[20] T. Nagashima, N. Shigematsu, R. Maruki et al., "Discovery of novel forkhead box O1 inhibitors for treating type 2 diabetes: improvement of fasting glycemia in diabetic *db/db* mice," *Molecular Pharmacology*, vol. 78, no. 5, pp. 961–970, 2010.

[21] P. Zou, L. Liu, L. Zheng et al., "Targeting FoxO1 with AS1842856 suppresses adipogenesis," *Cell Cycle*, vol. 13, no. 23, pp. 3759–3767, 2014.

[22] A. Wang, M. Liu, X. Liu et al., "Up-regulation of adiponectin by resveratrol: the essential roles of the Akt/FOXO1 and AMP-activated protein kinase signaling pathways and DsbA-L," *The Journal of Biological Chemistry*, vol. 286, no. 1, pp. 60–66, 2011.

[23] X. Liang, M. Hu, C. Q. Rogers, Z. Shen, and M. You, "Role of SIRT1-FoxO1 signaling in dietary saturated fat-dependent upregulation of liver adiponectin receptor 2 in ethanol-administered mice," *Antioxidants & Redox Signaling*, vol. 15, no. 2, pp. 425–435, 2011.

[24] A. Tsuchida, T. Yamauchi, Y. Ito et al., "Insulin/Foxo1 pathway regulates expression levels of adiponectin receptors and

adiponectin sensitivity," *Journal of Biological Chemistry*, vol. 279, no. 29, pp. 30817–30822, 2004.

[25] L. K. Hasseine, C. Hinault, P. Lebrun, N. Gautier, R. Paul-Bellon, and E. van Obberghen, "miR-139 impacts FoxO1 action by decreasing *FoxO1* protein in mouse hepatocytes," *Biochemical and Biophysical Research Communications*, vol. 390, no. 4, pp. 1278–1282, 2009.

[26] J. J. Kim, P. Li, J. Huntley, J. P. Chang, K. C. Arden, and J. M. Olefsky, "FoxO1 haploinsufficiency protects against high-fat diet-induced insulin resistance with enhanced peroxisome proliferator-activated receptor γ activation in adipose tissue," *Diabetes*, vol. 58, no. 6, pp. 1275–1282, 2009.

[27] D. Jin, J. Sun, J. Huang et al., "Peroxisome proliferator-activated receptor γ enhances adiponectin secretion via up-regulating DsbA-L expression," *Molecular and Cellular Endocrinology*, vol. 411, pp. 97–104, 2015.

[28] S.-M. Kim, J. P. Grenert, C. Patterson, and M. A. Correia, "CHIP$^{-/-}$-mouse liver: adiponectin-AMPK-FOXO-activation overrides CYP2E1-elicited JNK1-activation, delaying onset of NASH: therapeutic implications," *Scientific Reports*, vol. 6, no. 1, article 29423, 2016.

[29] G. J. P. L. Kops, T. B. Dansen, P. E. Polderman et al., "Forkhead transcription factor FOXO3a protects quiescent cells from oxidative stress," *Nature*, vol. 419, no. 6904, pp. 316–321, 2002.

[30] C. Diep, N. Charles, C. Blake Gilks, S. Kalloger, P. Argenta, and C. A. Lange, "Progesterone receptors induce FOXO1-dependent senescence in ovarian cancer cells," *Cell Cycle*, vol. 12, no. 9, pp. 1433–1449, 2014.

[31] H. Li, W. Yao, Z. Liu et al., "Hyperglycemia abrogates ischemic postconditioning cardioprotection by impairing AdipoR1/Caveolin-3/STAT3 signaling in diabetic rats," *Diabetes*, vol. 65, no. 4, pp. 942–955, 2016.

[32] Q. Wu, T. Wang, S. Chen et al., "Cardiac protective effects of remote ischaemic preconditioning in children undergoing tetralogy of fallot repair surgery: a randomized controlled trial," *European Heart Journal*, vol. 39, no. 12, pp. 1028–1037, 2018.

[33] Z. Cheng and M. F. White, "The AKTion in non-canonical insulin signaling," *Nature Medicine*, vol. 18, no. 3, pp. 351–3, 2012.

[34] Y. Ma, Y. Liu, S. Liu et al., "Dynamic alteration of adiponectin/adiponectin receptor expression and its impact on myocardial ischemia/reperfusion in type 1 diabetic mice," *American Journal of Physiology Endocrinology and Metabolism*, vol. 301, no. 3, pp. E447–E455, 2011.

[35] Z. Cheng, "FoxO1: mute for a tuned metabolism?," *Trends in Endocrinology and Metabolism*, vol. 26, no. 8, pp. 402-403, 2015.

[36] H. Li, W. Yao, M. G. Irwin et al., "Adiponectin ameliorates hyperglycemia-induced cardiac hypertrophy and dysfunction by concomitantly activating Nrf2 and Brg1," *Free Radical Biology & Medicine*, vol. 84, pp. 311–321, 2015.

[37] J. Tam, G. Godlewski, B. J. Earley et al., "Role of adiponectin in the metabolic effects of cannabinoid type 1 receptor blockade in mice with diet-induced obesity," *American Journal of Physiology. Endocrinology and Metabolism*, vol. 306, no. 4, pp. E457–E468, 2014.

[38] Y. Arita, S. Kihara, N. Ouchi et al., "Paradoxical decrease of an adipose-specific protein, adiponectin, in obesity. 1999," *Biochemical and Biophysical Research Communications*, vol. 425, no. 3, pp. 560–564, 2012.

[39] X. Xie and Z. Xia, "Enhancement of adiponectin ameliorates non-alcoholic fatty liver disease via inhibition of FoxO1 in type I diabetic rats," *FASEB Journal*, vol. 32, no. 1, 2018.

8

Choroidal Thickness and Ganglion Cell Complex in Pubescent Children with Type 1 Diabetes without Diabetic Retinopathy Analyzed by Spectral Domain Optical Coherence Tomography

Joanna Gołębiewska,[1] Andrzej Olechowski,[1] Marta Wysocka-Mincewicz,[2] Marta Baszyńska-Wilk,[2] Artur Groszek,[2] Agnieszka Czeszyk-Piotrowicz,[1] Mieczysław Szalecki,[2,3] and Wojciech Hautz[1]

[1]*Department of Ophthalmology, The Children's Memorial Health Institute, Aleja Dzieci Polskich 20, Warsaw, Poland*
[2]*Department of Diabetology and Endocrinology, The Children's Memorial Health Institute, Aleja Dzieci Polskich 20, Warsaw, Poland*
[3]*Department of Medicine and Health Sciences, UJK, Kielce, Poland*

Correspondence should be addressed to Joanna Gołębiewska; joanna.golebiewska@wp.pl

Academic Editor: Steven F. Abcouwer

Aim. To assess the retinal and choroidal thickness and ganglion cell complex (GCC) in pubescent children with type 1 diabetes (T1D) without diabetic retinopathy (DR), using spectral domain optical coherence tomography (SD-OCT). *Materials and Method.* Sixty-four right eyes of 64 subjects with T1D and 45 right eyes of 45 age-matched healthy volunteers (control group) were enrolled in this study. The mean age of the subjects and controls was 15.3 ($\pm SD = 2.2$) and 14.6 ($\pm SD = 1.5$), respectively. SD-OCT was performed using RTVue XR Avanti. Ganglion cell complex (GCC), GCC focal loss volume (FLV), GCC global loss volume (GLV), choroidal thickness (CT), foveal (FT) and parafoveal thickness (PFT), and foveal (FV) and parafoveal volume (PFV) data were analyzed. *Results.* There was no significant difference between subjects and controls in the CT in the fovea and nasal, temporal, superior, and inferior quadrants of the macula. There were no significant correlations between CT, duration of diabetes, and HbA1C level ($p = 0.272$ and $p = 0.197$, resp.). GCC thickness did not differ significantly between the groups ($p = 0.448$), but there was a significant difference in FLV ($p = 0.037$). Significant differences between the groups were found in the PFT and PFV ($p = 0.004$ and $p = 0.005$, resp.). There was a significant negative correlation between PFT, PFV, and HbA1C level ($p = 0.002$ and $p = 0.001$, resp.). *Conclusions.* Choroidal thickness remains unchanged in children with T1D. Increased GCC FLV might suggest an early alteration in neuroretinal tissue. Parafoveal retinal thickness is decreased in pubescent T1D children and correlates with HbA1C level. OCT can be considered a part of noninvasive screening in children with T1D and a tool for early detection of retinal and choroidal abnormalities. Further OCT follow-up is needed to determine whether any of the discussed OCT measurements are predictive of future DR severity.

1. Introduction

Diabetes mellitus (DM) is the third most common chronic disease in children. The majority of cases are type 1 diabetes (T1D), but the global obesity epidemic contributes to the increasing incidence of type 2 diabetes (T2D) in children and adolescents [1–3]. Most previous studies focused on diabetic retinopathy (DR) as an increasingly prevalent disease and the leading cause of blindness in working-age individuals in industrialized countries [4–6]. Far less attention has been paid to choroidal vasculopathy, despite clinical and experimental findings implicating choroidal blood flow in the pathogenesis of diabetic retinopathy [7–9]. Macular choroidal thickness (CT) is considered a putative measure of choroidal blood flow. Some researchers found decreased choroidal thickness in diabetic patients, whereas others reported increased or unchanged CT in various stages of DR [10–14]. Thus, the status of the choroid in patients with DM remains controversial.

Various studies using electroretinography, colour vision, and contrast sensitivity testing reported neural tissue loss, in particular affecting retinal ganglion cells, apoptosis of retinal glial and neural cells, and decreased thickness of inner retinal layers before DR becomes clinically detectable [15–17]. The exact mechanism for inner retinal loss is not clear and some authors investigated the relationship between diabetic peripheral neuropathy (DPN) and retinal tissue thickness [18, 19]. Therefore, early detection of choroidal vasculopathy and neuropathy in T1D patients through screening programs may be crucial for commencing treatment before the onset of DR.

Indirect ophthalmoscopy and stereoscopic dilated fundus photography, a practice commonly used worldwide, offers high diagnostic accuracy in DR detection [20]. Optical coherence tomography is a noninvasive tool enabling the reproducible and quantitative assessment of the retinal layers, which currently remains the most precise method to measure retinal and choroidal thicknesses *in vivo*. To date, there is a number of studies to discuss OCT findings in adults with diabetes mellitus and only a few reports to discuss OCT findings in DM pediatric population [21–27].

The aim of our study was to assess retinal and choroidal thickness and ganglion cell complex in pubescent T1D children.

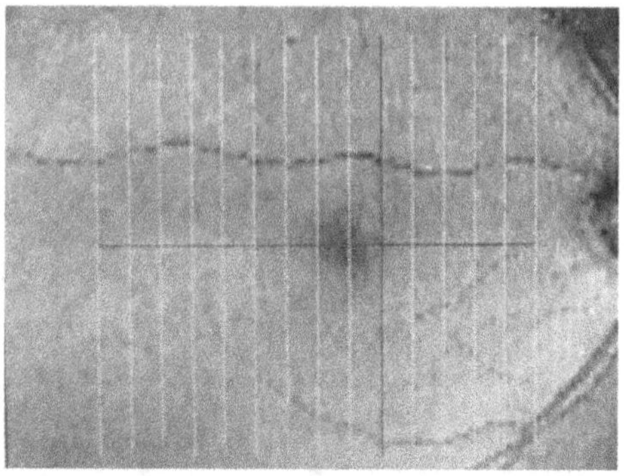

FIGURE 1: The ganglion cell complex scan pattern (7 × 7 mm) consists of 15 vertical and 1 horizontal scan lines.

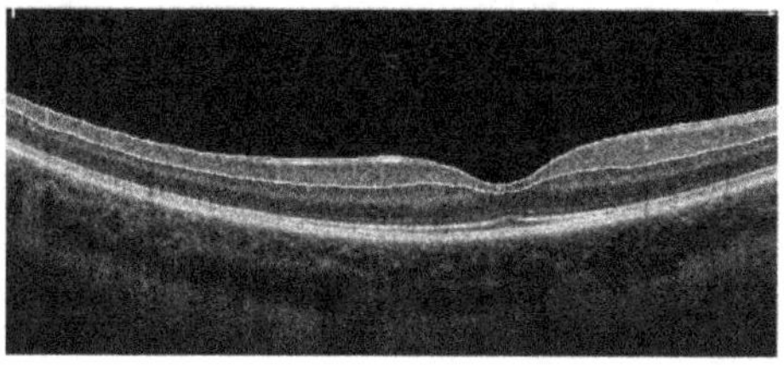

FIGURE 2: An example of horizontal macular OCT cross section in a T1D patient. The GCC thickness is automatically measured as the distance between the ILM and the outer IPL boundary.

2. Material and Methods

This cross-sectional study was approved by the Institutional Review Board and followed the tenets of the Declaration of Helsinki. After explanation of the nature and possible consequences of the study, a written informed consent was obtained from the patient's legal guardian and from patients above 16 years of age.

Sixty-four T1D children at the age of 11–18 years, without signs of DR and with diabetes duration of 1 year or more, were enrolled in the study. Exclusion criteria were history of prematurity and other concomitant retinal pathologies, such as hereditary retinal dystrophies, vitreoretinal diseases, as well as uveitis, glaucoma, history of peripheral neuropathy, and high refractive error (spheric equivalent > +/−3.00 diopters). Eyes with poor-quality scans, due to unstable fixation, were also excluded. Controls were defined as having a normal finding in ocular examination and no history of diabetes. They were age- and sex-matched to the patients.

Every patient underwent a complete ocular examination, including best-corrected visual acuity (BVCA), slit lamp biomicroscopy, dilated fundus examination, and colour fundus photography. Clinical data recorded for each diabetic subject included duration of diabetes, systolic and diastolic blood pressure, mean and actual levels of glycated hemoglobin (HbA1C), daily urine creatinine excretion, serum creatinine levels, as well as mean and actual levels of daily urine albumin excretion.

SD-OCT was performed in both subjects and controls using a commercially available RTVue XR Avanti (Optovue, Fremont, CA, USA). Foveal thickness (FT) (μm), parafoveal thickness (PFT) (μm), foveal volume (FV) (mm^3), and parafoveal volume (PFV) data were obtained from retinal maps, using the same device. All acquired images were inspected, and if automatic segmentation errors occurred or resulted in measurement artifacts, manual segmentation was performed. All OCT scans with motion artifacts were excluded.

GCC scan protocol (formerly called MM7 scan), which consists of one horizontal line with a 7 mm scan length (934 A scans) and 15 vertical lines with a 7 mm scan length and a 0.5 mm interval (800 A scans) centered at 1 mm temporally to the fovea, was used in all participants. GCC thickness, defined as the distance from the internal limiting membrane to the outer boundary of the inner plexiform layer, was calculated automatically by the device (Figures 1 and 2).

Eyes were divided into two sectors, superior and inferior. GCC was expressed as the average thickness of both sectors (Avg GCC) and separately as the thickness of the superior (Sup GCC) and inferior (Inf GCC) sector. Furthermore, the RTVue SD-OCT device is equipped with software enabling the analysis of diffuse and focal GCC defects by calculating global loss volume (GLV) and focal loss volume (FLV), respectively. These parameters, developed and introduced by Tan et al., provide a quantitative measurement of change in the GCC volume [28]. The GLV measures the average amount of GCC volume loss over the entire recorded GCC field and corresponds to the mean deviation (MD) values in

Table 1: Study sample characteristics.

Variable	M	SD	95% CI	Min.–max.
Age (years)				
Diabetic patients	15.3	2.2	14.7–15.8	11.3–18.5
Nondiabetic patients	14.6	1.6	14.1–15.0	13.0–18.0
Diabetes duration (years)	6.3	3.4	5.5–7.2	1.0–14.4
Age at onset (years)	8.9	3.8	8.0–9.0	2.3–16.5
Glycated hemoglobin – actual level (%)	8.2	1.2	7.9–8.5	6.4–13.3
Glycated hemoglobin – mean level (%)	8.1	1.1	7.8–8.3	6.3–11.6
Actual level of daily urine albumin excretion (mg/d)	10.3	6.9	8.5–12.2	0.5–33.3
Mean level of daily urine albumin excretion (mg/d)	8.9	8.1	6.7–11.1	0.5–40.5
Serum creatinine (mg/dL)	0.69	0.16	0.65–0.73	0.42–1.12
Daily urine creatinine excretion (mg/d)	1.29	0.95	1.01–1.58	0.27–5.47
Systolic blood pressure (mmHg)	114	10.8	111.0–116.9	84–140
Diastolic blood pressure (mmHg)	68	10.5	65.3–71.1	40–91

M: mean; SD: standard deviation; CI: confidence interval.

visual field tests. The GLV can best detect diffuse ganglion cell loss. The FLV detects focal losses to correct for overall absolute changes and corresponds to the corrected pattern standard deviation in the visual field. GLV is calculated from the fractional deviation map showing the percentage of GCC thickness decrease at each pixel location compared with the expected or normal values. The FLV is determined based on a normalized pattern map by dividing GCC thickness values at each location by the average GCC thickness from the entire map for a given individual. All significant differences between the pattern map created for an individual and pattern map of the normative database yields the pattern deviation map.

A crossline scan was performed to obtain high-quality images of the retina and choroid. Choroidal thickness was measured manually using the built-in calipers in OCT software. Choroidal thickness, defined as the distance between the hyperreflective line corresponding to the outer boundary of the RPE and the hyperreflective line corresponding to the chorioscleral interface, was measured three times by two independent researchers. Mean values were recorded and included in the analysis. The measurements were obtained in the subfoveal region and at a distance of 1500 μm superiorly, inferiorly, nasally, and temporally from this site. All measurements were performed at the same time of the day (between 9:00 am and 11:00 am) in all children to avoid the effect of diurnal CT variation on the results. Only measurements from right eyes of both subjects and controls were included in the analysis.

3. Statistical Analysis

The variables were expressed as means, standard deviations, 95% confidence intervals, and ranges. The one-way multifactor analysis of variance (ANOVA) was used to determine the differences between patients and controls, if the assumptions of normality of distribution and homogeneity of variances were met, or generalized linear models with robust standard errors, when said assumptions were violated. Linear relationships between selected quantitative variables were assessed using the Pearson product-moment correlation coefficient. Glass's Δ traditionally estimated for experimental case-control studies using a control group standard deviation rather than a pooled standard deviation was used as a measure of effect size [29]. A standard deviation from the nondiabetic group was chosen due to its lower variability and better stability. A level of $p < 0.05$ was considered statistically significant for all comparisons. All statistical computations were carried out using Stata/ Special Edition, release 14.2 (StataCorp LP, College Station, Texas, USA).

4. Results

Sixty-four right eyes of 64 subjects with T1D and 45 right eyes of 45 age-matched healthy volunteers (controls) were enrolled in this study. The mean age in the study group was 15.3 ($\pm$SD = 2.2) years and in the control group 14.6 ($\pm$SD = 1.5) years. All subjects had 20/20 vision and normal colour fundus photographs. The in-depth descriptive characteristics of the entire cohort are shown in Table 1.

Table 2 shows descriptive measures of the choroidal thickness (μm) in the studied patients by presence of T1D. CT in the fovea and nasal, temporal, superior, and inferior quadrants of the macula did not differ statistically between the study groups: $p = 0.134$, $p = 0.270$, $p = 0.691$, $p = 0.504$, and $p = 0.862$, respectively.

However, regardless of the prevalence of T1D in the studied children, the CT was significantly thicker in girls than in boys, except for the superior quadrant Figure 3.

There were no significant correlations between CT, duration of diabetes, and HbA1C level ($r = -0.16$, $p = 0.272$ and $r = -0.22$, $p = 0.197$, resp.).

GCC thickness did not differ significantly between the groups ($p = 0.448$), but there was a significant difference between FLV ($p = 0.037$) (Table 3).

TABLE 2: Descriptive statistics for choroidal thickness (CT, μm) in individual retinal quadrants (diabetic patients versus nondiabetic).

Variable	Study group	*M*	SD	95% CI	Range	*p*
Central choroidal thickness, CT (μm)	Diabetic	355.65	77.50	335.09–376.21	187–585	0.081
	Nondiabetic	327.98	66.02	307.66–248.29	179–479	
CT—nasal quadrant (μm)	Diabetic	282.32	76.59	261.99–302.64	138–542	0.427
	Nondiabetic	267.16	68.68	246.03–288.30	130–398	
CT—temporal quadrant (μm)	Diabetic	338.88	71.18	319.99–357.76	190–515	0.338
	Nondiabetic	324.07	70.17	302.47–345.66	155–512	
CT—superior quadrant (μm)	Diabetic	342.40	76.48	321.72–363.08	149–534	0.418
	Nondiabetic	328.70	70.11	307.12–350.27	169–453	
CT—inferior quadrant (μm)	Diabetic	352.35	82.17	330.13–374.56	185–599	0.813
	Nondiabetic	354.56	78.15	330.51–378.61	184–539	

M: mean; SD: standard deviation; CI: confidence interval.

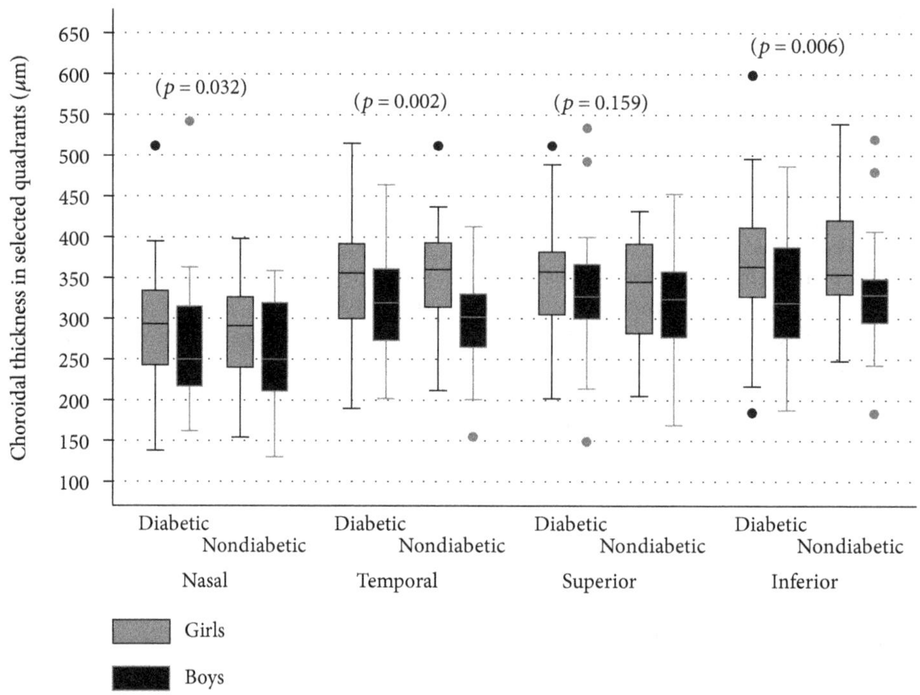

FIGURE 3: Central tendency and dispersion for the choroidal thickness (μm) in selected retinal quadrants in the study sample by T1D status and gender.

TABLE 3: Descriptive statistics of GCC parameters in the studied patients by presence of type 1 diabetes mellitus.

Variable	Study group	*M*	SD	95% CI	Range	*p*
Ganglion cell complex—total	Diabetic	97.51	6.77	95.77–99.24	80.97–118.39	0.448
	Nondiabetic	98.08	6.03	96.25–99.92	87.23–111.94	
GCC—superior quadrant	Diabetic	96.05	10.45	93.38–98.73	30.88–117.00	0.371
	Nondiabetic	97.42	6.56	95.42–99.41	86.46–111.43	
GCC—inferior quadrant	Diabetic	98.05	8.49	95.88–100.23	81.69–138.14	0.401
	Nondiabetic	98.74	5.74	96.99-100.48	88.00–112.47	
Focal loss volume (%)	Diabetic	0.512	0.756	0.313–0.711	0.000–4.420	**0.037**
	Nondiabetic	0.275	0.434	0.142–0.407	0.000–2.202	
Global loss volume (%)	Diabetic	2.349	2.926	1.580–3.118	0.000–14.402	0.282
	Nondiabetic	1.842	1.909	1.262–2.422	0.003–8.265	

M: mean; SD: standard deviation; CI: confidence interval.

TABLE 4: Descriptive statistics foveal/parafoveal thickness (μm) and volume (mm^3) in the studied patients by presence of type 1 diabetes mellitus.

Variable	Study group	M	SD	95% CI	Range	p
Foveal thickness (μm)	Diabetic	257.82	21.37	252.44–263.21	200–308	$p = 0.206$
	Nondiabetic	262.63	20.07	256.45–268.80	221–324	
Parafoveal thickness (μm)	Diabetic	315.90	17.95	311.38–320.42	270–360	$\mathbf{p = 0.004}$
	Nondiabetic	325.26	15.37	320.47–330.05	289–360	
Foveal volume (mm^3)	Diabetic	0.202	0.017	0.198–0.207	0.157–0.242	$p = 0.197$
	Nondiabetic	0.206	0.016	0.201–0.211	0.173–0.254	
Parafoveal volume (mm^3)	Diabetic	1.985	0.112	1.957–2.014	1.698–2.261	$\mathbf{p = 0.005}$
	Nondiabetic	2.043	0.096	2.013–2.073	1.818–2.261	

*Patient age and gender were considered in the multivariate analyses.

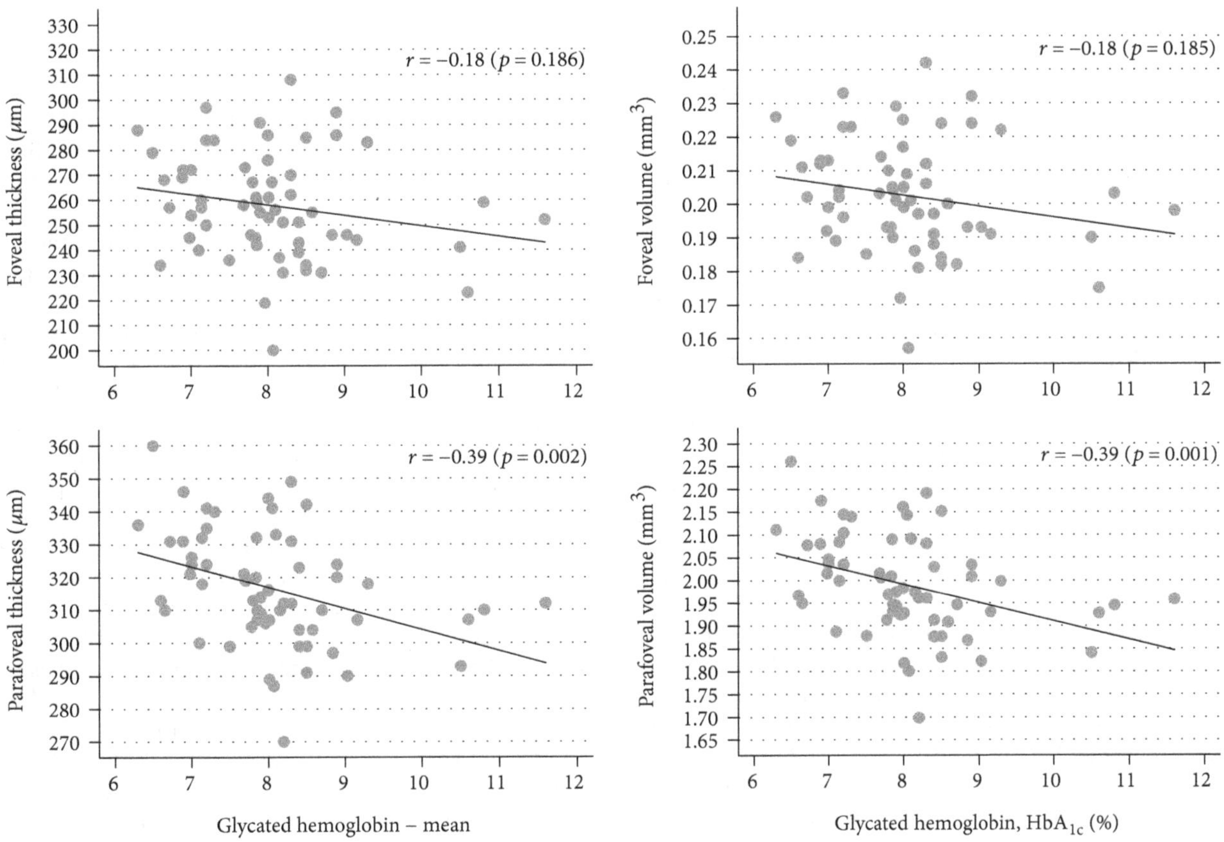

FIGURE 4: Correlations between the level of glycated hemoglobin (HbA_{1c}, %) and foveal/parafoveal thickness (μm) and volume (mm^3) in the studied patients with type 1 diabetes mellitus.

Effect size measures

(i) FLV, Glass's $\Delta = -0.548$ (95% CI: -0.953 to -0.136).

There was no significant correlation between GCC and duration of diabetes ($r = -0.05$, $p = 0.696$). There were no significant differences in foveal thickness and foveal volume between the study groups ($p = 0.206$ and $p = 0.197$, resp.).

Statistically significant differences were found in the PFT and PFV between the groups ($p = 0.004$ and $p = 0.005$, resp.) (Table 4).

Effect size measures

(i) parafoveal thickness, Glass's $\Delta = 0.609$ (95% CI: 0.194–1.018),

(ii) parafoveal volume, Glass's $\Delta = 0.601$ (95% CI: 0.186–1.009).

There was a significant correlation between PFT, PFV, and HbA1C level (Figure 4).

5. Discussion

Several studies over the past 20–30 years have shown a declining incidence of DR in children with diabetes, from 49% in the early 1990s to about 12–20% in the 2000s. This may be the result of more effective treatment, the use of the insulin pumps, and better education of the affected children and their families [30, 31]. In our study group, no child had any signs of diabetic retinopathy on fundus examination and colour fundus photography. The risk of developing retinopathy in youths is low before puberty. Adolescents with type 1 diabetes are faced with the significant challenge of regulating their blood sugar levels. Olsen et al. noted that the risk of DR increases twice in postpubertal years as compared to prepubertal years, which may be due to increasing hemoglobin A1c levels during puberty [32]. Since a group of pubescent children has a higher risk of developing DR, we decided to choose them for our research.

To the best of our knowledge, this is the first study to evaluate OCT data, which focused only on pubescent T1D children. Histological studies show loss of choriocapillaries in patients with DM, which results in reduced choroidal blood flow, retinal tissue hypoxia, as well as retinal pigment epithelium and photoreceptor dysfunction and death [10]. Regatieri et al. showed a significant decrease in CT in patients with diabetic macular oedema and those treated for proliferative diabetic retinopathy as compared to healthy volunteers. They concluded that reduced CT may have been related to the severity of retinopathy [21]. Sheth et al. found a significant reduction in CT in the eyes with ischemic diabetic maculopathy as compared to nonischemic DR and diabetic population without DR, which may explain the visual loss in ischemic maculopathy [33]. Our results do not support these findings, as we did not find significant differences in choroidal thickness between the groups. It should be noted, though, that whereas the former studies were carried out in adults, ours was carried out in children. Sayin et al. proved that CT of diabetic children is similar to healthy controls and is not affected by HbA1c, age, or duration of diabetes [27]. Their results, consistent with ours, might suggest unaffected choroidal blow flow in T1D children, without DR. Furthermore, in our study, girls had significantly thicker choroid than boys, regardless of T1D prevalence. The significance of this finding remains uncertain at the moment. Other authors suggested a biological explanation of this phenomenon, linked to a different hormonal exposure between males and females. The previous studies proved that sex and hormonal status influence the choroidal blood flow, probably due to the vascular effect of oestrogens and progestins [34, 35]. Further follow-up of these children is necessary in order to assess the clinical significance of these findings and to determine their potential effect on the DR onset. The exact relationship between DR and diabetic retinal neuropathy has not been fully explained yet. Some researchers have found that retinal neurodegeneration may occur in DM before any microcirculatory abnormalities become detectable [24]. They are also likely to occur in an independent manner [36–40]. The mechanism for inner retinal loss in DM patients may be explained by lower perfusion and higher metabolic demands of the inner retina, which is vulnerable to disease-induced metabolic stress [41]. Objective assessment of GCC finds importance in detection of inner retinal loss in patients with DM. Several studies reported GCC thinning in patients with DM without DR [23, 24]. Our results are consistent with Srinivasan, who found an abnormality in GCC FLV in affected subjects and confirmed that the loss of neural tissue begins in the early stages of diabetes as an independent predictor of diabetic peripheral neuropathy [39]. El-Fayoumi reported significant reduction in the average GCC thickness at the macula in 46 children with T1D with normal fundus examination. Similarly, in our study, there was no correlation between GGC thickness and HbA1c, duration of DM, and the age of DM onset [26]. Pierro et al. found decreased GCC and choroidal thickness only in patients with T2D, not T1D and suggested that insulin resistance might be one of the causes of neurodegeneration [41]. Most reports reveal that the retina becomes thinner in DR [13, 22, 40]. We confirm these results, as there were significant differences in PFT and PFV between the groups. However, unlike most previous studies, which show that macular thickness decreases due to neural tissue loss, the decreased PFT and PFV are not related to the decreased GCC thickness in our group of T1D patients. We agree with Srinivasan et al. who hypothesise that microglial changes, which can occur prior to neuronal cell death may be the reason of decreased PFT and thinner parafovea may proceed detectable changes in neuroretinal layer thickness [40]. The short duration of diabetes in our adolescent patients is a likely explanation for the absence of significant GCC thinning. The measurements of PFT and PFV, albeit of secondary importance to our study, appear interesting and require further research in a larger number of eyes. In the present study, pubescent youths with T1D presented with significantly fewer objective signs of retinal and choroidal structure impairment than diabetic adults as previously reported [10–13, 36–38, 41]. We are hoping to continue the follow-up of these young patients to monitor the status of their retinas and choroids.

The limitation of the current study is poor sample representativeness. It is a single-center study with monoracial background, as all subjects were Caucasian, and the uniformity of this clinical population may not exactly reflect the entire cohort of diabetic children worldwide.

6. Conclusions

Choroidal thickness remains unchanged in children with T1D. Furthermore, it is significantly thicker in girls than in boys, regardless of the prevalence of T1D. Increased GCC FLV might suggest an early alteration in neuroretinal tissue in these patients. Parafoveal retinal thickness is decreased in pubescent T1D children and correlates with HbA1C level. Based on these findings, OCT can be considered a part of noninvasive screening in children with T1D and a tool for early detection of retinal and choroidal abnormalities. Further OCT follow-up is needed to determine whether any of the discussed OCT measurements are predictive of future DR severity.

Conflicts of Interest

The authors declare that there is no conflict of interest regarding the publication of this paper.

References

[1] S. Wild, G. Roglic, A. Green, R. Sicree, and H. King, "Global prevalence of diabetes. Estimates for the year 2000 and projections for 2030," *Diabetes Care*, vol. 27, no. 5, pp. 1047–1053, 2004.

[2] SEARCH Study Group, "SEARCH for diabetes in youth: a multicenter study of the prevalence, incidence and classification of diabetes mellitus in youth," *Controlled Clinical Trials*, vol. 25, no. 5, pp. 458–471, 2004.

[3] M. B. Sultan, C. Starita, and K. Huang, "Epidemiology, risk factors and management of paediatric diabetic retinopathy," *The British Journal of Ophthalmology*, vol. 96, no. 3, pp. 312–317, 2012.

[4] M. Kubin, P. Tossavainen, V. Hannula, S. Lahti, N. Hautala, and A. Falck, "Prevalence of retinopathy in Finnish children and adolescents with type 1 diabetes: a cross-sectional population-based retrospective study," *Archives of Disease in Childhood*, vol. 96, no. 10, pp. 963–968, 2011.

[5] P. Massin, A. Erginay, I. Mercat-Caudal et al., "Prevalence of diabetic retinopathy in children and adolescents with type-1 diabetes attending summer camps in France," *Diabetes & Metabolism*, vol. 33, no. 4, pp. 284–289, 2007.

[6] S. Y. Wang, C. A. Andrews, W. H. Herman, T. W. Gardner, and J. D. Stein, "Incidence and risk factors for developing diabetic retinopathy among youths with type 1 or type 2 diabetes throughout the United States," *Ophthalmology*, vol. 124, no. 4, pp. 424–430, 2017.

[7] J. Cao, S. McLeod, C. A. Merges, and G. A. Lutty, "Choriocapillaris degeneration and related pathologic changes in human diabetic eyes," *Archives of Ophthalmology*, vol. 116, no. 5, pp. 589–597, 1998.

[8] S. H. Lee, J. Kim, H. Chung, and H. C. Kim, "Changes of choroidal thickness after treatment for diabetic retinopathy," *Current Eye Research*, vol. 39, no. 7, pp. 736–744, 2014.

[9] A. A. Hidayat and B. S. Fine, "Diabetic choroidopathy: light and electron microscopic observations of seven cases," *Ophthalmology*, vol. 92, no. 4, pp. 512–522, 1985.

[10] T. Nagaoka, N. Kitaya, R. Sugawara et al., "Alteration of choroidal circulation in the foveal region in patients with type 2 diabetes," *British Journal of Ophthalmology*, vol. 88, no. 8, pp. 1060–1063, 2004.

[11] F. Yülek, N. Uğurlu, E. D. Önal et al., "Choroidal changes and duration of diabetes," *Seminars in Ophthalmology*, vol. 29, no. 2, pp. 80–84, 2014.

[12] S. Galgauskas, G. Laurinavičiūtė, D. Norvydaitė, S. Stech, and R. Ašoklis, "Changes in choroidal thickness and corneal parameters in diabetic eyes," *European Journal of Ophthalmology*, vol. 26, no. 2, pp. 163–167, 2016.

[13] U. Yolcu, E. Cagiltay, S. Toyran, F. Akay, S. Uzun, and F. C. Gundogan, "Choroidal and macular thickness changes in type 1 diabetes mellitus patients without diabetic retinopathy," *Postgraduate Medicine*, vol. 128, no. 8, pp. 755–760, 2016.

[14] J. Xu, L. Xu, K. F. Du et al., "Subfoveal choroidal thickness in diabetes and diabetic retinopathy," *Ophthalmology*, vol. 120, no. 10, pp. 2023–2028, 2013.

[15] S. Sokol, A. Moskowitz, B. Skarf, R. Evans, M. Molitch, and B. Senior, "Contrast sensitivity in diabetics with and without background retinopathy," *Archives of Ophthalmology*, vol. 103, no. 1, pp. 51–54, 1985.

[16] A. J. Barber, E. Lieth, S. A. Khin, D. A. Antonetti, A. G. Buchanan, and T. W. Gardner, "Neural apoptosis in the retina during experimental and human diabetes: early onset and effect of insulin," *The Journal of Clinical Investigation*, vol. 102, no. 4, pp. 783–791, 1998.

[17] A. J. Barber, "A new view of diabetic retinopathy: a neurodegenerative disease of the eye," *Progress in Neuro-Psychopharmacology and Biological Psychiatry*, vol. 27, no. 2, pp. 283–290, 2003.

[18] L. Salvi, P. Plateroti, S. Balducci et al., "Abnormalities of retinal ganglion cell complex at optical coherence tomography in patients with type 2 diabetes: a sign of diabetic polyneuropathy, not retinopathy," *Journal of Diabetes and its Complications*, vol. 30, no. 3, pp. 469–476, 2016.

[19] S. Srinivasan, N. Pritchard, D. Vagenas et al., "Retinal tissue thickness is reduced in diabetic peripheral neuropathy," *Current Eye Research*, vol. 41, no. 10, pp. 1359–1366, 2016.

[20] R. Chakrabarti, C. A. Harper, and J. E. Keeffe, "Diabetic retinopathy management guidelines," *Expert Review of Ophthalmology*, vol. 7, no. 5, pp. 417–439, 2012.

[21] C. V. Regatieri, L. Branchini, J. Carmody, J. G. Fujimoto, and J. S. Duker, "Choroidal thickness in patients with diabetic retinopathy analyzed by spectral-domain optical coherence tomography," *Retina*, vol. 32, no. 3, pp. 563–568, 2012.

[22] C. Biallosterski, M. E. J. van Velthoven, R. P. J. Michels, R. O. Schlingemann, J. H. DeVries, and F. D. Verbraak, "Decreased optical coherence tomography-measured pericentral retinal thickness in patients with diabetes mellitus type 1 with minimal diabetic retinopathy," *The British Journal of Ophthalmology*, vol. 91, no. 9, pp. 1135–1138, 2007.

[23] E. B. Rodrigues, M. G. Urias, F. M. Penha et al., "Diabetes induces changes in neuroretina before retinal vessels: a spectral-domain optical coherence tomography study," *International Journal of Retina and Vitreus*, vol. 1, no. 1, p. 4, 2015.

[24] R. Dhasmana, S. Sah, and N. Gupta, "Study of retinal nerve fibre layer thickness in patients with diabetes mellitus using Fourier domain optical coherence tomography," *Journal of Clinical and Diagnostic Research*, vol. 10, no. 7, pp. NC05–NC09, 2016.

[25] A. Verma, P. K. Rani, R. Raman et al., "Is neuronal dysfunction an early sign of diabetic retinopathy? Microperimetry and spectral domain optical coherence tomography (SD-OCT) study in individuals with diabetes, but no diabetic retinopathy," *Eye*, vol. 23, no. 9, pp. 1824–1830, 2009.

[26] D. El-Fayoumi, N. M. Badr Eldine, A. F. Esmael, D. Ghalwash, and H. M. Soliman, "Retinal nerve fiber layer and ganglion cell complex thicknesses are reduced in children with type 1 diabetes with no evidence of vascular retinopathy," *Investigative Ophthalmology & Visual Science*, vol. 57, no. 13, pp. 5355–5360, 2016.

[27] N. Sayin, N. Kara, D. Pirhan et al., "Evaluation of subfoveal choroidal thickness in children with type 1 diabetes mellitus: an EDI-OCT study," *Seminars in Ophthalmology*, vol. 29, no. 1, pp. 27–31, 2014.

[28] O. Tan, V. Chopra, A. T. H. Lu et al., "Detection of macular ganglion cell loss in glaucoma by Fourier-domain optical coherence tomography," *Ophthalmology*, vol. 116, no. 12, pp. 2305–2314.e2, 2009.

[29] M. L. Smith and G. V. Glass, "Meta-analysis of psychotherapy outcome studies," *American Psychologist*, vol. 32, no. 9, pp. 752–760, 1977.

[30] E. Downie, M. E. Craig, S. Hing, J. Cusumano, A. K. F. Chan, and K. C. Donaghue, "Continued reduction in the prevalence of retinopathy in adolescents with type 1 diabetes," *Diabetes Care*, vol. 34, no. 11, pp. 2368–2373, 2011.

[31] D. Dabelea, E. J. Mayer-Davis, S. Saydah et al., "Prevalence of type 1 and type 2 diabetes among children and adolescents from 2001 to 2009," *JAMA*, vol. 311, no. 17, pp. 1778–1786, 2014.

[32] B. S. Olsen, A. K. Sjølie, P. Hougaard et al., "The significance of the prepubertal diabetes duration for the development of retinopathy and nephropathy in patients with type 1 diabetes," *Journal of Diabetes and its Complications*, vol. 18, no. 3, pp. 160–164, 2004.

[33] J. U. Sheth, A. Giridhar, B. Rajesh, and M. Gopalakrishnan, "Characterization of macular choroidal thickness in ischemic and nonischemic diabetic maculopathy," *Retina*, vol. 37, no. 3, pp. 522–528, 2017.

[34] M. Centofanti, S. Bonini, G. Manni, C. Guinetti-Neuschüler, M. G. Bucci, and A. Harris, "Do sex and hormonal status influence choroidal circulation?," *The British Journal of Ophthalmology*, vol. 84, no. 7, pp. 786-787, 2000.

[35] C. Mapelli, L. Dell'Arti, G. Barteselli et al., "Choroidal volume variations during childhood," *Investigative Ophthalmology & Visual Science*, vol. 54, no. 10, pp. 6841–6845, 2013.

[36] H. W. van Dijk, F. D. Verbraak, P. H. Kok et al., "Decreased retinal ganglion cell layer thickness in patients with type 1 diabetes," *Invest Ophthalmol Vis Sci*, vol. 51, no. 7, pp. 3660–3665, 2010.

[37] H. W. van Dijk, P. H. B. Kok, M. Garvin et al., "Selective loss of inner retinal layer thickness in type 1 diabetic patients with minimal diabetic retinopathy," *Investigative Ophthalmology & Visual Science*, vol. 50, no. 7, pp. 3404–3409, 2009.

[38] H. W. van Dijk, F. D. Verbraak, P. H. B. Kok et al., "Early neurodegeneration in the retina of type 2 diabetic patients," *Investigative Ophthalmology & Visual Science*, vol. 53, no. 6, pp. 2715–2719, 2012.

[39] S. Srinivasan, N. Pritchard, G. P. Sampson et al., "Focal loss volume of ganglion cell complex in diabetic neuropathy," *Clinical and Experimental Optometry*, vol. 99, no. 6, pp. 526–534, 2016.

[40] S. Srinivasan, N. Pritchard, G. P. Sampson et al., "Retinal thickness profile of individuals with diabetes," *Ophthalmic & Physiological Optics*, vol. 36, no. 2, pp. 158–166, 2016.

[41] L. Pierro, L. Iuliano, M. V. Cicinelli, G. Casalino, and F. Bandello, "Retinal neurovascular changes appear earlier in type 2 diabetic patients," *European Journal of Ophthalmology*, vol. 27, no. 3, pp. 346–351, 2018.

9

Neurophysiological Evidence for a Compensatory Activity during a Simple Oddball Task in Adolescents with Type 1 Diabetes Mellitus

Tereza Vitvarová,[1] David Neumann,[1] Radka Šimáková,[2] and Jan Kremláček[3]

[1]*Department of Pediatrics, University Hospital Hradec Kralove, Faculty of Medicine in Hradec Kralove, Charles University, Hradec Kralove, Czech Republic*
[2]*Philosophy Faculty, Palacky University Olomouc, Olomouc, Czech Republic*
[3]*Department of Pathological Physiology, Faculty of Medicine in Hradec Kralove, Charles University, Hradec Kralove, Czech Republic*

Correspondence should be addressed to Jan Kremláček; jan.kremlacek@lfhk.cuni.cz

Academic Editor: Marco Songini

Objective. The poor metabolic control in type 1 diabetes mellitus (T1D) has a negative impact on the developing brain. Hyperglycemia and glycemic fluctuations disrupt mainly executive functions. To assess a hypothesized deficit of the executive functions, we evaluated visual processing and reaction time in an oddball task. *Methods*. Oddball visual event-related potentials (ERPs), reaction time, and pattern-reversal visual evoked potentials (VEPs) were examined in a cohort of twenty-two 12- to 18-year-old T1D patients without diabetic retinopathy at normal glycemia and in nineteen 10- to 21-year-old healthy controls. *Results*. The P100 peak time of the VEPs was significantly prolonged in T1D patients compared with the control group ($p < 0.017$). In contrast to the deteriorated sensory response, the area under the curve of the P3b component of the ERPs was significantly larger ($p = 0.035$) in patients, while reaction time in the same task did not differ between groups ($p = 0.713$). *Conclusions*. The deterioration on a sensory level, enhanced activity during cognitive processing, and balanced behavioral response support the view that neuroplasticity counterbalances the neural impairment by enhanced cognitive processing to achieve normal behavioral performance in T1D adolescents.

1. Introduction

Executive functions (EFs) have a pivotal role in controlling adaptive behavior, activating motivation, and maintaining or changing the direction of action, thereby influencing various life activities, for example, school readiness and school success [1]. Altered EFs are thought to contribute to suboptimal adherence to treatment regimens in type 1 diabetes mellitus (T1D) [2–4], and neurodevelopmental problems are assumed to precede poor metabolic control [5].

Consequently, hypoglycemia and prolonged periods of hyperglycemia have a negative impact on the developing nervous system and can harm cognitive processes [6].

Such interrelated processes could send the patient's condition into a spiral of deterioration; therefore, an understanding of EFs in T1D is clinically important.

Various performance measures and rating inventories are widely used to assess EFs [7]. Aside from these neuropsychological approaches, objective neurophysiological methods offer noninvasive evaluation of the EFs via brain activity recording. The widely used oddball electrophysiological test presents two types of stimuli with different probabilities [8]. To succeed in the oddball task, one must follow the stream of stimuli for approximately 5 minutes, differentiate between rare and frequent stimuli, and respond selectively to the rare, or target, stimulus. On the neurobiological level, such behavior requires not only effective sensory and motor processing but also attention as part of inhibitory control, as well as working memory, both of which are core elements of executive functioning [1]. On a neural level, the response to the target stimuli evokes the P3b component of an event-related potential (ERP) [9, 10]. P3b originates from the activation of many regions of the neocortex and limbic system. It can be recorded noninvasively from the scalp as a positive potential with a maximum in the centroparietal area [11]. In the oddball test, a choice reaction time can also be recorded as a behavioral measure.

Adolescents with T1D constitute a risk group for suboptimal glycemic control. In the present study, we investigated whether the generally observed drop in therapy adherence in these patients is linked to a prolonged or delayed P3b component as an electrophysiological marker of EF impairment.

2. Methods

2.1. Study Design. In our observational case-control study, we compared a group of adolescents with T1D to an age- and gender-matched control group. The study was approved by the Ethical Committee of the University Hospital Hradec Kralove (numbers 201511 S10P and 201511S 2sP) and conducted according to the principles of the Declaration of Helsinki [12]. Patients were invited to join the study during regular visits to their diabetologist, and each invited patient was asked to bring a friend as a control subject. Attention-deficit/hyperactivity disorder, learning disorders, and retinopathy or other visual deficit were study exclusion criteria. After being informed about the study, all participants and their parents signed informed consent documents.

2.2. Participants, Diabetes, and Glycemic History. For the study, we recruited twenty-two adolescent patients with T1D, preferably with a known long-term history of poor compliance with therapy, older than eleven years of age, with disease duration over two years. All of them were frequently consulted on an outpatient and inpatient basis, alone, with parents, or in a group of peers, to improve their glycemic control. T1D duration, school performance (excellent, modest, and inferior), serious T1D complications (diabetic ketoacidosis with hospital admission, severe hypoglycemia, and long-lasting glycemic excursions), insulin regimen (human insulin, insulin analogs, and continuous subcutaneous insulin infusion), and mode of blood glucose monitoring were recorded, along with therapy-related measures of hemoglobin A1c (HbA1c) in a one-year period before testing and glycemia when tested.

2.3. HbA1c and Glycemia Assessment. Glycated hemoglobin was measured by an automated high-performance liquid chromatography gradient elution analyzer (Arkray Adams A1c HA-8180, Arkray Inc., Japan). Long-lasting glycemic variability was expressed as the coefficient of variability of HbA1c [13]. To determine mean and variability of the glycated hemoglobin, we used three or four measurements recorded over at least one year before the experiment. Actual glycemia just before the electrophysiological procedure was determined using personal glucose meters conforming to the ISO 15197:2013 standard. For post hoc evaluation, we calculated an exposure score as the sum of the z-transformed duration of T1D and glycemic control [14].

2.4. Electrophysiological Procedures. Landolt rings (EN ISO 8596) and the hole-in-the-card test determined subjects' visual acuity and ocular dominance, respectively. Subjects used their dominant eye in all tests.

Pathology in the sense of prolonged latency or decreased amplitude of P3b may be caused by an impairment of sensory processing. Since we used a visual oddball paradigm, we also evaluated visual acuity and recorded visual evoked potentials (VEPs) using equipment described below to assess sensory processing. In particular, we measured the pattern-reversal P100 peak, reflecting primary visual cortex activation [15].

ERP and VEP measurements were performed in a darkened, sound-attenuated, electromagnetically shielded room with a background luminance of 0.1 cd/m^2. During experiments, the subjects sat in a comfortable dental chair with a neck support to reduce muscle artifacts. A near-infrared camera monitored correct fixation. All stimuli were presented on a 21″ computer monitor (Vision Master Pro 510, Iiyama, Japan) subtending $37^\circ \times 28^\circ$ of the visual field from an observing distance of 0.6 m. Stimuli for VEPs were presented using the Visual Stimulus Generator 2/5 (CRS Ltd., UK) at a vertical refresh frequency of 105 Hz. The ERP stimuli were presented by Psychtoolbox-3 [16] at a vertical refresh frequency of 75 Hz. Recorded epochs were synchronized with a backward trace of the monitor's electron beam just before the first video frame of an appropriate stimulus change.

VEPs/ERPs were recorded from six unipolar derivations (O_Z, P_Z, C_Z, F_Z, and O_L; O_R—5 cm left and right from the O_Z) with a right earlobe reference (A_2). The minimum set of recording derivations was chosen on the basis of a previous topographical study concerning the scalp distribution of ERPs [9] and VEPs [17]. The ground electrode was connected to the reference. All electrode impedances were kept below 10 kΩ. The signal was amplified in the frequency band of 0.3–100 Hz (PSYLAB, System 5, Contact Precision Instruments, USA).

2.5. Cognitive Event-Related Potentials. ERPs were recorded during the visual oddball test in which the white letter X (frequent nontarget stimulus with a probability of 75%) and Arabic digits 1–9 (rare target stimuli with a probability of 25%) appeared pseudorandomly. The "X" or the digit, subtending $5.7^\circ \times 6.3^\circ$, was displayed for 500 ms in the center of the black stimulus field, followed by a blank screen with a fixation point displayed for 500 ms. The mean luminance was 1 cd/m^2. The subjects were instructed to press a handheld button as soon as possible whenever a rare stimulus appeared. This arrangement enabled an evaluation of the latency and amplitude of the main ERP peak P3b and the reaction time. Subjects learned the experimental task in a short training session before the test.

Twenty poststimulus EEG epochs of 1000 ms after target stimuli and 20 randomly selected epochs after nontarget stimuli were sampled at 250 Hz frequency. Epochs with absolute amplitude exceeding 70 μV were rejected. The rest of the responses were smoothed with a second-order polynomial Savitzky-Golay filter across 21 samples. The mean interpeak amplitudes (P3b − (N2 + N3)/2), the peak time of the P3b response, and the reaction times were evaluated offline.

Table 1: Demographic and diabetes-related characteristics of participating adolescents. Values in the table are expressed as the median and the first and third quartiles.

	T1D patients	Control group	p
Number of subjects	22 (10 males, 12 females)	19 (8 males, 11 females)	
Age (years)	15.5 (14.0–16.0)	16.0 (14.5–17.0)	0.231[a]
Visual acuity, logMAR (–)	0.00 (−0.10–0.00)	0.00 (−0.05–0.00)	0.217[a]
Age of T1D diagnosis (years)	8.0 (5.0–10.0)		
Duration of illness (years)	8.0 (5.0–10.8)		
HbA1c IFCC standard (mmol/mol)	68.5 (63.7–76.3)		
HbA1c NGSP (%)	8.4 (8.0–9.1)		
HbA1c coef. variability (%)	7 (5–10)		
Exposure (–)	0.07 (−1.12–0.73)		

[a]Wilcoxon rank-sum test.

2.6. Pattern-Reversal Visual Evoked Potentials. Forty reversals of a high-contrast black and white checkerboard pattern within 20 seconds evoked pattern-reversal VEPs. Two checkerboard stimulations with check sizes of 40 arcmin (PR-VEP 40′) and 20 arcmin (PR-VEP 20′) were used. The mean luminance of 17 cd/m^2 stayed constant. The subjects were instructed to keep their gaze on the fixation point during the recording. EEG poststimulus epochs of 440 ms duration were sampled at 500 Hz. Epochs with absolute amplitudes larger than 70 μV were rejected. The rest of the responses were smoothed with a second-order polynomial Savitzky-Golay filter across 21 samples. The number of samples was determined empirically to remove high-frequency noise. Both VEP variants were examined twice. The mean interpeak amplitudes (P100 − (N75 + N145)/2) and the peak time of P100 were evaluated offline.

2.7. Analysis and Statistics. Signal filtering, extraction of the parameters of interest, and data plotting were conducted in MATLAB Release 2017a (MathWorks, USA). Statistical analysis was performed with the "nortest" package in the software R 3.4.0 [18]. The normality of the data distribution was assessed by the Anderson-Darling test. To compare variables between groups, we used a Wilcoxon rank-sum test or a t-test for data with a nonnormal or normal distribution, respectively. The results are presented as the median and interquartile range. Relationships between continuous clinical, behavioral, and EF markers of interest were calculated using Pearson's correlation coefficient or Spearman's rank correlation, depending on the normality or nonnormality of the data distribution. Differences among groups defined by categorical variables (sex, insulin regimen, T1D complications, and school performance) were evaluated using ANOVA with post hoc t-tests corrected for multiple comparisons. Gender representation was compared between groups by Fisher's exact test. The level of statistical significance was preset to $p < 0.05$.

3. Results

Twenty-two adolescents with T1D (12 girls and 10 boys aged 12–18 years) were selected. The control group consisted of 19 age-matched healthy friends of patients (11 girls and 8 boys aged 10–21 years). Table 1 lists characteristics of the study groups. Patients were treated on fixed insulin regimens with either insulin applicators (10 patients) or insulin pumps (12 patients). They used personal glucometers as their standard monitoring devices and were familiar with occasional measurement by glucose sensors. In the T1D group, electrophysiological testing was performed at a blood glucose level of 3.9 to 10.0 mmol/l. There was no apparent retinopathy within our group, which urges absence of microvascular changes [19].

Brain reactions to stimuli in the oddball paradigm and other sensory responses were reliably recorded in all subjects (see Figure 1). There were no differences between the group of adolescents with T1D and the controls in age ($p = 0.231$), gender ($p = 1.0$), visual acuity ($p = 0.217$), or amplitudes of sensory responses ($p > 0.066$) (see Table 2). Nevertheless, in the T1D group, we found a significant delay in the P100 peak time in PR-VEP 40′ and PR-VEP 20′ (T1D subjects (median, interquartile range): 107, 105–113 ms; 110, 108–114 ms, resp.; controls: 104, 103–106 ms; 108, 106–110 ms, resp.); $p = 0.017$ and $p = 0.012$.

In the P3b component, neither the peak time difference of 16 ms between groups (T1D group: 384, 365–396 ms; controls: 368, 348–386 ms) ($p = 0.181$) nor the difference in P3b amplitude at the peak maximum (T1D subjects: 27.1, 21.2–33.5 μV; controls: 23.6, 19.7–28.8 μV) ($p = 0.331$) were significant.

However, the increase in P3b amplitude in the T1D group became prominent after the peak maximum (see Figure 2). The area under the curve (AUC) for the interval from 360 to 500 ms was significantly larger in the T1D group (2994; 2541–4047 μV·ms) than in the control group (2446; 1838–2987 μV·ms), $p = 0.035$.

In clinical diagnostics, a significant difference between groups is not directly usable; therefore, we assessed the discriminative potential of statistically significant parameters by an ROC (receiver operating characteristic) analysis [20]. Each threshold was determined as the point of maximal sensitivity and specificity [21]. The thresholds were as follows: P3b AUC, 2487 μV ms; P100 peak in PR-VEP 40′, 105 ms; and P100 peak in PR-VEP 20′, 109 ms. For those thresholds, the ROCs showed sensitivity of 53, 58, and 68%,

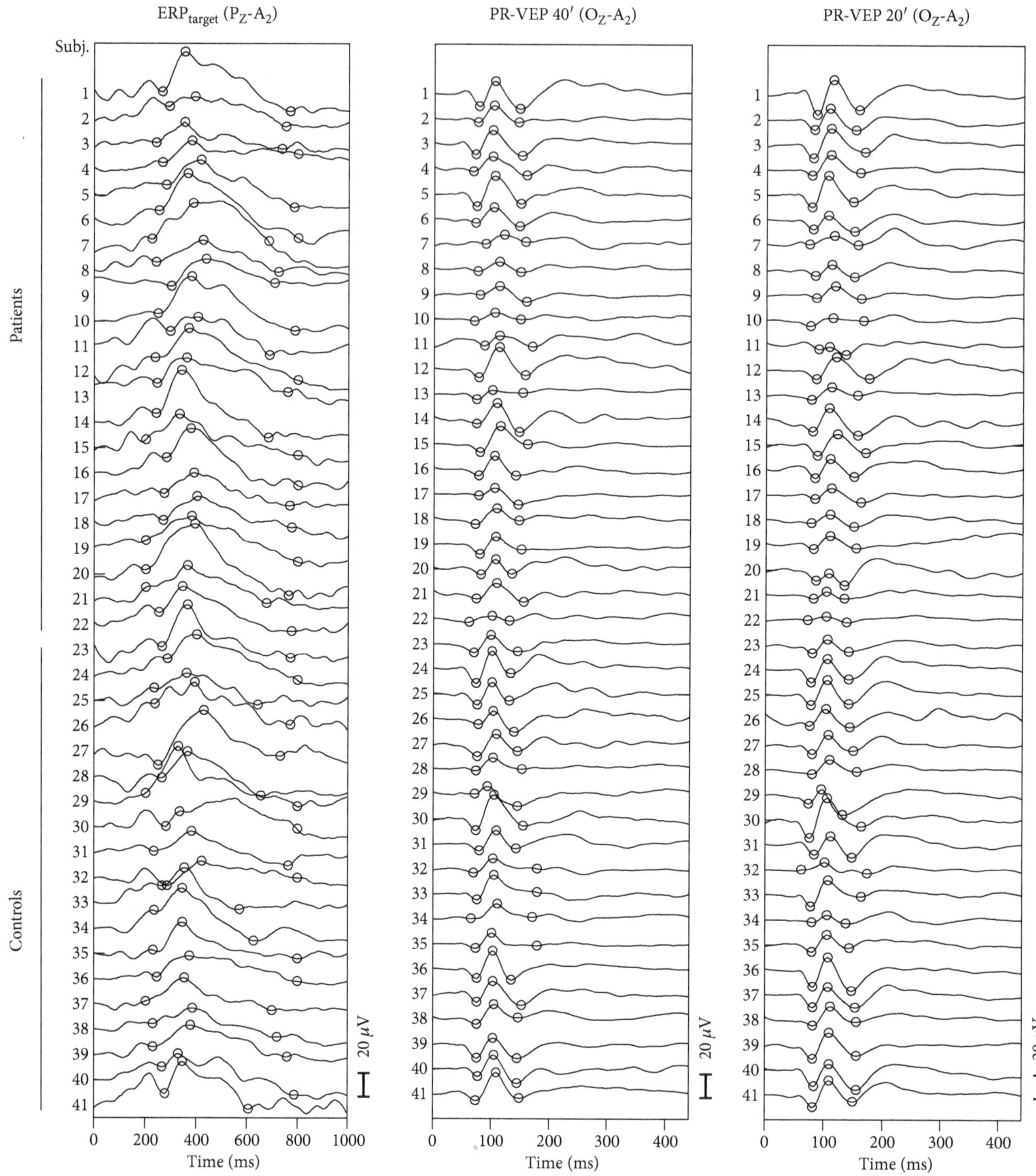

FIGURE 1: Individual ERP and VEP traces. Single subjects' ERPs and VEPs are plotted as thick or thin lines for patients and controls, respectively. The columns correspond to the selected derivation of examined ERP/VEPs, and the subjects' responses form the rows. The marked peaks were used for the statistical analysis. For the latency assessment, we used the middle marker; for amplitude, an average of two interpeak values (see Methods). There is an apparent increase in the area under curve of the P3b peak in the target ERP for patients, as we confirmed in the intergroup comparison ($p = 0.035$). Further, there is a slight but significant ($p < 0.016$) time shift of the middle marker of the pattern-reversal VEPs—the P100 peak—for both stimulation patterns (PR-VEP 40′ and 20′).

respectively, and specificity of 77, 73, and 64%, respectively. The control group was used to define a set of high-specificity (99.8%) reference limits. For P3b AUC, PR-VEP 40′ P100 latency, and PR-VEP 20′ P100 latency, respectively, 27% (6 patients), 27% (6), and 41% (9) of patients were outside these reference limits.

TABLE 2: Electrophysiological markers: comparisons between the T1D and control groups. The P3b component recorded in response to the visual oddball test was used to assess executive functions. Listed are the values for the target stimulus evaluated from the parietal derivation (P_Z–A_2). The sensory responses from the primary visual cortex were recorded in response to luminance reversal of checkerboard patterns with 40 arcmin and 20 arcmin squares, and peak P100 amplitude and latency were determined in the occipital derivation (O_Z–A_2). Values in the table are expressed as the median and the first and third quartiles.

	T1D patients $n = 22$	Control group $n = 19$	p
Responses related to executive functions			
P3b peak time (ms)	384 (365–396)	368 (348–386)	0.181[b]
P3b amplitude (μV)	27.1 (21.2–33.5)	23.6 (19.7–28.8)	0.331[b]
P3b area under the curve Amplitude × time (μV × ms)	2994 (2541–4047)	2446 (1838–2987)	**0.035** [b]
Reaction time (ms)	354 (333–384)	348 (332–372)	0.713[b]
The sensory responses of the primary visual cortex			
R40′ peak time (ms)	107 (105–113)	104 (103–106)	**0.017** [b]
R40′ amplitude (μV)	12.7 (8.6–17.2)	15.7 (12.2–18.9)	0.085[b]
R20′ peak time (ms)	110 (108–114)	108 (105–107)	**0.012** [a]
R20′ amplitude (μV)	10.0 (7.84–16.9)	16.0 (13.0–19.2)	0.066[b]

[a]Wilcoxon rank-sum test, [b]Student's t-test.

On the behavioral level, neither the reaction times (T1D subjects: 354, 333–384 ms; controls: 348, 332–372 ms), $p = 0.714$, nor the accuracy of the discrimination (median for both groups was 100%), $p = 0.24$, differed.

4. Post Hoc Analysis of EFs in T1D Subjects

4.1. Age of Onset and Duration of Diabetes. Subjects with T1D onset before 6 years ($n = 11$) showed no difference in age compared with those with T1D onset after 6 years and controls ($p = 0.179$). Subgroup comparison of P3b markers did not differ ($p > 0.393$).

4.2. Glycemic Control. The correlation analysis did not show any relationship between P3b markers (peak time, amplitude, and AUC) and HbA1c ($p > 0.146$) or HbA1c variability ($p > 0.317$); however, exposure score showed a significant relationship with P3b peak time (Pearson $r = -0.45$, $p = 0.034$). We did not find any significant correlation between P3b markers and T1D duration ($p > 0.130$) or age of its onset ($p > 0.303$).

When we grouped T1D patients by insulin regimen (insulin pump, $n = 12$; long-acting human insulins, $n = 6$; combination of short- and long-acting analogs, $n = 3$; human insulin/NPH insulin (excluded from comparison because of the small number of patients), $n = 1$), we found significant ($p = 0.038$) differences in the variability of the P3b peak time. The post hoc t-tests did not confirm ($p = 0.091$) shorter P3b latencies for long-acting analogs (366; 352–366 ms) than for insulin pump therapy (388; 383–405 ms) owing to correction for multiple comparisons. P3b amplitude and P3b AUC did not vary among therapies ($p > 0.09$). ANOVA also did not show any significant differences in the variability of P3b markers among patients grouped by T1D complications ($p > 0.427$) or school performance ($p > 0.463$).

In an attempt to reveal any possible dependency of P3b markers on clinical parameters, we conducted multiple linear regression analysis using age of T1D onset, disease duration, and average HbA1c as predictors. The linear models did not show any significant relation ($p > 0.164$).

5. Discussion

We compared behavioral performance and electrophysiological brain response during a simple discrimination task between a group of adolescents with T1D and age-matched controls to objectively evaluate the impairment of the executive control suggested by self-reported inventories [22, 23]. We expected a delayed peak time and a lower amplitude for the P3b component or a slower reaction time in adolescents with T1D as similar findings were described formerly [6, 24].

Although the T1D and control groups did not differ significantly in P3b peak time, we observed a trend toward a delayed P3b peak time in the T1D group as found in previous studies [6, 24]. In contrast to our expectations, however, we found that the P3b amplitude was larger in the patients, which confirmed the results of our statistical analysis for the AUC of the P3b component. The present study contrasts with a study by Shehata and Eltayeb [6] describing a drop in N2-P3b amplitude in 40 children (11.7 ± 2.3 years) during an auditory oddball task. We speculate it was likely disease severity that causes this disparity; while 95% of their patients experienced ketoacidosis, the proportion was just 27% among the patients in our study. Shehata and Eltayeb [6] note that the ketoacidosis was a significant factor that negatively correlated with almost all facets of cognitive performance they evaluated. Further, ketoacidosis causes significant morphological and functional brain changes in T1D patients compared to those without ketoacidosis [25].

Similar to our results, Überall et al., studying 29 adolescents with T1D (15.8 ± 3.1 years), did not find any significant

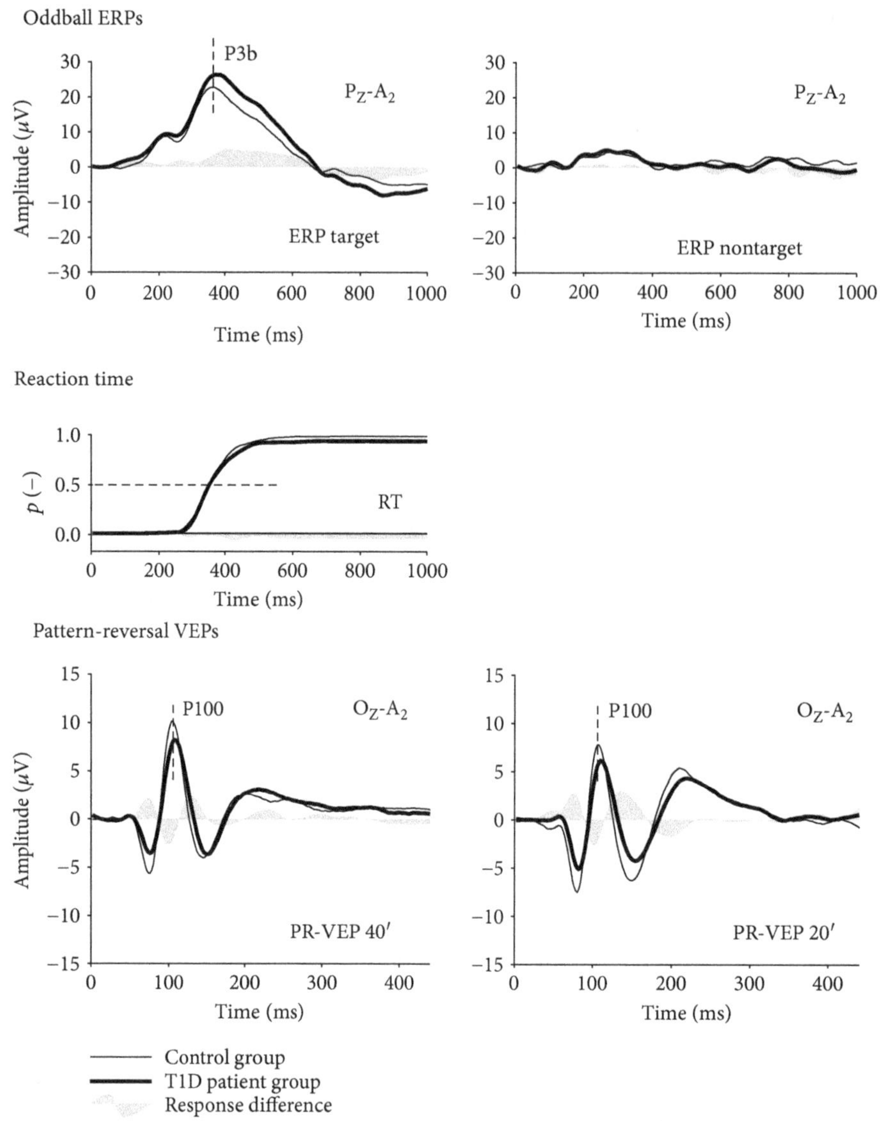

FIGURE 2: ERP and VEP grand averages in patients and controls. The patient and control grand average ERPs are plotted as the thick and thin lines, respectively; the between-group ERP difference is the gray area in the whole figure. The two horizontal gray lines show the level of variability, pointwise calculated as the mean plus 2.5 times the standard deviation of values in the first 60 ms for ERPs and 30 ms for VEPs. The first row depicts ERPs to target (left plot) and nontarget (right plot) stimuli in the oddball cognitive task, evaluated from the parietal derivation. The second row shows the cumulative distribution function of pressing the response button—the reaction time in response to the target stimulus. The pattern-reversal VEP PR-VEP 40′ (left plot) and PR-VEP 20′ (right plot), recorded in the central occipital derivation, are shown in the third row; motion-onset VEPs from the periphery (M-VEP 20°, left plot) and the central visual field (M-VEP C8°, right plot), recorded from the parietal derivation, are shown in the fourth row.

difference between them and the control group in the P3b amplitude recorded during visual oddball stimuli [24]; moreover, the grand average of patients' P3b component in their study apparently had a larger AUC than the grand average for controls (see Figure 2 in [24]).

The observed P3b amplitude augmentation in our study is consistent with a recent fMRI work by Gallardo-Moreno et al. [26]. They showed different activation of a brain network involved in a visuospatial working memory task in young adult T1D patients versus controls. Gallardo-Moreno et al. found extended and augmented BOLD signal in the inferior prefrontal cortex, basal ganglia, posterior cerebellum, and substantia nigra. These activation changes occurred without any difference in behavioral performance, consistent with our data and a study by Perantie et al. of young (5–16 years) T1D patients in the go/no-go task [14].

Considering the sensory-processing deficit on the way from the retina up to the primary visual area as indicated by the delayed P100 peak time of the pattern reversal VEPs, we assume that the enhancement of the P3b component reflects compensatory brain activity enabling to achieve a normal behavioral reaction in our T1D subjects.

A similar brain mechanism that can be interpreted as a compensatory response has also been described for adult T1D patients with retinitis in an fMRI study by Wessels et al. [27]. The compensatory neuroplasticity represents a general mechanism described for various pathological (e.g., cognitive load in multiple sclerosis [28]) and physiological (e.g., change detection in aging [29]) conditions involving neural disturbances, and we assume it is the most likely explanation for our results.

Comparing to clinical data, we did not find any relation between the P3b markers and the age of T1D diagnosis (2–16 years), disease duration (2–13 years), or HbA1c (6.5–13.6%), similar to the study of Überall and his colleagues [24].

The used oddball paradigm incorporates a motoric response, which is reflected in prestimulus (readiness potential and negative slope potential) and poststimulus ERP components (motoric potential followed by reafferent sensory response); for review, see [30]. These components might modulate the P3b response. In a further exploration, an evaluation of the motor-related cortical potentials could bring more answers about the compensatory activity we observed.

We emphasize that the selective reaction time and brain responses to oddball stimuli present a response to a rather simple task, and as such, it might not capture the exhaustion and maladaptation of children and adolescents with T1D under the demanding circumstances of T1D treatment and life. The difference between evaluation of EFs by ERPs and multilevel assessment by inventories is worth noting. The second measures broad real-life interplay, taking into account quality of life, treatment adherence, or parental EFs [31]. It shows the frequent failure of EFs in T1D adolescents [4, 32] with a bidirectional consequence for glycemic control and an increased level of T1D-related risk. ERPs analyze EF processing far away from the complexity of life. However, the method reflects, with millisecond accuracy, key elements of executive control such as attention, short-term visual working memory, and decision-making. There is no straightforward relationship between the results of the two approaches, and this situation is not unique, as performance-based measures score different facets of EFs compared with rating measures [33].

6. Conclusions

The behavioral performance of adolescents with T1D in a simple oddball test of executive functions was fully comparable with that of the control group; however, the AUC increase of the P3b component suggests a neural mechanism compensating for a subclinical visual impairment manifested by the delayed P100 peak time of pattern-reversal VEPs.

Further research on how adolescents with T1D make their self-management decisions based on EFs should follow two questions: first, whether they have diminished, normal, or advanced functional neurophysiological abilities for such decisions and, additionally, why their life outcomes drop back compared with adolescents without T1D.

Abbreviations

ANOVA: Analysis of variance
AUC: Area under the curve
BOLD: Blood oxygenation level-dependent
EFs: Executive functions
ERPs: Event-related potentials
fMRI: Functional magnetic resonance imaging
HbA1c: Hemoglobin A1c
N145: Negative peak of pattern-reversal VEPs
N2: Negative peak of oddball ERPs
N75: Negative peak of pattern-reversal VEPs
P100: Positive peak of pattern-reversal VEPs
P3b: Positive component of the oddball ERPs
PR-VEP 20′: VEPs to pattern reversal of 20 arcmin checkerboard
PR-VEP 40′: VEPs to pattern reversal of 40 arcmin checkerboard
ROC: Receiver operating characteristic
T1D: Type 1 diabetes mellitus
VEPs: Visual evoked potentials.

Conflicts of Interest

The authors declare that they have no conflict of interest.

Acknowledgments

This work was supported by MH CZ—DRO (UHHK, 00179906) and by the Charles University project PROGRES Q40/07.

Supplementary Materials

Table 1: demographic, clinical, behavioral, and electrophysiological data used for statistical evaluation. The first row describes variables as follows: ID: subject identification number; Group: T1D (patients), CON (controls); Sex: 1 (female), 0 (male); Age: age at the time of examination; T1D duration: illness duration; Recorded eye: dominant eye examined; Visual Acuity: fraction 1~4/4 (measured from 4 meters); HbA1c_actual: hemoglobin A1c at time of examination; HbA1c_avg: average hemoglobin A1c; HbA1c_var: variability of hemoglobin A1c; R40_latency: implicit time of dominant peak P100 of pattern-reversal VEPs evoked by reversing chessboard with checks of 40′; R20_latency: similar to preceding but evoked with checks 20′; M20_latency: peak time of dominant peak N2 of motion-onset VEPs evoked by radial motion outside of central 20°; C8_latency: similar to preceding but evoked by motion in central 8°; P300_latency: peak time of dominant peak P300 of ERPs recorded during oddball test; R40_amplitude, R20_amplitude, M20_amplitude, C8_amplitude, and P300_amplitude: amplitudes for appropriate VEP/ERP peaks; P300_auc: area under curve of the peek P300; Reaction_time: reaction time recorded during the oddball test. For details of determining single variables, see Methods. Every row from the third to 43th lists subjects' data.

References

[1] A. Diamond, "Executive functions," *Annual Review of Psychology*, vol. 64, no. 1, pp. 135–168, 2013.

[2] D. C. Duke and M. A. Harris, "Executive function, adherence, and glycemic control in adolescents with type 1 diabetes: a literature review," *Current Diabetes Reports*, vol. 14, no. 10, p. 532, 2014.

[3] K. K. Hood, C. M. Peterson, J. M. Rohan, and D. Drotar, "Association between adherence and glycemic control in pediatric type 1 diabetes: a meta-analysis," *Pediatrics*, vol. 124, no. 6, pp. e1171–e1179, 2009.

[4] K. M. Perez, N. J. Patel, J. H. Lord et al., "Executive function in adolescents with type 1 diabetes: relationship to adherence, glycemic control, and psychosocial outcomes," *Journal of Pediatric Psychology*, vol. 42, pp. 636–646, 2017.

[5] C. Nylander, H. Toivonen, S. Nasic, U. Söderström, Y. Tindberg, and E. Fernell, "Children and adolescents with type 1 diabetes and high HbA1c—a neurodevelopmental perspective," *Acta Paediatrica*, vol. 102, no. 4, pp. 410–415, 2013.

[6] G. Shehata and A. Eltayeb, "Cognitive function and event-related potentials in children with type 1 diabetes mellitus," *Journal of Child Neurology*, vol. 25, no. 4, pp. 469–474, 2010.

[7] L. B. Smith, B. B. Kugler, A. B. Lewin, D. C. Duke, E. A. Storch, and G. R. Geffken, "Executive functioning, parenting stress, and family factors as predictors of diabetes management in pediatric patients with type 1 diabetes using intensive regimens," *Children's Health Care*, vol. 43, no. 3, pp. 234–252, 2014.

[8] R. West, H. Schwarb, and B. N. Johnson, "The influence of age and individual differences in executive function on stimulus processing in the oddball task," *Cortex*, vol. 46, no. 4, pp. 550–563, 2010.

[9] C. C. Duncan, R. J. Barry, J. F. Connolly et al., "Event-related potentials in clinical research: guidelines for eliciting, recording, and quantifying mismatch negativity, P300, and N400," *Clinical Neurophysiology*, vol. 120, no. 11, pp. 1883–1908, 2009.

[10] J. Polich and K. L. Herbst, "P300 as a clinical assay: rationale, evaluation, and findings," *International Journal of Psychophysiology*, vol. 38, no. 1, pp. 3–19, 2000.

[11] J. Polich, "Updating P300: an integrative theory of P3a and P3b," *Clinical Neurophysiology*, vol. 118, no. 10, pp. 2128–2148, 2007.

[12] World Medical Association, "World Medical Association Declaration of Helsinki. Ethical principles for medical research involving human subjects," *JAMA*, vol. 310, no. 20, pp. 2191–2194, 2013.

[13] C. Gorst, C. S. Kwok, S. Aslam et al., "Long-term glycemic variability and risk of adverse outcomes: a systematic review and meta-analysis," *Diabetes Care*, vol. 38, no. 12, pp. 2354–2369, 2015.

[14] D. C. Perantie, A. Lim, J. Wu et al., "Effects of prior hypoglycemia and hyperglycemia on cognition in children with type 1 diabetes mellitus," *Pediatric Diabetes*, vol. 9, no. 2, pp. 87–95, 2008.

[15] F. Di Russo, S. Pitzalis, G. Spitoni et al., "Identification of the neural sources of the pattern-reversal VEP," *NeuroImage*, vol. 24, no. 3, pp. 874–886, 2005.

[16] D. H. Brainard, "The psychophysics toolbox," *Spatial Vision*, vol. 10, no. 4, pp. 433–436, 1997.

[17] J. V. Odom, M. Bach, M. Brigell et al., "ISCEV standard for clinical visual evoked potentials: (2016 update)," *Documenta Ophthalmologica*, vol. 133, no. 1, pp. 1–9, 2016.

[18] R Development Core Team, *R: A Language and Environment for Statistical Computing*, R Foundation for Statistical Computing, 2017.

[19] R. Broe, "Early risk stratification in pediatric type 1 diabetes," *Acta Ophthalmologica*, vol. 93, no. 5, p. 490, 2015.

[20] X. Robin, N. Turck, A. Hainard et al., "pROC: an open-source package for R and S+ to analyze and compare ROC curves," *BMC Bioinformatics*, vol. 12, no. 1, p. 77, 2011.

[21] W. J. Youden, "Index for rating diagnostic tests," *Cancer*, vol. 3, no. 1, pp. 32–35, 1950.

[22] C. M. Ryan, E. van Duinkerken, and C. Rosano, "Neurocognitive consequences of diabetes," *The American Psychologist*, vol. 71, no. 7, pp. 563–576, 2016.

[23] A. Cato and T. Hershey, "Cognition and type 1 diabetes in children and adolescents," *Diabetes Spectrum*, vol. 29, no. 4, pp. 197–202, 2016.

[24] M. Überall, C. Renner, S. Edl, E. Parzinger, and D. Wenzel, "VEP and ERP abnormalities in children and adolescents with prepubertal onset of insulin-dependent diabetes mellitus," *Neuropediatrics*, vol. 27, no. 2, pp. 88–93, 1996.

[25] F. J. Cameron, S. E. Scratch, C. Nadebaum et al., "Neurological consequences of diabetic ketoacidosis at initial presentation of type 1 diabetes in a prospective cohort study of children," *Diabetes Care*, vol. 37, no. 6, pp. 1554–1562, 2014.

[26] G. B. Gallardo-Moreno, A. A. Gonzalez-Garrido, E. Gudayol-Ferre, and J. Guardia-Olmos, "Type 1 diabetes modifies brain activation in young patients while performing visuospatial working memory tasks," *Journal of Diabetes Research*, vol. 2015, Article ID 703512, 9 pages, 2015.

[27] A. M. Wessels, S. A. R. B. Rombouts, S. Simsek et al., "Microvascular disease in type 1 diabetes alters brain activation: a functional magnetic resonance imaging study," *Diabetes*, vol. 55, no. 2, pp. 334–340, 2006.

[28] B. Audoin, D. Ibarrola, J. P. Ranjeva et al., "Compensatory cortical activation observed by fMRI during a cognitive task at the earliest stage of multiple sclerosis," *Human Brain Mapping*, vol. 20, no. 2, pp. 51–58, 2003.

[29] E. T. Sciberras-Lim and A. J. Lambert, "Attentional orienting and dorsal visual stream decline: review of behavioral and EEG studies," *Frontiers in Aging Neuroscience*, vol. 9, p. 246, 2017.

[30] F. Di Russo, M. Berchicci, C. Bozzacchi, R. L. Perri, S. Pitzalis, and D. Spinelli, "Beyond the "Bereitschaftspotential": action preparation behind cognitive functions," *Neuroscience & Biobehavioral Reviews*, vol. 78, pp. 57–81, 2017.

[31] E. R. Goethals, M. de Wit, N. van Broeck et al., "Child and parental executive functioning in type 1 diabetes: their unique and interactive role toward treatment adherence and glycemic control," *Pediatric Diabetes*, vol. 19, no. 3, pp. 520–526, 2018.

10

Teens with Type 1 Diabetes: How Does Their Nutrition Measure Up?

Eleanor Race Mackey,[1,2] Lyndsay O'Brecht,[2] Clarissa S. Holmes,[3,4] Marni Jacobs,[1,2] and Randi Streisand[1,2]

[1]*Children's National Health System, Psychology, Washington, DC, USA*
[2]*University of Toronto, Toronto, Ontario, Canada*
[3]*Virginia Commonwealth University, Pediatrics, Richmond, VA, USA*
[4]*Georgetown University, Psychiatry, Washington, DC, USA*

Correspondence should be addressed to Eleanor Race Mackey; emackey@cnmc.org

Academic Editor: Aila Ahola

Objective. To characterize the intake of macronutrient and fiber in adolescents with type 1 diabetes (T1D) and examine their association with health indicators. *Methods.* Baseline data from an RCT were examined. Adolescent-parent dyads ($n = 257$, mean age 12 ± 1.2 years, 49.4% girls) reported dietary intake via two separate 24-hour recall interviews during a two-week period. Demographic and medical variables were abstracted from questionnaires and medical charts. *Results.* Controlling for demographic and diet variables, a higher percentage of daily energy intake from fats was associated with poorer HbA1c. In contrast, an association between higher percent of energy intake from proteins and carbohydrates was found with higher systolic and diastolic BP, respectively. *Conclusions.* Many early adolescents with T1D did not meet diabetes nutritional guidelines. Lower adherence to nutritional guidelines, specifically more than recommended energy intake from fats, was associated with poorer HbA1c. Addressing nutritional guidelines and increasing adherence as part of treatment may improve health outcomes for youth with T1D.

1. Introduction

Type 1 diabetes (T1D), one of the most common childhood chronic illnesses, requires adherence to a complex daily routine for proper management [1, 2]. Poorer diabetes management and glycemic control increase risk for poorer outcomes, both concurrently and later in life [3]. However, adolescence is characterized by a period of poor adherence and glycemic control, in part due to the developmental task of establishing independence from caregivers, which often has negative consequences for diabetes management [4, 5].

Adhering to diabetes-specific guidelines for percentage of daily energy intake of macronutrients (i.e., carbohydrates, proteins, and fats), as well as intake of dietary fiber, is especially important for individuals with T1D to promote good ambient glycemic control and to prevent long-term consequences including cardiovascular disease [5–9]. Adolescents may choose to exert independence through their food choices, which, in turn, can be associated with the declines in glycemic control frequently found during this developmental period [1, 10]. Therefore, examination of the nutritional behaviors of adolescents with T1D and the connection between macronutrient and fiber intake and critical health indicators linked to diabetes-related complications and cardiovascular disease is important.

The dietary composition of adolescents with T1D is not likely to significantly differ from the general population, which is generally related to high fat consumption (e.g., [11]); however, the stakes are clearly higher for those with T1D due to the increased likelihood of poor health outcomes secondary to T1D. Additionally, research specifically comparing youth with and without diabetes found that youth with diabetes have higher fat intake [12]. Dietary research with adults who have type 1 diabetes also indicates difficulty adhering to nutrition guidelines (e.g., [13, 14]). Given the importance of dietary intake to glycemic control and to the health of youth with T1D, the nutritional content and behaviors of this population merit careful investigation.

Nutritional guidelines based on both the American Diabetes Association (ADA; [15]) and the International Society for Pediatric and Adolescent Diabetes (ISPAD; [7]) support using medical nutritional therapy (MNT) in order to optimize the metabolic profiles (i.e., lower LDL plasma levels) of individuals with diabetes and to offset risk factors for cardiovascular disease [4, 5, 9]. Specifically, MNT recommends provision of individualized nutrition plans as an essential component of disease management for type 1 diabetes. MNT can include counseling about carbohydrate counting, as well as specific recommendations for nutritional intake and associated behavioral strategies [15, 16]. Moreover, planning should take into account insulin regimen and personal and familial food preferences [7, 15]. For example, nutrition recommendations may vary based on insulin regimen. Conventional insulin therapy generally refers to a more structured insulin regimen in which youth have a set range of carbohydrate intakes per meal and fewer injections (e.g., 2–3 per day). Individuals on flexible/basal bolus therapy (administered via multiple injections or a pump) are able to use an insulin-to-carbohydrate ratio for food intake to tailor their insulin administration to what they choose to eat [9]. Flexible insulin regimens are associated with better glycemic control [17], yet they may inadvertently facilitate consumption of unhealthy foods and use of processed/packaged foods. The latter approach, in particular, may be appealing to the adolescent because it simplifies carbohydrate counting [18].

Few studies have explored specific macronutrient and fiber intake in adolescents with T1D. Initial evidence of suboptimal nutrition and its adverse relation to metabolic control has been demonstrated [19–23]. Although dietary intake is generally associated with concurrent glycemic control measured via continuous glucose monitoring [22], a direct intervention to improve dietary behaviors in youth did not result in improved glycemic control [24], suggesting that adherence to nutritional guidelines may be necessary for improved glycemic control, but not sufficient on its own. However, dietary behaviors also relate to other health indicators. For example, dietary intake, specifically low consumption of vegetables and fish, is related to retinal problems in youth with T1D [25]. Higher fiber intake is associated with reduced inflammation and lower mortality risk in adults with T1D [26, 27].

Given the association of dietary intake with health outcomes, the first aim of the current study is to describe the macronutrient and fiber intake of early adolescents with T1D. The second goal is to evaluate the association of macronutrient and fiber intake with important health indicators including glycemic control (hemoglobin A1c; HbA1c), obesity as indicated by body mass index, dyslipidemia as indexed by levels of plasma LDL, and hypertension as indexed by systolic and diastolic blood pressure (BP). It is hypothesized that only a small percentage of early adolescents with T1D will meet diabetes-specific nutritional guidelines and that macronutrient and fiber intake, as well as adherence to guidelines, will be associated with health indicators.

2. Methods

2.1. Participants. Early adolescents, aged 11 to 14, and their parents participated in a randomized controlled trial (RCT) at two mid-Atlantic children's hospitals. Participation in the RCT entailed completion of four brief sessions of behavioral intervention or diabetes education in conjunction with quarterly diabetes clinic visits over the course of 1 to 1 and 1/2 years. The intervention and outcomes are described in greater detail in a previously published paper [28]. The data for the current study were drawn from the baseline assessments of all of participants in the RCT with at least one completed dietary interview.

Eligibility requirements of the RCT included diabetes duration of at least 1 year, absence of severe complications (e.g., retinopathy and nephropathy) or other medical diagnoses (e.g., cancer and asthma), and English fluency. The sample consisted of 257 dyads composed of one adolescent with T1D (49% girls) and one parent (91% mothers). Mean age at baseline was 12.8 years (SD = 1.2), mean illness duration was 5.1 years (SD = 3.1), and mean HbA1c was 73 mmol/mol (SD = 4). Two-thirds (64%) of the samples were prescribed a flexible insulin regimen, i.e., ≥4 injections or basal/bolus injections, or continuous subcutaneous insulin infusion/pump. Participant characteristics are summarized in Table 1.

2.2. Procedures. Institutional review boards from each institution approved the larger study. Eligible families were identified from clinic lists and were mailed an informational letter. These families then received a follow-up telephone call from trained research assistants. At regularly scheduled diabetes clinic visit, each participant and his/her parent provided consent and assent, completed self-report questionnaires, and participated in separate parent and child 24-hour nutrition and diabetes self-care interviews. A second 24-hour retrospective dietary interview was completed over the telephone within two weeks of the baseline assessment. Completion of questionnaires took approximately 45 minutes, and each interview was approximately 15 minutes. Families received a $25 gift card in appreciation of their time. Of the 404 eligible families successfully contacted, 285 consented to participate (71%). Those who declined consent primarily cited lack of interest or time as the reason. Completed baseline data were provided by 257 parent-adolescent dyads (89%).

2.3. Measures

2.3.1. Background Information. Demographic and medical information was obtained via questionnaire and a retrospective review of the medical charts. Socioeconomic status (SES) was calculated based on parental occupation and education [29], with higher scores related to lower SES. Coding was completed by research assistants. When there was not a clear category for a current career, the research assistant discussed

Table 1: Demographic and baseline characteristics.

	Mean (SD) or %	Range
Demographic		
Youth age (years)	12.8 (1.2)	11–15.3
Youth sex, % girls	49.4	
Youth ethnicity, % Caucasian	69.5	
Hollingshead SES, % level 1 or 2	53.8	
Medical		
Diabetes duration (years)	5.1 (3.1)	1–13.6
Insulin regimen		
2–3 injections per day (%)	35.3	
Basal/bolus (≥4 shots per day, %)	20.4	
CSII insulin pump (%)	44.3	
Nutrition intake		
% energy from carbohydrates (DI)	49.6 (8.3)	19.8–74.0
% energy from fats (DI)	35.3 (7.4)	12.8–55.0
% energy from proteins (DI)	15.9 (4.0)	6.7–29.8
Dietary fiber (g/1000 kcal (g/4184 kJ), DI)	14.7 (6.3)	3.8–38.3
Health indicators		
HbA1c (mmol/mol)	73 (4)	37–130
Systolic blood pressure (mmHg)	113.8 (10.6)	85–148
Diastolic blood pressure (mmHg)	64.0 (8.1)	44–94
LDL cholesterol (mg/dL)	89.3 (28.9)	6.0–187.0
BMI percentile	69.4 (24.5)	3–99

Note: SES = socioeconomic status; DI = dietary interview; BMI=body mass index.

with a senior study staff member and a joint decision was made. Insulin regimen was categorized as conventional (2–3 fixed injections/day) or flexible (≥4 injections, basal/bolus or pump) therapy. Parents reported the type of their child's nutrition plan (i.e., carbohydrate counting and exchanges) and the percentage of time their child adhered to his/her nutrition plan on average (i.e., ≤25% of the time, 26–50% of the time, 51–75% of the time, and >75% of the time). HbA1c and LDL cholesterol concentration were measured via blood assay at regular clinic visits and extracted from the medical record to represent metabolic control and lipid profile, respectively. HbA1c was assessed with the same measurement technology at each site (DCA 2000, 4.3–5.7%, Bayer Inc., Tarrytown, NY, USA). Height and weight also were measured at the baseline clinic visit, and body mass index (BMI) for age and gender percentile was calculated. Blood pressure (BP) also was measured and recorded.

2.3.2. Nutrition. To assess macronutrient and fiber intake, youth and one parent separately completed the 24-hour diabetes interview (DI) [30]. The DI is a diary-like interview in which parents and adolescents separately describe the completion of diabetes self-care tasks and nutritional intake over the previous 24 hours. Parents and adolescents each completed the DI on the same day on two different occasions within a two-week span. The responses of each parent and youth report were combined for each interview using a formula created by the research team [31] and scored using the Food Processor® Nutrition Software (ESHA Research, Salem, OR, USA). A combination of the two reports via decision rules overcomes common parent-child discrepancies and reduces bias and source error [30]. To further increase reliability, an average score of the two interviews was analyzed. For the current analyses, percentage of energy intake composed of carbohydrates, proteins, and fats, as well as grams dietary fiber, was evaluated. The 24-hour dietary recall method is a reliable, valid, well-established measure of diabetes self-care behavior [32, 33], energy, and nutritional intake.

Parent- and youth-reported dietary intake was compared to current nutritional recommended guidelines (Table 2) for adolescents with T1D provided by the American Diabetes Association (ADA). The International Society for Pediatric and Adolescent (ISPAD) guidelines also were consulted as a secondary source when specific guidelines did not exist by the ADA [4, 9]. These guidelines differ from standard guidelines in that recommended ranges are similar, but narrower for adolescents with diabetes than in the general population (e.g., % of energy intake from carbohydrates is recommended at 45–65% for healthy adolescents and 50–55% for adolescents with diabetes) [34].

2.4. Data Analytic Plan. Analyses were conducted using SAS software, version 9.3 (SAS Institute Inc., Cary, NC). One of the 257 parent-adolescent dyads who completed baseline questionnaires was excluded from dietary analysis because they did not report dietary intake. To quantify the portion of the sample that met nutritional guidelines, each nutritional variable was recoded into dichotomous variables based on the cutoff recommended level for each nutrient (i.e., 0 = did not meet guidelines; 1 = met guidelines). Next, bivariate associations between dietary intake, demographic variables, metabolic control, blood pressure, and lipid profile were assessed with general linear regression. Nonlinear relationships between significant nutrition variables and health indicators also were explored by including exponential variables in linear models. Following bivariate analyses, in order to evaluate the overall and unique contributions of hypothesized predictors to outcomes, multivariable linear regression models were conducted by including demographic variables associated with a health indicator at $p \leq 0.10$ in Step 1. Step 2 added nutrition variables associated with a health indicator at $p \leq 0.10$ to Step 1 (model 2). Finally, a fully saturated model was tested that included demographic and nutrition variables associated with any health indicator at $p \leq 0.10$ (model 3). Health indicators not associated with any nutrition variables were not included in the model testing. Continuous nutrition variables were given preference over categorized variables; however, significant categorized variables were explored in secondary models. Variables associated with health indicators at $p \leq 0.05$ were considered significant in all models, and R^2 was used to assess the amount of variance accounted for by the addition of nutrition variables to the model.

Table 2: Frequency of participants meeting nutritional recommendations.

	Recommendation	Insulin regimen Conventional (%)	Flexible (%)
Nutritional intake			
% energy from carbohydrates	50–55[1]	24.7	26.6
% energy from proteins	15–20[2]	48.8	44.7
% energy from fats	<35[1]	35.6	46.1
Cholesterol (mg/day)	<200[2]	54.4	57.6
Dietary fiber (g/1000 kcal (g/4184 kJ))	14[1]	37.8	52.9*
Health indicators			
HbA1c (mmol/mol)	≤58[2]	14.1	25.2*
BMI (normal, %)	5th–85th[2]	58.9	68.5
Systolic BP (mmHg)	<130/80 (or <90th %)[2]	93.0	91.9
Diastolic BP (mmHg)	<130/80 (or <90th %)[2]	97.7	96.9
LDL cholesterol (mg/dL (mmol/L))	<100 (2.6)[2]	62.5	52.1

[1]Recommendation from the International Society for Pediatric and Adolescent Diabetes. [2]Recommendation from the American Diabetes Association. *Values significantly different between regimens.

3. Results

3.1. Nutritional Recommendations. The proportion of participants who met nutritional recommendations by category and by type of regimen is summarized in Table 2. Only 25.8% of the samples met the guidelines for the percentage of their energy intake comprised of carbohydrates, 51.2% ate less than recommended, and 23.8% ate more than recommended. Only 45.9% of participants achieved recommendations for percentage of their energy intake from proteins, 44.7% ate less than recommended, and 9.3% ate more than recommended. Only 42% of youth met the guidelines for percent of energy intake as fats, and 51.6% of participants consumed more fats than recommended. Only 47.6% met the minimum guidelines for intake of dietary fiber. Participants on a flexible insulin regimen were significantly more likely to meet dietary fiber guidelines as compared to those on a conventional regimen ($\chi^2(1) = 5.23$, $p = 0.02$).

3.2. Adherence. Approximately half of parents (51.7%) reported that their child followed their nutrition plan less than 75% of the time. Using 75% of the time as a cutoff, parents of youth on a flexible regimen were significantly more likely to report that their child followed their nutrition plan the majority of time than those on a conventional regimen ($\chi^2(1) = 13.65$, $p < 0.001$).

3.3. Health Recommendations. Targets for HbA1c were met more frequently by those participants on a flexible regimen versus conventional regimen ($\chi^2(1) = 4.03$, $p = 0.05$). Of the health outcomes evaluated, only 21.3% achieved an HbA1c below 58 (mmol/mol) and was within the glycemic goal target range. Consideration of weight revealed 64.8% had a BMI percentile within the normal range, although 21.4% were classified as overweight and 13.6% had obesity. Moreover, 64.5% of participants had measured LDL cholesterol levels less than 100 mg/dL (2.59 mmol/L). Approximately 90% had measured blood pressure below 130/80 mmHg. These health indicators did not differ significantly by type of insulin regimen (χ^2 all $p > 0.05$).

3.4. Bivariate Associations. Bivariate associations between demographic and nutrition variables and all health indicators are presented in Table 3. Demographic associations were quite varied, with longer duration of disease associated with higher systolic BP ($\beta = 0.46$, $p = 0.04$) and higher LDL ($\beta = 1.53$, $p = 0.03$). Lower SES category was related to poorer HbA1c ($\beta = 0.61$, $p < 0.001$), as was a conventional insulin regimen ($\beta = 0.69$, $p = 0.002$). Non-Caucasian ethnicity and older age were each associated with every poorer health indicator except BMI percentile, which was not statistically significantly related to either non-Caucasian ethnicity or age. A higher percentage of energy intake from proteins was the only nutrient associated with higher systolic BP ($\beta = 0.42$, $p = 0.01$), whereas a higher percentage of energy intake from carbohydrates was significantly associated with higher diastolic BP ($\beta = 0.13$, $p = 0.04$). The majority of nutritional variables were associated with HbA1c including fats ($\beta = 0.05$, $p < 0.001$), carbohydrates ($\beta = -0.05$, $p < 0.001$), and dietary fiber ($\beta = -0.04$, $p = 0.02$). No significant nutrition associations were noted for BMI percentile or LDL, and no evidence of nonlinear associations were seen.

3.5. Regressions Predicting Health Indicators. Results of regression analyses are shown in Table 4. Overall, in Step 1, demographic variables accounted for 9% of the variance in systolic BP, with older age ($\beta = 2.09$, $p < 0.001$) and longer diabetes duration ($\beta = 0.43$, $p < 0.05$) significantly contributing to the model predicting systolic BP. The addition of nutritional variables in Step 2 increased the variance explained by 2% points. Specifically, controlling for relevant demographic factors, a higher percentage of energy intake from proteins was significantly associated with higher systolic BP ($\beta = 0.36$, $p = 0.03$). Although nutritional variables were not significantly associated with diastolic BP

TABLE 3: Bivariate associations among demographic and nutritional variables and all health measures.

	Systolic BP		Diastolic BP		HbA1C		BMI%		LDL	
	β	p value	β	p value	β	p value	β	p value	β	p value
Age	**2.18**	**<0.0001**	**0.92**	**0.03**	**0.17**	**0.05**	0.63	0.62	**4.46**	**0.007**
Sex (boys vs. girls)[1]	0.47	0.73	−0.72	0.49	0.09	0.68	−4.72	0.13	−2.20	0.59
Duration	**0.46**	**0.04**	0.18	0.31	0.003	0.82	−0.15	0.77	**1.53**	**0.03**
SES	1.17	0.14	0.68	0.27	**0.61**	**<0.0001**	1.86	0.32	2.13	0.37
Ethnicity (non-Caucasian vs. Caucasian)[2]	**2.96**	**0.04**	**2.78**	**0.01**	**0.84**	**0.0003**	5.53	0.10	**8.77**	**0.04**
Insulin regimen[3]	−0.85	0.55	1.41	0.19	**0.69**	**0.002**	5.29	0.10	3.82	0.37
Fats (% energy)	0.0001	0.99	−0.14	0.06	**0.05**	**0.0002**	−0.02	0.92	−0.28	0.33
Carbohydrates (% energy)	−0.05	0.51	**0.13**	**0.04**	**−0.05**	**0.0004**	0.10	0.58	0.07	0.78
Proteins (% energy)	**0.42**	**0.01**	0.14	0.28	0.05	0.07	0.31	0.42	0.78	0.12
Dietary fiber	−0.09	0.42	−0.12	0.13	**−0.04**	**0.02**	−0.21	0.39	−0.38	0.22
Fats (in range versus)										
Less than recommended	1.14	0.69	0.20	0.93	−0.24	0.60	−2.21	0.74	12.46	0.12
More than recommended	1.86	0.19	−0.60	0.58	**0.70**	**0.001**	1.35	0.67	−0.52	0.90
Carbohydrates (in range versus)										
Less than recommended	−0.41	0.80	−0.08	0.95	**0.74**	**0.003**	−2.21	0.56	−3.76	0.44
More than recommended	−1.43	0.46	1.29	0.38	0.01	0.97	−4.43	0.32	−0.88	0.88
Proteins (in range versus)										
Not in range	1.17	0.39	−1.12	0.28	0.21	0.34	−4.91	0.11	2.78	0.50
Dietary fiber (in range versus)										
Not in range	−2.22	0.64	**−7.07**	**0.05**	0.61	0.42	−14.89	0.18	4.19	0.75

Estimates based on linear regression analysis. Bold = $p < 0.05$. [1]Boys coded as 0. [2]Caucasian coded as 1. [3]Flexible regimen coded as 1.

TABLE 4: Multivariable associations between demographic and nutritional variables and nutrition-associated health measures.

	Systolic BP			Diastolic BP			HbA1C		
R^2	Model 1 0.09	Model 2 0.11	Model 3 0.12	Model 1 0.04	Model 2 0.06	Model 3 0.08	Model 1 0.14	Model 2 0.20	Model 3 0.21
	β	β	β	β	β	β	β	β	β
Demographic variables									
Age	2.14‡	2.09‡	2.05‡	0.92*	0.92*	0.66	0.19*	0.17*	0.17*
Duration	0.42*	0.43*	0.37	—	—	0.11	—	—	0.009
SES[2]	—	—	1.32	—	—	0.26	0.50‡	0.44‡	0.46‡
Ethnicity[3]	2.94*	2.51	2.39	2.77†	2.89†	1.85	0.36	0.44	0.42
Insulin regimen[4]	—	—	−2.40	—	—	1.03	0.35	0.26	0.26
Nutrition variables									
Fats (% energy intake)	—	—	0.11	—	−0.03	0.09	—	0.05^{*,5}	0.05*
Carbohydrates (% energy intake)	—	—	0.11	—	0.11	0.27*	—	0.005^5	0.004
Proteins (% energy intake)	—	0.36*	0.47*	—	—	0.31	—	0.04	0.04
Dietary fiber	—	—	−0.00	—	—	−0.12	—	−0.02	−0.02

[1]Estimates based on linear regression analysis. Model 1 includes demographic variables significant at $p < 0.10$ in bivariate models. Model 2 includes variables in model 1 + nutrition variables significant at $p < 0.10$ in bivariate models. Model 3 is a fully saturated model that includes all variables significant for any outcome in bivariate models. [2]SES: categorical with lower categories indicating higher SES. [3]Non-Caucasian coded as 0 vs. Caucasian coded as 1. [4]Conventional coded as 0 vs. flexible coded as 1. [5]Categorical "not in range" or "less/more than recommended" as 0 vs. "in range" as 1. $^*p < 0.05$; $^†p \leq 0.01$; $^‡p \leq 0.001$.

controlling for relevant demographic factors, inclusion of nutritional variables marginally improved R^2 (6% vs. 4%), showing contribution to the variance in diastolic BP. In Step 3, a higher percentage of energy intake from carbohydrates was associated with higher diastolic BP ($\beta = 0.27$, $p < 0.05$)

The health indicator most highly associated with study variables was HbA1c, as 20% of the variance in outcome was accounted for by the model including relevant demographic and nutrition variables. A higher percentage of energy intake from fats was associated with higher HbA1c controlling for all other variables in the model ($\beta = 0.05$, $p = 0.02$). Fully saturated models did not alter these conclusions or improve percentage of variance explained.

4. Discussion

The current study reveals that many primarily middle-class early adolescents with T1D do not meet national nutritional guidelines set by the American Diabetes Association [4]. Nevertheless, most health indicators are relatively favorable and within normal limits at this age, despite suboptimal glycemic control. Perhaps more importantly, the current study provides evidence that adherence to nutritional guidelines for macronutrient intake is associated with better glycemic control, consistent with prior research. Additionally, this study demonstrates a link between higher percentage of energy intake from fats and poorer glycemic control in a young adolescent T1D sample, above and beyond the contribution of demographic and other dietary variables. Finally, longer diabetes duration was related to higher systolic blood pressure and higher LDL in the current pediatric sample, consistent with the increased risk of hyperlipidemia in diabetes [35, 36].

A higher percentage of energy intake from fats was related to poorer glycemic control after accounting for other study demographic, disease, and nutritional factors. Taken together, demographic variables and diet variables explained 20% of the variance in glycemic control, consistent with existing T1D research [22, 37]. In contrast, a higher percentage of energy intake from proteins was associated with higher systolic BP and a higher percentage of energy intake from carbohydrates related to higher diastolic BP. In the current sample, nutritional intake was not associated with BMI percentile or LDL cholesterol. Further, insulin regimen, conventional versus flexible, did not distinguish groups on the basis of nutritional intake or health indicators, with the exception of HbA1c, for which a higher percentage of participants on a flexible regimen met the guidelines. These findings are slightly different from previous research [37] that found variation in nutrition and health status by insulin regimen.

The current study illustrates that a sizable majority of youth did not meet ADA or ISPAD nutritional guidelines and may be at risk for cardiovascular disease and other health complications later in life. Early inklings of this risk are found in the present association between longer disease duration and higher LDL cholesterol and higher systolic blood pressure. Diabetes carries a known morbidity for hyperlipidemia, and therefore, youth may benefit from close monitoring of health status and macronutrient intake, particularly saturated fats, to prevent onset of cardiovascular disease [38]. Parents were aware that their adolescents were not following their nutritional plan, as over half (51%) reported that their adolescent followed their specific nutrition plan less than 75% of the time. However, parents of youth on flexible regimens were more likely to report that their adolescents were following nutrition guidelines. In support of our findings, existing studies have reported that adolescents with T1D do not meet the recommended ADA guidelines [39, 40].

Our study adds to the literature by finding an association between dietary intake and health indicators of glycemic control and blood pressure in early adolescents. That is, specific dietary components in the present study had a direct relation to established health indicators, beyond the contribution of demographic factors and general nutritional status which were controlled statistically. Previous work has examined the association between nutrition and health status in Chinese adults with T1D, whose diets likely are dissimilar to those of American adolescents [41]. Nevertheless, links were found among dietary patterns with HbA1c and LDL cholesterol in this Asian sample. Work in youth with T1D indicates that carbohydrate intake, when examined alone, is associated with lipid profiles, BMI, and HbA1c [20] and saturated fat intake is associated with HbA1c [19]. The current study not only supports these findings but also adds new information through examination of multiple demographic and nutritional variables simultaneously, regardless of insulin regimen. Adolescents and their parents may perceive that improved insulin delivery and dosing systems allow more freedom in food choices, but these data indicate that a heart-healthy diet has ramifications beyond traditional short- and long-term cardiac status and, in fact, directly relates to level of glycemic control.

A novel direct association also was found between macronutrient consumption and BP, although BP was not elevated overall in the current sample. Specifically, consumption of a higher percentage of energy from proteins related to higher systolic BP and a higher percentage of energy intake from carbohydrates related to diastolic BP. Importantly, evidence of dietary links to glycemic control and BP status based on just two samples of nutritional intake from two days is compelling and requires further study. More subtle associations may be found with more extensive sampling and other methods of assessing dietary intake. With an average disease duration in the present sample of just five years, the importance of understanding the dietary correlates of glycemic and cardiac status is underscored by the fact that longer diabetes duration was associated with higher LDL levels, a known risk factor for cardiovascular disease [42].

Consistent with previous literature [43, 44], Table 3 shows that demographic variables were associated with nutrition behaviors and diabetes health indicators. Specifically, older age places youth at risk for poorer health indicators overall. However, age was not associated with patterns of nutritional intake. Longer disease duration was associated with higher systolic BP and LDL. Non-Caucasian adolescents with T1D reported similar nutritional intake to Caucasians but were more likely to have overall poorer health indicators, suggesting that factors other than nutritional behaviors may place minority youth at greater risk for cardiovascular disease. Consistent with previous literature, low SES was associated with higher HbA1c values (e.g., [45]). Differences in disease-related variables, such as duration of illness and insulin regimen, may place early adolescents at different levels of risk for a confluence of poorer nutritional behaviors and health indicators. For example, longer duration of illness was associated with a higher systolic BP leading to a potential risk of hypertension and was associated with higher LDL, which potentiates for dyslipidemia. Adolescents on flexible regimens may have higher intake of carbohydrates and lower intake of proteins than peers on conventional regimens, which could be important for dieticians counseling adolescents on flexible regimens regarding the importance of adhering to nutrition guidelines.

5. Clinical Implications

When youth with T1D are first diagnosed, especially as younger children, their care and management fall solely to their parents. At the time of diagnosis, most families receive "survival skills" training, which incorporates nutrition guidelines and medical nutrition therapy. However, early adolescence represents a period of increased independence and self-management, as well as greater freedom in food choices. Early adolescents may not be routinely included in initial diabetes education such that they may be unaware of the importance of balanced nutrition to manage their HbA1c and to prevent future health risk. The present study's findings underscore the ADA recommendation of yearly meetings with a registered dietician such that nutrition counseling is a routine and frequent part of diabetes education and management. Particularly pressing is the need to help early adolescents understand the importance of adherence to nutrition recommendations to optimize their glycemic control and to decrease their risk for future cardiovascular disease [5, 9].

Given that education alone is not always sufficient to produce changes in behavior, for optimal efficacy, nutrition counseling could include focus on individual and cultural preferences, motivation, and self-efficacy to make healthful choices, as well as familial financial considerations. When adolescents and families have difficulty adhering to nutritional guidelines, clinical psychologists may be a critical component of care in order to promote adherence. Integration of technology may be an appealing facet of diabetes care to engage adolescents and promote self-monitoring behaviors as a means to support healthful decision-making. Technology may represent a fruitful avenue to keep nutritional education and reeducation updated and enjoyable.

6. Limitations

The current study is strengthened by the use of multimethod and multisource data at multiple time points. However, the cross-sectional nature of the study makes it impossible to determine casual relations among demographic, nutritional, and health variables. Moreover, the number of analyses increases risk for type 1 error. Future research should examine these relationships longitudinally, particularly as adolescents reach young adulthood and beyond. Moreover, although parents and youth reported their nutritional intake at two different time points using the gold standard for assessment of dietary intake, self-report of food intake is often underreported [32] and may not accurately represent actual consumption. Future research should incorporate other methods, such as direct observation or innovative technologies such as remote food photography method [46]. Other factors that affect glycemic control, such as meal timing, physical activity, and insulin dosing, should be simultaneously evaluated. Although the current sample is representative of the two institutions from which it was drawn, it may not be representative of all youth with type 1 diabetes.

7. Conclusions

Overall, many early adolescents with T1D did not meet guidelines for nutritional intake. Nonadherence to nutritional guidelines, above and beyond the influence of demographic variables, was associated with poorer HbA1c and places youth at risk for later health complications. Regular nutritional education, particularly for early adolescents, along with behavioral adherence to the guidelines may prove crucial for maintenance of better glycemic control and prevention of future cardiovascular disease.

Conflicts of Interest

The authors declare that they have no conflict of interest.

Acknowledgments

The authors would like to acknowledge the NIH/NIDDK for the funding to perform the current study (5R01DK070917-04 awarded to CH). The authors would also like to thank the W.T. Gill, Jr., Summer Fellowship for the support for a summer project to complete the paper (educational scholarship awarded to Lyndsay O'Brecht). They would also like to thank the research staff who contributed to the data collection and analysis.

References

[1] J. S. Borus and L. Laffel, "Adherence challenges in the management of type 1 diabetes in adolescents: prevention and intervention," *Current Opinion in Pediatrics*, vol. 22, no. 4, pp. 405–411, 2010.

[2] J. Silverstein, G. Klingensmith, K. Copeland et al., "Care of children and adolescents with type 1 diabetes: a statement of the American Diabetes Association," *Diabetes Care*, vol. 28, no. 1, pp. 186–212, 2005.

[3] D. M. Nathan, P. A. Cleary, J. Y. Backlund et al., "Intensive diabetes treatment and cardiovascular disease in patients with type 1 diabetes," *The New England Journal of Medicine*, vol. 353, no. 25, pp. 2643–2653, 2005.

[4] American Diabetes Association, "11. Children and adolescents," *Diabetes Care*, vol. 38, Supplement 1, pp. S70–S76, 2015.

[5] J. L. Chiang, M. S. Kirkman, L. M. Laffel, A. L. Peters, and Type 1 Diabetes Sourcebook Authors, "Type 1 diabetes through the life span: a position statement of the American Diabetes Association," *Diabetes Care*, vol. 37, no. 7, pp. 2034–2054, 2014.

[6] Diabetes Control and Complications Trial/Epidemiology of Diabetes Interventions and Complications, L. M. Delahanty, D. M. Nathan et al., "Association of diet with glycated hemoglobin during intensive treatment of type 1 diabetes in the diabetes control and complications trial," *The American Journal of Clinical Nutrition*, vol. 89, no. 2, pp. 518–524, 2009.

[7] K. Lange, P. Swift, E. Pankowska, T. Danne, and ISPAD clinical practice consensus guidelines 2014, "Diabetes education in children and adolescents," *Pediatric Diabetes*, vol. 15, Supplement 20, pp. 77–85, 2014.

[8] N. C. Overby, H. D. Margeirsdottir, C. Brunborg, L. F. Andersen, and K. Dahl-Jorgensen, "The influence of dietary intake and meal pattern on blood glucose control in children and adolescents using intensive insulin treatment," *Diabetologia*, vol. 50, no. 10, pp. 2044–2051, 2007.

[9] C. E. Smart, F. Annan, L. P. Bruno, L. A. Higgins, and C. L. Acerini, "ISPAD clinical practice consensus guidelines 2014. Nutritional management in children and adolescents with diabetes," *Pediatric Diabetes*, vol. 15, Supplement 20, pp. 135–153, 2014.

[10] S. R. Patton, "Adherence to diet in youth with type 1 diabetes," *Journal of the American Dietetic Association*, vol. 111, no. 4, pp. 550–555, 2011.

[11] E. C. Banfield, Y. Liu, J. S. Davis, S. Chang, and A. C. Frazier-Wood, "Poor adherence to US dietary guidelines for children and adolescents in the National Health and Nutrition Examination Survey population," *Journal of the Academy of Nutrition and Dietetics*, vol. 116, no. 1, pp. 21–27, 2016.

[12] V. S. Helgeson, L. Viccaro, D. Becker, O. Escobar, and L. Siminerio, "Diet of adolescents with and without diabetes: Tting candy for potato chips?," *Diabetes Care*, vol. 29, no. 5, pp. 982–987, 2006.

[13] K. A. K. Davison, C. A. Negrato, R. Cobas et al., "Relationship between adherence to diet, glycemic control and cardiovascular risk factors in patients with type 1 diabetes: a nationwide survey in Brazil," *Nutrition Journal*, vol. 13, no. 1, pp. 1–11, 2014.

[14] S. S. Soedamah-Mutu, N. Chaturvedi, J. H. Fuller, M. Toeller, and EURODIAB, "Do European people with type 1 diabetes consume a high atherogenic diet? 7-year follow-up of the EURODIAB prospective complications study," *European Journal of Nutrition*, vol. 52, no. 7, pp. 1701–1710, 2013.

[15] American Diabetes Association, J. P. Bantle, J. Wylie-Rosett, C. M. Apovian, N. G. Clark, and M. J. Franz, "Nutrition recommendations and interventions for diabetes: a position statement of the American Diabetes Association," *Diabetes Care*, vol. 31, Supplement 1, pp. S61–S78, 2008.

[16] American Diabetes Association, "3. Foundations of care and comprehensive medical evaluation," *Diabetes Care*, vol. 39, Supplement 1, pp. S23–S35, 2016.

[17] M. A. Testa, J. Gill, M. Su, R. R. Turner, L. Blonde, and D. C. Simonson, "Comparative effectiveness of basal-bolus versus premix analog insulin on glycemic variability and patient-centered outcomes during insulin intensification in type 1 and type 2 diabetes: a randomized, controlled, crossover trial," *The Journal of Clinical Endocrinology and Metabolism*, vol. 97, no. 10, pp. 3504–3514, 2012.

[18] A. J. Rovner and T. R. Nansel, "Are children with type 1 diabetes consuming a healthful diet?: a review of the current evidence and strategies for dietary change," *The Diabetes Educator*, vol. 35, no. 1, pp. 97–107, 2009.

[19] C. Maffeis, A. Morandi, E. Ventura et al., "Diet, physical, and biochemical characteristics of children and adolescents with type 1 diabetes: relationship between dietary fat and glucose control," *Pediatric Diabetes*, vol. 13, no. 2, pp. 137–146, 2012.

[20] T. Meissner, J. Wolf, M. Kersting et al., "Carbohydrate intake in relation to BMI, HbA1c and lipid profile in children and adolescents with type 1 diabetes," *Clinical Nutrition*, vol. 33, no. 1, pp. 75–78, 2014.

[21] S. F. Michaliszyn, G. Q. Shaibi, L. Quinn, C. Fritschi, and M. S. Faulkner, "Physical fitness, dietary intake, and metabolic control in adolescents with type 1 diabetes," *Pediatric Diabetes*, vol. 10, no. 6, pp. 389–394, 2009.

[22] T. R. Nansel, L. M. Lipsky, and A. Liu, "Greater diet quality is associated with more optimal glycemic control in a longitudinal study of youth with type 1 diabetes," *American Journal of Clinical Nutrition*, vol. 104, no. 1, pp. 81–87, 2016.

[23] M. Saito, H. Kuratsune, H. Nitta et al., "Plasma lipid levels and nutritional intake in childhood- and adolescence-onset young type 1 diabetic patients in Japan," *Diabetes Research and Clinical Practice*, vol. 73, no. 1, pp. 29–34, 2006.

[24] T. R. Nansel, L. M. B. Laffel, D. L. Haynie et al., "Improving dietary quality in youth with type 1 diabetes: randomized clinical trial of a family-based behavioral intervention," *International Journal of Behavioral Nutrition and Physical Activity*, vol. 12, no. 1, p. 58, 2015.

[25] S. Keel, C. Itsiopoulos, K. Koklanis, M. Vukicevic, F. Cameron, and L. Brazionis, "Prevalence and risk factors for diabetic retinopathy in a hospital-based population of Australian children and adolescents with type 1 diabetes," *Journal of Pediatric Endocrinology and Metabolism*, vol. 29, no. 10, pp. 1135–1142, 2016.

[26] F. S. R. Bernaud, M. Beretta, C. do Nascimento et al., "Fiber intake and inflammation in type 1 diabetes," *Diabetology & Metabolic Syndrome*, vol. 6, no. 1, pp. 66–10, 2014.

[27] D. A. J. M. Schoenaker, the EURODIAB Prospective Complications Study Group, M. Toeller, N. Chaturvedi, J. H. Fuller, and S. S. Soedamah-Muthu, "Dietary saturated fat and fibre and risk of cardiovascular disease and all-cause mortality among type 1 diabetic patients: the EURODIAB prospective complications study," *Diabetologia*, vol. 55, no. 8, pp. 2132–2141, 2012.

[28] C. S. Holmes, R. Chen, E. Mackey, M. Grey, and R. Streisand, "Randomized clinical trial of clinic-integrated, low-intensity treatment to prevent deterioration of disease care in adolescents with type 1 diabetes," *Diabetes Care*, vol. 37, no. 6, pp. 1535–1543, 2014.

[29] A. A. Hollingshead, *Four-Factor Index of Social Status*, Yale University, New Haven, CT, 1974, Unpublished manuscript.

[30] S. B. Johnson, J. Silverstein, A. Rosenbloom, R. Carter, and W. Cunningham, "Assessing daily management in childhood diabetes," *Health Psychology*, vol. 5, no. 6, pp. 545–564, 1986.

[31] C. S. Holmes, R. Chen, R. Streisand et al., "Predictors of youth diabetes care behaviors and metabolic control: a structural equation modeling approach," *Journal of Pediatric Psychology*, vol. 31, no. 8, pp. 770–784, 2006.

[32] A. Freund, S. B. Johnson, J. Silverstein, and J. Thomas, "Assessing daily management of childhood diabetes using 24-hour recall interviews: reliability and stability," *Health Psychology*, vol. 10, no. 3, pp. 200–208, 1991.

[33] A. L. Quittner, A. C. Modi, K. L. Lemanek, C. E. Ievers-Landis, and M. A. Rapoff, "Evidence-based assessment of adherence to

medical treatments in pediatric psychology," *Journal of Pediatric Psychology*, vol. 33, no. 9, pp. 916–936, 2008.

[34] US Department of Health and Human Services & US Department of Agriculture, "2015–2020 Dietary Guidelines for Americans," 2015, 8th edition, http://health.gov/dietaryguidelines/2015/guidelines/.

[35] The Diabetes Control and Complications Trial/Epidemiology of Diabetes Interventions and Complications (DCCT/EDIC) Study Research Group, "Intensive diabetes treatment and cardiovascular disease in patients with type 1 diabetes," *New England Journal of Medicine*, vol. 353, no. 25, pp. 2643–2653, 2005.

[36] K. O. Schwab, J. Doerfer, W. Hecker et al., "Spectrum and prevalence of atherogenic risk factors in 27,358 children, adolescents, and young adults with type 1 diabetes: cross-sectional data from the German diabetes documentation and quality management system (DPV)," *Diabetes Care*, vol. 29, no. 2, pp. 218–225, 2006.

[37] M. L. Katz, S. Mehta, T. Nansel, H. Quinn, L. M. Lipsky, and L. M. B. Laffel, "Associations of nutrient intake with glycemic control in youth with type 1 diabetes: differences by insulin regimen," *Diabetes Technology & Therapeutics*, vol. 16, no. 8, pp. 512–518, 2014.

[38] J. B. Buse, H. N. Ginsberg, G. L. Bakris et al., "Primary prevention of cardiovascular diseases in people with diabetes mellitus: a scientific statement from the American Heart Association and the American Diabetes Association," *Diabetes Care*, vol. 30, no. 1, pp. 162–172, 2007.

[39] E. J. Mayer-Davis, M. Nichols, A. D. Liese et al., "Dietary intake among youth with diabetes: the SEARCH for Diabetes in Youth Study," *Journal of the American Dietetic Association*, vol. 106, no. 5, pp. 689–697, 2006.

[40] N. C. Overby, V. Flaaten, M. B. Veierod et al., "Children and adolescents with type 1 diabetes eat a more atherosclerosis-prone diet than healthy control subjects," *Diabetologia*, vol. 50, no. 2, pp. 307–316, 2007.

[41] L. M. Jaacks, J. Crandell, M. A. Mendez et al., "Dietary patterns associated with HbA1c and LDL cholesterol among individuals with type 1 diabetes in China," *Journal of Diabetes and its Complications*, vol. 29, no. 3, pp. 343–349, 2015.

[42] P. W. F. Wilson, R. B. D'Agostino, D. Levy, A. M. Belanger, H. Silbershatz, and W. B. Kannel, "Prediction of coronary heart disease using risk factor categories," *Circulation*, vol. 97, no. 18, pp. 1837–1847, 1998.

[43] V. S. Helgeson, L. Siminerio, O. Escobar, and D. Becker, "Predictors of metabolic control among adolescents with diabetes: a 4-year longitudinal study," *Journal of Pediatric Psychology*, vol. 34, no. 3, pp. 254–270, 2009.

[44] J. J. Jacobsen, M. H. Black, B. H. Li, K. Reynolds, and J. M. Lawrence, "Race/ethnicity and measures of glycaemia in the year after diagnosis among youth with type 1 and type 2 diabetes mellitus," *Journal of Diabetes and its Complications*, vol. 28, no. 3, pp. 279–285, 2014.

[45] S. Zilioli, D. A. Ellis, J. M. Carre, and R. B. Slatcher, "Biospychosocial pathways linking subjective socioeconomic disadvantage to glycemic control in youths with type 1 diabetes," *Psychoneuroendocrinology*, vol. 78, pp. 222–228, 2017.

[46] C. K. Martin, J. B. Correa, H. Han et al., "Validity of the remote food photography method (RFPM) for estimating energy and nutrient intake in near real-time," *Obesity*, vol. 20, no. 4, pp. 891–899, 2012.

11

Association of PD-1 and PD-L1 Genetic Polymorphyisms with Type 1 Diabetes Susceptibility

Chenyue Qian,[1] Heming Guo,[2] Xiaohong Chen,[2] Aiming Shi,[1] Sicheng Li,[2] Xin Wang,[3] Jie Pan,[1] and Chen Fang[2]

[1]*Department of Pharmacy, The Second Affiliated Hospital of Soochow University, Suzhou 215004, China*
[2]*Department of Endocrinology, The Second Affiliated Hospital of Soochow University, Suzhou 215004, China*
[3]*Department of Endocrinology, Jiangsu Province Hospital of TCM, 155 Hanzhonglu, Jiangsu Nanjing 210029, China*

Correspondence should be addressed to Jie Pan; pankypan@163.com and Chen Fang; afa9911@sina.com

Academic Editor: Marco Songini

Aims. The programmed death- (PD-) 1/PD-1 ligand (PD-L) pathway plays an important role in regulating T cell activation and maintaining peripheral tolerance. Accumulated studies showed that PD-1/PD-L1 pathway was involved in the development of type 1 diabetes (T1DM). Since the genetic background of type 1 diabetes differs greatly among the different population, we aim to investigate the association of genetic polymorphisms in PD-1 and PD-L1 with T1DM susceptibility in Chinese population. *Methods.* In total, 166 T1DM patients and 100 healthy controls were enrolled into the study. Genomic DNA was extracted from 4 mL peripheral blood samples collected from each subject. Genotyping of 8 selected SNPs of PD-1 and PD-L1 was carried out by the pyrosequencing PSQ 24 System using PyroMark Gold reagents (QIAGEN). *Results.* SNP rs4143815 in PD-L1 was significantly associated with T1DM. People carrying the C allele of rs4143815 suffering less risk of T1DM and T1DM patients with G/G genotype showed higher levels of autoantibody (AAB) positive incidence compared with C allele carriers. No significant associations were found in other SNPs. *Conclusions.* Our results indicate that rs4143815 of PD-L1 is significantly associated with T1DM and may serve as a new biomarker to predict the T1DM susceptibility.

1. Introduction

The increased prevalence of diabetes mellitus is considered one of the greatest public health challenges nowadays. Type 1 diabetes mellitus (T1DM), a polygenic autoimmune disease, is resulted from both genetic and environmental factors [1]. Although T1DM has a lower prevalence compared with type 2 diabetes mellitus (T2DM), it is the most common form of diabetes in childhood and has a greater impact on the quality of living life.

Programmed cell death 1 (PD-1) is an immunoinhibitory factor belonging to the CD28/B7 family. It plays a vital role in regulating T cell activation and maintaining peripheral tolerance as a core costimulatory molecule [2, 3]. Recently, PD-1 has been widely studied as an immune checkpoint that is applied to the treatment of numerous advanced cancers [4–6]. Programmed death ligand-1 (PD-L1) has been shown to be overexpressed in many cancers, including gastric cancer [7], esophageal cancer, pancreatic cancer, and other human gastrointestinal tumors [8]. Accumulated studies showed that blockage of the interaction between PD-1 and PD-L1 can help with better prognosis in various malignant tumors [6, 9, 10]. However, autoimmune diabetes has been reported after receiving anti-PD-1 therapy for tumor in both mouse models and human cases [11–13]. Thus, we assume that there may be a connection between PD-1/PD-L1 pathway and autoimmune diabetes.

Increasing studies had been committed to the association with PD-1/PD-L1 and autoimmune disease, including systemic lupus erythematosus, ankylosing spondylitis, allergic bronchial asthma, and autoimmune diabetes [14–17]. The role of PD-1 in T1DM has been studied using animal models. As a costimulatory molecule that inhibits T cell proliferation, PD-1 deficiency was shown to increase the risk of T1DM in nonobese diabetic (NOD) mice [18]. Studies had shown that low PD-1 might increase T cell proliferation and activation which lead to the destruction of beta cells, providing a possible mechanism for T1DM. Lower PD-1 expression was proposed to have associations with the development of T1DM in mouse models [19]. PD-L1 recently had been found expressed in the islets of people with type 1 diabetes [20], and we also found that PD-L1 was significantly reduced in the serum of T1DM patients [21]. Since single nucleotide polymorphisms (SNPs) play vital roles in the transcription and translation of genes and have associations with the occurrence and development of diseases, studies had been devoted to the associations between gene polymorphisms with T1DM susceptibility. Existing researches pointed out that PD-1 and PD-L1 SNPs were associated with T1DM susceptibility in different populations [21–23].

However, there is only a few studies focus on the associations between PD-1/PD-L1 gene polymorphisms and T1DM in Chinese population. Therefore, in the present study we investigated 8 selected SNPs of PD-1 and PD-L1 to ascertain whether PD-1 and PD-L1 SNPs influence the T1DM susceptibility.

2. Materials and Methods

2.1. Study Population. A total of 166 T1DM patients and 100 healthy controls were recruited for the study (Table 1). Blood samples were collected after overnight fasting from patients at the Endocrinology Department in the Second Affiliated Hospital of Soochow University, Suzhou, China, between 2013 and 2017. All the T1DM patients were diagnosed following the criteria of the American Diabetes Association (reference from Diabetes Care published by ADA). Samples from healthy blood donors, self-report healthy, were chosen as matched controls. Prior to commencing this study, the approval from the Ethics Review Board of the Second Affiliated Hospital of Soochow University was granted.

2.2. Selection of SNPs and Genotyping. Eight SNPs in 2 genes (PD-1 and PD-L1) were selected from the National Center for Biotechnology Information (NCBI) database (Table 2). All of the SNPs satisfied the following criteria: (1) SNPs that are associated with autoimmune disease occurrence or development according to the results of existing research; (2) SNPs that may influence function or expression of PD-1 and PD-L1 by NCBI; (3) minor allele frequency (MAF) $\geq 5\%$ in Chinese Han population.

4 mL peripheral blood samples was collected in EDTA anticoagulant tubes for each patient. Genomic DNA was extracted using Genomic DNA Purification Kit according to the standard protocols. Genotyping of each polymorphism in the PD-1 and PD-L1 genes was carried out by the pyrosequencing PSQ 24 System using PyroMark Gold reagents (QIAGEN). Primers were designed using Pyrosequencing™ Assay Design Software and Primer Premier 5. The genomic region of interest was amplified by polymerase chain reaction (PCR) using one regular primer and one biotinylated primer; PCR products were sequenced using sequencing primer on PSQ 24 System. All the primers used in the present study were shown in Table 3.

Table 1: Characteristics of T1DM patients and normal controls in this study.

Characteristic	All	Type 1 diabetes	Control
Total number	266	166	100
Gender			
Female (n)	146	82	64
Male (n)	120	84	36
Age (year)	34.1 ± 15.9	25.9 ± 12.3	47.7 ± 11.1
Diabetes duration (year)	—	7.3 ± 6.5	—
HbA1c (%)	—	8.7 ± 2.8	—
Presence of AABs (IAA, ICA, and GADA)	—	97	—

Data are mean—standard deviation (SD); HbA1c: glycated hemoglobin; AABs: subjects tested for autoantibodies; IAA: insulin autoantibody; ICA: islet cell autoantibody; GADA: glutamic acid decarboxylase autoantibody.

2.3. Statistical Analysis. The chi-squared test was used to evaluate the Hardy-Weinberg equilibrium for allele frequencies of all SNPs. Unconditional logistic regression was conducted to calculate the adjusted odds ratio (OR) and 95% confidence intervals (95% CI). The associations between genotypes and T1DM susceptibility were tested using logistic regression analysis with Plink under additive, dominant, and recessive models. The test of significance was set at two-tailed $P = 0.05$.

The secondary structure of the mRNA was simulated using online webserver RNAfold (http://rna.tbi.univie.ac.at/cgi-bin/RNAWebSuite/RNAfold.cgi), which is a recognized software providing structure prediction service [24].

3. Results

166 T1DM patients and 100 healthy controls were listed into the present study. All subjects were Chinese and had a mean (SD) age of 34.1 ± 15.9 at the time of recruitment. 8 SNPs were genotyped in these subjects, only five of which conformed to Hardy-Weinberg equilibrium ($P > 0.05$) (shown in Table 2). Thus, we took rs2227981, rs34819629, rs4143815, rs2297136, and rs2297137 into final analyses. The results were summarized in Table 4.

There was a significant association between the PD-L1 SNP rs4143815 and T1DM susceptibility in the additive model (OR 0.50; $P = 0.003$), dominant model (OR 0.31; $P = 0.012$), and the recessive model (OR 0.46; $P = 0.028$). No significant association was observed between other SNPs and T1DM susceptibility. Considering multiple-testing correction, we calculated the P value for the SNPs by false detection rate (FDR) for correction. According to these results, rs4143815 remained significant in the additive model ($P = 0.045$).

In an exploratory analysis, clinical characteristics related to T1DM were compared among different genotypes of PD-L1 rs4143815 (shown in Table 5). Age, gender, HbA1c, LDL, and HDL did not vary considerably among genotypes

Table 2: Eight single nucleotide polymorphisms examined in the present study.

Gene	SNP	Chromosome	Position	Mutation	MAF	HWE
PDCD1	rs34819629	2:241852468	Intron	G/A	A = 0.44	$P = 0.170$
	rs11568821	2:241851760	Intron	C/T	C = 1.0	$P < 0.001$
	rs10204525	2:241850169	Intron	C/T	C = 0.50	$P = 0.002$
	rs2227982	2:241851281	Intron	G/A	A = 0.60	$P < 0.001$
	rs2227981	2:241851121	Intron	G/T	T = 0.25	$P = 0.758$
PD-L1	rs2297136	9:5467955	3′UTR	A/G	G = 0.16	$P = 0.197$
	rs4143815	9:5468257	3′UTR	C/G	C = 0.46	$P = 0.752$
	rs2297137	9:5465732	Intron	G/A	A = 0.49	$P = 0.845$

SNP: single nucleotide polymorphism; MAF: minor allele frequency; HWE: Hardy-Weinberg equilibrium.

Table 3: All the primers used in the present study.

rs Number	Primer	Sequence
rs34819629	F	GTCCTGCACCTGGGGAATG
	R-Biotin	TCTGGAAGGGCACAAAGGTC
	Sequencing primer	ACCTGGGGAATGGTG
rs11568821	F	CCCCAGGCAGAACCTCAAT
	R-Biotin	GACCGCAGGCAGGCACATAT
	Sequencing primer	CCCCAGCCCACCTGC
rs10204525	F-Biotin	CTGACTCCCTCTCCCTTTCTC
	R	AAATCCAGCTCCCCATAGTCC
	Sequencing primer	GAGAACACAGGCACG
rs2297137	F	GCAAAGGCATTCCACTGTTC
	R-Biotin	ACCCCTTACGCTTCATCTTCAC
	Sequencing primer	GCATTCCACTGTTCAA
rs2227981	F	TTTCCAGTGGCGAGAGAAGA
	R-Biotin	GGCCAAGAGCAGTGTCCA
	Sequencing primer	CCGCCCGCAGGGGCT
rs2297136	F	ACGTAATCCAGCATTGGAACTT
	R-Biotin	TTCAGTGCTTGGGCCTTTTAA
	Sequencing primer	CAAGAGGAAGGAATGG
rs4143815	F	CTTTGCCTCCACTCAATGC
	R-Biotin	TACTGTCCCGTTCCAACACTG
	Sequencing primer	ACTCAATGCCTCAATTT
rs2227982	F	GGTTCGGTGCCGGTACTG
	R-Biotin	GGTCTTCTCTCGCCACTGGA
	Sequencing primer	CAAAGAAGGAGGACCC

of the rs4143815 SNP. However, the presence of subjects tested for autoantibodies (AABs) was higher in T1DM patients who were homozygous for the rs4143815G/G genotype compared with C allele carriers ($P = 0.033$).

We also simulated the secondary structure of partial PD-L1 3′UTR mRNA with different allele carrier using RNAfold (Figure 1). Different allele carrier of rs4143815 makes a great difference to the stem-loop structure of PD-L1 3′UTR, and this may account for its different binding force between miR-570 and mRNA leading to altered expression of PD-L1 protein and different susceptibility to T1DM.

4. Discussion

For the past few years, increasing studies had been committed to the associations with gene polymorphisms and T1DM susceptibility. The present study was made to investigate whether genetic polymorphisms in immune checkpoints could predict the onset of T1DM. In total, 266 subjects were included in the present study. With 8 selected SNPs genotyped, PD-L1 SNP rs4143815 remained significantly associated with T1DM susceptibility after FDR correction (additive model: $P = 0.045$). No significant associations were

Table 4: Association of five single nucleotide polymorphisms with type 1 diabetes susceptibility in all subjects.

Gene	SNP	Model	OR (95% CI)	*P* value
PD-1	rs2227981	ADD	1.05 (0.64 ~ 1.72)	0.846
		DOM	0.98 (0.52 ~ 1.84)	0.941
		REC	1.45 (0.41 ~ 5.12)	0.563
	rs34819629	ADD	0.74 (0.48 ~ 1.13)	0.163
		DOM	0.62 (0.30 ~ 1.27)	0.190
		REC	0.70 (0.34 ~ 1.43)	0.326
PD-L1	rs4143815	ADD	0.50 (0.31 ~ 0.79)	0.003*
		DOM	0.31 (0.13 ~ 0.77)	0.012*
		REC	0.46 (0.23 ~ 0.92)	0.028*
	rs2297136	ADD	0.83 (0.48 ~ 1.43)	0.504
		DOM	0.76 (0.39 ~ 1.48)	0.421
		REC	1.00 (0.21 ~ 4.76)	0.995
	rs2297137	ADD	0.82 (0.53 ~ 1.28)	0.388
		DOM	0.61 (0.29 ~ 1.30)	0.203
		REC	0.97 (0.46 ~ 2.05)	0.930

ADD: additive model; DOM: dominant model; REC: recessive model; additive model: comparing the minor allele with major allele subjects; dominant model: comparing carriers of the minor allele with the major homozygous subjects; recessive model: comparing carriers of the major allele with the minor homozygous subjects.

Table 5: Clinical characteristics of T1DM patients in different genotype of rs4143815.

	PD-L1 rs4143815			
	G/G ($n = 43$)	G/C ($n = 85$)	C/C ($n = 34$)	*P* value
Age (years)	25.7 ± 11.6	26.8 ± 13.5	24.5 ± 10.5	0.661
Gender (% males)	46.5	55.3	44.1	0.447
HbA1c (%)	9.0 ± 2.5	8.6 ± 2.8	8.6 ± 2.7	0.737
LDL	2.7 ± 1.2	2.6 ± 0.7	2.6 ± 0.6	0.565
HDL	1.5 ± 0.5	1.6 ± 0.6	1.6 ± 0.4	0.212
Presence of AABs (IAA, ICA, GADA) (%)	72.1	49.4	67.6	0.033*

Data are mean—standard deviation (SD); HbA1c: glycated hemoglobin; LDL: low-density lipoprotein; HDL: high-density lipoprotein; AABs: subjects tested for autoantibodies; IAA: insulin autoantibody; ICA: islet cell autoantibody; GADA: glutamic acid decarboxylase autoantibody.

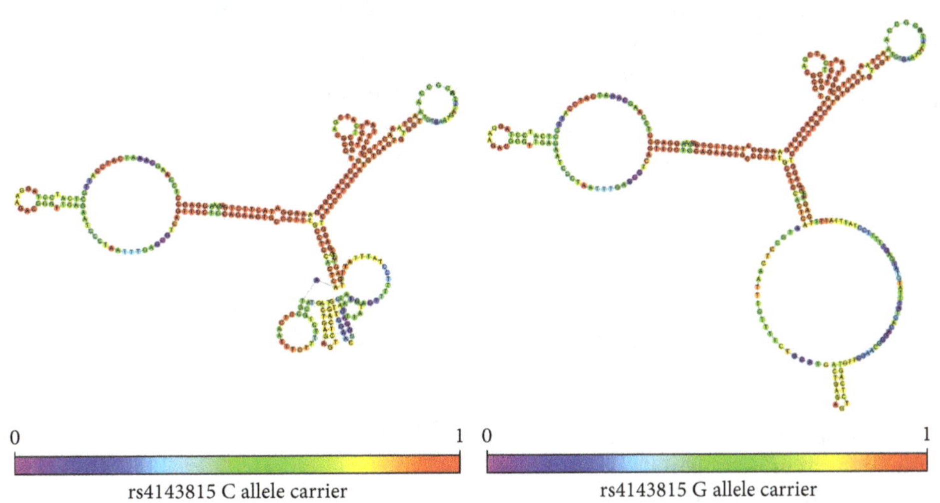

Figure 1: The secondary structure of partial PD-L1 3′UTR mRNA with different allele carrier of rs4143815 using RNAfold (http://rna.tbi.univie.ac.at/cgi-bin/RNAWebSuite/RNAfold.cgi).

observed with other SNPs. Furthermore, T1DM patients homozygous for the rs4143815 G/G genotype showed higher levels of AAB positive incidence compared with C allele carriers ($P = 0.033$).

PD-1 is a core costimulatory molecule expressed by T cells that interact with its ligands PD-L1 and PD-L2 on antigen-presenting cells. PD-L1 was shown to be overexpressed in human gastrointestinal tumors [8]. PD-L1 negatively regulated immune response by interacting with PD-1 on T cells and therefore promoting T cell apoptosis [25]. Anti-PD-1 antibody treatment has been applied to the treatment of numerous advanced cancers; however, insulin-dependent diabetes had been reported during the anti-PD-1 immunotherapy process in both mouse models and human cases [11–13].

Increasing studies had been committed to the association with PD-1/PD-L1 and type 1 diabetes; low serum level of PD-1 and PD-L1 was reported being associated with T1DM in Japanese and Chilean patients [3, 21]. Association of polymorphisms of the PD-1and PD-L1 with T1DM has been evaluated previously in other countries [21–23]. Nevertheless, the genetic background of type 1 diabetes differs greatly among the different population.

In the present study, rs4143815 was found being associated with T1DM susceptibility. People carrying the C allele of rs4143815 suffering less risk of T1DM and T1DM patients with G/G genotype showed higher levels of AAB positive incidence compared with C allele carriers. Since the level of AABs has high associations of T1DM, the results of AABs reinforce the importance of rs4143815. People carrying the C allele of rs4143815 suffer lower AAB level and less risk of T1DM. However, HbA1c did not vary considerably among genotypes of the rs4143815 SNP. Since HbA1c is an important indicator for glycemic control and has little relevance to the susceptibility of the disease, this may be induced by the different treatment stage of T1DM patients.

It had been reported that rs4143815 was associated with the increased risk of gastric cancer [26, 27] and non-small-cell lung cancer [28, 29], possibly resulted from the suppression of immunological tumor surveillance by increased PD-L1 expression [30]. rs4143815 was also found being associated with the risk of T1DM in Chile [21]. This previous study comprised 205 T1DM patients and 205 normal children; however, the HWE equilibrium of rs4143815 for T1DM was 0.006. Our results use pyrosequencing to genotype all the SNPs, and the HWE equilibrium of rs4143815 is 0.752. With proper HWE equilibrium and advanced genotyping method, our results reinforce the importance of rs4143815 in T1DM susceptibility in Chinese population.

The rs4143815 is located in the 3′UTR of PD-L1 and binds to miR-570 [26]. Different allele may change the secondary structure of PD-L1 3′UTR. RNAfold was used to predict the secondary structure of PD-L1 3′UTR; G allele carrier shows a bigger stem-loop structure compared with C allele (shown in Figure 1) which may increase the interaction between PD-L1 3′UTR and miR-570 leading to lower PD-L1 expression. Lee et al. found that rs4143815 G allele exhibited a decreased transcription activity compared with C allele though luciferase report [31] which accords with our previous prediction.

Several studies had been committed to the association with PD-1 and autoimmune disease. PD 1.2, PD1.3, PD1.5, and PD1.9 were found being associated with systemic lupus erythematosus, ankylosing spondylitis, and allergic bronchial asthma [14–17]. However, our results showed that there are no associations between PD-1 polymorphisms and T1DM susceptibility. This may be due to different pathogenesis between T1DM and other autoimmune diseases.

Our study has some limitations. With limited SNPs and small sample size, the final result may have a certain deviation. We will select more typical SNPs and increase the sample size in the next step, and we will use gene chip and conduct multicenter studies to revalidate our results in the future.

5. Conclusion

In this study, our results indicate that rs4143815 of PD-L1 is significantly associated with T1DM susceptibility. Importantly, this SNP remained significantly after FDR correction. Furthermore, the presence of AABs is higher in T1DM patients homozygous for the rs4143815 G/G genotype compared with C allele carriers.

Conflicts of Interest

The authors declare that they have no conflict of interest.

Authors' Contributions

Chenyue Qian and Heming Guo contributed equally to this work.

Acknowledgments

This study was funded by grants from the National Natural Science Foundation of China (Grant no. 81471041 to Ji Hu, 81600607 to Chen Fang, and 81502865 to Yun Huang). This work was also supported by the Open Research Project of Shanghai Key Laboratory of Diabetes Mellitus (SHKLD-KF-1604) and Ministry of Science and Technology of China under Award Number 2016YFC1305202. This work was also supported by Second Affiliated Hospital of Soochow University Science Foundation (no. SDFEYQN1604) and Suzhou Science Foundation (no. SYSD2016148).

References

[1] J. Tian, Y. Liu, Y. Liu, K. Chen, and S. Lyu, "Cellular and molecular mechanisms of diabetic atherosclerosis: herbal medicines as a potential therapeutic approach," *Oxidative Medicine and Cellular Longevity*, vol. 2017, Article ID 9080869, 16 pages, 2017.

[2] B. T. Fife and J. A. Bluestone, "Control of peripheral T-cell tolerance and autoimmunity via the CTLA-4 and PD-1 pathways," *Immunological Reviews*, vol. 224, no. 1, pp. 166–182, 2008.

[3] R. Fujisawa, F. Haseda, C. Tsutsumi et al., "Low programmed cell death-1 (PD-1) expression in peripheral CD4$^+$ T cells in Japanese patients with autoimmune type 1 diabetes," *Clinical & Experimental Immunology*, vol. 180, no. 3, pp. 452–457, 2015.

[4] E. Nolan, P. Savas, A. N. Policheni et al., "Combined immune checkpoint blockade as a therapeutic strategy for *BRCA1*-mutated breast cancer," *Science Translational Medicine*, vol. 9, no. 393, article eaal4922, 2017.

[5] A. Bang, T. J. Wilhite, L. R. G. Pike et al., "Multicenter evaluation of the tolerability of combined treatment with PD-1 and CTLA-4 immune checkpoint inhibitors and palliative radiation therapy," *International Journal of Radiation Oncology, Biology, Physics*, vol. 98, no. 2, pp. 344–351, 2017.

[6] S. Marwitz, S. Scheufele, S. Perner, M. Reck, O. Ammerpohl, and T. Goldmann, "Epigenetic modifications of the immune-checkpoint genes *CTLA4* and *PDCD1* in non-small cell lung cancer results in increased expression," *Clinical Epigenetics*, vol. 9, no. 1, p. 51, 2017.

[7] C. Wu, Y. Zhu, J. Jiang, J. Zhao, X. G. Zhang, and N. Xu, "Immunohistochemical localization of programmed death-1 ligand-1 (PD-L1) in gastric carcinoma and its clinical significance," *Acta Histochemica*, vol. 108, no. 1, pp. 19–24, 2006.

[8] W. Zou and L. Chen, "Inhibitory B7-family molecules in the tumour microenvironment," *Nature Reviews Immunology*, vol. 8, no. 6, pp. 467–477, 2008.

[9] Q. Li, J. F. Gao, and B. L. Qi, "PDCD1 strengthens the sensitivity of ovarian cancer to cisplatin chemotherapy by promoting apoptosis," *Journal of Balkan Union of Oncology*, vol. 22, no. 3, pp. 746–756, 2017.

[10] J. Y. Kim, E. Lee, K. Park et al., "Immune signature of metastatic breast cancer: identifying predictive markers of immunotherapy response," *Oncotarget*, vol. 8, no. 29, pp. 47400–47411, 2017.

[11] M. J. I. Ansari, A. D. Salama, T. Chitnis et al., "The programmed death-1 (PD-1) pathway regulates autoimmune diabetes in nonobese diabetic (NOD) mice," *Journal of Experimental Medicine*, vol. 198, no. 1, pp. 63–69, 2003.

[12] J. Hughes, N. Vudattu, M. Sznol et al., "Precipitation of autoimmune diabetes with anti-PD-1 immunotherapy," *Diabetes Care*, vol. 38, no. 4, pp. e55–e57, 2015.

[13] J. Martin-Liberal, A. J. S. Furness, K. Joshi, K. S. Peggs, S. A. Quezada, and J. Larkin, "Anti-programmed cell death-1 therapy and insulin-dependent diabetes: a case report," *Cancer Immunology, Immunotherapy*, vol. 64, no. 6, pp. 765–767, 2015.

[14] S. Dai, R. Jia, X. Zhang, Q. Fang, and L. Huang, "The PD-1/PD-Ls pathway and autoimmune diseases," *Cellular Immunology*, vol. 290, no. 1, pp. 72–79, 2014.

[15] E. V. Dmitrieva-Zdorova, M. V. Gabaeva, Y. A. Seregin, N. V. Bodoev, and O. E. Voronko, "PDCD1 PD-1.3 polymorphism and allergic bronchial asthma in Russian and Buryat patients," *Journal of Asthma*, vol. 54, no. 1, pp. 46–52, 2017.

[16] K. Chua, L. Lian, X. Sim, T. Cheah, and T. Lau, "Association between *PDCD1* gene polymorphisms and risk of systemic lupus erythematosus in three main ethnic groups of the Malaysian population," *International Journal of Molecular Sciences*, vol. 16, no. 12, pp. 9794–9803, 2015.

[17] M. Yang, Y. Zou, Y. Bai, and M. Li, "The programmed cell death 1 gene polymorphisms (PD 1.3 G/A, PD 1.5 C/T and PD 1.9 C/T) and susceptibility to ankylosing spondylitis: a meta-analysis," *Journal of Orthopaedic Science*, vol. 20, no. 1, pp. 55–63, 2015.

[18] B. Zhang, Y. Li, X. Zhong, W. Huang, L. Nie, and W. Zhang, "Establishment of retinoblastoma model in NOD-SCID mice and study of metastasis," *Yan Ke Xue Bao*, vol. 21, no. 3, pp. 185–191, 2005.

[19] J. Wang, T. Yoshida, F. Nakaki, H. Hiai, T. Okazaki, and T. Honjo, "Establishment of NOD-*Pdcd1*$^{-/-}$ mice as an efficient animal model of type I diabetes," *Proceedings of the National Academy of Sciences of the United States of America*, vol. 102, no. 33, pp. 11823–11828, 2005.

[20] M. L. Colli, J. L. E. Hill, L. Marroquí et al., "PDL1 is expressed in the islets of people with type 1 diabetes and is up-regulated by interferons-α and-γ via IRF1 induction," *EBioMedicine*, vol. 36, pp. 367–375, 2018.

[21] C. Pizarro, D. F. García-Díaz, E. Codner, F. Salas-Pérez, E. Carrasco, and F. Pérez-Bravo, "PD-L1 gene polymorphisms and low serum level of PD-L1 protein are associated to type 1 diabetes in Chile," *Diabetes/Metabolism Research and Reviews*, vol. 30, no. 8, pp. 761–766, 2014.

[22] Y. H. Lee, S. C. Bae, J. H. Kim, and G. G. Song, "Meta-analysis of genetic polymorphisms in programmed cell death 1. Associations with rheumatoid arthritis, ankylosing spondylitis, and type 1 diabetes susceptibility," *Zeitschrift für Rheumatologie*, vol. 74, no. 3, pp. 230–239, 2015.

[23] Y. Hiromine, H. Ikegami, T. Fujisawa et al., "Trinucleotide repeats of programmed cell death-1 gene are associated with susceptibility to type 1 diabetes mellitus," *Metabolism*, vol. 56, no. 7, pp. 905–909, 2007.

[24] R. B. Denman, "Using RNAFOLD to predict the activity of small catalytic RNAs," *BioTechniques*, vol. 15, no. 6, pp. 1090–1095, 1993.

[25] H. Dong, S. E. Strome, D. R. Salomao et al., "Tumor-associated B7-H1 promotes T-cell apoptosis: a potential mechanism of immune evasion," *Nature Medicine*, vol. 8, no. 8, pp. 793–800, 2002.

[26] W. Wang, F. Li, Y. Mao et al., "A miR-570 binding site polymorphism in the *B7-H1* gene is associated with the risk of gastric adenocarcinoma," *Human Genetics*, vol. 132, no. 6, pp. 641–648, 2013.

[27] L. H. Tao, X. R. Zhou, F. C. Li et al., "A polymorphism in the promoter region of PD-L1 serves as a binding-site for SP1 and is associated with PD-L1 overexpression and increased occurrence of gastric cancer," *Cancer Immunology, Immunotherapy*, vol. 66, no. 3, pp. 309–318, 2017.

[28] W. Du, J. Zhu, Y. Chen et al., "Variant SNPs at the microRNA complementary site in the B7-H1 3′-untranslated region increase the risk of non-small cell lung cancer," *Molecular Medicine Reports*, vol. 16, no. 3, pp. 2682–2690, 2017.

[29] T. Nomizo, H. Ozasa, T. Tsuji et al., "Clinical impact of single nucleotide polymorphism in PD-L1 on response to nivolumab

for advanced non-small-cell lung cancer patients," *Scientific Reports*, vol. 7, no. 1, article 45124, 2017.

[30] X. L. Shi, S. Mancham, B. E. Hansen et al., "Counter-regulation of rejection activity against human liver grafts by donor PD-L1 and recipient PD-1 interaction," *Journal of Hepatology*, vol. 64, no. 6, pp. 1274–1282, 2016.

[31] S. Y. Lee, D. K. Jung, J. E. Choi et al., "Functional polymorphisms in *PD-L1* gene are associated with the prognosis of patients with early stage non-small cell lung cancer," *Gene*, vol. 599, pp. 28–35, 2017.

12

Skeletal Status, Body Composition, and Glycaemic Control in Adolescents with Type 1 Diabetes Mellitus

Elzbieta Wierzbicka,[1] **Anna Swiercz**,[2] **Pawel Pludowski**,[3] **Maciej Jaworski**,[3] **and Mieczyslaw Szalecki**[2,4]

[1]*Department of Human Nutrition, Warsaw University of Life Sciences (SGGW), Warsaw, Poland*
[2]*Department of Endocrinology and Diabetology, The Children's Memorial Health Institute, Warsaw, Poland*
[3]*Department of Biochemistry, Radioimmunology, and Experimental Medicine, The Children's Memorial Health Institute, Warsaw, Poland*
[4]*Faculty of Medicine and Health Sciences, Jan Kochanowski University, Kielce, Poland*

Correspondence should be addressed to Elzbieta Wierzbicka; elzbieta_wierzbicka@sggw.pl

Academic Editor: Paolo Fiorina

Background. Disturbed bone turnover, osteoporosis, and increased fracture risk are late complications of insulin-dependent diabetes mellitus. Little is known about how far and to what extent can glycaemic control of type 1 diabetes mellitus (T1DM) prevent disturbances of bone health and body composition during the growth and maturation period. *Objective.* The aim of this cross-sectional study was to compare the skeletal status outcomes and body composition between patients stratified by glycaemic control (1-year HbA1c levels) into well- and poorly-controlled subgroups in a population of T1DM adolescents, that is, <8% and ≥8%, respectively. *Subjects and Methods.* Skeletal status and body composition were evaluated in 60 adolescents with T1DM (53.3% female; mean aged: 15.1 ± 1.9 years; disease duration: 5.1 ± 3.9 years) using dual energy X-ray absorptiometry (GE Prodigy). The results were compared to age- and sex-adjusted reference values for healthy controls. The calculated Z-scores of different metabolic control subgroups were compared. Clinical data was also assessed. *Results.* As evidenced by Z-scores, patients with T1DM revealed a significantly lower TBBMD (total body bone mineral density), TBBMC (total body bone mineral content), S24BMD (bone mineral density of lumbar spine L2–L4), and TBBMC/LBM ratio (total body bone mineral content/lean body mass), but higher FM (fat mass) and FM/LBM ratio (fat mass/lean body mass) values compared to an age- and sex-adjusted general population. The subset (43.3% patients) with poor metabolic control (HbA1c ≥ 8%) had lower TBBMD, TBBMC, and LBM compared to respective values noted in the HbA1c < 8% group, after adjusting for confounders (mean Z-scores: −0.74 vs. −0.10, $p = 0.037$; −0.67 vs. +0.01, $p = 0.026$; and −0.45 vs. +0.20, $p = 0.043$, respectively). Additionally, we found a significant difference in the TBBMC/LBM ratio (relative bone strength index) between the metabolic groups (−0.58 vs. −0.07; $p = 0.021$). A statistically significant negative correlation between 1-year HbA1c levels and Z-scores of TBBMD, TBBMC, and LBM was also observed. In patients with longer disease duration, a significant negative correlation was established only for TBBMD, after adjusting for confounders. The relationships between densitometric values and age at onset of T1DM and sex were not significant and showed no relation to any of the analysed parameters of the disease course. *Conclusion.* Findings from this study of adolescents with T1DM indicate that the lower Z-scores of TBBMD, TBBMC, and LBM as well as the TBBMC/LBM ratio are associated with increased HbA1c levels. Their recognition can be crucial in directing strategies to optimise metabolic control and improve diabetes management for bone development and maintenance in adolescents with T1DM.

1. Introduction

Type 1 diabetes mellitus (T1DM) is one of the most common chronic childhood diseases, the prevalence of which is rising globally [1, 2]. In Poland, a recent epidemiological study confirmed this trend and demonstrated an increased incidence of diabetes in the paediatric population [3, 4]. Type 1 DM is a chronic systemic autoimmune-mediated disease characterised by hyperglycaemia, due to progressive absolute insulin deficiency, as a result of the destruction of the pancreatic β-cells [1, 5]. In the majority of patients, the disease develops during childhood and patients are therefore exposed to the deleterious effects of insulin deficiency and hyperglycaemia for a long time, causing micro- and macrovascular complications [6, 7]. It is apparent that the skeleton has been recognised as an organ that is also adversely affected by a diabetic condition [8–12]. The reported results indicate that diabetic bone disease with fragility is another complication of a long-standing disease in patients with T1DM [13, 14]. There is evidence confirming an association between glucose utilisation and bone-fat tissue interaction [15–18], as well as the muscle-bone crosstalk [19–21]. The risk of fracture among adult patients with long-standing T1DM is higher compared with an age- and sex-matched non-diabetic control population [22–24], while no relevant data exist on childhood type 1 DM. Notably, one study reported, for the first time, a higher fracture incidence in young males and females with T1DM (aged < 20 years) compared to subjects without T1DM, as assessed by hazard ratio (HR) — 1.14 (95% CI 1.01–1.29) and 1.35 (95% CI 1.12–1.63), respectively [25]. On the other hand, recent studies have reported low rates of non-vertebral fractures in aging individuals with long-standing T1DM [26]. However, this study described an association between the presence of cardiovascular disease and low bone mineral density at the femoral neck. Other studies, looking specifically at adolescents [27] and young women [28] as well as adult T1DM patients [29, 30], identified microvascular complications as a factor of skeletal deficits and decreased bone quality.

Childhood and adolescence are the most critical periods for growth and bone mineral accrual [31–33]. Importantly, the onset of the disease often starts at a time when peak bone mass is not yet achieved; thus, it is likely that it impairs bone accrual during this period of bone growth [34]. In children with T1DM, abnormal bone accrual (density and quality) [10–12] can also be associated with alterations of the growth hormone/insulin like growth factor-1 (GH/IGF-1) axis [35]. Since the maximum bone mineral accrual occurs during the first two decades of life [31, 32], the reduced bone mineral mass gain during these critical periods can lead to serious consequences, in particular, osteoporosis and bone fracture risk in later in life [33]. In type 1 DM, a failure of bone cells in high-glucose conditions [36] is associated with abnormal activities of neighbouring cells in bone, such as adipocytes, mesenchymal cells, and endothelial progenitor cells [37], and may increase influence on adipocyte differentiation and fat accumulation [16–18], as well as increased bone marrow adiposity [15, 38]. Adipose tissue is a metabolically dynamic organ [39] that is also an endocrine organ, capable of producing cytokines and adipokines that may regulate bone metabolic homeostasis [10, 13, 14]. Due to the fact that adipose tissue distribution affects bone mass, the relationship between adipose and bone tissue is notable [15, 16, 18]. On the other hand, deteriorated muscle function [40] might result in adverse effects on skeletal status [19–21]. Poor glycaemic control, as seen in hyperglycaemia, is a known risk factor for bone disorders [36, 37]. Many substantial studies in patients with T1DM described an association with reduced bone mineral density and osteoporosis [8, 9]. Bone mass and density deficits in T1DM patients most likely reflect the defects in bone formation with osteoblastic dysfunction [10, 11], as alterations of bone microarchitectures are involved in reducing bone quality and strength [12–14]. This, in turn, increases the risk of fractures in later life [22–25]. It is important to note that in children and adolescents with T1DM such data is limited and inconsistent [34].

In this context, the hypothesis of this study is that inadequate glycaemic control is an important variable associated with insufficient bone mineral accrual, and that this association is related to decreased muscle mass and increased fat stores, which may be an important factor in bone development in childhood type 1 DM.

The aim of this cross-sectional study was to compare the skeletal status outcomes, body composition, and relative bone strength between patients stratified by glycated haemoglobin levels (%HbA1c) into two study subgroups, that is, relatively well- and poorly-controlled in a population based on T1DM adolescents.

2. Material and Methods

2.1. Study Population. The purposive cross-sectional study population was composed of 60 Caucasian adolescent patients (aged 15.1 ± 1.9 years) with type 1 insulin-dependent diabetes mellitus (T1DM), admitted for a regular check-up to the Department of Endocrinology and Diabetology of the Children's Memorial Health Institute in Warsaw, Poland. Participants were selected based on the following criteria: age of 12–18 years, males and females (1 : 1 ratio), diagnosis of T1DM according to ISPAD criteria, duration of diabetes and received medical services in the clinic for at least six months, treated by continuous subcutaneous insulin infusion, complete data for the glycated haemoglobin (A1c) values, and the DXA measurements performed. The exclusion criteria for patients were as follows: history of any acute (severe hypoglycaemia, diabetic ketoacidosis) or chronic (retinopathy, neuropathy, and nephropathy) complications of diabetes, the presence of any associated metabolic bone or musculoskeletal diseases, and any chronic illness other than diabetes as well as any medications other than insulin.

The study was approved by the local ethics committee (Warsaw, Poland) and was conducted in accordance with the World Medical Association Declaration of Helsinki. Written informed consent was obtained from the parents of all the patients at the initial enrolment in this study.

2.2. Data Collection. For all study participants, a medical record review was undertaken. The following information was collected and recorded using a standardised questionnaire: demographics, physical activity (including school-based physical activity), age at diabetes onset, duration of diabetes, insulin delivery system, daily insulin dose (units per kilogram of body weight), general medical history, and clinical characteristics, as well as data related to metabolic control of diabetes, including the glycated haemoglobin (HbA1c) level in a 1-year period.

Each patient underwent a comprehensive examination that included a measurement of skeletal and body composition using dual-energy X-ray absorptiometry (DXA), allowing the assessment of three tissue compartments (bone, lean, and fat tissue). Anthropometric measurements of the patients were obtained together with densitometry during a single visit. The adolescents' height and weight Z-scores were calculated using national reference data. The subjects' pubertal stage was assessed by a physical examination performed by a trained paediatrician using the Tanner classification.

Blood samples were obtained in the morning after an overnight fast. Glycated haemoglobin A1c (HbA1c) was analysed in a whole blood sample by a direct turbidimetric inhibition immunoassay (Roche Diagnostics, Germany) that determines HbA1c as a percentage of total haemoglobin (HbA1c, %), performed according to IFCC guidelines. The serum levels of calcium and inorganic phosphorous were measured spectrophotometrically using commercially available test kits (Roche Diagnostics, Germany). Serum total 25(OH)D and PTH (iPTH) were measured by a chemiluminescence immunoassay (ECLIA, Roche Diagnostics, Germany), according to the manufacturer's instructions.

2.3. Assessment of Glycaemic Control. Glycaemic control was evaluated on the basis of %HbA1c levels in the past year. These were calculated as an average of data collected at least three times in a 1-year period. Based on HbA1c levels, T1DM patients with different metabolic control states were divided into subgroups. For this purpose, patients with HbA1c < 8% (<64 mmol/mol) were considered as having relatively good glycaemic control, while those with HbA1c ≥ 8% (≥64 mmol/mol) as having poor glycaemic control.

2.4. Assessment of Skeletal Status and Body Composition — DXA Data. In all investigated patients, skeletal data, that is, total body bone mineral density (TBBMD, g/cm^2), total body bone mineral content (TBBMC, g), and both bone mineral density (S24BMD, g/cm^2) and bone mineral content (S24BMC, g) at the lumbar spine L2–L4, as well as body composition (lean mass and fat mass of the total body) were measured by dual-energy X-ray absorptiometry (DXA), using the Prodigy Advance device (General Electric™) with paediatric software ver. 14. For the calibration of a densitometer, a daily quality control procedure was performed. Additionally, anthropomorphic spine phantom was scanned at least twice a week. Measurement error (CV%) was 0.33% for L2–L4 BMD and 0.35% for L2–L4 BMC in the whole study period.

Moreover, the fat mass/lean body mass ratio (FM/LBM ratio) was calculated from DXA data. Also, relative bone strength index, estimated as the total body bone mineral content/lean body mass ratio (TBBMC/LBM ratio), and bone mineral content of lumbar spine L2–L4/lean body mass (S24BMC/LBM ratio) were considered as the muscle-bone relationship indicator.

Absolute densitometric data were compared with sex- and age-adjusted reference values established in healthy counterparts [41, 42], and the Z-scores were calculated using the following formula: Z-score = [(result for a subject) – (age- and gender-matched mean in reference subjects)]/(age- and gender-matched standard deviation in reference subjects). Low bone mass or bone mineral density was defined as Z-scores lower than or equal to −2.0 standard deviation [43].

2.5. Statistical Analysis. For the purposes of this study, multiple analyses were performed. In the first one, the results were referred to the norms according to age and sex and presented as Z-score (corresponding abbreviations are preceded by the letter "Z"). Deviations from the normal distribution were verified by the Shapiro-Wilk test. Z-score values were evaluated by one-sample Student's *t*-test with the hypothetic value "0", assumed to reflect expected data in healthy control subjects. Only for fat mass (FM) was the non-parametric one-sample Wilcoxon test used. Association tests (Student's *t*-test or Mann–Whitney's *U* test) were performed to compare the quantitative variables in both subgroups. The differences in descriptive values were estimated using the Chi-square test for categorical variables. Pearson's correlation coefficient or nonlinear association Spearman's correlation coefficient were calculated to assess the relationships between skeletal and body composition parameters and clinical data. Correlation analysis was also performed between disease duration, insulin requirement, glycemic control (%HbA1c levels), and skeletal and body composition Z-score values (for age- and sex-dependent reference data for healthy subjects). Partial correlation coefficients were calculated for these parameters, using age, sex, pubertal stage, height, weight, and physical activity level as confounders. The second analysis consisted of comparison of Z-score values for bone density and body composition parameters, between the two subgroups of different metabolic control, that is, HbA1c < 8% and ≥8%. Analysis of covariance (ANCOVA) was used to compare skeletal and body parameters between subgroups of good and poor metabolic control, adjusting for disease duration, age, sex, pubertal stage, insulin dose, height, weight, and physical activity level. The analyses were performed using software Statistica v.13 and IBM SPSS Statistics v.25. Data were presented as mean ± SD (standard deviation) and SE (standard error of the mean) or number (%) unless specified, and a p-value ≤ 0.05 was considered to indicate statistical significance.

3. Results

3.1. Characteristics of the Studied Group. The study included 60 adolescents with type 1 diabetes (53.3% female) (mean ± SD) aged 15.0 ± 1.9 years with a disease duration of 5.1 ± 3.9 years and patients with young-onset diabetes of 9.9 ± 3.9 years. Of all DM patients, 56.7% of the patients were categorised as relativity well-controlled (HbA1c < 8%;

Table 1: Demographic and clinical characteristics of patients with T1DM.

Variable[/1]	Total $n = 60$	HbA1c < 8% $n = 34$	HbA1c ≥ 8% $n = 26$	p^*
Clinical, metabolic and anthropometric characteristics				
Females (%)	32 (53.3)	17 (50.0)	15 (57.7)	NS
Age (y)	15.1 ± 1.9	14.4 ± 1.8	16.0 ± 1.7	0.001
Age at diagnosis (y)	9.9 ± 3.9	10.5 ± 3.3	9.4 ± 4.6	NS
Diabetes duration (y)	5.1 ± 3.9	3.9 ± 3.1	6.7 ± 4.3	0.005
Insulin dose (U/kg/d)	0.75 ± 0.21	0.67 ± 0.16	0.86 ± 0.22	0.001
Pubertal (Tanner stage)	3.7 ± 0.9	3.4 ± 0.9	4.0 ± 0.8	NS
HbA_{1c} (%), 1-year period	7.9 ± 1.4	6.9 ± 0.6	9.2 ± 1.0	0.001
Serum 25(OH)D (ng/mL)	15.3 ± 7.0	17.2 ± 7.9	12.8 ± 4.7	0,015
Serum iPTH (pg/mL)	30.4 ± 16.4	27.0 ± 12.6	34.8 ± 19.8	NS
Serum Ca (mmol/L)	2.44 ± 0.09	2.45 ± 0.10	2.44 ± 0.08	NS
Serum P (mmol/L)	1.39 ± 0.19	1.41 ± 0.21	1.35 ± 0.20	NS
Body height (cm)	166.5 ± 11.5	167.2 ± 12.4	166.2 ± 10.3	NS
Body height (SD score)[/2]	0.07 ± 1.12	0.38 ± 1.10	−0.34 ± 1.02	0.012
Body weight (kg)	58.9 ± 11.9	58.1 ± 13.6	60.0 ± 9.4	NS
Body weight (SD score)[/2]	0.29 ± 1.16	0.39 ± 1.32	0.16 ± 0.93	NS
Physical exercise (hours in school/week)	3.3 ± 1.3	3.3 ± 1.1	3.4 ± 1.5	NS
DXA parameters				
TBBMD (g/cm^2)	1.064 ± 0.093	1.055 ± 0.104	1.074 ± 0.077	NS
TBBMC (g)	2271 ± 516	2252 ± 581	2297 ± 429	NS
LBM (kg)	42.8 ± 10.3	42.8 ± 11.0	42.7 ± 9.7	NS
FM (kg)	13.7 ± 7.4	13.0 ± 8.0	14.6 ± 6.7	NS
S24BMD (g/cm^2)	1.039 ± 0.166	1.005 ± 0.170	1.084 ± 0.154	NS
S24BMC (g)	43.3 ± 11.9	42.1 ± 12.5	44.8 ± 11.2	NS
S24BMC/LBM (ratio)	1.019 ± 0.197	0.984 ± 0.185	1.063 ± 0.207	NS
TBBMC/LBM (ratio)	0.054 ± 0.007	0.053 ± 0.006	0.055 ± 0.008	NS
FM/LBM (ratio)	0.343 ± 0.198	0.324 ± 0.202	0.370 ± 0.194	NS

[/1]Data are expressed as mean ± SD; [/2]SD-scores calculated according to age- and sex-dependent reference data for healthy subjects; *p-values for differences between subgroups were calculated with independent Student's t-test, or Chi-square test for categorical variables; NS — not significant. TBBMD — total body bone mineral density; TBBMC — total body bone mineral content; LBM — lean body mass FM — fat mass; S24BMD — bone mineral density, lumbar spine L2–L4; S24BMC — bone mineral content, lumbar spine L2–L4; S24BMC/LBM — bone mineral content, lumbar spine L2–L4/lean body mass ratio; TBBMC/LBM — total body bone mineral content/lean body mass ratio; FM/LBM — fat mass/lean body mass ratio.

64 mmol/mol) and 43.3% of the patients as poorly-controlled (HbA1c ≥ 8%; 64 mmol/mol). The basic characteristics of both DM subgroups are given in Table 1.

Overall, the mean HbA1c value (in a 1-year period) was 7.9 ± 1.4% (Table 1). The highest HbA1c levels were observed in the uncontrolled DM subgroup (9.2 ± 1.0%), while the well-controlled DM subgroup showed the lowest HbA1c levels (6.9 ± 0.6%); $p = 0.001$. Patients from both subgroups had a similar age at the diagnosis of about 10 years; there were no statistically significant differences. The group of adolescents with poor glycaemic control was characterised by significantly longer diabetes duration (6.7 ± 4.3 vs. 3.9 ± 3.1 years, $p = 0.005$), higher insulin dose (0.86 ± 0.22 vs. 0.67 ± 0.16 U/kg bw/d, $p = 0.005$) which is strictly connected with HbA1c levels, older age (16.0 ± 1.7 vs. 14.4 ± 1.8 years, $p = 0.001$), and lower body height values (SD score) (i.e., −0.34 ± 1.02 vs. +0.38 ± 1.10, $p = 0.012$), compared to patients with good glycaemic control. Both studied groups revealed low 25(OH)D serum levels of 15.3 ± 7.0 ng/mL, below the optimal values of 30–50 ng/mL (Table 1). Significantly increased serum levels of 25(OH)D levels (17.2 ± 7.9 ng/mL vs. 12.8 ± 4.4 ng/mL; $p = 0.015$) were found in the well-controlled patients compared to those found in the uncontrolled DM subgroup. The serum calcium, iPTH, and inorganic phosphorus levels were within the normal range in both groups ($p > 0.05$).

Among the studied subgroups (Table 1), no significant differences were found in the remaining analysed clinical and other anthropometric data. Similarly, no differences were found in DXA parameters (Table 1), expressed as absolute values. In contrast, the analysis of the skeletal status and body composition in comparison with Z-scores, calculated according to age- and gender-dependent reference data for the healthy subject, revealed statistically significant differences between the examined groups of subjects (Table 2).

3.2. Skeletal Status and Body Composition. Skeletal status and body composition of T1DM patients, as a whole group, as

Table 2: The Z-score values for DXA parameters in T1DM patients with well or poorly controlled glycaemia.

Variable (Z-scores)[/1]	$x \pm SD$	SE	95% CI	p^*
$n = 60$				
Z TBBMD	−0.38 ± 0.95	0.12	−0.63; −0.14	0.003
Z TBBMC	−0.29 ± 0.97	0.13	−0.54; −0.03	0.027
Z LBM	−0.08 ± 0.90	0.12	−0.32; +0.15	0.483
Z S24BMD	−0.30 ± 1.06	0.14	−0.58; −0.03	0.031
Z S24BMC	−0.09 ± 0.99	0.13	−0.35; +0.16	0.461
Z TBBMC/LBM	−0.29 ± 0.97	0.13	−0.54; −0.04	0.025
Z S24BMC/LBM	+0.29 ± 1.16	0.15	−0.01; +0.59	0.055
Z FM[/2]	+0.38 ± 1.27	0.16	+0.05; +0.70	0.025
Z FM/LBM	+0.31 ± 0.99	0.13	+0.63; +0.57	0.018
$n = 34$ (*HbA1c* < 8%)				
Z TBBMD	−0.10 ± 0.97	0.17	−0.44; +0.23	0.535
Z TBBMC	+0.01 ± 1.02	0.18	−0.35; +0.37	0.959
Z LBM	+0.20 ± 0.90	0.15	−0.11; +0.52	0.197
Z S24BMD	−0.20 ± 1.16	0.20	−0.61; +0.20	0.321
Z S24BMC	+0.09 ± 1.06	0.18	−0.28; +0.46	0.618
Z TBBMC/LBM	−0.07 ± 0.96	0.17	−0.41; +0.27	0.677
Z S24BMC/LBM	+0.44 ± 1.20	0.21	+0.02; +0.86	0.039
Z FM[/2]	+0.36 ± 1.44	0.25	−0.14; +0.86	0.153
Z FM/LBM	+0.20 ± 1.05	0.18	−0.16; +0.57	0.266
$n = 26$ (*HbA1c* ≥ 8%)				
Z TBBMD	−0.74 ± 0,80	0.16	−1.07; −0.42	0.001
Z TBBMC	−0.67 ± 0.77	0.15	−0.98; −0.37	0.001
Z LBM	−0.45 ± 0.77	0.15	−0.77; −0.14	0,006
Z S24BMD	−0.43 ± 0.91	0.18	−0.80; −0.07	0.022
Z S24BMC	−0.34 ± 0.85	0.17	−0.68; +0.01	0.053
Z TBBMC/LBM	−0.58 ± 0.92	0.18	−0.95; −0.20	0.004
Z S24BMC/LBM	+0.10 ± 1.10	0.22	−0.35; +0.54	0.652
Z FM[/2]	+0.40 ± 1.03	0.20	−0.02; +0.81	0.060
Z FM/LBM	+0.45 ± 0.90	0.18	+0.09; +0.82	0.018

$x \pm SD$: mean ± standard deviation; SE: standard error of the mean; 95% CI: confidence interval; *p-values were calculated with one-sample t-test compared to the hypothetical values of 0 (expected in healthy subjects); [/1]Z-scores for DXA parameters calculated according to age- and sex-dependent reference data for healthy subjects; [/2]Wilcoxon test TBBMD — total body bone mineral density; TBBMC — total body bone mineral content; LBM — lean body mass; FM — fat mass; S24BMD — bone mineral density, lumbar spine L2–L4; S24BMC — bone mineral content, lumbar spine L2–L4; S24BMC/LBM — bone mineral content, lumbar spine L2–L4/lean body mass ratio; TBBMC/LBM — total body bone mineral content/lean body mass ratio; FM/LBM — fat mass/lean body mass ratio.

well as in the well-controlled subgroup (HbA1c < 8%) and the poorly-controlled subgroup (HbA1c ≥ 8%), were referenced to their age- and gender-matched healthy counterparts, as shown in Table 2. As indicated in Table 2, T1DM patients as a whole had slightly decreased Z-scores for bone mass and density of the whole skeleton (TBBMD, TBBMC) and slightly decreased bone density in the lumbar spine (S24BMD) region, compared to the value of zero (expected in healthy counterparts). In contrast, the HbA1c ≥ 8%

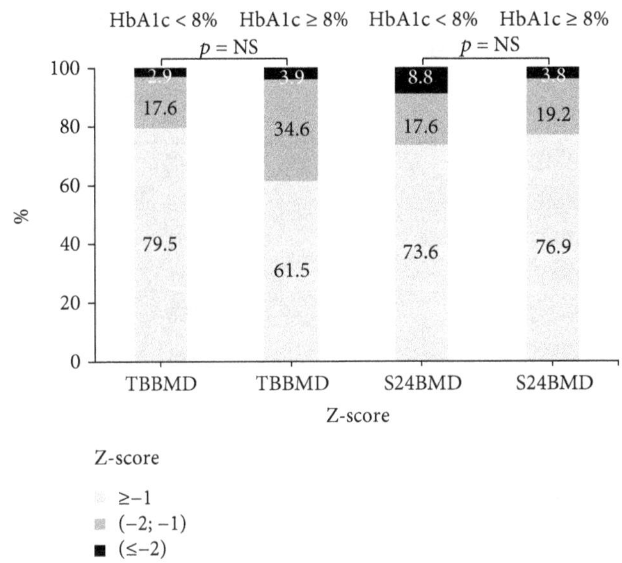

Figure 1: The stacked bar of frequency distribution (%) of the bone mineral density of the whole skeleton and of the lumbar spine bone mineral density in T1DM patients with well- or poorly controlled glycaemia. TBBMD — total body bone mineral density; S24BMD — bone mineral density, lumbar spine L2–L4.

subgroup (Table 2) revealed decreased Z-scores for bone density of both whole skeleton and lumbar spine (TBBMD Z-score of -0.74 ± 0.80, $p < 0.01$ and S24BMD Z-score of -0.43 ± 0.91, $p < 0.05$). Bone mineral content appeared decreased in the whole skeleton (TBBMC Z-score) but normal in the lumbar spine (S24BMC Z-score).

Figure 1 shows BMD Z-score distribution in relation to glycaemic control. As shown in Figure 1, the majority of cases, irrespective of %HbA1c value or region of the skeleton, had a BMD Z-score above the value of −2.00.

Lean body mass (an estimate of muscle mass) Z-score values (Table 2) calculated for the whole group appeared normal (mean LBM Z-score of -0.08 ± 0.90), but FM and the distributed relationship between FM and LBM as assessed by the FM/LBM ratio were slightly higher (FM Z-scores of $+0.38 \pm 1.27$, $p < 0.05$; FM/LBM Z-scores of $+0.31 \pm 0.99$; $p < 0.05$) when compared to the value of zero (expected in healthy counterparts). The HbA1c ≥ 8% subgroup had decreased LBM Z-score values of -0.45 ± 0.77 ($p < 0.05$), normal FM (FM Z-score of $+0.40 \pm 1.03$, $p = 0.060$), and statistically increased FM/LBM Z-score values of $+0.45 \pm 0.90$ ($p < 0.05$) (Table 2).

Relative bone strength was estimated as the total body bone mineral content/lean body mass ratio. Patients with T1DM had TBBMC/LBM ratio Z-scores slightly lower than expected in healthy subjects, but S24BMC/LBM ratio Z-scores were normal compared to their age- and gender-matched healthy reference (Table 2). Furthermore, when HbA1c (%) was controlled for, the subgroup with HbA1c < 8% showed physiological values for all DXA measured parameters, and S24BMC/LBM Z-score was even slightly higher than expected in the healthy subjects. In contrast, the HbA1c ≥ 8% subgroup revealed decreased Z-scores for the whole skeleton (TBBMC Z-score) but normal in the

TABLE 3: Relationship between disease duration, insulin requirement, glycaemic control, and skeletal and body composition Z-score values (for age- and sex- dependent reference data for healthy subjects) in T1DM patients.

Variable (Z-scores)[/1]	Diabetes duration		Insulin requirement		HbA1c	
	r	p	r	p	r	p
Z TBBMD	−0.260*	0.049	−0.423*	0.001	−0.283*	0.031
Z TBBMC	−0.253	0.056	−0.302*	0.021	−0.331*	0.011
Z S24BMD	−0.163	0.221	−0.324*	0.013	−0.133	0,321
Z S24BMC	−0.121	0.356	−0.242	0.067	−0.246	0.063
Z TBBMC/LBM	−0.158	0.238	−0.386*	0.003	−0.182	0.171
Z S24BMC/LBM	−0.094	0.481	−0.272*	0.039	−0.129	0.334
Z LBM	−0.246	0.062	−0.110	0.410	−0.345*	0.008
Z FM	0.046	0.731	−0.111	0.408	0.013	0.921
Z FM/LBM	0.123	0.359	−0.115	0.390	0.054	0.689
Diabetes duration (y)	—	—	0.303*	0.021	0.265*	0.045
Insulin requirement (U/kg/d)	0.303*	0.021	—	—	0.626*	0.001
HbA1c (%)	0.265*	0.045	0.626	0.001*	—	—

Results are expressed as correlation coefficient (r) and two-tailed statistical significance (p); p-values adjusted for age, sex, pubertal stage, height, weight, and physical activity level; *p-value ≤ 0.05; [/1]Z-scores for DXA parameters calculated according to age- and sex-dependent reference data for healthy subjects; TBBMD — total body bone mineral density; TBBMC — total body bone mineral content; LBM — lean body mass; FM — fat mass; S24BMD — bone mineral density, lumbar spine L2–L4; S24BMC — bone mineral content, lumbar spine L2–L4; S24BMC/LBM — bone mineral content, lumbar spine L2–L4/lean body mass ratio; TBBMC/LBM — total body bone mineral content/lean body mass ratio; FM/LBM — fat mass/lean body mass ratio.

lumbar spine (S24BMC Z-score) and had decreased LBM Z-scores. In these patients, there was a significant relationship between BMC and LBM, where the TBBMC/LBM ratio value was lower than the value of zero, as assessed by the ratio Z-score of -0.58 ± 0.92 ($p < 0.05$), but the S24BMC/LBM ratio Z-score was normal and not significant (Table 2).

3.3. Effect of Disease Duration, Insulin Requirement, and HbA1c Levels. We explored the effects of disease-related factors, such as disease duration, insulin requirement, and HbA1c (%), on skeletal and body composition parameters (Z-scores) by carrying out a partial correlation analysis (controlled for age, sex, pubertal stage, height, weight, and physical activity level). As shown in Table 3, we detected no effect of disease duration on the studied DXA parameters, except for TBBMD Z-score value ($p < 0.05$). Moreover, TBBMC and LBM Z-scores tended to be lower as the disease duration increased ($p = 0.056$ and r, respectively). In contrast, diabetes duration was positively related to insulin requirement and HbA1c levels ($p < 0.05$). As presented in Table 3, the insulin requirement dose was negatively associated with Z-scores for TBBMD, TBBMC, TBBMC/LBM, S24BMD, and 24TBBMC/LBM ($p < 0.05$). Mean 1-year HbA1c levels (%) were also negatively related to the Z-scores for bone mass and density of the whole skeleton (TBBMD, TBBMC) and LBM ($p < 0.05$).

As shown in Figure 2, HbA1c (%) levels correlated negatively with Z-scores for TBBMD, TBBMC, and LBM ($r = -0.27$, -0.30, and -0.32; $p < 0.05$, respectively) as well as Z-scores for absolute TBBMC ($r = -0.28$, $p = 0.038$) and LBM ($r = -0.27$, $p = 0.040$) (data not shown). No significant relationships were found between HbA1c levels (%) and other DXA parameters as well as Z-scores and absolute data ($p > 0.05$).

3.4. Skeletal Status and Body Composition in Relation to Glycaemic Control. As shown in Figures 3 and 4, skeletal and body composition parameters were compared between the HbA1c < 8% and HbA1c ≥ 8% subgroups. After adjusting for disease duration, age, sex, pubertal stage, insulin dose, height, weight, and physical activity level, significantly lower Z-scores were noted in the HbA1c ≥ 8% subgroup for TBBMD and TBBMC, as well as for the TBBMC/LBM ratio (Figure 3). In the lumbar spine, the Z-score values showed that, in T1DM patients with HbA1c0> 8%, S24BMD and S24BMC/LBM were slightly lower when compared with the HbA1c < 8% subgroup; however, the differences were not significant ($p > 0.05$). Moreover, S24BMC Z-scores tended to be lower in HbA1c ≥ 8% than in the HbA1c < 8% subgroup ($p = 0.098$). In the comparison of body composition parameters (Figure 4), we found that only Z-scores of LBM in the HbA1c ≥ 8% subgroup were lower than those with good metabolic control ($p < 0.05$). There were no significant relationships found between DXA values and age at T1DM diagnosis and sex ($p > 0.05$).

4. Discussion

To the best of our knowledge, this study for the first time provided comprehensive analyses of skeletal status, body composition, and estimates of relative bone strength in adolescents with T1DM using the DXA method as well as the normative reference data of a nationally representative group of healthy adolescents in applying the DXA system. Moreover, our results enabled us to evaluate the possible impact of glycaemic control on the three main compartments of the human body: bone, fat, and muscle mass, as

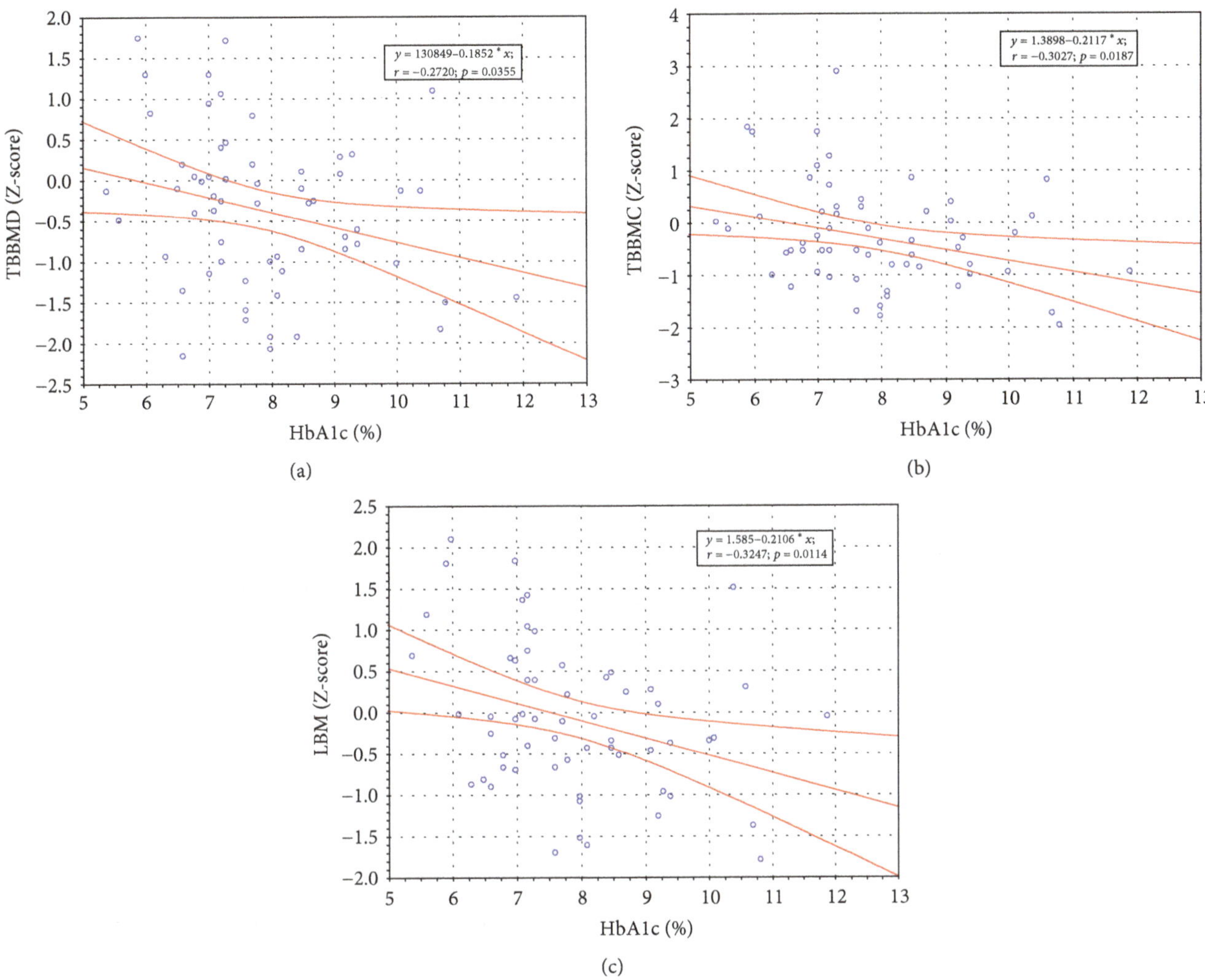

FIGURE 2: HbA1c (%) levels in relation to Z-score values of (a) the total body bone mineral density, (b) total bone mineral content, and (c) lean body mass in patients with T1DM. TBBMD — total body bone mineral density; TBBMC — total body bone mineral content; LBM — lean body mass.

well as the functional relationships between the abovementioned tissues.

Glycated haemoglobin A1c (HbA1c, %) is currently used as a measure of longer-term glycaemic control. This value reflects average blood glucose levels over a period of two to three months, and is an indicator for overall glucose exposure integrating both fasting and postprandial blood glucose levels. Regular HbA1c measurement is recommended by international guidelines for the assessment of glycaemic control as it provides information on long-term glycaemic status [5]. Several studies confirmed a link between elevated HbA1c levels and development of microvascular and macrovascular complications [6, 7]. Therefore, achieving low HbA1c levels is an important therapeutic target in the management of diabetes [5]. To investigate whether metabolic control is associated with skeletal status outcomes, body composition, and relative bone strength in adolescents with T1DM, two subgroups of patients were identified as having good (HbA1c < 8%) or poor glycaemic control (HbA1c ≥ 8%). The concept of stratifying the patients into these two groups is based on the fact that HbA1c levels impact the presence of diabetic complication [7]. The maintenance of glycaemic control levels under the 8% value in this study was utilised in an attempt to examine the effects of glycaemic management on the skeletal status and body composition in patients with T1DM. It was hypothesised that improved glycaemic control would prevent the negative effects of T1DM on bone, muscle, and fat tissues in adolescents with T1DM. While poorer glycaemic control and bone complications have already been described in the literature [8–12], the evidence examining the skeletal status and body composition in adolescents with T1DM is limited [16, 17, 20, 27, 34].

In the present study, it was proven that adolescents with T1DM in the poor metabolic control group had significantly lower BMD and BMC Z-score values for the total skeleton and lower BMD Z-score values for the lumbar spine. Several previous studies in T1DM children and adolescents also investigated this association and found similar results. In particular, multiple cross-sectional studies using DXA-based outcomes reported that bone mineral density and/or bone mineral content were significantly lower in T1DM patients when compared to non-diabetic subjects [44–53].

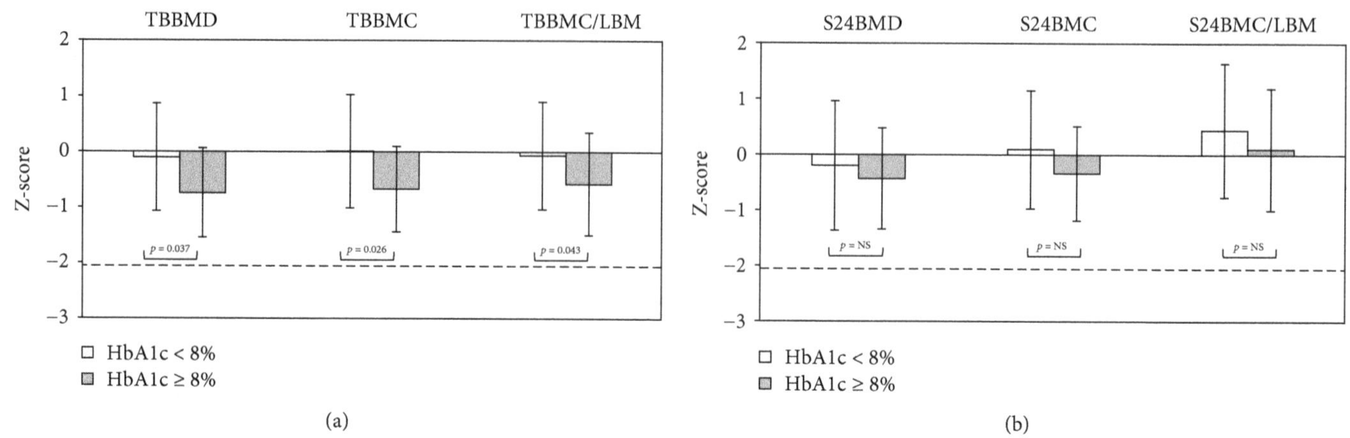

FIGURE 3: Comparison of DXA parameters expressed as the mean (±SD) Z-score values (calculated according to age- and gender-dependent data for healthy subjects), including (a) bone mineral density and bone mineral content of the whole skeleton, relative bone strength ratio (TBBMC/LBM ratio), and (b) bone mineral density and bone mineral content of the lumbar spine, between T1DM patients with well-controlled glycaemia versus those with poorly controlled glycaemia. The dotted line represents the lowest level of the acceptable range of value in healthy subjects (Z-score = −2.0). p-Value indicates significant differences between studied subgroups, adjusted for age, sex, disease duration, pubertal stage, insulin dose, height, weight, and physical activity level; NS, not significant. TBBMD — total body bone mineral density; TBBMC — total body bone mineral content; TBBMC/LBM — total body bone mineral content/lean body mass ratio; S24BMD — bone mineral density, lumbar spine L2–L4; S24BMC — bone mineral content, lumbar spine L2–L4; S24BMC/LBM — bone mineral content, lumbar spine L2–L4/lean body mass ratio.

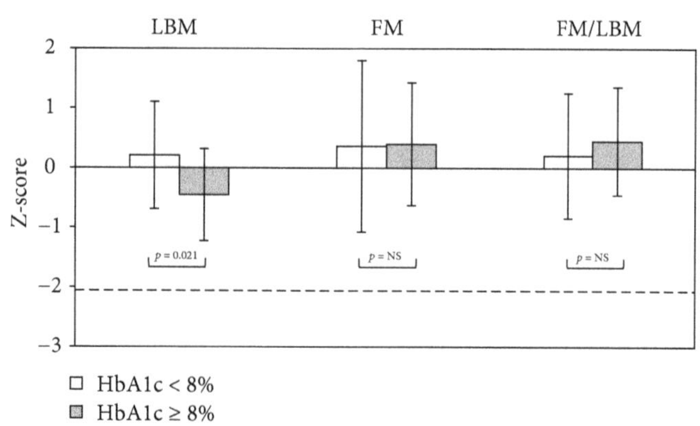

FIGURE 4: Comparison of body composition parameters expressed as the mean (±SD) Z-score values (calculated according to age- and gender-dependent data for healthy subjects), including lean body mass, fat body mass, and FM/LBM ratio, between T1DM patients with well-controlled glycaemia versus those with poorly controlled glycaemia. The dotted line represents the lowest level of the acceptable range of value in healthy subjects (Z-score = −2.0). p-Value indicates significant differences between the studied subgroup adjusted for age, sex, disease duration, pubertal stage, insulin dose, height, weight, and physical activity levels; NS, not significant. LBM — lean body mass; FM — fat mass; FM/LBM — fat mass/lean body mass ratio.

However, in other studies, the DM-associated skeletal disorders were not confirmed relative to the non-diabetic population [54–56]. Impaired GH/IGF-1 axis [27, 35] and decreased bone turnover during the period of skeletal growth in adolescents with type 1 diabetes may attenuate formation during this period of bone growth [46–48]. Some other studies conducted in T1DM patients, also showed deficits in bone size, bone strenght and/or lower trabecular and cortical vBMD, compared to healthy controls [57–60]. However, another study found normal levels of bone size [61]. A study in young adults utilising MRI-based measures reported that T1DM patients had deficits in trabecular bone microarchitecture [28], and using the HR-pQCT method found deficits in cortical and trabecular bone [29]. Moreover, these studies identified an association between the presence of microvascular disease and skeletal deficits in patients with T1DM [28, 29]. Uncontrolled T1DM is a known risk factor for bone disease [8–12]. Numerous studies among children and adolescents with T1DM have shown that poorly controlled diabetes may have a negative effect on bone outcomes [49–53].

Body composition significantly influences bone health during diabetic childhood. This study showed that patients with poor glycaemic control (HbA1c > 8%) had a significant impairment of the relationship between the fat and muscle tissue (FM/LBM). Moreover, an increased Z-FM was coupled with decreased lean body mass Z-LBM and Z-TBBMC/LBM ratio (relative bone strength index). It is worth noting that the impairment of the relationship between these components is an important factor in the development of the bone fragility [14, 15] and increased risk of fractures [22–25]. Moreover, other studies showed abnormalities of bone microarchitecture, intra-abdominal fat content, and bone fat marrow [18]. Also regarding the detection of poor glycaemic control, our study observed negative correlations of total body BMD, BMC, and LBM (Z-scores) with increased HbA1c in type 1 diabetes patients. We suggested that the reduced relative bone strength and the high risk of fractures later in life, associated with it, would be higher in these patients. Adolescence is considered a critical period for bone mass accrual. Impaired bone acquisition during this period can lead to alterations in peak bone mass [34, 35, 44, 45], and increase the risk of fractures, but the number of studies corresponding to adolescents is small [25].

In our study, for parameters concerning the lumbar spine, a trend towards decreased BMD and BMC was seen in the group of HbA1c ≥ 8%, but differences were not statistically significant. We have also demonstrated a significant correlation between total body BMC and metabolic control. Similar results were found in a comparison of bone density in T1DM children with the norms of the age- and sex-adjusted general population [51]. However, in this analysis BMD was significantly lower for the lumbar spine as well. The greater difference in BMD and BMC for total skeleton than for lumbar vertebrae between studied groups can evidence an important contribution of decreased mineral density in the peripheral skeleton in T1DM children. This hypothesis should be confirmed in peripheral bone examination by the pQCT method. The use of this imaging technique would allow an assessment of the volumetric BMD, a separate measurement of cortical and trabecular bone, and determination of bone strength.

In this study, in further confirmation of the skeletal and body compartments' assessment, reduced relative bone strength reveals deterioration in the TBBMC/LBM ratio in T1DM patients, suggesting a deterioration of the muscle-bone relationship. BMC is highly influenced by mechanical stimulation from skeletal muscle, consistent with the functional bone-muscle unit theory [43]. The proper muscle-bone interaction during the growth period is an important factor for skeletal adaptation towards changing loads [43]. The decreased BMC and LBM could play an important role in decreased bone strength [31–33]. Our results also demonstrate reduced BMC or BMD Z-scores and an impairment of the relationship between the fat and muscle tissue. Several previous studies also investigated this association and found similar results [16–18, 20, 21, 29, 44–46, 58, 59]. Our observations of reduced relative bone strength of T1DM patients, and more so in the poor metabolic control patients, have led us to speculate that maintaining such status may be associated with increased risk of fractures later in life. Importantly, increased fracture incidence in young patients with T1DM aged <20 years, compared with their control counterparts without T1DM, was observed in a large population-based cohort study [25].

Our study showed that patients with poor glycaemic control (HbA1c > 8%) also had a significant impairment of the relationship between the fat and muscle tissue (FM/LBM). Moreover, an increased fat mass was coupled with decreased lean body mass Z-LBM and Z-TBBMC/LBM (relative bone strength index). It is worth noting that the impairment of the relationship between these components is an important factor in bone fragility [13, 14]. Based on the analysis conducted in the group of patients with good metabolic control, no deficiencies related to bone mineral content or density were found. Also, no impairment in the relationship between the bone and muscle tissue was noted. Interestingly, the value of the TBBMC/LBM parameter (Z-score) in the lumbar spine was higher for patients in this group (HbA1c < 8%). Skeletal development of diabetics during adolescence is also impacted by the metabolic control. Some studies have also shown that poor glycaemic control has negative effects on the circulating IGF system in patients with T1DM [27, 35, 46–48]. Other studies conclude that osteocalcin levels are inversely associated with HbA1c [62, 63], and can be involved in the regulation of glucose and energy metabolism [64]. In this way, the skeleton is a metabolically active organ, and recent studies suggest that there is cross-talk between bone and other tissues [15–17, 22], and osteocalcin plays an important role in the regulation of glucose metabolism [64].

There are many factors that are suggested to impair bone mass accrual in patients with T1DM. In the present study, we found that duration of disease, at a similar age of onset was significantly higher in the poor metabolic group (HbA1c ≥ 8%) compared with the good metabolic group. In the former subgroup, significantly lower Z-TBBMD, Z-TBBMC, and Z-TBBMC/LBM were observed. Although the duration of diabetes was negatively correlated with skeletal outcome, a significant correlation could only be established between longer disease duration and Z-TBBMD, adjusted for confounders. A longer duration of diabetes implies a longer period of elevated glucose levels, and when associated with poor metabolic control, it can have a negative impact on bone mass accrual at an early age [34, 35]. In the pubertal period, fast body weight and height gain takes place [31–33], which in children with T1DM often results in a worsening of metabolic control parameters [5–7]. Indeed, a negative association between disease duration and bone or muscle parameters in adolescents with T1DM has been previously reported [19, 20, 45, 46, 51, 52, 65, 66]. However, other studies have reported normal or minimal deterioration of skeletal outcomes [17, 27, 44, 47, 53, 55, 56, 60, 67]. Of all age groups, adolescents are currently the farthest from achieving HbA1c targets, reflecting the diabetes mismanagement that frequently accompanies the increased independence in diabetes self-care [5].

Several factors could explain the results of our analyses. During the course of type 1 DM, various mechanisms may interact to determine skeletal disorders and impaired bone quality. T1DM is characterised as a state of low bone turnover [68], as determined by osteoblast dysfunction [65–67]. Of note is that insulin deficiency and insulin-like growth factor-1 (IGF-1) reduction [27, 46–48] and hyperglycaemia-induced oxidative stress and accumulation of advanced glycation end-products (AGEs) that compromise collagen properties [69, 70], low osteocalcin levels [62, 63], and/or Wnt signalling pathway [71, 72] seem to be causing these changes, resulting in a reduction in the mature osteoblast numbers and thus bone formation, leading to low peak bone mass at a young age [31–34]. Other factors such as inflammatory systemic diseases are characterised by increased levels of proinflammatory cytokines [73] that uncouple the bone remodelling cycle, also interfering with bone mass acquisition [35]. Consequently, these factors are likely to also have adverse effects on muscle and bone cells and the impaired bone-muscle relationship [20, 21, 40]. Disturbed body composition such as decreased lean muscle mass and increased fat stores [16–18, 38, 39] are a known risk factor of skeletal disorders in DM patients.

To achieve the primary goal of preventing or minimising diabetes complications, it is imperative, among others, to keep blood sugar levels within certain ranges [5]. It is well-recognised that micro- and macrovascular complications are associated with long-term diabetes duration and poor glycaemic control [6, 7]. Close adherence to the dietary balancing of carbohydrate intake and insulin levels [74], healthy eating behaviours as well as a healthy lifestyle are associated with better glycaemic control [75]. Thus, it is necessary to achieve good metabolic control in childhood diabetes in order to ensure appropriate growth and development. The present study aimed at determining the potential benefit of good metabolic control on various skeletal parameters and body composition in T1DM patients. Our results demonstrate that a physiologically relevant well-controlled T1DM in young patients can improve the development of bone mass and that long-term HbA1c < 8% levels are beneficial to bones. Moreover, the effects of vitamin D deficiency on skeletal muscle functioning usually also accompany diabetes, and may be an important factor responsible for decreased muscle mass [76, 77]. As previously reported in the same study population [78], T1DM patients displayed low 25(OH)D serum levels compared to healthy controls (15.3 ± 7.0 vs. 17.9 ± 9.3 ng/mL), but the difference was not significant ($p > 0.05$). Furthermore, higher HbA1c levels coincided with lower 25(OH)D levels. In our previous report, we also showed a close relationship between the altered body composition outcomes and poor glycaemic control in T1DM adolescents. Moreover, we found that increased fat stores (FM Z-score) and reduced lean body mass (LBM Z-score) were inversely associated with 25(OH)D levels in T1DM [78]. Our patients with T1DM showed reduced levels of 25(OH)D compared with the healthy controls. Consistently, in other studies it has been reported that patients with T1DM displayed vitamin D deficiency [11, 20, 28, 47, 54, 59], and that insulin gene expression in pancreatic β-cells may also be modulated by vitamin D [20, 35, 37, 76]. Vitamin D also modulates muscle and bone-derived hormones, hormones, including GH-IGF-1 axis and sex hormones, facilitating cross-talk between these tissues [77].

The management of diabetes mellitus in adolescents, in particular with poor metabolic control, is essential. Effective prevention of poor glycaemic control needs comprehensive management [5–7], including healthy lifestyle and adequate nutrition [79, 80], with sufficient vitamin D intake from food and supplements [78]. Some dietary components can impact the mechanisms leading to loss of bone density, skeletal muscle mass, or function, especially if calcium and vitamin D intakes are not adequate. Calcium and vitamin D are well established as essential for bone health as is protein for skeletal muscle, but there are also other nutrients that are integral to bone and muscle physiology and are a key factor in achieving peak bone mass during childhood [31–33]. Thus, optimisation of bone health is critical in paediatric patients, particular for children and adolescents with T1DM. Recommended is an adequate intensive treatment with continuous subcutaneous insulin infusion, balanced healthy diet and self-monitoring of blood glucose, and increasing physical activity. A primary goal of care in adolescent patients with T1DM is the optimisation of glycaemic control for the prevention of bone complications, especially in case of longer disease duration.

Our study has several strengths and weaknesses. The study's strengths are the novelty of studying the skeletal status, body composition, and relative bone strength in the paediatric type 1 diabetes and the comparison of results obtained using the DXA method with a nationally representative group of healthy adolescents, which increases the generalisability of the study findings. The main limitation of this study is its cross-sectional design with respect to establishing temporality in assessing a causal relationship, and other factors such as relatively small sample size, and reliance on a single clinic for the conduct of the work, so the associations of diverse variables should be considered with caution.

Future multicentre, long-term studies are required to verify our results. Future studies should examine this further by increasing the number of patients with T1DM and ensuring a longer study period of glycaemic control. Many factors that link metabolic control and skeletal and body composition have been investigated in the past. A very interesting and still not fully discovered factor impacting bone health as well as type 1 diabetes is the gut microbiome. In the course of diabetes, alterations in the gut microbiome may trigger inflammation of the intestinal mucosa and reduce absorption of essential nutrients. The functional changes of the gastrointestinal tract and gut microbiome in relation to diabetes complications [81] and the interplay between the gut microbiome with the immune system are a highly interesting field of research. Remission prolongation, alleviation of disease, and improving the quality of a patient's life have been highlighted as important objectives in the last years. These could be addressed through a new, promising, therapeutic approach of islet cell transplantation, which has a beneficial impact of restoring partial β-cell function [82]. In line with this finding, the new therapy has shown to have a positive impact on diabetes complications. Further development of this innovative approach could benefit patients with T1DM.

5. Conclusion

In conclusion, our results showed that adolescent patients with T1DM had lower physiological values of TBBMD, TBBMC, and S24BMD and worse relative bone strength index (TBBMC/LBM ratio), coinciding with higher FM and FM/LBM ratio values compared to age- and sex-adjusted generally healthy counterparts. These observations were further reinforced by decreased LBM values in patients with poor glycaemic control. In contrast, most DXA-assessment parameters appeared to be normal in the well-controlled metabolic group when adjusted for healthy control subjects. Adolescent patients with T1DM should be monitored in terms of their skeletal status and body composition, especially in conditions of poor metabolic control and longer duration of disease. Early recognition of developing abnormalities in skeletal status and body composition is important for bone status in young adulthood when peak bone mass is achieved.

Abbreviations

TBBMD:	Total body bone mineral density
TBBMC:	Total body bone mineral content
LBM:	Lean body mass
FM:	Fat mass
S24BMD:	Bone mineral density, lumbar spine L2–L4
S24BMC:	Bone mineral content, lumbar spine L2–L4
S24BMC/LBM:	Bone mineral content, lumbar spine L2–L4/lean body mass ratio
TBBMC/LBM:	Total body bone mineral content/lean body mass ratio
FM/LBM:	Fat mass/lean body mass ratio
HbA1c:	Glycated haemoglobin A1c.

Conflicts of Interest

The authors declare that they have no conflicts of interest.

Acknowledgments

The study was supported by the National Science Centre, Poland (Grant no. N N312 433140).

References

[1] M. E. Craig, C. Jefferies, D. Dabelea, N. Balde, A. Seth, and K. C. Donaghue, "Definition, epidemiology, and classification of diabetes in children and adolescents," *Pediatric Diabetes*, vol. 15, no. S20, pp. 4–17, 2014.

[2] C. Patterson, L. Guariguata, G. Dahlquist, G. Soltész, G. Ogle, and M. Silink, "Diabetes in the young — a global view and worldwide estimates of numbers of children with type 1 diabetes," *Diabetes Research and Clinical Practice*, vol. 103, no. 2, pp. 161–175, 2014.

[3] M. Szalecki, M. Wysocka-Mincewicz, A. Ramotowska et al., "Epidemiology of type 1 diabetes in Polish children: a multicentre cohort study," *Diabetes/Metabolism Research and Reviews*, vol. 34, no. 2, article e2962, 2018.

[4] A. Chobot, J. Polanska, A. Brandt et al., "Updated 24-year trend of type 1 diabetes incidence in children in Poland reveals a sinusoidal pattern and sustained increase," *Diabetic Medicine*, vol. 34, no. 9, pp. 1252–1258, 2017.

[5] M. J. Rewers, K. Pillay, C. de Beaufort et al., "Assessment and monitoring of glycemic control in children and adolescents with diabetes," *Pediatric Diabetes*, vol. 15, no. S20, pp. 102–114, 2014.

[6] K. C. Donaghue, R. P. Wadwa, L. A. Dimeglio et al., "Microvascular and macrovascular complications in children and adolescents," *Pediatric Diabetes*, vol. 15, no. S20, pp. 257–269, 2014.

[7] S. A. Virk, K. C. Donaghue, Y. H. Cho et al., "Association between HbA1c variability and risk of microvascular complications in adolescents with type 1 diabetes," *The Journal of Clinical Endocrinology & Metabolism*, vol. 101, no. 9, pp. 3257–3263, 2016.

[8] J. Starup-Linde and P. Vestergaard, "Diabetes and osteoporosis — cause for concern?," *European Journal of Endocrinology*, vol. 5, no. 3, pp. 93–99, 2015.

[9] C. Hamann, S. Kirschner, K. P. Günther, and L. C. Hofbauer, "Bone, sweet bone—osteoporotic fractures in diabetes mellitus," *Nature Reviews Endocrinology*, vol. 8, no. 5, pp. 297–305, 2012.

[10] L. R. McCabe, "Understanding the pathology and mechanisms of type I diabetic bone loss," *Journal of Cellular Biochemistry*, vol. 102, no. 6, pp. 1343–1357, 2007.

[11] V. V. Zhukouskaya, A. P. Shepelkevich, and I. Chiodini, "Bone health in type 1 diabetes: where we are now and how we should proceed," *Advances in Endocrinology*, vol. 2014, Article ID 982129, 12 pages, 2014.

[12] H. A. Keenan and E. Maddaloni, "Bone microarchitecture in type 1 diabetes: it is complicated," *Current Osteoporosis Reports*, vol. 14, no. 6, pp. 351–358, 2016.

[13] F. S. Hough, D. D. Pierroz, C. Cooper, S. L. Ferrari, and The IOF CSA Bone and Diabetes Working Group, "Mechanisms in endocrinology: mechanisms and evaluation of bone fragility in type 1 diabetes mellitus," *European Journal of Endocrinology*, vol. 174, no. 4, pp. R127–R138, 2016.

[14] N. Napoli, M. Chandran, D. D. Pierroz et al., "Mechanisms of diabetes mellitus-induced bone fragility," *Nature Reviews Endocrinology*, vol. 13, no. 4, pp. 208–219, 2017.

[15] B. Lecka-Czernik and C. J. Rosen, "Energy excess, glucose utilization, and skeletal remodeling: new insights," *Journal of Bone and Mineral Research*, vol. 30, no. 8, pp. 1356–1361, 2015.

[16] A. Wędrychowicz, M. Stec, K. Sztefko, and J. Starzyk, "Associations between bone, fat tissue and metabolic control in children and adolescents with type 1 diabetes mellitus," *Experimental and Clinical Endocrinology & Diabetes*, vol. 122, no. 8, pp. 491–495, 2014.

[17] S. M. Abd El Dayem, A. M. El-Shehaby, A. Abd El Gafar, A. Fawzy, and H. Salama, "Bone density, body composition, and markers of bone remodeling in type 1 diabetic patients," *Scandinavian Journal of Clinical and Laboratory Investigation*, vol. 71, no. 5, pp. 387–393, 2011.

[18] N. Abdalrahaman, C. McComb, J. E. Foster et al., "The relationship between adiposity, bone density and microarchitecture is maintained in young women irrespective of diabetes status," *Clinical Endocrinology*, vol. 87, no. 4, pp. 327–335, 2017.

[19] S. K. Coleman, I. A. Rebalka, D. M. D'Souza, and T. J. Hawke, "Skeletal muscle as a therapeutic target for delaying type 1 diabetic complications," *World Journal of Diabetes*, vol. 6, no. 17, pp. 1323–1336, 2015.

[20] K. Maratova, O. Soucek, J. Matyskova et al., "Muscle functions and bone strength are impaired in adolescents with type 1 diabetes," *Bone*, vol. 106, pp. 22–27, 2018.

[21] S. Balducci, M. Sacchetti, G. Orlando et al., "Correlates of muscle strength in diabetes. The study on the assessment of determinants of muscle and bone strength abnormalities in diabetes (SAMBA)," *Nutrition, Metabolism and Cardiovascular Diseases*, vol. 24, no. 1, pp. 18–26, 2014.

[22] D. E. Sellmeyer, R. Civitelli, L. C. Hofbauer, S. Khosla, B. Lecka-Czernik, and A. V. Schwartz, "Skeletal metabolism, fracture risk, and fracture outcomes in type 1 and type 2 diabetes," *Diabetes*, vol. 65, no. 7, pp. 1757–1766, 2016.

[23] J. Starup-Linde, M. Frost, P. Vestergaard, and B. Abrahamsen, "Epidemiology of fractures in diabetes," *Calcified Tissue International*, vol. 100, no. 2, pp. 109–121, 2017.

[24] V. N. Shah, C. S. Shah, and J. K. Snell-Bergeon, "Type 1 diabetes and risk of fracture: meta-analysis and review of the literature," *Diabetic Medicine*, vol. 32, no. 9, pp. 1134–1142, 2015.

[25] D. R. Weber, K. Haynes, M. B. Leonard, S. M. Willi, and M. R. Denburg, "Type 1 diabetes is associated with an increased risk of fracture across the life span: a population-based cohort study using The Health Improvement Network (THIN)," *Diabetes Care*, vol. 38, no. 10, pp. 1913–1920, 2015.

[26] E. Maddaloni, S. D'Eon, S. Hastings et al., "Bone health in subjects with type 1 diabetes for more than 50 years," *Acta Diabetologica*, vol. 54, no. 5, pp. 479–488, 2017.

[27] M. A. AboElAsrar, N. S. Elbarbary, D. E. Elshennawy, and A. M. Omar, "Insulin-like growth factor-1 cytokines cross-talk in type 1 diabetes mellitus: relationship to microvascular complications and bone mineral density," *Cytokine*, vol. 59, no. 1, pp. 86–93, 2012.

[28] N. Abdalrahaman, C. McComb, J. E. Foster et al., "Deficits in trabecular bone microarchitecture in young women with type 1 diabetes mellitus," *Journal of Bone and Mineral Research*, vol. 30, no. 8, pp. 1386–1393, 2015.

[29] V. V. Shanbhogue, S. Hansen, M. Frost et al., "Bone geometry, volumetric density, microarchitecture, and estimated bone strength assessed by HR-pQCT in adult patients with type 1 diabetes mellitus," *Journal of Bone and Mineral Research*, vol. 30, no. 12, pp. 2188–2199, 2015.

[30] C. Eller-Vainicher, V. V. Zhukouskaya, Y. V. Tolkachev et al., "Low bone mineral density and its predictors in type 1 diabetic patients evaluated by the classic statistics and artificial neural network analysis," *Diabetes Care*, vol. 34, no. 10, pp. 2186–2191, 2011.

[31] A. B. Sopher, I. Fennoy, and S. E. Oberfield, "An update on childhood bone health: mineral accrual, assessment and treatment," *Current Opinion in Endocrinology & Diabetes and Obesity*, vol. 22, no. 1, pp. 35–40, 2015.

[32] C. M. Weaver, C. M. Gordon, K. F. Janz et al., "The National Osteoporosis Foundation's position statement on peak bone mass development and lifestyle factors: a systematic review and implementation recommendations," *Osteoporosis International*, vol. 27, no. 4, pp. 1281–1386, 2016.

[33] R. Rizzoli, M. L. Bianchi, M. Garabédian, H. A. McKay, and L. A. Moreno, "Maximizing bone mineral mass gain during growth for the prevention of fractures in the adolescents and the elderly," *Bone*, vol. 46, no. 2, pp. 294–305, 2010.

[34] M. L. Bianchi, M. B. Leonard, S. Bechtold et al., "Bone health in children and adolescents with chronic diseases that may affect the skeleton: the 2013 ISCD pediatric official positions," *Journal of Clinical Densitometry*, vol. 17, no. 2, pp. 281–294, 2014.

[35] M. Raisingani, B. Preneet, B. Kohn, and S. Yakar, "Skeletal growth and bone mineral acquisition in type 1 diabetic children; abnormalities of the GH/IGF-1 axis," *Growth Hormone & IGF Research*, vol. 34, pp. 13–21, 2017.

[36] E. Kalaitzoglou, I. Popescu, R. C. Bunn, J. L. Fowlkes, and K. M. Thrailkill, "Effects of type 1 diabetes on osteoblasts, osteocytes, and osteoclasts," *Current Osteoporosis Reports*, vol. 14, no. 6, pp. 310–319, 2016.

[37] N. Napoli, R. Strollo, A. Paladini, S. I. Briganti, P. Pozzilli, and S. Epstein, "The alliance of mesenchymal stem cells, bone, and diabetes," *International Journal of Endocrinology*, vol. 2014, Article ID 690783, 26 pages, 2014.

[38] T. Y. Kim and A. L. Schafer, "Diabetes and bone marrow adiposity," *Current Osteoporosis Reports*, vol. 14, no. 6, pp. 337–344, 2016.

[39] E. E. Kershaw and J. S. Flier, "Adipose tissue as an endocrine organ," *The Journal of Clinical Endocrinology & Metabolism*, vol. 89, no. 6, pp. 2548–2556, 2004.

[40] G. Karsenty and P. Mera, "Molecular bases of the crosstalk between bone and muscle," *Bone*, vol. 155, pp. 43–94, 2018.

[41] P. Płudowski, H. Matusik, M. Olszaniecka, M. Lebiedowski, and R. S. Lorenc, "Reference values for the indicators of skeletal and muscular status of healthy Polish children," *Journal of Clinical Densitometry*, vol. 8, no. 2, pp. 164–177, 2005.

[42] P. Pludowski, M. Jaworski, H. Matusik, M. Kobylinska, P. Klimek, and R. S. Lorenc, "The evaluation of consistency between body composition assessments in pediatric population using pencil beam and fan beam dual-energy X-ray absorptiometers," *Journal of Clinical Densitometry*, vol. 13, no. 1, pp. 84–95, 2010.

[43] N. J. Crabtree, A. Arabi, L. K. Bachrach et al., "Dual-energy X-ray absorptiometry interpretation and reporting in children and adolescents: the revised 2013 ISCD pediatric official positions," *Journal of Clinical Densitometry*, vol. 17, no. 2, pp. 225–242, 2014.

[44] J. Heap, M. A. Murray, S. C. Miller, T. Jalili, and L. J. Moyer-Mileur, "Alterations in bone characteristics associated with glycemic control in adolescents with type 1 diabetes mellitus," *The Journal of Pediatrics*, vol. 144, no. 1, pp. 56–62, 2004.

[45] L. J. Moyer-Mileur, S. B. Dixon, J. L. Quick, E. W. Askew, and M. A. Murray, "Bone mineral acquisition in adolescents with type 1 diabetes," *The Journal of Pediatrics*, vol. 145, no. 5, pp. 662–669, 2004.

[46] L. J. Moyer-Mileur, H. Slater, K. C. Jordan, and M. A. Murray, "IGF-1 and IGF-binding proteins and bone mass, geometry, and strength: relation to metabolic control in adolescent girls with type 1 diabetes," *Journal of Bone and Mineral Research*, vol. 23, no. 12, pp. 1884–1891, 2008.

[47] J. Léger, D. Marinovic, C. Alberti et al., "Lower bone mineral content in children with type 1 diabetes mellitus is linked to female sex, low insulin-like growth factor type I levels, and high insulin requirement," *The Journal of Clinical Endocrinology & Metabolism*, vol. 91, no. 10, pp. 3947–3953, 2006.

[48] K. S. C. de Souza, M. A. G. Ururahy, Y. M. da Costa Oliveira et al., "Low bone mineral density in patients with type 1 diabetes: association with reduced expression of *IGF1*, *IGF1R* and *TGFB1* in peripheral blood mononuclear cells," *Diabetes/Metabolism Research and Reviews*, vol. 32, no. 6, pp. 589–595, 2016.

[49] M. B. Loureiro, M. A. G. Ururahy, F. P. Freire-Neto et al., "Low bone mineral density is associated to poor glycemic control and increased OPG expression in children and adolescents with type 1 diabetes," *Diabetes Research and Clinical Practice*, vol. 103, no. 3, pp. 452–457, 2014.

[50] K. Heilman, M. Zilmer, K. Zilmer, and V. Tillmann, "Lower bone mineral density in children with type 1 diabetes is associated with poor glycemic control and higher serum ICAM-1

and urinary isoprostane levels," *Journal of Bone and Mineral Metabolism*, vol. 27, no. 5, pp. 598–604, 2009.

[51] G. Valerio, A. Del Puente, A. Esposito-del Puente, P. Buono, E. Mozzillo, and A. Franzese, "The lumbar bone mineral density is affected by long-term poor metabolic control in adolescents with type 1 diabetes mellitus," *Hormone Research*, vol. 58, no. 6, pp. 266–272, 2002.

[52] M. O. Çamurdan, P. Ciaz, A. Bideci, and F. Demirel, "Role of hemoglobin A_{1c}, duration and puberty on bone mineral density in diabetic children," *Pediatrics International*, vol. 49, no. 5, pp. 645–651, 2007.

[53] A. P. Chobot, A. Haffke, J. Polanska et al., "Bone status in adolescents with type 1 diabetes," *Diabetologia*, vol. 53, no. 8, pp. 1754–1760, 2010.

[54] A. Onder, S. Cetinkaya, O. Tunc, and Z. Aycan, "Evaluation of bone mineral density in children with type 1 diabetes mellitus," *Journal of Pediatric Endocrinology and Metabolism*, vol. 26, no. 11-12, pp. 1077–1081, 2013.

[55] N. Soto, R. Pruzzo, F. Eyzaguirre et al., "Bone mass and sex steroids in postmenarcheal adolescents and adult women with type 1 diabetes mellitus," *Journal of Diabetes and its Complications*, vol. 25, no. 1, pp. 19–24, 2011.

[56] A. Salvatoni, G. Mancassola, R. Biasoli et al., "Bone mineral density in diabetic children and adolescents: a follow-up study," *Bone*, vol. 34, no. 5, pp. 900–904, 2004.

[57] M. T. Saha, H. Sievänen, M. K. Salo, S. Tulokas, and H. H. Saha, "Bone mass and structure in adolescents with type 1 diabetes compared to healthy peers," *Osteoporosis International*, vol. 20, no. 8, pp. 1401–1406, 2009.

[58] S. Bechtold, I. Dirlenbach, K. Raile, V. Noelle, W. Bonfig, and H. P. Schwarz, "Early manifestation of type 1 diabetes in children is a risk factor for changed bone geometry: data using peripheral quantitative computed tomography," *Pediatrics*, vol. 118, no. 3, pp. e627–e634, 2006.

[59] R. Franceschi, S. Longhi, V. Cauvin et al., "Bone geometry, quality, and bone markers in children with type 1 diabetes mellitus," *Calcified Tissue International*, vol. 102, no. 6, pp. 657–665, 2018.

[60] I. Roggen, I. Gies, J. Vanbesien, O. Louis, and J. De Schepper, "Trabecular bone mineral density and bone geometry of the distal radius at completion of pubertal growth in childhood type 1 diabetes," *Hormone Research in Pædiatrics*, vol. 79, no. 2, pp. 68–74, 2013.

[61] S. Bechtold, S. Putzker, W. Bonfig, O. Fuchs, I. Dirlenbach, and H. P. Schwarz, "Bone size normalizes with age in children and adolescents with type 1 diabetes," *Diabetes Care*, vol. 30, no. 8, pp. 2046–2050, 2007.

[62] T. Neumann, S. Lodes, B. Kästner et al., "Osteocalcin, adipokines and their associations with glucose metabolism in type 1 diabetes," *Bone*, vol. 82, pp. 50–55, 2016.

[63] E. Maddaloni, L. D'Onofrio, A. Lauria et al., "Osteocalcin levels are inversely associated with Hba1c and BMI in adult subjects with long-standing type 1 diabetes," *Journal of Endocrinological Investigation*, vol. 37, no. 7, pp. 661–666, 2014.

[64] M. L. Zoch, T. L. Clemens, and R. C. Riddle, "New insights into the biology of osteocalcin," *Bone*, vol. 82, pp. 42–49, 2016.

[65] A. Pater, G. Sypniewska, and O. Pilecki, "Biochemical markers of bone cell activity in children with type 1 diabetes mellitus," *Journal of Pediatric Endocrinology and Metabolism*, vol. 23, no. 1-2, pp. 81–86, 2010.

[66] F. R. Brandao, E. J. Vicente, C. H. Daltro, M. Sacramento, A. Moreira, and L. Adan, "Bone metabolism is linked to disease duration and metabolic control in type 1 diabetes mellitus," *Diabetes Research and Clinical Practice*, vol. 78, no. 3, pp. 334–339, 2007.

[67] A. B. Maggio, S. Ferrari, M. Kraenzlin et al., "Decreased bone turnover in children and adolescents with well controlled type 1 diabetes," *Journal of Pediatric Endocrinology and Metabolism*, vol. 23, no. 7, pp. 697–707, 2010.

[68] K. Hygum, J. Starup-Linde, T. Harsløf, P. Vestergaard, and B. L. Langdahl, "Diabetes mellitus, a state of low bone turnover—a systematic review and meta-analysis," *European Journal of Endocrinology*, vol. 176, no. 3, pp. 137–157, 2017.

[69] M. Yamamoto and T. Sugimoto, "Advanced glycation end products, diabetes, and bone strength," *Current Osteoporosis Reports*, vol. 14, no. 6, pp. 320–326, 2016.

[70] D. Farlay, L. A. G. Armas, E. Gineyts, M. P. Akhter, R. R. Recker, and G. Boivin, "Nonenzymatic glycation and degree of mineralization are higher in bone from fractured patients with type 1 diabetes mellitus," *Journal of Bone and Mineral Research*, vol. 31, no. 1, pp. 190–195, 2016.

[71] C. Tsentidis, D. Gourgiotis, L. Kossiva, A. Marmarinos, A. Doulgeraki, and K. Karavanaki, "Increased levels of Dickkopf-1 are indicative of Wnt/β-catenin downregulation and lower osteoblast signaling in children and adolescents with type 1 diabetes mellitus, contributing to lower bone mineral density," *Osteoporosis International*, vol. 28, no. 3, pp. 945–953, 2017.

[72] M. F. Faienza, A. Ventura, M. Delvecchio et al., "High sclerostin and dickkopf-1 (DKK-1) serum levels in children and adolescents with type 1 diabetes mellitus," *The Journal of Clinical Endocrinology & Metabolism*, vol. 102, no. 4, pp. 1174–1181, 2017.

[73] S. S. Pereira and J. I. Alvarez-Leite, "Low-grade inflammation, obesity, and diabetes," *Current Obesity Reports*, vol. 3, no. 4, pp. 422–431, 2014.

[74] S. N. Mehta, N. Quinn, L. K. Volkening, and L. M. B. Laffel, "Impact of carbohydrate counting on glycemic control in children with type 1 diabetes," *Diabetes Care*, vol. 32, no. 6, pp. 1014–1016, 2009.

[75] C. Maffeis, E. Fornari, A. Morandi et al., "Glucose-independent association of adiposity and diet composition with cardiovascular risk in children and adolescents with type 1 diabetes," *Acta Diabetologica*, vol. 54, no. 6, pp. 599–605, 2017.

[76] K. M. Thrailkill and J. L. Fowlkes, "The role of vitamin D in the metabolic homeostasis of diabetic bone," *Clinical Reviews in Bone and Mineral Metabolism*, vol. 11, no. 1, pp. 28–37, 2013.

[77] J. E. Gunton, C. M. Girgis, P. A. Baldock, and P. Lips, "Bone muscle interactions and vitamin D," *Bone*, vol. 80, pp. 89–94, 2015.

[78] E. Wierzbicka, M. Szalecki, P. Pludowski, M. Jaworski, and A. Brzozowska, "Vitamin D status, body composition and glycemic control in Polish adolescents with type 1 diabetes," *Minerva Endocrinologica*, vol. 41, no. 4, pp. 445–455, 2016.

[79] S. N. Balk, D. A. J. M. Schoenaker, G. D. Mishra et al., "Association of diet and lifestyle with glycated haemoglobin in type 1 diabetes participants in the EURODIAB prospective complications study," *European Journal of Clinical Nutrition*, vol. 70, no. 2, pp. 229–236, 2016.

[80] T. R. Nansel, L. M. Lipsky, and A. Liu, "Greater diet quality is associated with more optimal glycemic control in a longitudinal study of youth with type 1 diabetes," *The American Journal of Clinical Nutrition*, vol. 104, no. 1, pp. 81–87, 2016.

[81] F. D'Addio and P. Fiorina, "Type 1 diabetes and dysfunctional intestinal homeostasis," *Trends in Endocrinology & Metabolism*, vol. 27, no. 7, pp. 493–503, 2016.

[82] R. Bassi and P. Fiorina, "Impact of islet transplantation on diabetes complications and quality of life," *Current Diabetes Reports*, vol. 11, no. 5, pp. 355–363, 2011.

Markers of Anemia in Children with Type 1 Diabetes

Ewa Rusak,[1] Anna Rotarska-Mizera,[2] Piotr Adamczyk,[3] Bogdan Mazur,[3] Joanna Polanska,[2] and Agata Chobot[4]

[1]*Department of Pediatrics and Children's Diabetology, Medical University of Silesia, 40-752 Katowice, Poland*
[2]*Data Mining Division, Faculty of Automatic Control, Electronics, and Computer Science, Silesian University of Technology, 44-100 Gliwice, Poland*
[3]*Department of Pediatrics, School of Medicine with the Division of Dentistry in Zabrze, Medical University of Silesia, 40-752 Katowice, Poland*
[4]*Department of Pediatric Gastroenterology and Hepatology, Clinical Hospital No. 1, 41-800 Zabrze, Poland*

Correspondence should be addressed to Ewa Rusak; rusakewa@gmail.com

Academic Editor: Ulrike Rothe

Aim. The aim of the study was to assess markers of anemia in type 1 diabetes (T1D) children, compare them to results obtained in the control group, and estimate their relation to BMI SDS. *Methods.* 94 (59% ♀) T1D children without other autoimmune disorders, aged 12.5 ± 4.1 years, T1D duration: 4.2 ± 3.6 years, HbA1c $7.3 \pm 1.5\%$ (57 ± 12.6 mmol/mol). Sex- and age-matched controls (43 children). In all children, anthropometric measurements, the blood count, iron turnover parameters, and vitamin B12 concentration were taken. *Results.* T1DM children had significantly higher red cell distribution width (RDW) (13.6 versus 12.6%; $p < 0.001$), hepcidin (0.25 versus 0.12 ng/ml; $p < 0.001$), and vitamin B12 concentrations (459 versus 397 pg/ml; $p < 0.01$) and lower TIBC (59.09 versus 68.15 μmol/l; $p < 0.001$) than in the control group. Logistic regression revealed that RDW, TIBC (both $p < 0.001$), and hepcidin ($p < 0.05$) significantly differentiated both groups. In T1DM children, BMI SDS negatively correlated with vitamin B12 ($p < 0.01$) concentration and mean corpuscular hemoglobin concentration ($p < 0.05$) and positively with TIBC ($p < 0.01$) and HbA1c ($p < 0.001$). *Conclusions.* Patients and controls differed especially in terms of RDW and TIBC. In studied T1DM children, BMI SDS was associated to iron metabolism parameters and vitamin B12 concentration.

1. Introduction

Type 1 diabetes (T1D), because of the rising incidence, remains a challenge for diabetologists as well as for pediatricians and general practitioners, who more and more often face the challenge to take optimal care for young patients with this disease [1, 2]. With time, systemic consequences such as anemia may develop in children with T1D. In order to diagnose this condition, it is enough to perform a simple blood count and to search for its causes; besides the standard assessment of the iron serum concentration, it is worth to broaden the diagnostics by the assessment of the parameters of iron metabolism. The interpretation of such results is not easy. Anemia in T1D may have a complex, multifactorial background [3]. Among the most common causes of anemia in the course of T1D in children is iron deficiency, which will present as anemia with microcytosis in the blood count. Its prevalence is higher among T1D patients in comparison to people without diabetes [4]. However, anemia that accompanies inflammation may also present with microcytosis [5]. On the other hand, in cases of diabetic nephropathy, because of insufficient erythropoietin production, normocytic anemia develops [6]. If diagnostic procedures rule out the most common causes, cooccurrence of other autoimmune diseases (thyroiditis, celiac disease, Addison's disease, and autoimmune atrophic gastritis) that may be accompanied by anemia of various morphologies should be taken into account [3]. The variability of causes and their mutual overlapping significantly impedes the interpretation of the obtained results, but the proper diagnosis conditions optimal treatment and allows avoiding systemic complications. Additionally, adequate interpretation of the HbA1c measurement, that is routinely performed during diabetes control visits, requires also to know the patient's serum iron concentration, because the presence of iron deficiency anemia correlates with higher HbA1c values [7]. It is interesting that even though the value of a performed blood count is well known as well as the multiplicity of information it gives, there are no recommendations whether and when it should be carried out in T1D patients—neither in the guidelines published by Diabetes Poland (2018) nor those of the International Society for Pediatric and Adolescent Diabetes [8, 9]. Until present, there have been a few publications assessing the blood count, iron metabolism parameters, and vitamin B12 levels in children with T1D, which most often use other T1D individuals as a control group. To our knowledge comparisons to healthy peers are lacking.

According to our research hypothesis, children with T1D differ from healthy peers in terms of blood count, iron metabolism parameters, and vitamin B12 levels. Therefore, the aim of the study was to assess the abovementioned parameters in T1D pediatric patients with no other autoimmune diseases and compare them to results obtained in a group of healthy children as well as estimate their relation to chosen factors, among others: anthropometric measurements, sex, glycemic control, and disease duration. Confirming the research hypothesis would be a strong premise to monitor red blood cell parameters and—depending on the results—adequate broadening of the diagnostic tests.

2. Material and Methods

2.1. Patients. The study group included 94 children with T1D (55 females) (Diabetic Outpatient Clinic, Upper Silesian Centre for Child's Health in Katowice, Poland). The blood samples were collected during the routine control visit in the Outpatient Clinic. Their mean age at study time was 12.5 ± 4.1 years (SD) (ranging from 3 to 19 years). Mean duration of T1D was 4.2 ± 3.6 years (SD) (0.08–15.7 years). For the purposes of statistical analysis, the percent of life with diabetes was calculated (ratio of disease duration to age, expressed in %). The mean glycated hemoglobin A1c (HbA1c) at the day of the study is equaled to $7.3 \pm 1.5\%$ (57 ± 12.6 mmol/mol).

In all patients, physical examination with auxological assessment was performed. Routine laboratory tests (screening for autoimmune concomitant diseases and complications) were performed according to recent Diabetes Poland and ISPAD guidelines [8, 9].

Patients with clinical and/or laboratory signs of other than T1D autoimmune diseases (celiac disease, thyroiditis) or infection were excluded from the study. Furthermore, children enrolled for this study, according to their medical records, did not have chronic diabetes complications.

2.2. Controls. The control group comprised 43 children (24 females, 19 males) that were age- and sex-matched to the individuals from the study group. They were recruited from patients admitted to the Clinical Hospital No. 1 in Zabrze for nocturnal enuresis or arterial hypertension diagnostics in whom hospital observation and diagnostic procedures allowed to exclude any organic disease that could influence the parameters assessed in this project. These children had no infection, autoimmune diseases, or family history of such diseases.

2.3. Anthropometric Assessment. Anthropometric measurements carried out in all children included weight (kg) and height (cm). Using these values, the body mass index (BMI) was calculated using the standard equation (the body mass in kilograms divided by the square of the body height in meters). To allow comparisons, weight, height, and BMI were expressed as standard deviation scores (SDS).

2.4. Laboratory Measurements. Patients and controls had blood samples taken to perform the blood count (1.6 ml) and carry out biochemical measurements (5 ml)—iron, ferritin, transferrin, hepcidin, vitamin B12 concentrations, and total iron-binding capacity (TIBC). Additionally, children with T1D had their HbA1c and fetal hemoglobin (HbF) measured (capillary blood 10 μg). The blood samples were taken between 7 and 9 am while the children were on fasting. Peripheral blood count (RBC: red blood cells ($10 > 6/\mu l$), MCV: mean corpuscular volume (fl), MCHC: mean corpuscular hemoglobin concentration (g/dl), HGB: hemoglobin (g/dl), HCT: hematocrit (%), RDW: red cell distribution width (%) measured using Sysmex XT-2000i (Kobe, Japan)) and biochemical parameters (by means of immunochemical methods using commercial sets (Roche Diagnostics GmbH, Mannheim, Germany) and the cobas 6000 device (Hitachi, Japan)) were measured in the Central Laboratory of the Clinical hospital No. 1 in Zabrze, Poland. Normal ranges, lower limits of detection (LLD), indirect precision (IP), and repeatability (R) of the measured biochemical parameters are the following: vitamin B12 > 150 pg/ml (LLD 100 pg/ml, IP 4.5%, R 3.5%), transferrin 2–3.6 g/l (0.1 g/l, IP 3.0%, R 1.5%), ferritin 20–200 μg/l (LLD 5 μg/l, IP 2.2%, R 1.2%), iron 5.83–24.5 μmol/l (LLD 0.90 μmol/l, IP 1.5%, R 1.0%), and TIBC 55–75 μmol/l (LLD 6 μmol/l, IP 4.8%, R 1.2%). Hepcidin concentration was determined using an enzyme-linked immunosorbent assay (EIA Science Co., Wuhan, China); normal range: 0.187 to 12 ng/ml (LLD 0.00625 ng/ml, IP 9.8%, R 6.1%). HbA1c assessment was carried out using a DCCT (Diabetes Control and Complications Trial) reference method; normal range < 6% (<42 mmol/mol).

Anemia was defined as reduction in hemoglobin concentration and/or red blood cells compared to norms adopted for a specific child's age and gender.

The project was carried out between August 2014 and June 2015 as a part of the MNiSW grant number IP2012 007672. The study and its protocol obtained a positive opinion of the Ethical Committee of the Medical University of Silesia in Katowice, Poland. Parents or lawful caregivers and patients aged 16 years or more gave written consent for the abovementioned diagnostic procedures and for participation in this research project.

2.5. Statistical Analysis. Statistical analyses were performed using the R software (http://www.bioconductor.org/).

TABLE 1: Age, clinical parameters related to type 1 diabetes (T1D), complete blood count and serum parameters results in all patients with T1D and in the control group. Parameters are expressed as mean value and its 95% confidence interval.

		T1D ($N = 94$)	Controls ($N = 43$)
Clinical parameters	Age (yrs)	12.9 (12.1, 13.8)	13.1 (12.0, 14.3)
	Age at T1D diagnosis (yrs)	8.7 (7.9, 9.5)	
	T1D duration (yrs)	4.2 (3.5, 4.9)	
	HbA1c (%)	7.34 (7.02, 7.65)	
Complete blood count	RBC ($10^6/\mu l$)	4.72 (4.64, 4.79)	4.76 (4.64, 4.89)
	MCV (fl)	86.5 (85.7, 87.3)	85.5 (84.2, 86.8)
	MCHC (g/dl)	33.8 (33.7, 34.0)	34.0 (33.7, 34.3)
	Hemoglobin (g/dl)	13.79 (13.58, 13.99)	13.83 (13.46, 14.21)
	Hematocrit (%)	40.8 (40.0, 41.4)	40.7 (39.7, 41.7)
	RDW (%)	13.6 (13.3, 13.8)*	12.6 (12.4, 12.9)*
Serum parameters	Iron (μmol/l)	17.34 (16.19, 18.49)	16.40 (14.19, 18.60)
	TIBC (μmol/l)	59.09 (57.51, 60.67)*	68.15 (65.29, 71.02)*
	Ferritin (μg/l)	48.51 (41.93, 55.08)	45.87 (35.21, 56.53)
	Transferrin (g/l)	3.01 (2.47, 3.56)	3.01 (2.83, 3.19)
	Vitamin B12 (pg/ml)	459 (419, 500)*	397 (356, 437)*
	Hepcidin (ng/ml)	0.25 (0.20, 0.29)*	0.12 (0.10, 0.14)*

T1D: type 1 diabetes, HbA1c: glycated hemoglobin A1c, RBC: red blood cells, MCV: mean corpuscular volume, MCHC: mean corpuscular hemoglobin concentration, RDW: red blood cell distribution width, TIBC: total iron-binding capacity. *Significant difference between T1D and controls (RDW $p < 0.001$; vitamin B12 $p < 0.01$; hepcidin $p < 0.001$; TIBC $p < 0.001$).

For all of the analyzed parameters, the following descriptive statistics were determined: number (N), median, upper and lower quartile (Q1 and Q3), minimal (min) and maximal (max) value, mean, and standard deviation (SD).

Tukey's criterion was used to identify outlying values. Lilliefors parametric test was used to assess the normality of the distribution. The variance homogeneity hypothesis was tested by means of F or Bartlett statistic. Comparative analysis of normally distributed variables was carried out by analysis of variance (ANOVA) or Student's t-test depending on the group number. In cases of other types of distribution, the nonparametric ANOVA Kruskal-Wallis and Mann–Whitney U test were employed. For post hoc comparisons, we used the Tukey-Kramer test or its nonparametric alternative. The logistic regression technique with the forward feature selection procedure was applied during the construction of the binary classifier. Akaike information criterion supported by Bayes factor principle adjudged on the final model (BF > 3.1623) [10]. Correlations between two continuous variables were assessed by means of the Pearson's or Spearman's correlation coefficients. To identify the most influential explanatory variables and estimate the adjusted model coefficients, the multivariate linear regression method combined with forward feature selection algorithm and likelihood ratio test (LRT) were used. Discrete variables were analyzed using the χ^2 or likelihood ratio G test. Statistical significance was considered at $p < 0.05$.

3. Results

In patients as well as in controls, the mean values of all blood count, iron metabolism parameters, and vitamin B12 results were within normal range—mean values and their 95% confidence intervals are presented in Table 1. Despite that both studied groups differed in terms of the RDW, which was significantly higher in children with T1D (13.6 (95% Cl 13.3, 13.8) versus 12.6 (95% Cl 12.4, 12.9) $p < 0.001$) (Table 1). Analysis of biochemical parameters revealed higher hepcidin (0.25 (95% Cl 0.20, 0.29) versus 0.12 (95% Cl 0.10, 0.14) $p < 0.001$) and vitamin B12 concentrations (459 (95% Cl 419, 500) versus 397 (95% Cl 356, 437) $p < 0.01$) as well as significantly lower TIBC values (59.09 (95% Cl 57.51, 60.67) versus 68.15 (95% Cl 65.29, 71.02) $p < 0.001$) in T1D patients (Table 1). Logistic regression allowed to determine RDW, TIBC (for both $p < 0.001$), and hepcidin ($p < 0.05$) as parameters significantly differentiating the study and the control group with 89% sensitivity and 77% specificity (Tables 2 and 3).

Among patients with T1D, hepcidin correlated positively with RDW ($r = 0.27$, $p < 0.01$). There was also a negative relation between RDW and HGB ($r = -0.24$, $p < 0.05$) and positive correlation between iron concentration and age ($r = 0.28$, $p < 0.01$). HbA1c was positively associated with MCV ($r = 0.31$, $p < 0.01$) and negatively with MCHC ($r = -0.33$, $p < 0.001$). Additionally, statistical analysis revealed some significant correlations of the analyzed biochemical and blood count parameters with BMI SDS in T1D patients. Vitamin B12 concentration ($r = -0.27$, $p < 0.01$) (Figure 1) and MCHC ($r = -0.23$, $p < 0.05$) were inversely related to BMI SDS. Furthermore, a positive correlation was determined with TIBC ($r = 0.28$, $p < 0.01$) (Figure 2) and HbA1c ($r = 0.37$, $p < 0.001$).

Neither T1D duration nor the percent of life with T1D was found to be related to BMI SDS.

TABLE 2: Logistic regression—final model (controls versus T1D). Columns 2–4 present coefficient estimates, their standard error, and p value; columns 5-6 adjusted odds ratio (OR) and its 95% confidence interval (CI).

Final model components	β estimate	Standard error	p value	OR	95% CI
Intercept	−4.42	4.85	0.3621		
RDW	1.08	0.37	0.0034	2.94	(1.43; 6.06)
Hepcidin	11.24	4.41	0.0108	$7.6e+04$	(13.38; $4.3e+08$)
TIBC	−0.17	0.04	$3.4e-06$	0.85	(0.79; 0.91)

TABLE 3: Logistic regression—final model (controls versus T1D)—indices of prediction quality.

(a)

Index	True positive TP	True negative TN	False negative FN	False positive FP	Total
Classification results	84	33	10	10	137

(b)

Index	Sensitivity	Specificity	Accuracy
Classification results	89.4%	76.7%	85.4%

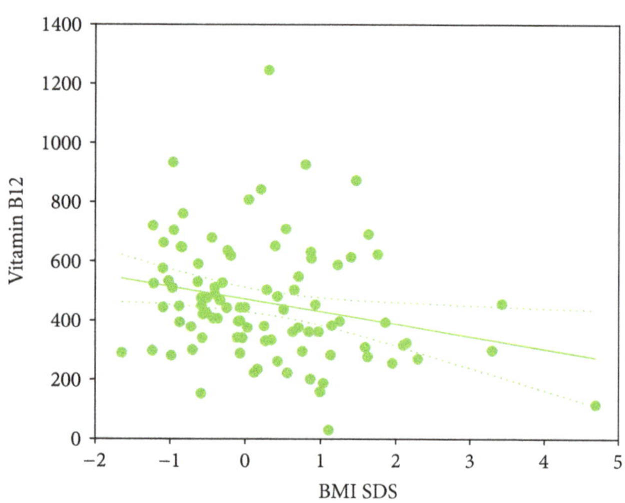

FIGURE 1: Correlation between serum vitamin B12 concentration (pg/ml) and body mass index standard deviation score (BMI SDS) in type 1 diabetes children ($r = -0.27$, $p < 0.01$).

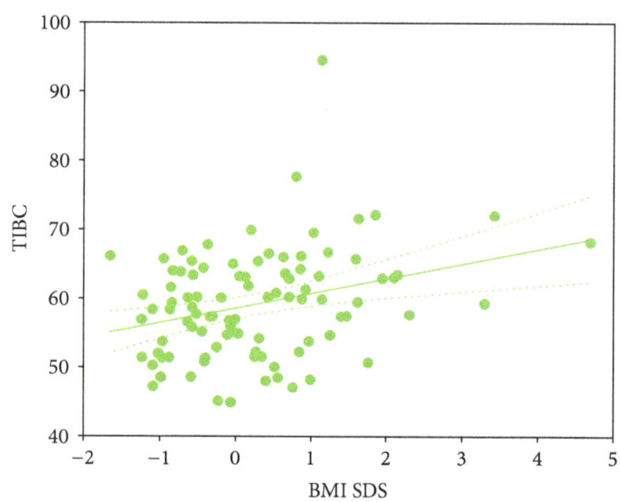

FIGURE 2: Correlation between total iron-binding capacity (TIBC) (μmol/l) and body mass index standard deviation score (BMI SDS) in type 1 diabetes children ($r = 0.28$, $p < 0.01$).

4. Discussion

Until present, there have not been many studies assessing the prevalence of anemia among children with T1D. There is a range of publications regarding patients with type 2 diabetes and anemia, usually accompanying renal complications [11, 12].

None of the investigated children in this study had anemia. Thomas et al. estimated that the prevalence of anemia (based on the hemoglobin concentration) in a group of adults having T1D for a mean of 20 years is equaled to 14%. Risk factors included disturbed renal function and albuminuria (anemia was present in 52% of patients with macroalbuminuria, 24% with microalbuminuria, and only <8% of individuals with normal albumin secretion) [13]. The mentioned study included adults with long lasting diabetes, in which renal complications had already developed. In the pediatric population, disturbances of renal function are rare. Children remain under strict parental and specialist medical care. Regular control visits and glycemic control (HbA1 measurements) as well as education allow achieving optimal diabetes control and avoiding renal complications. Children enrolled for this study according to their medical records did not have diagnosis of micro- or macroalbuminuria. Although urine albumin secretion was not measured at the day when blood for laboratory test was drawn, all patients are followed in the outpatient clinic according to the recommendations of Diabetes Poland and have serum creatinine and urine albumin measured every 1-2 years and blood pressure at every control visit.

In an analysis of 200 children with T1D conducted in Egypt, anemia was diagnosed in 37% of cases. Among patients with anemia, 54.7% had iron deficiency, 18.7% had folic acid deficiency, 18.7% were diagnosed with thalassemia minor, 4% with celiac disease, and in 24% anemia developed as a consequence of a parasitic infestation [14]. Mean age of the analyzed patients (11.2 years) and the duration of T1D (mean 4 years) are similar to that of our patients. However, such high prevalence of anemia in Egyptian children may result from a different socioeconomic situation of this region leading to cases of nutritional deficits (folic acid and/or iron deficiency) and hygienic negligence (parasitic infestations). Such frequent cases of thalassemia minor is related to its general higher prevalence in the region of the Mediterranean Sea.

In another investigation, coming from Poland, patients with newly diagnosed T1D revealed a tendency for iron deficiency anemia in comparison to children with longer lasting T1D (>1 year) [15].

The mean values of iron concentration, iron metabolism parameters, and vitamin B12 levels were within normal ranges in our patients. Normal vitamin B12 and iron concentrations in children with T1D were also described by other authors [14, 16].

Adequate blood count results, iron concentrations, iron metabolism parameters, and vitamin B12 levels in our patients can be explained by optimal nutrition and regular control visits at the outpatient clinic as well as continuous reeducation. Despite results remaining within normal ranges, we revealed statistically significant differences in terms of RDW, TIBC, and hepcidin in comparison to the control subjects, which partially confirms the initial research hypothesis. RDW is a sensitive indicator of a developing anemia. Its normal value reflects isocytosis. Increased RDW (anisocytosis) occurs not only in cases of iron deficiency but also in anemia related to inflammation, although the values are higher in iron deficiency anemia [17]. Hepcidin is a systemic regulator of iron homeostasis. It is produced in the liver as a result of iron stimulation as well as in inflammatory states (IL-6 stimulation). Its role is to stop iron in the intracellular poll and decrease iron absorption from the gastrointestinal tract. As a result serum iron concentration decreases. In inflammatory states caused by infection, this is a beneficial defensive mechanism, which hides iron from being used by bacteria. Nevertheless, in chronic inflammation, it may lead to inflammation-related anemia [5]. Higher RDW in comparison to the control group, higher hepcidin concentration, and lower TIBC may suggest a trend towards typical changes of observed anemia subsequent to chronic inflammation. It could be hypothesized/speculated that in these children there was an occult, asymptomatic, and chronic inflammation or such changes in the measured parameters are a consequence of other unidentified factors. This requires further investigation and possibly also a follow-up to see whether this trend of parameter results is sustained.

Because of the increasing global problem concerning improper body weight in children, also those with T1D [18], as well as higher prevalence of overweight and obesity among young adults with T1D (aged 20–40 years old) in comparison to healthy individuals [19], we analyzed the correlations between BMI SDS and the assessed red blood cell and biochemical parameters. Frequency of overweight in children with T1D in past publications was approximated as high as 30% [20, 21]. In our patients with T1D, BMI SDS > 1 SDS was revealed in 21% of cases. The publications concerning the relationship between overweight and anemia in children with T1D, according to our knowledge, are lacking. However, studies on the obese population are available. In our study BMI SDS values correlated negatively with vitamin B12 concentrations. This is unequivocal with the results of analyses of 1252 patients of an obesity clinic, who were diagnosed with severe obesity (BMI > 40 kg/m^2) [22]. The authors revealed also a negative association of BMI and vitamin B12 levels. In the mentioned study, vitamin B12 deficiency was revealed in as many as 20.9%. It is interesting that iron deficiency in this group of patients was present in only 9.8% subjects [22]. Taking into consideration the above information in obese patients, in the first line, not iron deficiency but rather vitamin B12 deficiency should be suspected. This is probably related to improper dietary habits of the obese patients—ingestion of foods with high carbohydrate and fat content and restriction of consumption of valuable products. In our study, iron and vitamin B12 concentrations were within normal ranges. This fact may result from a much smaller number of obese individuals in our study group. Additionally, none of our patients had severe obesity. T1D children are under parental care, and a balanced diet is crucial part of diabetes therapy. Nevertheless, the inverse association could be confirmed. We did not reveal a direct relation between BMI SDS and iron concentration, which is similar to the results of other publications [22]. The results revealed, however, a positive association of BMI SDS and TIBC, a parameter often used in iron metabolism disorders, and an inverse relation with MCHC. These associations are not surprising, as the results of a meta-analysis confirmed a strong relation of obesity and iron deficiency [23].

It is also a known fact that T1D patients with improper body weight often do not have optimal glycemic control [24, 25]. In our study, it is reflected by a positive correlation of BMI SDS and HbA1c.

Expanded diagnostic tests conducted in a representative group of children and adolescents with T1D allowed to construct a reliable database. Another strength of this study is the enrollment of patients without other concomitant autoimmune diseases which could interfere the final results as well as the comparison with a healthy control group. The analysis of the iron metabolism parameters was precise and complex, including the assessment of hepcidin, which is not often measured in T1D children. As a limitation, the quite wide range of diabetes duration (recently diagnosed to long lasting) should be mentioned.

5. Conclusions

The assessed blood count, iron metabolism parameters, and vitamin B12 results remained in the studied patients within normal ranges. Therefore, single assays of the abovementioned basic parameters may not be sufficient indicators of anemia in children with T1D.

However, results remaining within reference ranges do not exclude a patient with T1D from being at risk of the development of anemia. Basing on statistically significant differences among respective parameters of the blood count and iron metabolism in children with T1D as compared with the control group, it is indicated to monitor trends, and the interpretation of results should be holistic and simultaneous.

In the schedule of the health care of children with T1D, in addition to monitoring development of celiac disease and thyroid dysfunction, it should also be considered to follow alteration in the blood count, iron metabolism, and vitamin B12 status.

Moreover, in children with T1D and abnormal body weight, coexisting deficiencies of vitamin B12 and iron should be taken into account.

Conflicts of Interest

The authors declare that there is no conflict of interest regarding the publication of this paper.

Acknowledgments

The authors would like to thank Professor Przemysława Jarosz-Chobot for the support on the project and constructive suggestions. The authors would also like to express their gratitude to Maria Kalina, M.D., PhD, for valuable discussions, advice, and assistance that greatly improved the manuscript. Joanna Polanska received financial support from Silesian University of Technology (Grant BK-204/RAU1/2017/9).

References

[1] G. J. Kahaly and M. P. Hansen, "Type 1 diabetes associated autoimmunity," *Autoimmunity Reviews*, vol. 15, no. 7, pp. 644–648, 2016.

[2] C. C. Patterson, G. G. Dahlquist, E. Gyürüs, A. Green, and G. Soltész, "Incidence trends for childhood type 1 diabetes in Europe during 1989–2003 and predicted new cases 2005–20: a multicentre prospective registration study," *The Lancet*, vol. 373, no. 9680, pp. 2027–2033, 2009.

[3] A. Angelousi and E. Larger, "Anaemia, a common but often unrecognized risk in diabetic patients: a review," *Diabetes & Metabolism*, vol. 41, no. 1, pp. 18–27, 2015.

[4] A. T. Soliman, V. De Sanctis, M. Yassin, and N. Soliman, "Iron deficiency anemia and glucose metabolism," *Acta Bio Medica Atenei Parmensis*, vol. 88, no. 1, pp. 112–118, 2017.

[5] T. Jackowska and J. Wójtowicz, "Niedokrwistość chorób przewlekłych," *Postępy Nauk Medycznych*, vol. 27, no. 10B, pp. 26–33, 2014.

[6] P. Cotroneo, B. Maria Ricerca, L. Todaro et al., "Blunted erythropoietin response to anemia in patients with type 1 diabetes," *Diabetes/Metabolism Research and Reviews*, vol. 16, no. 3, pp. 172–176, 2000.

[7] A. L. Christy, P. A. Manjrekar, R. P. Babu, A. Hegde, and M. S. Rukmini, "Influence of iron deficiency anemia on hemoglobin A1c levels in diabetic individuals with controlled plasma glucose levels," *Iranian Biomedical Journal*, vol. 18, no. 2, pp. 88–93, 2014.

[8] M. E. Craig, C. Jefferies, D. Dabelea, N. Balde, A. Seth, and K. C. Donaghue, "ISPAD clinical practice consensus guidelines 2014. Definition, epidemiology, and classification of diabetes in children and adolescents," *Pediatric Diabetes*, vol. 15, no. S20, Supplement 20, pp. 4–17, 2014.

[9] Clinical Diabetology, "2018 guidelines on the management of diabetic patients. A position of Diabetes Poland," *Clinical Diabetology*, vol. 7, no. 1, pp. 1–90, 2018.

[10] H. Jeffreys, *The Theory of Probability*, Oxford University Press, Oxford, UK, 1961.

[11] H. Ito, Y. Takeuchi, H. Ishida et al., "Mild anemia is frequent and associated with micro- and macroangiopathies in patients with type 2 diabetes mellitus," *Journal of Diabetes Investigation*, vol. 1, no. 6, pp. 273–278, 2010.

[12] C. E. Ezenwaka, A. Jones-LeCointe, E. Nwagbara, D. Seales, and F. Okali, "Anaemia and kidney dysfunction in Caribbean type 2 diabetic patients," *Cardiovascular Diabetology*, vol. 7, no. 1, p. 25, 2008.

[13] M. C. Thomas, R. J. MacIsaac, C. Tsalamandris et al., "Anemia in patients with type 1 diabetes," *The Journal of Clinical Endocrinology & Metabolism*, vol. 89, no. 9, pp. 4359–4363, 2004.

[14] N. Salah, F. A. el Hamid, S. Abdelghaffar, and M. el Sayem, "Prevalence and type of anaemia in young Egyptian patients with type 1 diabetes mellitus," *Eastern Mediterranean Health Journal*, vol. 11, no. 5-6, pp. 959–967, 2005.

[15] R. W. Wójciak, E. Mojs, and M. Stanisławska-Kubiak, "The occurrence of iron-deficiency anemia in children with type 1 diabetes," *Journal of Investigative Medicine*, vol. 62, no. 6, pp. 865–867, 2014.

[16] G. Forte, B. Bocca, A. Peruzzu et al., "Blood metals concentration in type 1 and type 2 diabetics," *Biological Trace Element Research*, vol. 156, no. 1–3, pp. 79–90, 2013.

[17] M. A. Johnson, "Iron: nutrition monitoring and nutrition status assessment," *The Journal of Nutrition*, vol. 120, Supplement 11, pp. 1486–1491, 1990.

[18] E. E. Frohlich-Reiterer, J. Rosenbauer, S. Bechtold-Dalla Pozza et al., "Predictors of increasing BMI during the course of diabetes in children and adolescents with type 1 diabetes: data from the German/Austrian DPV multicentre survey," *Archives of Disease in Childhood*, vol. 99, no. 8, pp. 738–743, 2014.

[19] A. Szadkowska, A. Madej, K. Ziółkowska et al., "Gender and age-dependent effect of type 1 diabetes on obesity and altered body composition in young adults," *Annals of Agricultural and Environmental Medicine*, vol. 22, no. 1, pp. 124–128, 2015.

[20] W. Łuczyński, A. Szypowska, B. Głowińska-Olszewska, and A. Bossowski, "Overweight, obesity and features of metabolic syndrome in children with diabetes treated with insulin pump therapy," *European Journal of Pediatrics*, vol. 170, no. 7, pp. 891–898, 2011.

[21] W. Luczyński, A. Szypowska, A. Bossowski et al., "Overweight, obesity and metabolic syndrome in children with type 1 diabetes mellitus," *Pediatric Endocrinology, Diabetes, and Metabolism*, vol. 16, no. 2, pp. 83–88, 2010.

[22] M. Arshad, S. Jaberian, A. Pazouki, S. Riazi, M. A. Rangraz, and S. Mokhber, "Iron deficiency anemia and megaloblastic anemia in obese patients," *Romanian Journal of Internal Medicine*, vol. 55, no. 1, pp. 3–7, 2017.

[23] L. Zhao, X. Zhang, Y. Shen, X. Fang, Y. Wang, and F. Wang, "Obesity and iron deficiency: a quantitative meta-analysis," *Obesity Reviews*, vol. 16, no. 12, pp. 1081–1093, 2015.

[24] L. P. Jose, A. Cardoso-Demartini Ade, R. D. Liberatore Junior et al., "Clinical and laboratory profile of pediatric and adolescent patients with type 1 diabetes," *Jornal de Pediatria*, vol. 85, no. 6, pp. 490–494, 2009.

[25] M. Wysocka-Mincewicz, H. Kołodziejczyk, E. Wierzbicka, and M. Szalecki, "Overweight, obesity and lipids abnormalities in adolescents with type 1 diabetes," *Pediatric Endocrinology Diabetes and Metabolism*, vol. 21, no. 2, pp. 70–81, 2015.

14

Women with Type 1 Diabetes Mellitus: Effect of Disease and Psychosocial-Related Correlates on Health-Related Quality of Life

Syed Wasif Gillani,[1] Irfan Altaf Ansari,[2] Hisham A. Zaghloul,[1] Mohi Iqbal Mohammad Abdul,[1] Syed Azhar Syed Sulaiman,[3] Mirza R. Baig,[4] and Hassaan Anwar Rathore[3]

[1]*College of Pharmacy, Taibah University, Al Madinah Al Munawarah, Saudi Arabia*
[2]*Department of Pathology, College of Medicine, Taibah University, Al Madinah Al Munawarah, Saudi Arabia*
[3]*School of Pharmaceutical Sciences, Universiti Sains Malaysia (USM), Penang, Malaysia*
[4]*Dubai Pharmacy College, Dubai, UAE*

Correspondence should be addressed to Syed Wasif Gillani; wasifgillani@gmail.com

Academic Editor: Patrizio Tatti

Background. This study is aimed at investigating the various disease-specific and health-related psychosocial concepts of HRQOL among insulin-dependent diabetes mellitus (IDDM) and understanding the gender differences in HRQOL among IDDM patients. *Methods.* A cross-sectional observational study was conducted to assess the effect of health-related and psychosocial correlates on HRQOL of IDDM patients in Penang, Malaysia. The participants were recruited from five governmental diabetic clinics. Patients with insulin use only, IDDM diagnosed at least 1 year earlier, were identified from clinical registers. The sample was then age stratified for 20–64 years, and severe complications (e.g., end-stage renal failure, hemodialysis, and liver cirrhosis) were excluded; a total of 1003 participants were enrolled in the study. Multivariate regression analysis was used to predict the response. *Results.* A total of 853 (100%) participants were enrolled and completed the study. Women exhibited significantly higher/better mental health ($p < 0.013$) and health perception scores ($p < 0.001$) despite high prevalence of impaired role (49.2%), social (24.2%), and physical (40.5%) functionings as compared to men. Women with longer diabetes exposure and uncontrolled glycemic levels (HbA1c) have poorer HRQOL. Availability of social support showed no significant association with either HRQOL or diabetes distress levels. Diabetes distress levels remained not associated with social support. Women also showed significantly higher association with health perception (15% versus 13% men, $p < 0.001$) and mental health (13% versus 11% men, $p < 0.001$) in diabetes-specific psychosocial factors. Thus, among women alone, diabetes-related specific and psychosocial factors explained 15% and 13% of variations in HRQOL extents, respectively. *Conclusion.* Women exhibit extensive and significant patterns with health-related factors and diabetes-specific psychosocial factors (self-efficacy, social support, and DLC) to improve HRQOL. Also, women have significantly high reported distress levels and low social functioning compared to men.

1. Introduction

Diabetes mellitus (DM) is a metabolic disorder categorized with relative (type 2) and absolute (type 1) deficiency of glucose regulatory hormone—insulin [1]. More than three hundred fifty million people were recognized with DM by 2011 and estimated to be doubled by 2030 [2]. Insulin-dependent diabetes mellitus (IDDM/type 1 DM) is presented with either lacking or reducing of insulin segregation or completely depletion of pancreatic cells responsible for producing insulin. Thus, the relevant patients required daily parenteral dosing of insulin to maintain glycemic levels. Disease progression rate is directly related to glycemic control; poor glycemic control leads to rapid disease progression and therefore involves in serious complications: nephropathy, retinopathy, macrovascular diseases, etc. [3, 4]. Thus, treatment of IDDM is based on monitoring and delaying harmful effects by controlling glycemic levels and improving relative quality of life (QOL) of the patient.

Self-care is the one of the important factor for achieving optimal glycemic levels among patients with IDDM [2, 3]. Diabetes patients are responsible for their daily care, such as self-monitoring blood glucose (SMBG), diet management, and insulin dose adjustments [5, 6]. Diabetes affects the daily life functioning therefore, lowering the health status and QOL among patients [1, 2]. Such factors cause treatment failure and poor glucose tolerance which in turn leads to poorer health quality of life (HRQOL) [7].

Treatment success or failure also based on patient's satisfaction to different aspects of disease domains [1, 6]. Diabetes is often examined in terms of compliance and metabolic outcomes. Clinical comorbidities play an important role in diabetes progression and also provide sufficient information for patient-treatment adjustments [8]. Therefore, in recent years, the scientific literature focused on evaluating HRQOL among patients with chronic disorders.

HRQOL is a multidimensional construct [9] comprising of physical, social, and psychosocial domains. Also, the core feature of HRQOL is the self-evaluation of patient regarding his health-related quality of life [1, 4, 6]. Studies have suggested that adequate self-care will improve the glycemic control [1, 3]. Certainly, internal locus of control of having a belief that life events are resultant of past own actions would help and beneficial for patient's active disease coping [1, 7]. Social/peer support also considered as an important factor in controlling disease-related psychosocial problems and improving health literacy together with modified psychosocial factors such as beliefs about disease and treatment [4, 10]. Thus, to prevent future diabetic complications, it is necessary to understand the factors relating to the HRQOL among patients with chronic illnesses to reduce the risk of severe functional limitations.

The aim of this study was to investigate the various disease-specific and health-related psychosocial concepts of HRQOL among IDDM patients, especially on social support, diabetes-related psychosocial factors, and self-care behavior and practices to understand the gender differences in HRQOL among IDDM patients.

2. Methodology

2.1. Ethical Approval. Approvals were made prior to conducting the study from Ministry of Health, Malaysia and Clinical Research Committee (CRC), registration ID: NMRR-17-776-6941.

2.2. Study Design, Location, and Duration. A cross-sectional observational study was conducted to assess the effect of health-related and psychosocial correlates on HRQOL of IDDM patients in Penang, Malaysia. The participants were recruited from five governmental diabetic clinics. Participant recruitment process was done from February to March 2017, data collection from April to June 2017, and analysis from July to September 2017. Written consent forms were obtained from all the participants.

2.3. Recruitment Process. Patients with insulin use only, IDDM diagnosed at least 1 year earlier, were identified from clinical registers. The sample was then age stratified for 20–64 years, and severe complications (e.g., end-stage renal failure, hemodialysis, and liver cirrhosis) were excluded; a total of 1526 participants were eligible to participate. Out of them, 1344 patients were approached/agreed to participate by post, mail, telephone, or during follow-up visits. The recruitment process is briefly explained in Figure 1. A total of 853 participants' data were used to analyze the hypothesis of the study from the eligible sample (1344). Participants with missing data and nonrespondents were analyzed to evaluate the differences between age, gender, comorbidities, and glycemic control values (recent) from the clinical records. No significant difference was found in these variables (data is not presented).

This study presented the subsample of participants with age 20–64 years old, insulin treatment only, without severe complication (no effect of HRQOL), attended the clinic for clinical assessments (HbA1c), and completed/returned all the questionnaires for the study.

3. Instruments

3.1. Dependent Measures. Health-related quality of life (HRQOL) was measured by the prevalidated Malaysian version of the medical outcome study (MOS-SF-20 [11, 12]) health survey questionnaire. There are six self-reported subscales; higher value indicates better well-being. A pilot study ($n = 68$) among Malaysian IDDM s was conducted to validate subscales as health perception (5 items, Cronbach's α coefficient = 0.89), physical functioning (6 items, $\alpha = 0.85$), role functioning (2 items, $\alpha = 0.94$), mental health (5 items, $\alpha = 0.91$), social functioning (1 item), and pain (1 item). Reported physical functioning was used as a control variable in this study.

3.2. Independent Measures. Demographics: the variables were age, marital status, education, and occupation status.

Health-related factors: diabetes exposure, comorbidities, glycemic control (HbA1c), and physical functioning reported at MOS-SF-20.

Social support: the measure for general support was adopted from the literature [13]. Participants have to assess the support with adequacy and/or availability. Internal consistencies for the composite scales were 0.71 and 0.88 with adequacy and availability.

Diabetes-related specific support [14, 15]: the original 16-item scale was modified for this study on the basis of measures with supportive family behavior only (excluding peer/friends). The alpha coefficient values were constructed by using factor analysis (component analysis-varimax rotation). Supportive behaviors: (9-items, $\alpha = 0.79$ and criticizing behavior: 7 items, $\alpha = 0.75$. The diabetes-related specific support measure was then modified by subtracting the criticizing behavior from composites.

Diabetes-related health beliefs [16, 17]: perceived benefits of the regimen (8 items, $\alpha = 0.89$).

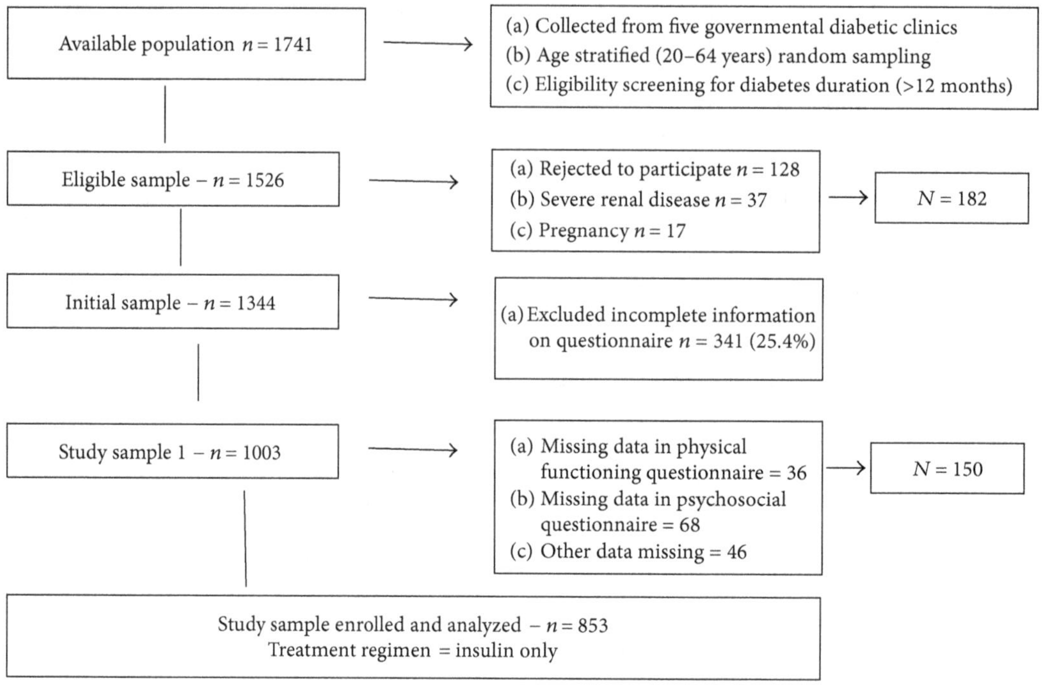

FIGURE 1: Recruitment process and the study.

Susceptibility scale [18, 19]: participants estimated the likelihood of a diabetes-related health hazards (e.g., eye disease, pain in feet, kidney disease, and ambulation). Each measures on 5-point Likert scale ($\alpha = 0.91$). Severity of these complications was estimated on 7-point Likert scale ($\alpha = 0.88$).

Diabetes locus of control (DLC) [20]: a 27-item scale with four subscales was used; internal DLC ($\alpha = 0.79$), chance DLC ($\alpha = 0.76$), professional DLC ($\alpha = 0.80$), and other DLCs ($\alpha = 0.71$).

Self-efficacy scale [21]: a 13-item measure for perceived competence in self-care with overall alpha coefficient ($\alpha = 0.86$) was used to evaluated self-report on dietary habits, frequency of exercise, and self-monitoring blood glucose (SMBG).

Problem areas in diabetes (PAID) [22]: a 20-item measure ($\alpha = 0.93$) was used to estimate the participants' response on a 5-point Likert scale. Total score ranges between 0 and 100; higher value indicates high distress.

N.B.: construction and psychometric validation of health beliefs, susceptibility, DLC, self-efficacy, and PAID scales were evaluated in the pilot study as mentioned earlier.

3.3. Statistical Analysis. Bivariate and multivariate models were used to determine the association between gender and demographic factors and independent variables. Hierarchical regression analysis was used to determine the predictive association of diabetes-related psychosocial factors on HRQOL. Health beliefs, mental health status, and diabetes distress associated with HRQOL were evaluated with logistic regression modelling. Also, role and social functioning and pain measures were dichotomized for logistic regression analysis because of the skewed distribution pattern.

The stepwise multiple regression analysis was used in the following order: step 1: sociodemographic, step 2: health-related factors, step 3: social support, step 4: diabetes-related support, step 5: diabetes-related health beliefs, and step 6: self-care practices. The final regression model was presented after adjustment of background factors. Initial logistic model starts with steps 1–4 and then followed by subsequent steps.

4. Results and Findings

4.1. Sample/Participants' Characteristics. A total of 853 (100%) participants were enrolled and completed the study; Table 1 presented the sample characteristics. Men to women ratio was 1.05 : 1. Women showed significantly higher mean age ($p < 0.001$) with low duration of diabetes exposure (years) ($p < 0.021$) than men. Findings also suggested that women exhibited significantly higher/better mental health ($p < 0.013$) and health perception scores ($p < 0.001$) despite high prevalence of impaired role (49.2%), social (24.2%), and physical (40.5%) functionings as compared to men. In contrast, women (64.9%) reported pain was significantly ($p < 0.001$) higher than men (43.1%). Also, the diabetes distress scale score showed that women have significantly higher ($p < 0.011$) mean score (48.1) than men (36.4) which reflects emotional burnout.

4.2. Sociodemographic Characteristics and HRQOL: Association/Pattern. In the analysis, both genders reported a similar pattern with age, as increase in age significantly related with reduced/poorer HRQOL in health perception ($p < 0.05$) and pain ($p < 0.001$). Women showed more difficulty in role ($p < 0.01$) and social ($p < 0.05$) functionings as compared to men. Women who were not currently

Table 1: Participants' characteristics of type I diabetes ($n = 853$).

Characteristics	Men ($n = 436$)¯ 51.1%	Women ($n = 417$)¯ 48.9%	Difference p value
Age*, mean (years) ± SD	34.7 ± 7.4	36.1 ± 6.4	0.001
Marital status, n (%)			
Single	41 (9.40)	24 (5.8)	0.643
Married	299 (68.6)	297 (71.2)	
Widow	71 (16.3)	29 (7.0)	
Separated	25 (5.7)	67 (16.1)	
Education status, n (%)			
Primary	80 (18.3)	22 (5.3)	0.021
Intermediate	129 (29.6)	69 (16.5)	
Secondary	201 (16.1)	207 (49.6)	
University	26 (6.0)	159 (38.1)	
Occupation, n (%)			
Government	95 (21.8)	101 (24.3)	0.77
Private	87 (20.0)	84 (20.1)	
Business	254 (85.2)	232 (55.6)	
Diabetes exposure, mean (years) ± SD	15.5 ± 4.3	12.9 ± 6.8	0.001
Glycosylated hemoglobin, mean ± SD	9.3 ± 0.8	8.9 ± 1.3	0.485
Comorbidity, n (%)			
Congestive heart failure	147 (33.7)	284 (68.1)	0.001
Hyperlipidemia	239 (54.8)	113 (27.1)	
Mild renal disease	11 (2.6)	7 (1.7)	
None	39 (8.9)	13 (3.1)	
Mental health‡, mean ± SD	5.73 ± 2.14	6.98 ± 1.71	0.013
Health perception≠, mean ± SD	4.11 ± 1.22	6.46 ± 1.53	0.001
Role functioning, n (%)			
Impaired	140 (32.1)	205 (49.2)	0.189
Normal	296 (67.9)	212 (50.8)	
Social functioning, n (%)			
Impaired	96 (22.0)	101 (24.2)	0.014
Normal	340 (78.0)	316 (75.8)	
Physical functioning			
Impairments	138 (31.7)	169 (40.5)	0.017
No impairments	298 (68.3)	248 (59.5)	
Pain, n (%)—yes	188 (43.1)	271 (64.9)	0.001
Problem areas in diabetes (PAID) (diabetes distress scale), mean ± SD†	36.4 ± 11.83	48.1 ± 10.51	0.011

*Age range = 20–63 years, ‡Range = 0–10, ≠Range = 0–10, †Range = (0–100), ¯Participants scoring ≥ 40 predicts "emotional burnout" in contrast participants with drop to ≤10 indicative for denial.

in married status have more difficulty in physical functioning ($p < 0.001$) and also lower mental health scores ($p < 0.05$). Findings also suggested that the lower education status of women relates to high distress levels ($p < 0.001$), pain ($p < 0.001$), and role functioning ($p < 0.01$). The longer diabetes exposure and uncontrolled glycemic levels (HbA1c) of women are related to poorer HRQOL with health perception ($p < 0.01$), mental health ($p < 0.001$), physical ($p < 0.01$), and social ($p < 0.001$) functionings and increase distress levels ($p < 0.001$). Bivariate analysis is provided in Table 2.

4.3. Social Support and HRQOL. Availability of social support showed no significant association with either HRQOL or diabetes distress levels. However, perceived adequacy of social support showed significant association with HRQOL in all subvariables except role and social functionings. Diabetes distress levels remained not associated with social support.

4.4. Disease-Related Psychosocial Factors and HRQOL. Younger age women with married status correlates increase self-efficacy ($p < 0.001$) in diabetes management and strong diabetes social support ($p < 0.001$) with reduce diabetes

TABLE 2: Hierarchical regression analysis to evaluate patterns of health perception, mental health, and PAID on HRQOL.

Characteristics	Health perception[1] (β^2)		Mental health[1] (β^2)		PAID[3] (β^2)	
	Men	Women	Men	Women	Men	Women
Age	−0.15*	−0.13*	−0.05	−0.03	0.05	0.09*
Marital status	−0.08	−0.05	0.03	0.08*	0.02	0.07
Education	0.07$\Delta R^2 = 0.13$	0.09 $\Delta R^2 = 0.11$	0.09 $\Delta R^2 = 0.10$	0.09 $\Delta R^2 = 0.010$	0.10 $\Delta R^2 = 0.09$	0.15 $\Delta R^2 = 0.12$**
Occupation	0.031	0.054	−0.02	−0.09	0.12**	0.06
Diabetes exposure	−0.02	0.18**	−0.12*	−0.19***	−0.09	−0.08
Glycemic control (HbA1c)	−0.04*	−0.011*	0.07	0.11*	−0.21***	−0.35***
Comorbidities	−0.21***	−0.26***	−0.13**	−0.21***	−0.02	0.09
Physical functioning	0.38 $\Delta R^2 = 0.24$**	0.41 $\Delta R^2 = 0.35$**	−0.12 $\Delta R^2 = 0.11$**	−0.25 $\Delta R^2 = 0.23$**	0.24 $\Delta R^2 = 0.19$**	0.29 $\Delta R^2 = 0.25$***
Self-care behaviors						
Diet management	−0.09 $\Delta R^2 = 0.01$*	−0.13 $\Delta R^2 = 0.09$*	−0.03 $\Delta R^2 = 0.00$	−0.11 $\Delta R^2 = 0.09$**	—	—
Self-monitoring blood glucose	0.13*	0.17**	0.02	−0.05	—	—
Social support						
Availability	−0.03	−0.06	−0.03	−0.17**	−0.11*	−0.19**
Adequacy	0.14 $\Delta R^2 = 0.10$*	0.19 $\Delta R^2 = 0.17$**	−0.28 $\Delta R^2 = 0.25$**	−0.31 $\Delta R^2 = 0.29$**	0.21 $\Delta R^2 = 0.20$**	0.29 $\Delta R^2 = 0.26$***
Diabetes-related psychosocial factors						
Self-efficacy	0.24**	0.39***	0.16	0.24***	−0.19*	−0.31***
Diabetes social support	0.14*	0.17***	0.11*	0.35***	−0.12	−0.23**
DLC (others)	−0.09	−0.13*	—	—	—	—
Severity	−0.03 $\Delta R^2 = 0.02$	−0.09 $\Delta R^2 = 0.10$*	—	—	—	—
R^2/R^2 adjusted	0.56/0.54**	0.68/0.67***	0.41/0.39***	0.57/0.55***	0.44/0.41**	0.61/0.63***

[1]Higher score indicates good health-related quality of life, [2]Standardized coefficient, —Not entered in the stepwise procedure, [3]Higher score indicates emotion distress. *$p < 0.05$, **$p < 0.01$, ***$p < 0.001$.

distress score ($p < 0.001$) than men; in contrast, older age (regardless of marital status) women's longer diabetes exposure and increase comorbidities are related with poorer HRQOL in health perception ($p < 0.001$), role functioning ($p < 0.05$), social functioning ($p < 0.001$), pain ($p < 0.001$), and increased diabetes distress levels ($p < 0.001$). Education was not related to HRQOL only slight difference was observed among low education status women with diabetes distress levels. Multivariate analysis also showed association as age with health perception and mental health, gender with social and physical functionings, and marital status with pain, self-care behavior, and distress levels. Findings suggested that physical functioning has strong predictor effect on health perception, mental health, pain, distress levels, and social functioning. Tables 2 and 3 present the results of multivariate models.

4.5. Impact of DLC and Diet on HRQOL. Women showed better mental health status with net benefits of the regimen than men ($p < 0.001$). Results showed that strong internal DLC is significantly related with less pain, improved social functioning, and reduced distress levels. While low significant association was found with beliefs in other DLCs on poor health perception ($p < 0.05$).

Regular diet showed significant association with poorer health perception and mental health. Women with proper diet management exhibits better perceived health, mental health, and reduce pain exposures.

4.6. Glycemic Control (HbA1c) and HRQOL. Earlier, we found that women with longer duration of diabetes and uncontrolled glycemic levels have impact on HRQOL factors; however, to evaluate the close relationship between glycemic levels and HRQOL, further analysis was made by factorizing the variable with three categories: consistent control (HbA1c < 6%), moderate control (HbA1c 6–8%), and poor control (HbA1c > 8%). Both pain ($p < 0.01$) and role functioning ($p < 0.001$) were found significant with the glycemic level. Findings showed no gender difference in the pattern suggesting that problems in role functioning and pain experiences were more frequent among poor glycemic control participants than the consistent control group. Thus, it strongly predicts that longer diabetes exposure is strongly related to poorer HRQOL. Tables 2 and 3 present the results of multivariate models.

4.7. Physical Functioning and HRQOL. The ratio between reported good to impaired physical functioning among participants was 1.8 : 1. The percentage variances were calculated

Table 3: Hierarchical logistic regression analysis for social and role functioning and pain experiences among participants.

Characteristics	Pain Odds (95% CI)		Impaired social functioning Odds (95% CI)		Impaired role functioning Odds (95% CI)	
	Men	Women	Men	Women	Men	Women
Age	1.03 (0.96–1.09)	1.05 (0.97–1.07)	1.08 (1.01–1.15)*	1.11 (0.85–1.43)	1.05 (0.98–1.17)	1.07 (0.63–1.21)
Marital status	1.13 (1.01–1.19)	2.41 (1.23–4.70)***	0.72 (0.28–1.86)	0.75 (0.41–1.00)	0.41 (0.21–0.65)	0.44 (0.13–0.73)
Education	1.01 (.57–1.61)	1.03 (0.67–1.55)	0.94 (0.47–1.86)	0.91 (0.56–1.28)	1.01 (0.71–1.32)	1.06 (0.81–1.19)
Occupation	0.79 (0.44–1.41)	0.83 (0.59–1.47)	0.30 (0.12–0.63)	0.47 (0.17—0.98)	1.36 (1.10–1.29)	1.39 (1.01–1.93)*
Diabetes exposure	1.00 (0.94–1.06)	1.34 (1.13–2.61)**	0.95 (0.79–1.01)	0.98 (0.62–1.32)	0.99 (0.73–1.29)	0.88 (0.39–0.99)
Glycemic control (HbA1c)	0.98 (0.82–1.17)	1.27 (1.11–1.98)*	1.13 (0.86–1.45)	1.31 (1.11–1.99)*	0.98 (0.67–1.36)	0.81 (0.24–1.11)
Comorbidities	1.01 (0.91–0.19)	1.43 (1.13–2.86)**	2.32 (1.37–3.89)*	3.76 (2.01–5.77)**	1.41 (0.93–1.83)	1.67 (1.10–2.21)**
Physical functioning	6.14 (4.11–13.98)**	7.86 (4.23–14.49)**	34.51 (10.73–49.46)*	39.64 (10.11–43.4)**	7.07 (2.81–14.37)**	8.01 (2.96–18.69)***
Self-care behaviors						
Diet management	2.33 (1.26–5.44)*	6.23 (4.14–13.81)**	—	—	—	—
Self-monitoring blood glucose	7.27 (5.15–15.48)**	2.01 (0.86–3.16)	—	—	—	—
Social support						
Availability	0.96 (0.84–1.24)	1.01 (0.85–1.07)	1.07 (0.96–1.18)	1.13 (0.85–1.43)	1.09 (0.79–1.73)	1.18 (1.01–1.44)*
Adequacy	0.89 (0.76–1.33)	0.88 (0.71–1.49)	0.95 (0.82–1.67)	0.97 (0.81–1.23)	0.89 (0.43–1.21)	0.93 (0.66–1.00)
Diabetes-related psychosocial factors						
Self-efficacy	—	—	0.79 (0.48–0.99)	0.81 (0.51–1.03)	—	—
Diabetes social support	0.91 (0.43–1.19)	0.80 (0.54–1.13)	—	—	0.77 (0.61–0.99)	0.84 (0.55–1.01)
DLC (others)	—	—	—	—	—	—
Problems areas in diabetes (PAID)						
≥40 points (distress burnout)	1.43 (1.13–1.89)**	1.27 (1.01–1.94)**	4.36 (2.19–8.36)***	5.29 (3.38–10.42)***	10.11 (4.62–21.11)***	15.38 (5.32–23.3)***

— Not entered in the stepwise procedure. $^{*}p < 0.05$; $^{**}p < 0.01$; $^{***}p < 0.001$. N.B.: age: 40<, >40; marital: currently married/not; education: secondary<, >secondary; occupation: government, nongovernmental; diabetes exposure: <10, >10 years; glycemic control: <7, >7; comorbidities: yes/no.

to determine the contributions of each predictor variable in predicting health perception, mental health, and distress levels among normal and limited physical functioning (Table 4). In participants with good physical functioning (regardless of gender differences), the most predicting variable was diabetes-specific psychosocial factors both in health perception and mental health. However, women showed significantly higher association with health perception (15% versus 13% men, $p < 0.001$) and mental health (13% versus 11% men, $p < 0.001$) in diabetes-specific psychosocial factors. Thus, among women alone diabetes-related specific and psychosocial factors explained 15% and 13% of variations in HRQOL extents, respectively. However, participants with impaired physical functioning both health factors and diabetes-specific psychosocial factors among women with 15% and 14% in health perception. While social support was the only strongest predictor in mental health of women (13%). In contrast, among men participants with physical impairment, variance predicted with health factors was only 13% ($p < 0.01$) in health perception and 11% with social support in mental health.

4.8. Diabetes Distress Levels (PAID) and Physical Impairment. In multivariate analysis, PAID values were added to the model, it predicts regardless of physical functioning (impaired/good) and gender (man/woman) significantly and strongly predicts the effect of high distress levels with poorer HRQOL in health perception ($p < 0.001$), mental health ($p < 0.017$), social functioning ($p < 0.011$), and pain experiences ($p < 0.012$) (Table 4).

5. Discussion

The outcome measures of this study assessed HRQOL, which is more responsive to disease-specific psychosocial factors, social support, disease outcome, and disease distress levels than subjective factors. This study has reported a low nonresponse rate about 14.95% mainly with tediousness of the questionnaires and blood testing procedure, not influenced on the internal validity of the study. To be absolutely sure, we evaluated the demographic factors for nonresponse bias and it showed no significant findings. However, this does not apply to other factors like health-related and disease-specific psychosocial factors. Thus, demographic factors were controlled in the multivariate modelling procedure to increase the external validity of the study.

The study findings are consistent with the previous published literature, older participants [10–19, 23, 24] and respondents with low educational status [18–20, 23, 24] showed poorer HRQOL and social well-being. However, analysis showed that the health-related factors and disease-specific psychosocial factors mediated the association between sociodemographic and HRQOL; therefore, after adjusting these factors, there was no significant association reported between demographic and HRQOL. Several studies reported the role of cognitive factors in mediating the effect between demographic factors with health outcomes [25]. None of the previous literature reported the gender differences in multivariate analysis; only the present study focused on the effect of multidimensional factors on HRQOL including distress levels and also determined the gender differences in the five-relative domains.

Physical and social functionings are the determinants for the good perceived health status as well as well-being of the patient [17, 25]. The present study supports the literature and reports that both physical and social functionings had strong influence on perceived health, mental health, role functioning, pain, and also diabetes distress levels. Impact was also found with glycemic levels and duration of diabetes exposure but to lesser extent. Gender differences revealed significant findings with women, physical functioning, and diabetes distress levels compared to men. Further analysis also showed that reported diabetes comorbidities significantly lower the social and health well-being among patients with IDDM; these findings support the earlier findings as well [15–18, 22]. Glycemic control did not relate to HRQOL (all five dimensions) in the regression model; however, slight association was found among women in health perception and distress levels than men. Also, in poorer to consistent glycemic control groups, more frequent problems were reported with role functioning, physical functioning, pain, and high distress levels.

Social support, either general social support or diabetes-specific social support, reported beneficial outcomes among diabetes patients for lowering depression levels [19, 26]. Similarly, self-care behavior/self-efficacy also showed improvement in patient health-related outcomes and perceived diabetes distress status [27]. In concordance to these literature findings, our study reported better perceived HRQOL (except mental health and pain) with perceived adequacy of general social support. Lower distress levels also associated with perceived adequacy of support. In addition to these, we further analyzed the diabetes-specific social support factors and found significant association in modifying HRQOL among participants of this study. Improved social functioning, better health perception and mental health, and low distress levels were highly associated with strong perceived self-care behavior participants. Findings also showed that participants reported to receive strong self-efficacy/care related support were better well-bring in health perception, mental health, and low distress levels, even in controlling the general support factors. Both SMBG and diet showed marginal impact on HRQOL; however, gender differences revealed strong association of diet with women and SMBG among men participants. Usually diabetic diet (DASH) considered to be more public self-care than glucose self-monitoring, as diet significantly related to many more psychosocial factors. Sometime diabetic-specific diet may cause unwanted experiences, [25, 27] and this can heighten the role of illness in participant's life.

The health-related outcomes were generally better reported with perceived disease control [18, 19]. Also, patient education and counselling improves both health literacy and self-care behavior that will be beneficial to disease management [26, 27]. The present study reported moderate association of diabetes-control beliefs to HRQOL, particularly related with pain experiences and diabetes distress levels. The findings of this study identified several patterns that

TABLE 4: Variance (%) explained for health perception and mental health predictor[1] groups on reported physical functioning.

Characteristics	No physical impairment ($n = 546$) %		Physical impairment ($n = 307$) %	
	Men ($n = 298$)	Women ($n = 248$)	Men ($n = 138$)	Women ($n = 169$)
Health perception				
Demographics	3*	4**	3	4*
Health factors	4*	3*	13**	15***
Self-care behaviors	7***	6**	6*	8**
Social support	3	8***	7	4
Diabetes-specific psychosocial factors	13***	15***	1	14***
Mental health				
Demographics	1	3*	4	4
Health factors	3*	4**	3	4
Social support	8**	9***	11***	13**
Diabetes-specific psychosocial factors	11***	13***	6*	5*
Self-care behaviors	1	0	8*	3
Diabetes distress (PAID)	10**	13*	11***	15***

[1]Difference between R^2 of the complete model: R^2 of the model (after removing the predictor group). Demographics: age, marital status, education, and occupation. Health factors: diabetes exposure, glycemic control (HbA1c), comorbidities, and physical functioning. $^{*}p < 0.05$, $^{**}p < 0.01$, $^{***}p < 0.001$.

are significantly modifying HRQOL dimensions among IDDM patients. Also debated the gender differences to individualize the care plan on patient-specific characteristics. With the presence of comorbidities, physical impairment generally presented with lower/poorer HRQOL and high distress levels. In contrast, glycemic/metabolic control levels are not modifying HRQOL or distress levels except women who only call for attention. Diabetes-specific psychosocial factors, self-efficacy behavior, and social feedback would be modified and improved with education and intervening counseling.

5.1. Limitations of the Study

(1) Cross-sectional study design weakened the internal validity so the implication would be tentative rather than definitive.

(2) Lacking medical criteria for secondary clinical parameters determining diabetes mellitus related to comorbid conditions; for example, renal profiling, liver functioning, BMI, and hematological findings. Age criterion further limits the proportion of patients' sample and reduces the study population to 5–10%.

(3) SF-20 questionnaire measures pain and social functioning with a single domain, it would be better to use a more refined and detailed measurement tool for these dimensions.

(4) Self-care reporting particularly with self-perception may prod the diabetics to answer normatively.

6. Conclusion

This study concluded that there are various factors that affect the HRQOL among insulin-dependent diabetes patients. Women exhibit extensive and significant patterns with health-related factors and diabetes-specific psychosocial factors (self-efficacy, social support, and DLC) to improve HRQOL. Health-specific factors were more important among participants with physical impairment (regardless of age and gender). Also, women have significantly high reported distress levels and low social functioning compared to men.

6.1. Practice Implications. Practical implications of this study are focused on the subjective terms of HRQOL, social support, and disease distress levels rather than medical terms only. Strength of this study is the construct and correlational patterns of QOL as a multidimensional concept. The study provides sufficient information to develop a care plan on the basis of personal resources and life circumstances for individualized therapy. Lastly, the data from this study develop, promote, and support self-efficacy to improve disease factors with patient's self-care behavior.

Consent

Written consent forms were obtained from all the participants.

Conflicts of Interest

There is no conflict of interest among the authors.

Authors' Contributions

Syed Wasif Gillani worked as the principal investigator and drafted the manuscript. Irfan Altaf Ansari and Hisham A. Zaghloul were assigned in content analysis and data validation. Mohi Iqbal Mohammad Abdul and Syed Azhar Syed

Sulaiman participated in data collection and data analysis. Mirza R. Baig participated in study content analysis and helped to draft the manuscript. All authors read and approved the final manuscript.

Acknowledgments

The authors acknowledge the efforts of nursing staff for arranging patients' records and managing the scheduled follow-ups. The authors also express their gratitude to the College of Pharmacy Administration for the continued support on administrative approvals.

References

[1] S. W. Gillani, "Determining effective diabetic care; a multicentre - longitudinal interventional study," *Current Pharmaceutical Design*, vol. 22, no. 42, pp. 6469–6476, 2016.

[2] International Diabetes Federation (IDF), "About diabetes," 2013, May 2017, http://www.idf.org/about-diabetes.

[3] S. W. Gillani, S. A. S. Sulaiman, M. I. M. Abdul, and M. R. Baig, "Combined effect of metformin with ascorbic acid versus acetyl salicylic acid on diabetes-related cardiovascular complication; a 12-month single blind multicenter randomized control trial," *Cardiovascular Diabetology*, vol. 16, no. 1, p. 103, 2017.

[4] S. W. Gillani, E. Azeem, A. Siddiqui et al., "Oxidative stress correlates (OSC) in diabetes mellitus patients," *Current Diabetes Reviews*, vol. 12, no. 3, pp. 279–284, 2016.

[5] S. W. Gillani and M. I. M. Abdul, "Public health care system, a quasi-experimental study: acceptance and attitude to implicate clinical services," *Acta Pharmaceutica*, vol. 67, no. 1, pp. 71–83, 2017.

[6] S. W. Gillani, S. A. S. Sulaiman, M. I. M. Abdul, and S. Y. Saad, "A qualitative study to explore the perception and behavior of patients towards diabetes management with physical disability," *Diabetology & Metabolic Syndrome*, vol. 9, no. 1, p. 58, 2017.

[7] L. R. Vartanian, M. B. Schwartz, and K. D. Brownell, "Effects of soft drink consumption on nutrition and health: a systematic review and meta-analysis," *American Journal of Public Health*, vol. 97, no. 4, pp. 667–675, 2007.

[8] A. G. Tabák, M. Jokela, T. N. Akbaraly, E. J. Brunner, M. Kivimäki, and D. R. Witte, "Trajectories of glycaemia, insulin sensitivity, and insulin secretion before diagnosis of type 2 diabetes: an analysis from the Whitehall II study," *The Lancet*, vol. 373, no. 9682, pp. 2215–2221, 2009.

[9] L. G. Hemkens, U. Grouven, R. Bender et al., "Risk of malignancies in patients with diabetes treated with human insulin or insulin analogues: a cohort study," *Diabetologia*, vol. 52, no. 9, pp. 1732–1744, 2009.

[10] S. E. Inzucchi, R. M. Bergenstal, J. B. Buse et al., "Management of hyperglycemia in type 2 diabetes, 2015: a patient-centered approach: update to a position statement of the American Diabetes Association and the European Association for the Study of Diabetes," *Diabetes Care*, vol. 38, no. 1, pp. 140–149, 2015.

[11] Medical Outcome Study-Health Survey (MOS-SF-20), January 2017, https://www.rand.org/health/surveys_tools/mos/20-item-short-form/survey-instrument.html.

[12] R. D. Hays, C. D. Sherbourne, and R. Mazel, "User's manual for the medical outcomes study (MOS) core measures of health-related quality of life," RAND Corporation. Monograph Reports 1995. MR-162-RC-E-Book. https://www.rand.org/pubs/monograph_reports/MR162.html.

[13] L. M. Santos, L. D. A. F. Amorim, D. N. Santos, and M. L. Barreto, "Measuring the level of social support using latent class analysis," *Social Science Research*, vol. 50, pp. 139–146, 2015.

[14] A. M. La Greca and K. J. Bearman, "The diabetes social support questionnaire-family version: evaluating adolescents' diabetes-specific support from family members," *Journal of Pediatric Psychology*, vol. 27, no. 8, pp. 665–676, 2002.

[15] L. C. Schafer, K. D. McCaul, and R. E. Glasgow, "Supportive and nonsupportive family behaviors: relationships to adherence and metabolic control in persons with type I diabetes," *Diabetes Care*, vol. 9, no. 2, pp. 179–185, 1986.

[16] J. Chao, D. P. Nau, J. E. Aikens, and S. D. Taylor, "The mediating role of health beliefs in the relationship between depressive symptoms and medication adherence in persons with diabetes," *Research in Social & Administrative Pharmacy*, vol. 1, no. 4, pp. 508–525, 2005.

[17] S. O. Adejoh, "Diabetes knowledge, health belief, and diabetes management among the Igala, Nigeria," *SAGE Open*, vol. 4, 2014.

[18] R. Harris and M. W. Linn, "Health beliefs, compliance, and control of diabetes mellitus," *Southern Medical Journal*, vol. 78, no. 2, pp. 162–166, 1985.

[19] S. W. Gillani, I. A. Ansari, H. A. Zaghloul, M. I. M. Abdul, S. A. S. Sulaiman, and M. R. Baig, "Bridging glycated hemoglobin with quality of life and health state; a randomized case–control study among type 2 diabetes patients," *Diabetology & Metabolic Syndrome*, vol. 10, no. 23, pp. 1–10, 2018.

[20] L. A. Ferraro, J. H. Price, S. M. Desmond, and S. M. Roberts, "Development of a diabetes locus of control scale," *Psychological Reports*, vol. 61, no. 3, pp. 763–770, 1987.

[21] S. S. Bains and L. E. Egede, "Associations between health literacy, diabetes knowledge, self-care behaviors, and glycemic control in a low income population with type 2 diabetes," *Diabetes Technology & Therapeutics*, vol. 13, no. 3, pp. 335–341, 2011.

[22] G. W. Welch, A. M. Jacobson, and W. H. Polonsky, "The problem areas in diabetes scale: an evaluation of its clinical utility," *Diabetes Care*, vol. 20, no. 5, pp. 760–766, 1997.

[23] S. D. Persell, N. L. Keating, M. B. Landrum et al., "Relationship of diabetes specific knowledge to self-management activities, ambulatory preventive care, and metabolic outcomes," *Preventive Medicine*, vol. 39, no. 4, pp. 746–752, 2004.

[24] C. Y. Osborn and L. E. Egede, "Validation of an information–motivation–behavioral skills model of diabetes self-care (IMB-DSC)," *Patient Education and Counseling*, vol. 79, no. 1, pp. 49–54, 2010.

[25] M. Dømgaard, M. Bagger, N. A. Rhee, C. M. Burton, and B. Thorsteinsson, "Individual and societal consequences of

15

Predictors of Cardiovascular Autonomic Neuropathy Onset and Progression in a Cohort of Type 1 Diabetic Patients

M. Matta,[1] A. Pavy-Le Traon,[2,3] S. Perez-Lloret,[4] C. Laporte,[1] I. Berdugo,[1] N. Nasr,[2,3] H. Hanaire,[1] and J. M. Senard[3,5]

[1]*Service de Diabétologie et maladies métaboliques, CHU de Toulouse, 1 avenue Jean Poulhès, 31059 Toulouse Cedex 9, France*
[2]*Service de Neurologie, Hôpital Pierre-Paul Riquet, Place du Docteur Baylac-TSA 40031, 31059 Toulouse Cedex 9, France*
[3]*Institut des Maladies Métaboliques et Cardiovasculaires, INSERM, Université de Toulouse, 1 avenue Jean Poulhès, BP 84225, 31432 Toulouse Cedex 4, France*
[4]*Institute of Cardiology Research, University of Buenos Aires, National Research Council (CONICET-ININCA), Buenos Aires, Argentina*
[5]*Service de Pharmacologie Clinique, Faculté de Médecine, CHU de Toulouse, 37 allées Jules Guesde, 31000 Toulouse, France*

Correspondence should be addressed to J. M. Senard; jean-michel.senard@inserm.fr

Academic Editor: Norman Cameron

Aim. The prevalence of cardiovascular autonomic neuropathy (CAN) in diabetes mellitus is well documented. However, the rate and predictors of both the development and progression of CAN have been less studied. Hereby, we assessed the rate and the major risk factors for CAN initiation and progression in a cohort of type 1 diabetic patients followed over a three-year period. *Methods.* 175 type 1 diabetic patients (mean age: 50 ± 11 years; female/male: 76/99) with positive bedside screening for CAN were included and underwent 2 standardized autonomic testings using 4 standardized tests (deep breathing, Valsalva maneuver, 30/15 ratio, and changes in blood pressure during standing), separated by 3 ± 1 years. CAN staging was achieved according to the Toronto Consensus Panel on Diabetic Autonomic Neuropathy into 4 categories: absent, possible, confirmed, or severe CAN. *Results.* Out of the 175 patients included, 31.4% were free of CAN, 34.2% had possible CAN, 24.6% had confirmed CAN, and 9.7% exhibited severe CAN at the first assessment. Among the 103 patients with nonsevere CAN at inclusion, forty-one (39.8%) had an increase of at least one category when reassessed and 62 (60.2%) remained stable. A bivariate analysis indicated that only BMI and exposure to selective serotonin reuptake inhibitors (SSRIs) were significantly different in both groups. A multivariate analysis indicated that lower BMI (OR: 0.15, CI 95%: 0.05–0.48, $p = 0.003$) and SSRI exposure (OR: 4.18, CI 95%: 1.03–16.97, $p = 0.04$) were the sole predictors of CAN deterioration. In the 55 patients negative for CAN at the first laboratory assessment, 12 became positive at the second assessment. *Conclusion.* No clear predictive factor for CAN onset was identified. However, once present, CAN progression was related to low BMI and SSRI exposure.

1. Introduction

Cardiovascular autonomic neuropathy (CAN) is a common but often neglected diabetes mellitus complication. Based on the CAN Subcommittee of the Toronto Consensus Panel on Diabetic Neuropathy [1], CAN is defined as the impairment of cardiovascular autonomic control in patients with established diabetes mellitus following the exclusion of other causes. It is generally believed that CAN incidence is related to age, duration of diabetes, poor glycemic control, and microvascular disease [2–5]. Although unpredictable, CAN progression results in a significant cardiovascular morbidity and mortality [6].

A better understanding of predictive risk factors for CAN incidence and progression is crucial for the development of new strategies for follow-up as well as of novel therapeutic targets.

The purpose of the present study was to assess major risk factors of CAN onset and progression and to describe the time line changes in cardiac autonomic dysfunction in a cohort of type 1 diabetic patients over a mean period of 3 years.

2. Patients and Methods

2.1. Selection of Patients. 175 consecutive type 1 diabetic patients attending the Department of Diabetes and Metabolism of Toulouse University Hospital between July 2003 and June 2010 and who had a positive bedside screening for CAN were included. Patients on beta-blocker treatment at selection were not included. The screening for CAN included 3 cardiovascular reflex tests described by Ewing and Clarke [7]: the heart rate (HR) response to deep breathing, which assesses beat-to-beat HR variation (R-R variation) during paced deep breathing [expiration-to-inspiration ratio (E:I)]; the initial HR response to standing expressed as the 30 : 15 ratio (ratio of the longest R-R interval (around the 30th beat) to the shortest R-R interval (around the 15th beat)) elicited by a change from the horizontal to vertical position; and the blood pressure (BP) response to standing. A single abnormal result suffices to suspect the diagnosis of possible CAN. The study was performed according to the French law for clinical research.

2.2. Laboratory Autonomic Testing. All patients with a positive screening for CAN underwent more elaborated tests as previously described [8]. The autonomic laboratory evaluation was based on continuous digital BP (photoplethysmography, Nexfin) and computerized ECG recordings during the following tests: paced deep breathing test (6 cycles/min), Valsalva maneuver (40 mmHg, 15 sec) performed in supine position, a 5 min stand test, and a 3 min isometric exercise (hand grip, 30% of maximal force) performed in seated position. The Ewing score (ES) was based on the following parameters: HR changes with deep breathing, 30/15 ratio, Valsalva ratio (HR max during maneuver : HR min during recovery), BP response to active standing, and diastolic BP increase to hand grip. The response to each test was considered normal (0), borderline (0.5), or abnormal (1) according to the laboratory normal values for age. Orthostatic hypotension (OH) was defined as a reduction in systolic BP of at least 20 mmHg and/or diastolic BP of at least 10 mmHg within 3 minutes of standing. The Ewing score (ES) ranging from 0 (normal) to 5 (severe autonomic failure) represents the sum of the responses to the different tests. Further assessment was performed using the Toronto Consensus classification based on previous tests except isometric hand grip: absence of CAN (no abnormal response, score 0), possible (one abnormal cardiovagal test, score 1), confirmed (at least 2 abnormal cardiovagal tests, score 2), and severe (1 abnormal cardiovagal test plus orthostatic hypotension, score 3).

2.3. Selection of CAN Potential Predictors. At the time of CAN screening, the following clinical characteristics of the patients were recorded: age, weight, body mass index (BMI), HbA1c level, diabetes duration, insulin treatment (subcutaneous insulin infusion or multiple daily injection), and diabetes-related complications. Diabetic nephropathy was assessed using the estimated glomerular filtration rate (eGFR), which was calculated using the MDRD equation and the urinary albumin/creatinine ratio (ACR) of a single early morning urine. Stage 1 nephropathy was considered for ACR between 30 and 299 mg/g, and stage 2 nephropathy was considered for ACR $\geq$ 300 mg/g and/or an eGFR < 60 ml·min^{-1} per 1.73 m^2. Retinopathy stages included mild nonproliferative (NPR) (stage 1), moderate NPR (stage 2), and severe NPR or proliferative retinopathy and scatter laser treatment (stage 3). Knee and ankle reflexes, distal vibration perception, and pinprick tests were performed. Clinical distal peripheral neuropathy was diagnosed on at least one abnormal test. Associated cardiovascular risk factors such as arterial hypertension, hypercholesterolemia, and smoking were recorded. Silent myocardial ischemia was assessed using an exercise stress test or stress thallium myocardial perfusion imaging.

2.4. Statistical Analysis. Analyses were performed using STATA Version 10. Numerical variables with normal distribution are expressed as means ± SD and reported as median (interquartile range). Bivariate comparisons were performed by a chi-square test for categorical variables or by *t*-test for numerical variables (with adjustments for unequal variances when needed). A multivariate analysis was performed by logistic regression. All variables with bivariate p value < 0.10 were included. Numerical variables were categorized in tertiles for the exploration of the nonlinear relationship with the dependent variable. If present, the categorical variable was included in the multivariate model instead of the original numerical one. Multicolinearity was explored by correlation coefficients. Only participants with two complete and analyzable autonomic testings during the period of the study were included in the statistical analysis.

3. Results

3.1. Characteristics of the Studied Population. One hundred seventy-five (175) consecutive type 1 diabetic patients, who had a positive bedside screening for CAN (mean age: 50 ± 11 years, M/F: 1.30), were included in the study. One hundred fifty-eight out of 175 patients underwent a second complete and analyzable autonomic testing after a mean time interval of 3.0 ± 1.1 years.

The clinical and biochemical characteristics of the study population are depicted in Table 1. Mean BMI, duration of diabetes, and HbA1c level were 24.4 ± 3.0 kg/m^2, 26 ± 11 years, and 7.9 ± 1.2%, respectively. Forty-two percent (42%) of patients were on subcutaneous insulin infusion, 12% were on intraperitoneal insulin infusion, and 46% received multiple daily injections.

Prevalence rates of arterial hypertension, hypercholesterolemia, and current smoking were 40.0%, 33.1%, and 28.6%, respectively. Concerning diabetes-related complications, 30.8% had diabetic nephropathy, of which 11% were at stage 2 nephropathy (ACR $\geq$ 300 mg/g and or an eGFR < 60 ml·min^{-1} per 1.73 m^2). The prevalence of retinopathy at any stage was around 67.4%, of whom 38%

Table 1: Baseline characteristics of the cohort of type 1 diabetic patients.

	$N = 175$
Demographic characteristics	
Age (years)	50 ± 11
Women/men	76/99
Diabetes duration (years)	26 ± 11
HbA1c (%)	7.9 ± 1.2
BMI (kg/m^2)	24.4 ± 3
Complications and comorbidities	
Nephropathy	54 (31%)
Retinopathy	118 (67%)
Peripheral neuropathy	77 (44%)
Hypertension	70 (40%)
Dyslipidemia	58 (33%)
Tobacco smoking	50 (29%)
Silent myocardial ischemia	3 (2%)
Neurovegetative symptoms	
Cardiovascular	63 (36%)
Digestive	47 (27%)
Erectile dysfunction	51 (52%)
Bladder dysfunction	50 (29%)

were at stage 3 retinopathy. Peripheral neuropathy was found in 44%. 75% of the patients underwent screening for silent ischemic cardiac disease at the time of the first visit with only 3 positive screenings. The prevalence of neurovegetative disorders including gastrointestinal symptoms, bladder dysfunction, cardiovascular symptoms, and erectile dysfunction was found in 26.9%, 28.6%, 36.0%, and 29.1%, respectively.

According to Spallone et al. [1], fifty-five patients (31.4%) out of the 175 included did not have CAN at laboratory assessment. Sixty patients (34.2%) had possible CAN, 43 (24.6%) had a confirmed CAN, and 17 (9.7%) had severe CAN. An abnormal HR response to deep breathing was found in 61.2%, abnormal HR response to standing in 29.7%, abnormal Valsalva ratio or abnormal response to sustained hand grip in 12%, and, finally, orthostatic hypotension in 10.3%.

3.2. Risk Factors for CAN Progression over a Three-Year Period. One hundred and three (103) patients out of 158, with at least possible or more severe CAN at first laboratory assessment, had a second complete and analyzable testing. In sixty-two patients (51.7%), CAN severity remained stable or improved during the study period whereas worsening (change from possible to confirmed or from confirmed to severe CAN) was found in 41 patients (34.2%). The tests which became more frequently abnormal were the HR response to standing in 21% and the blood pressure response to sustained hand grip and Valsalva ratio in 14% and 15%, respectively. The blood pressure response to standing became abnormal in only 8% of the cases.

The characteristics of the two groups are shown in Table 2. A bivariate analysis indicates that age; gender; diabetes duration; cardiovascular-associated risk factors; morbidities including peripheral neuropathy, retinopathy, and nephropathy; and treatment modalities were not significantly different between the 2 groups. However, the mean BMI value was significantly lower ($p = 0.047$), and the exposure to selective serotonin reuptake inhibitors (SSRIs) was significantly higher (0.04) in patients from group II. In a multivariate analysis, both BMI and SSRI exposure were found to be independently related to CAN deterioration (Table 2).

3.3. Risk Factors for CAN Initiation over a Three-Year Period. Fifty-five (55) patients had no CAN at inclusion. Among them, 43 (78.2%) remained free from CAN at the end of the study, and 12 (21.8%) became positive on the second autonomic testing.

The clinical and biochemical characteristics of patients with persistent negative CAN and those who were positive for CAN upon the second reassessment were not statistically different (Table 3). A trend for higher exposure to diuretics in the group developing CAN ($n = 2$ patients) versus the group remaining free from CAN ($n = 1$ patient) was noticed but did not reach the level of significance ($p = 0.053$), and the very limited number of patients makes this finding nonrelevant.

4. Discussion

Previous studies provided information about cardiovascular autonomic neuropathy (CAN) prevalence in subjects with type 1 diabetes, but few of them raised the issue of the rate and predictors of CAN progression. The main results of the present study are that no clear risk factor was related to CAN onset and that factors associated with CAN progression from the mild stage are low BMI and SSRI exposure.

The interpretation of our results has to be made keeping in mind that the population included in this study is not representative of the global type 1 diabetic population. In fact, according to the strategy in our institution, and as recommended by French guidelines at the time of the study [9], only patients with at least one abnormal response to 3 bedside-performed screening tests were addressed for complete autonomic laboratory testing. Moreover, patients receiving beta-blockers, which could modify results of autonomic tests, were discarded, thus explaining the low rate of silent myocardial ischemia. Despite these potential biases, the observed frequency of CAN severity in this survey is coherent with previously published results [8, 10]. The selection strategy also explains that only a relatively reduced number of patients were free of cardiovascular autonomic neuropathy at the first assessment, thus making the evaluation of CAN incidence not realistic from our results. However, we observed that a reduced proportion of initially normal patients (21.8%) developed autonomic neuropathy within a 3-year period.

Our criterion for CAN progression was an increase of at least one point in the Spallone scoring. Indeed, very few studies investigated the progression rate of autonomic dysfunction in diabetes mellitus, and most of them concentrated on

Table 2: Baseline clinical and biochemical characteristics of type 1 diabetic patients with mild CAN who remained stable (group I) or had CAN worsening (group II) for over a mean period of 3 years.

	Group I ($n = 62$)	Group II ($n = 41$)	p value	Logistic regression OR (95% CI)
Age (years)	50.69 ± 1.36	47.63 ± 1.57	0.15	
Males	39 (63%)	22 (54%)	0.35	
Diabetes duration (years)	26.32 ± 1.45	26.12 ± 1.62	0.92	
≤20	21 (34%)	13 (32%)	0.8	
21–30	22 (35%)	13 (32%)		
>30	19 (31%)	15 (37%)		
BMI (kg/m^2)	25.07 ± 0.38	23.58 ± 0.5	0.018	
≤22.94	16 (26%)	20 (49%)	0.003	1
22.94–25.68	17 (27%)	15 (37%)		0.73 (0.28–1.95)
>25.68	29 (47%)	6 (15%)		0.15 (0.05–0.48)
HbA1c (%)	7.76 ± 0.13	8.08 ± 0.2	0.16	
≤7.4	23 (37%)	11 (27%)	0.25	
7.5–8.2	24 (39%)	14 (34%)		
>8.2	15 (24%)	16 (39%)		
DPN	27 (44%)	18 (44%)	0.97	
Nephropathy			0.72	
0	44 (71%)	26 (63%)		
1	11 (18%)	9 (22%)		
2	7 (11%)	6 (15%)		
Retinopathy			0.18	
0	22 (35%)	7 (17%)		
1	8 (13%)	8 (20%)		
2	10 (16%)	6 (15%)		
3	22 (35%)	20 (49%)		
Microalbuminuria (mg/24 h)	41 ± 12.32	163.16 ± 69.92	0.09	
≤7.0	23 (37%)	11 (27%)	0.44	
7.1–14.6	20 (32%)	13 (32%)		
>14.7	19 (31%)	17 (41%)		
Clearance (ml/min)	80.46 ± 2.02	79.26 ± 3.71	0.75	
≤73.87	20 (32%)	18 (44%)	0.37	
73.87–88.49	26 (42%)	12 (29%)		
>88.49	16 (26%)	11 (27%)		
Hypertension	25 (40%)	13 (32%)	0.37	
Tobacco smoking	18 (29%)	12 (30%)	0.91	
Dyslipidemia	17 (27%)	16 (39%)	0.21	
CSII			0.39	
0	28 (45%)	23 (56%)		
1	27 (44%)	16 (39%)		
2	7 (11%)	2 (5%)		
HMG-CoA inhibitors	16 (26%)	14 (34%)	0.36	
CEI/AT1 antagonists	26 (42%)	16 (39%)	0.76	
Antiaggregants	7 (11%)	5 (12%)	0.89	
Diuretics	5 (8%)	6 (15%)	0.27	
Calcium inhibitors	4 (6%)	3 (7%)	0.86	
SSRIs	4 (6%)	8 (20%)	0.04	4.18 (1.03–16.97)

Shown are means ± standard error of the mean. DPN: distal peripheral neuropathy; CV: cardiovascular; CSII: continuous subcutaneous and intraperitoneal insulin infusion; NC: not calculated. Data were analyzed according to Statistical Analysis.

TABLE 3: Baseline clinical and biochemical characteristics of type 1 diabetic patients without CAN at inclusion who remained stable (no CAN) or developed autonomic dysfunction (CAN) for over a mean period of 3 years.

	No CAN ($n = 43$)	CAN ($n = 12$)	p value	No CAN ($n = 43$) and not No CAN ($n = 43$)
Age (years)	52.12 ± 1.56	56.33 ± 3.56	0.23	
Males	27 (63%)	6 (50%)	0.42	
Diabetes duration (years)	25.47 ± 1.83	22.17 ± 2.66	0.38	
≤20	19 (44%)	6 (50%)	0.09	
21–30	8 (19%)	5 (42%)		
>30	16 (37%)	1 (8%)		
BMI (kg/m^2)	23.74 ± 0.67	24.27 ± 0.71	0.69	
≤22.94	12 (28%)	4 (33%)	0.87	
22.94–25.68	17 (40%)	5 (42%)		
>25.68	14 (33%)	3 (25%)		
HbA1c (%)	8.07 ± 0.18	7.57 ± 0.37	0.21	
≤7.4	14 (33%)	6 (50%)	0.53	
7.5–8.2	14 (33%)	3 (25%)		
>8.2	15 (35%)	3 (25%)		
DPN	16 (37%)	5 (42%)	0.79	
Nephropathy			0.13	
0	32 (74%)	11 (92%)		
1	10 (23%)	0 (0%)		
2	1 (2%)	1 (8%)		
Retinopathy			0.89	
0	19 (44%)	6 (50%)		
1	6 (14%)	2 (17%)		
2	6 (14%)	2 (17%)		
3	12 (28%)	2 (17%)		
Microalbuminuria (mg/24 h)	44.71 ± 27.74	7.76 ± 1.32	0.48	
≤7.0	17 (40%)	8 (67%)	0.25	
7.1–14.6	12 (28%)	2 (17%)		
>14.7	14 (33%)	2 (17%)		
Clearance (ml/min)	85.31 ± 2.32	81.1 ± 4.68	0.4	
≤73.87	9 (21%)	5 (42%)	0.34	
73.87–88.49	15 (35%)	3 (25%)		
>88.49	19 (44%)	4 (33%)		
Hypertension	17 (40%)	6 (50%)	0.48	
Tobacco smoking	10 (23%)	4 (33%)	0.5	
Dyslipidemia	16 (37%)	3 (25%)	0.43	
CSII			0.6	
0	16 (37%)	6 (50%)		
1	19 (44%)	5 (42%)		
2	8 (19%)	1 (8%)		
HMG-CoA inhibitors	9 (21%)	1 (8%)	0.31	
CEI/AT1 antagonists	19 (44%)	7 (58%)	0.38	
Antiaggregants	7 (16%)	0 (0%)	0.13	
Diuretics	1 (2%)	2 (17%)	0.053	
Calcium inhibitors	4 (9%)	0 (0%)	0.27	
SSRIs	4 (9%)	0 (0%)	0.27	

DPN: distal peripheral neuropathy; CV: cardiovascular; CSII: continuous subcutaneous and intraperitoneal insulin infusion; NC: not calculated. Data were analyzed according to Statistical Analysis.

the prevalence of CAN. In these studies, the usual minimal score to diagnose CAN is 2 abnormal responses to cardiovagal tests to discard the false positive assessment of CAN [1]. In fact, the response to the tests composing the autonomic battery we used is highly dependent on the quality of patient performance. The choice of a one-point increase in autonomic score to define CAN progression was made in order to detect minimal changes accounting for progression. However, special attention was paid to the conditions in which autonomic testing was performed. In fact, all testings were performed at entry and at study end in the same laboratory by the same persons, and exactly the same devices were used in order to reduce the variability of the measured parameters. However, we cannot exclude that, despite these cautions, our experimental design could have led to some overestimation of the progression of CAN.

Other confusion biases potentially accounting for changes in the autonomic score at the second testing could result from changes in diabetes treatment. However, our data showed that cardiac autonomic neuropathy in long-standing type 1 diabetic patients is associated with the progression of autonomic dysfunction. During the DCCT/EDIC study, diabetes duration and degree of glycemic control were the dominant determinants of the risk progression of microvascular complications in type 1 diabetic patients [3]. However, CAN prevalence increased in both intensive and conventionally treated groups even if it was significantly lower in the former intensive group than in the former conventional group (28.9% versus 35.2%; $p = 0.018$) [3], thus suggesting that hyperglycemia is not the sole mechanism involved in CAN progression.

Regarding the progression of CAN, the present study demonstrates that 39.8% of the patients with mild autonomic dysfunction progress to a more advanced stage over a three-year period and that progression is related to low BMI and SSRI exposure but not to HbA1c level, disease duration, retinopathy, peripheral neuropathy, or nephropathy. Despite previous studies postulating that the progression of CAN is slow [11, 12] and linked to diabetes duration, blood glucose control, and microangiopathic complications [13–15], the nature of CAN progression predictors remains controversial. The progression of CAN has been shown to be positively correlated with low BMI, but, in the contrary, several studies reported obesity as a positive predictive factor for CAN progression in nondiabetic and type 1 and 2 diabetic patients [2]. Since most evidences indicate that low BMI is a marker of uncontrolled diabetes and thus a risk factor for CAN deterioration, our results have to be taken with caution and will need confirmation in specific future studies. In our study, the HbA1c level was not statistically different between patients that deteriorate their CAN and those who did not. This might be explained by the fact that the HbA1c level was measured at a point time related to the first CAN screening and does only show the blood glucose control over the last three-month period. Another possibility is that HbA1c is not a good indicator of blood glucose variability promoting hypoglycemic stress that was associated in a recent study with reduced heart rate variability independent of glycemic control as assessed by HbA1c [16]. Thus, it could be suggested that glucose variability rather than glucose levels contributes to cardiovascular autonomic dysfunction among adults with type 1 diabetes.

Our findings are surprising since diabetic CAN has been repeatedly reported to associate with nephropathy and since autonomic neuropathy is encountered in approximatively 60% of the patients with chronic kidney disease. The relationship between CAN and nephropathy in diabetes is rather complex and unclear. In fact, on one hand, CAN may be an aggravating factor of nephropathy [14]. A faster rate over 1 year of the progression of renal dysfunction was suggested in type 1 diabetic patients with autonomic dysfunction [17]. Nephropathy was found to be an independent risk factor for CAN prevalence [18]. On the other hand, autonomic neuropathy was not considered to be a progression promoter in diabetic nephropathy in a prospective observational follow-up study including 388 type 1 diabetic patients with ($n = 197$) and without ($n = 191$) diabetic nephropathy followed for 10.1 years [19]; in this study, there was no relationship between CAN and a faster decline in GFR. Finally, several authors have hypothesized that CAN is indirectly involved in the pathogenesis of diabetic nephropathy, via hemodynamic changes such as lack of nocturnal BP dipping (causing increased intraglomerular pressure resulting in albuminuria) and diurnal postural falls in BP (resulting in lower intraglomerular pressure) and endothelial dysfunction [19]. Others suggested that CAN is a strong predictor of nephropathy and participates in the progression of chronic kidney disease through deficient erythropoietin production and anemia [20–22].

We found that serotonin reuptake inhibitor exposure was higher in patients with CAN progression. This finding first suggests an indirect link between SSRIs and CAN worsening. In fact, even if SSRIs are not first-line recommended drugs for diabetic neuropathic pain, antidepressants are often used in diabetes, and, globally, an association between their use and CAN worsening could be related to a higher frequency of depressive symptoms in worsening patients. In fact, our data indicate that there is a significant difference ($p = 0.04$; OR: 4.18 [1.03–16.97]) in the frequency of SSRI use in patients with neuropathy in both patients remaining stable (6%) and worsening ones (20%). Secondly, it could suggest that SSRI drugs worsen diabetes equilibrium, thus favoring CAN progression. However, on the one hand, no differences in diabetes characteristics, including HbA1c, were found between stable and worsening patients, and, on the other hand, data from literature about effects of SSRIs on diabetes remain controversial. In young patients with type 1 diabetes, SSRIs have been found to be associated with negative clinical outcomes, an effect ascribed to the impact of comorbid depression on the quality of diabetes treatment [23]. By contrast, other studies have reported lower insulin requirement for the control of type 1 diabetes in patients receiving SSRIs [24]. Finally, another hypothesis could be the negative impact of SSRIs on autonomic nervous system activity. Data from the literature converge on neutral effects of SSRIs on autonomic function when compared to older tricyclic antidepressants [25]. SSRIs have also been proposed for the management of vasovagal syncope

[26] or orthostatic hypotension in neurodegenerative disorders such as Parkinson's disease [27], but there are no data in orthostatic hypotension in diabetes mellitus.

5. Conclusion

Few studies raised the question about the initiation and progression of CAN in type 1 diabetic patients, which makes this paper original. The main findings are that no clear factors seem to be associated with CAN onset while its worsening is correlated with low BMI and SSRI exposure but not with classical clinical or biological disease parameters. Despite some limitations, resulting from the study design and the number of patients in subgroups which limit conclusions about any causal relation between CAN progression and other microvascular and macrovascular diabetes-related complications, these data suggest that mechanisms underlying the onset and worsening of autonomic dysfunction in type 1 diabetes are different. However, larger prospective studies with longer follow-up are needed to confirm these results.

Conflicts of Interest

The authors declare that there is no conflict of interest regarding the publication of this manuscript.

References

[1] V. Spallone, D. Ziegler, R. Freeman et al., "Cardiovascular autonomic neuropathy in diabetes: clinical impact, assessment, diagnosis, and management," *Diabetes/Metabolism Research and Reviews*, vol. 27, no. 7, pp. 639–653, 2011.

[2] P. Valensi, J. Paries, and J. R. Attali, "Cardiac autonomic neuropathy in diabetic patients: influence of diabetes duration, obesity, and microangiopathic complications—the French multicenter study," *Metabolism Clinical and Experimental*, vol. 52, no. 7, pp. 815–820, 2003.

[3] R. Pop-Busui, P. A. Low, B. H. Waberski et al., "Effects of prior intensive insulin therapy on cardiac autonomic nervous system function in type 1 diabetes mellitus: the Diabetes Control and Complications Trial/Epidemiology of Diabetes Interventions and Complications study (DCCT/EDIC)," *Circulation*, vol. 119, no. 22, pp. 2886–2893, 2009.

[4] P. Kempler, S. Tesfaye, N. Chaturvedi et al., "Autonomic neuropathy is associated with increased cardiovascular risk factors: the EURODIAB IDDM Complications Study," *Diabetic Medicine*, vol. 19, no. 11, pp. 900–909, 2002.

[5] C. L. Martin, J. W. Albers, R. Pop-Busui, and DCCT/EDIC Research Group, "Neuropathy and related findings in the Diabetes Control and Complications Trial/Epidemiology of Diabetes Interventions and Complications Study," *Diabetes Care*, vol. 37, no. 1, pp. 31–38, 2014.

[6] P. Valensi, R. N. Sachs, B. Harfouche et al., "Predictive value of cardiac autonomic neuropathy in diabetic patients with or without silent myocardial ischemia," *Diabetes Care*, vol. 24, no. 2, pp. 339–343, 2001.

[7] D. J. Ewing and B. F. Clarke, "9 – Autonomic neuropathy: its diagnosis and prognosis," *Clinics in Endocrinology and Metabolism*, vol. 15, no. 4, pp. 855–888, 1986.

[8] A. Pavy-Le Traon, S. Fontaine, G. Tap, B. Guidolin, J. M. Senard, and H. Hanaire, "Cardiovascular autonomic neuropathy and other complications in type 1 diabetes," *Clinical Autonomic Research*, vol. 20, no. 3, pp. 153–160, 2010.

[9] P. Valensi and J. R. Attali, "Why and how should cardiovascular autonomic neuropathy in the diabetic be researched? Recommendations of ALFEDIAM (French Language Association for the Study of Diabetes and Metabolic Diseases)," *Diabetes & Metabolism*, vol. 23, no. 4, pp. 351–356, 1997.

[10] D. Ziegler, K. Dannehl, H. Mühlen, M. Spüler, and F. A. Gries, "Prevalence of cardiovascular autonomic dysfunction assessed by spectral analysis, vector analysis, and standard tests of heart rate variation and blood pressure responses at various stages of diabetic neuropathy," *Diabetic Medicine*, vol. 9, no. 9, pp. 806–814, 1992.

[11] N. S. Levitt, K. B. Stansberry, S. Wynchank, and A. I. Vinik, "The natural progression of autonomic neuropathy and autonomic function tests in a cohort of people with IDDM," *Diabetes Care*, vol. 19, no. 7, pp. 751–754, 1996.

[12] M. J. Sampson, S. Wilson, P. Karagiannis, M. Edmonds, and P. J. Watkins, "Progression of diabetic autonomic neuropathy over a decade in insulin-dependent diabetics," *QJM*, vol. 75, no. 278, pp. 635–646, 1990.

[13] C. Voulgari, M. Psallas, A. Kokkinos, V. Argiana, N. Katsilambros, and N. Tentolouris, "The association between cardiac autonomic neuropathy with metabolic and other factors in subjects with type 1 and type 2 diabetes," *Journal of Diabetes and its Complications*, vol. 25, no. 3, pp. 159–167, 2011.

[14] A. J. Burger, J. A. D'Elia, L. A. Weinrauch, I. Lerman, and A. Gaur, "Marked abnormalities in heart rate variability are associated with progressive deterioration of renal function in type I diabetic patients with overt nephropathy," *International Journal of Cardiology*, vol. 86, no. 2-3, pp. 281–287, 2002.

[15] D. R. Witte, S. Tesfaye, N. Chaturvedi et al., "Risk factors for cardiac autonomic neuropathy in type 1 diabetes mellitus," *Diabetologia*, vol. 48, no. 1, pp. 164–171, 2005.

[16] M. Jaiswal, K. McKeon, N. Comment et al., "Association between impaired cardiovascular autonomic function and hypoglycemia in patients with type 1 diabetes," *Diabetes Care*, vol. 37, no. 9, pp. 2616–2621, 2014.

[17] L. A. Weinrauch, F. P. Kennedy, R. E. Gleason, J. Keough, and J. A. D'Elia, "Relationship between autonomic function and progression of renal disease in diabetic proteinuria: clinical correlations and implications for blood pressure control," *American Journal of Hypertension*, vol. 11, no. 3, pp. 302–308, 1998.

[18] A. Tahrani, K. Dubb, N. T. Raymond et al., "Cardiac autonomic neuropathy predicts renal function decline in patients with type 2 diabetes: a cohort study," *Diabetologia*, vol. 57, no. 6, pp. 1249–1256, 2014.

[19] A. S. Astrup, L. Tarnow, P. Rossing, B. V. Hansen, J. Hilsted, and H. H. Parving, "Cardiac autonomic neuropathy predicts cardiovascular morbidity and mortality in type 1 diabetic patients with diabetic nephropathy," *Diabetes Care*, vol. 29, no. 2, pp. 334–339, 2006.

[20] G. Sundkvist and B. Lilja, "Autonomic neuropathy predicts deterioration in glomerular filtration rate in patients with IDDM," *Diabetes Care*, vol. 16, no. 5, pp. 773–779, 1993.

[21] K. Iseki and K. Kohagura, "Anemia as a risk factor for chronic kidney disease," *Kidney International*, vol. 72, pp. S4–S9, 2007.

[22] R. Deicher and W. H. Horl, "Anaemia as a risk factor for the progression of chronic kidney disease," *Current Opinion in Nephrology and Hypertension*, vol. 12, no. 2, pp. 139–143, 2003.

[23] P. L. Plener, E. Molz, G. Berger et al., "Depression, metabolic control, and antidepressant medication in young patients with type 1 diabetes," *Pediatric Diabetes*, vol. 16, no. 1, pp. 58–66, 2015.

[24] M. J. Knol, H. J. Derijks, M. I. Geerlings et al., "Influence of antidepressants on glycaemic control in patients with diabetes mellitus," *Pharmacoepidemiology & Drug Safety*, vol. 17, no. 6, pp. 577–586, 2008.

[25] R. Noordam, M. E. van den Berg, M. N. Niemeijer et al., "Antidepressants and heart-rate variability in older adults: a population-based study," *Psychological Medicine*, vol. 46, no. 06, pp. 1239–1247, 2016.

[26] G. Vaddadi, S. J. Corcoran, and M. Esler, "Management strategies for recurrent vasovagal syncope," *Internal Medicine Journal*, vol. 40, no. 8, pp. 554–560, 2010.

[27] B. P. Grubb, D. Samoil, D. Kosinski, D. Wolfe, M. Lorton, and E. Madu, "Fluoxetine hydrochloride for the treatment of severe refractory orthostatic hypotension," *The American Journal of Medicine*, vol. 97, no. 4, pp. 366–368, 1994.

16

Detection of Islet Cell Immune Reactivity with Low Glycemic Index Foods: Is This a Concern for Type 1 Diabetes?

Datis Kharrazian,[1,2,3] Martha Herbert,[1,2] and Aristo Vojdani[3,4]

[1]*Harvard Medical School, Boston, MA, USA*
[2]*TRANSCEND Research, Department of Neurology, Massachusetts General Hospital, Charlestown, Boston, MA 02129, USA*
[3]*Department of Preventive Medicine, Loma Linda University School of Medicine, Loma Linda, CA, USA*
[4]*Immunosciences Laboratory, Inc., Los Angeles, CA, USA*

Correspondence should be addressed to Datis Kharrazian; datis_kharrazian@hms.harvard.edu

Academic Editor: Hiroshi Okamoto

Dietary management of autoimmune diabetes includes low glycemic foods classified from the glycemic index, but it does not consider the role that immunoreactive foods may play with the immunological etiology of the disease. We measured the reactivity of either monoclonal or polyclonal affinity-purified antibodies to insulin, insulin receptor alpha, insulin receptor beta, zinc transporter 8 (ZnT8), tyrosine phosphatase-based islet antigen 2 (IA2), and glutamic acid decarboxylase (GAD) 65 and 67 against 204 dietary proteins that are commonly consumed. Dietary protein determinants included unmodified (raw) and modified (cooked and roasted) foods, herbs, spices, food gums, brewed beverages, and additives. There was no immune reactivity between insulin or insulin receptor beta and dietary proteins. However, we identified strong to moderate immunological reactivity with antibodies against insulin receptor alpha, ZnT8, IA2, GAD-65, and GAD-67 with several dietary proteins. We also identified 49 dietary proteins found in foods classified as low glycemic foods with immune reactivity to autoimmune target sites. Laboratory analysis of immunological cross-reactivity between pancreas target sites and dietary proteins is the initial step necessary in determining whether dietary proteins may play a potential immunoreactive role in autoimmune diabetes.

1. Introduction

Diabetes mellitus, commonly called diabetes, is a group of metabolic diseases in which the body experiences unusually high blood sugar levels over an extended period of time. Diabetes is a leading cause of death and disability in the United States and affects more than 9.3% of the population [1]. The total cost of diabetes in the United States is estimated at more than $245 billion annually [2]. There are four broad recognized categories of diabetes:

(i) Type 1 diabetes (T1D) is a result of the pancreas' failure to produce sufficient insulin. The pancreas is a glandular organ that not only secretes digestive enzymes but also produces important hormones. These hormones are produced inside the pancreas by clumps of cells called islet cells. Of the five kinds of islet cells, alpha, beta, delta, gamma (PP), and epsilon, only beta islet cells produce the hormone insulin, which regulates blood sugar levels. In an autoimmune condition, the body's own immune system can mistakenly attack and damage or destroy beta islet cells, leading to a reduction of the insulin needed to regulate the body's blood sugar levels [3].

(ii) Type 2 diabetes is a condition in which the cells of the body fail to respond to insulin properly, usually caused by excessive body weight and lack of exercise. Lack of insulin may also develop as the disease progresses [3, 4].

(iii) Gestational diabetes occurs when pregnant women without a previous history of diabetes develop high blood sugar levels [3].

(iv) Other specific types are a collection of a few dozen different causes [5].

Many new cases of diabetes are due to an overlooked autoimmune etiology called latent autoimmune diabetes of adulthood (LADA), which is often misdiagnosed as type 2 diabetes [6]. In the early stages of LADA, progressive autoimmune destruction of islet cells leads to hyperglycemia that does not yet require insulin. As a result, it is commonly misdiagnosed as type 2 diabetes [7]. LADA accounts for 10% of all cases of diabetes and 50% of nonobese diabetes [8]. Despite the autoimmune pathophysiology of LADA, current medication and treatment approaches are focused solely on hyperglycemia control rather than clinical strategies to prevent progression of autoimmune destruction of islet cells [9]. Progression of islet cell destruction from autoimmunity leads to insulin therapy and associated complications of autoimmunity [10]. Experts have expressed the need to identify new therapeutic applications for individuals who are diagnosed with LADA, as the glucose-control model is not sufficiently effective with these patients [9]. The standard practice of using the glycemic index restriction diet for autoimmune diabetes does not consider dietary proteins that have the potential to immunologically cross-react with pancreatic islet cells.

LADA and juvenile type 1 diabetes are characterized by autoimmune destruction hyperglycemia. The pathogenic model in which antigens initiate and drive the process is currently under investigation [11, 12]. Other pathogenic organisms, such as rubella infection, enteroviruses, human cytomegalovirus, and rotavirus, have all been suggested to play a role in cross-reactivity leading to pancreatic islet cell destruction [13]. Cross-reactivity is thought to occur when antigens share amino acid sequence homology with self-tissue proteins in susceptible hosts and has been theorized as a trigger for tissue-specific autoimmune diseases [14–16]. Immunological cross-reactivity was first identified in 1942 when it was found that individuals sensitized to pollen allergens developed immune reactivity to specific fruits [17]. Further study found that cross-reactivity with pollen could also occur to human tissue target proteins [18].

Dietary protein cross-reactivity research has received limited attention in type 1 diabetes. Current research has mostly been limited to gluten and milk proteins as potential sources of pancreatic islet cell destruction. Cow's milk albumin has also been suggested in the etiology of type 1 diabetes due to milk peptide antibody (bovine serum albumin antibodies) binding to beta-cell-specific surface protein and promoting islet cell destruction [19–21]. Additionally, the prevalence of celiac disease in adult type 1 diabetic patients was found to be approximately 10.5% [22]. In one study, antibodies to the wheat storage globulin Glb1 were found in the serum of diabetic patients, but not in age-, sex-, nor HLA-DQ-matched controls. This provides a first candidate wheat protein that is not only antigenic in diabetic rats and human patients but also closely linked to autoimmune attack on the pancreas [23]. A review paper found that studies in animal models and infant exposure to gluten demonstrated diabetogenic potential of gluten exposure. Some studies now suggest a gluten-free diet that may preserve beta cell function [24].

It is possible that other food proteins play a role in pancreatic cell cross-reactivity leading to islet cell destruction. In this study, we evaluated the potential for dietary protein cross-reactivity with insulin and pancreatic target sites by evaluating immune reactivity between target-specific antibodies and purified dietary proteins shown in Table 1. We measured immune reactivity of either target-specific monoclonal or polyclonal antibodies for insulin, insulin receptor alpha (IR-A), insulin receptor beta (IR-B), zinc transporter 8 (ZnT8), islet antigen 2 (IA2), and glutamic acid decarboxylase (GAD) 65 and 67 antibodies against 204 food items that are commonly consumed. Insulin is a signaling hormone produced by the beta cells of the pancreatic islets that allows for the utilization of glucose across cell membranes for bioenergetics metabolism. Some dietary food proteins have been shown to promote autoimmunity to insulin via cross-reactivity [25]. Insulin receptors are tyrosine kinase receptors that play a key role in glucose homeostasis. There are two isomers of insulin receptors, alpha (IR-A) and beta (IR-B) [26, 27]. Antibodies reactive with islet cells have long been associated with T1D and are considered early markers for the disease [28]. Islet antigen 2 (IA2), formerly known as islet cell antigen 512 (ICA512), is a common tyrosine phosphatase-related autoantigen located in the insulin secretory granule membrane in beta cells [29]. Zinc transporter 8 (ZnT8) is the most consistent zinc transporter expressed by beta cells [29]. It has been found as an autoantigen in a high percentage of new-onset T1D patients [30]. Autoantibodies and T-cell responses against ZnT8 are produced in patients that develop autoimmune diabetes [29]. Glutamic acid decarboxylase (GAD) exists in two isoforms (GAD-65 and 67) and both are found in pancreatic tissue and support neuroendocrine modulation of insulin release [31–33].

The determination of food proteins that cross-react with islet cell antigens may identify dietary proteins that are potential triggers for a subset of individuals with autoimmune diabetes.

2. Materials and Methods

2.1. Polyclonal and Monoclonal Antibodies. Mouse monoclonal anti-insulin antibodies, affinity-purified rabbit polyclonal insulin receptor alpha (IR-A) antibodies, mouse monoclonal insulin receptor beta (IR-B) antibodies, affinity-purified rabbit polyclonal GAD-65 antibodies, and affinity-purified rabbit polyclonal GAD-67 antibodies were purchased from Abcam (Cambridge, MA, USA). Mouse monoclonal ZnT8 antibodies were purchased from Santa Cruz Biotechnology, Inc. (Dallas, TX, USA), and mouse monoclonal IA2 antibodies were purchased from ThermoFisher Scientific (Rockford, IL, USA).

2.2. Preparation of Dietary Antigens. Food antigens were prepared from products purchased from the supermarket in either raw, roasted, or cooked form. Cooked food proteins have different structural epitopes, and dietary protein preparation was conducted to reflect dietary proteins in either cooked or raw form as represented in typical human diets. For that preparation, 10 g of food product was put in a food

TABLE 1: Dietary proteins screened for immune reaction.

Dairy and eggs, modified	Flax seed	Seaweed	Imitation crab
Alpha-casein & beta-casein	Hazelnut, raw + roasted	Spinach + Aquaporin	Clam, boiled
Cow's milk	Macadamia nut, raw + roasted	Tomato + Aquaporin	Oyster, boiled
Chocolate milk	Mustard seed	Tomato paste	Scallops, seared
Egg white, boiled	Pecan, raw + roasted	Yam + Sweet potato, baked	Squid (Calamari), seared
Egg yolk, boiled	Peanut, roasted	Zucchini, boiled	Shrimp, seared
Goat's milk	Peanut butter	*Fruit, raw and modified*	Shrimp tropomyosin
Milk butyrophilin	Peanut agglutinin	Apple	Parvalbumin
Soft cheese + Hard cheese	Peanut oleosin	Apple cider	*Meat, modified*
Whey protein	Pistachio, raw + roasted	Apricot	Beef, boiled medium
Yogurt	Pumpkin seeds, roasted	Avocado	Chicken, boiled
Grains, raw and modified	Sesame albumin	Banana	Lamb, baked
Amaranth	Sesame oleosin	Banana, boiled	Pork, baked
Buckwheat	Sunflower seeds, roasted	Latex hevein	Turkey, baked
Casomorphin	Walnut	Blueberry	Gelatin
Oats	*Vegetables, raw and modified*	Cantaloupe + Honeydew melon	Meat glue
Quinoa	Artichoke, boiled	Cherry	*Herbs, raw*
Rice	Asparagus	Coconut, meat + milk	Basil
Rice, white + brown, boiled	Asparagus, boiled	Cranberry	Cilantro
Rice cake	Beet, boiled	Date	Cumin
Rice protein	Bell pepper	Fig	Dill
Rice endochitinase	Broccoli	Grape, red + green	Ginger
Rye, barley, spelt, polish wheat	Broccoli, boiled	Red wine	Oregano
Sesame	Brussels Sprouts, boiled	White wine	Parsley
Sorghum	Cabbage, red + green	Grapefruit	Rosemary
Tapioca	Cabbage, boiled	Kiwi	Thyme
Teff	Canola oleosin	Lemon + Lime	*Spices, raw*
Wild rice, boiled	Carrot	Mango	Cinnamon
Wheat + Alpha-gliadins	Carrot, boiled	Orange	Clove
Yeast miller	Cauliflower, boiled	Orange juice	Mint
Hemp	Celery	Papaya	Nutmeg
Beans, modified	Chili pepper	Peach + Nectarine	Paprika
Black bean, boiled	Corn + Aquaporin, boiled	Pear	Turmeric (Curcumin)
Bean agglutinins	Popped corn	Pineapple	Vanilla
Dark chocolate + Cocoa	Corn oleosin	Pineapple bromelain	*Gums*
Fava bean, boiled	Cucumber, pickled	Plum	Carrageenan

TABLE 1: Continued.

Garbanzo bean, boiled	Eggplant, boiled	Pomegranate	Gum guar
Kidney bean, boiled	Garlic	Strawberry	Gum tragacanth
Lentil, boiled	Garlic, boiled	Watermelon	Locust bean gum
Lentil lectin	Green Bean, boiled	*Fish and seafood, raw and modified*	Mastic gum + Gum arabic
Lima bean, boiled	Lettuce	Cod, baked	Xanthan gum
Pinto bean, boiled	Mushroom, raw + boiled	Halibut, baked	*Brewed beverages and additives*
Soybean agglutinin	Okra, boiled	Mackerel, baked	Coffee bean protein, brewed
Soybean oleosin + Aquaporin	Olive, green + black, pickled	Red Snapper, baked	Instant coffee
Soy Sauce, gluten-free	Onion + Scallion	Salmon	Black tea, brewed
Tofu	Onion + Scallion, boiled	Salmon, baked	Green tea, brewed
Nuts and seeds, raw and modified	Pea, boiled	Sardine + Anchovy, cooked	Honey, raw + processed
Almond	Pea protein	Sea bass, seared	Beta-glucan
Almond, roasted	Pea lectin	Tilapia, baked	Food coloring
Brazil nut, raw + roasted	Potato, white, baked	Trout, baked	
Cashew	Potato, white, fried	Tuna	
Cashew, roasted	Pumpkin + Squash, boiled	Tuna, seared	
Cashew vicilin	Radish	Whitefish, baked	
Chia seed	Safflower + Sunflower oleosin	Crab + Lobster, boiled	

processor using 0.1 M of phosphate buffer saline (PBS) at pH 7.4. The mixer was turned on and off for 1 hour and then kept on the stirrer overnight at 4°C. The food processor was decontaminated after each food product. After centrifugation at 20,000g for 15 minutes, the top layer, which contained oil bodies, was discarded. The liquid phase was removed and dialyzed against 0.01 M of PBS using dialysis bags, with a cut-off of 6000 kDa. Dialysis was repeated three times to ensure all small molecules were removed. After dialysis, protein concentrations were measured using a kit provided by Bio-Rad (Hercules, CA, USA).

2.3. Preparation of Dietary Oleosin Antigens. To purify the oleosin from peanuts, corn, safflower, sunflower, and soybean, the foods were prepared according to the method described above. A total of 100 mL of chloroform/methanol (2/1, *v*/*v*) was then added and blended for 2 minutes using a food processor. The mixture was put in a 50 mL tube and centrifuged at 14,000g for 5 minutes. The liquid in the upper phase was filtered through two layers of filter paper. The resultant filtrate was collected in multiple glass bottles and dried under a stream of air, with strong continuous agitation. The chloroform/methanol extraction step was repeated twice. A total of 20 mL of diethyl ether was then added, and the white, solid material stuck on the surface of the glass bottles was detached and resuspended in diethyl ether. At this point, 10 mL of water was added to each bottle, which was centrifuged at 20,000g for 5 minutes. The upper diethyl ether layer that contained lipids was removed, and the white, solid, interface material containing the oleosins was collected and transferred to microtubes with a minimum volume of water and diethyl ether. The microtubes were centrifuged at 20,000g for 5 minutes. The interfacial material was exposed to a stream of nitrogen to evaporate the remaining diethyl ether. One milliliter of chloroform/ethanol (95/5, *v*/*v*) was added to the interfacial material in each tube. The contents of each tube were quickly vortexed and transferred to a glass flask. To separate any protein contaminants from the oleosins, 10 mL of chloroform/methanol (95/5, *v*/*v*) was added, and the mixture was filtered through filter paper that was previously rinsed with chloroform/methanol. The filtrate was collected in a flask and dried under a stream of nitrogen. The dried oleosins were dissolved in chloroform/methanol and applied to a Sephadex LH-60 column (Bio-Rad, Hercules, CA, USA) using chloroform/methanol as the solvent. The collected fractions of oleosins were checked by sodium dodecyl sulfate- (SDS-) gel electrophoresis.

2.4. Preparation of Dietary Gum Antigens. Mastic gum, carrageenan, xanthan gum, guar gum, gum tragacanth, locust bean gum, and β-glucan were purchased from Sigma Aldrich (Saint Louis, MO, USA). Ten grams of each gum were extracted in 500 mL of buffer pH 4.6 by mixing them for 8 hours at 25°C on a magnetic stirrer. The solution was centrifuged at 20,000g, and supernatant was removed and concentrated by a factor of 10 using an Amicon filter. The protein concentration was measured using a kit provided by Bio-Rad (Hercules, CA, USA). All extracts were aliquoted and stored frozen at −20°C until used.

2.5. Enzyme-Linked Immunosorbent Assay (ELISA) for Demonstration of Immune Reactivity. Antigens and peptides were dissolved in PBS or methanol at a concentration of 1.0 mg/mL, then diluted 1 : 100 in 0.1 M carbonate-bicarbonate buffer (pH of 9.5). One hundred microliters was added to each well of the polystyrene flat-bottom ELISA plate. Plates were incubated overnight at 4 degrees Celsius and then washed three times with 200 μL Tris-buffered saline (TBS) containing 0.05% Tween 20 at a pH of 7.4. The nonspecific binding of immunoglobulins was prevented by adding a mixture of 1.5% bovine serum albumin (BSA) and 1.5% gelatin in TBS, and then incubated overnight at 4°C. Plates were washed as described above, and then monoclonal or polyclonal antibodies that had been diluted 1 : 500 in 0.1 M PBS Tween containing 2% BSA were added to duplicate wells and incubated for 1 hour at room temperature.

Plates were washed, and then enzyme-labeled anti-mouse or anti-rabbit IgG antibodies were added to each well; plates were incubated for an additional 1 hour at room temperature. They were then washed five times with TBS-Tween buffer. The enzyme reaction was started by adding 100 μL of paranitrophenylphosphate (PNPP) in 0.1 mL diethanolamine buffer 1 mg/mL containing 1 mM $MgCl_2$ and sodium azide at a pH of 9.8. The reaction was stopped 45 minutes later with 50 μL of 1N NaOH and the samples were ready for quantitative analysis by an ELISA reader. The OD was recorded at 405 nm by the microtiter reader to provide quantitative antibody reactivity levels and compared with control wells.

3. Results

3.1. Determination of Immune Reactivity Scale. Two hundred and four proteins were tested for seven target tissue antibodies in duplicate, leading to 2856 antigen-antibody OD measurements. The results of each duplicate OD were averaged together for one OD value. Of the 2856 OD measurements, the mean OD measurement was 0.25 with a standard deviation (SD) of 0.14. The OD of 0.53 represented two SD from the mean, the OD of 0.67 represented three SD from the mean, and an OD of 0.81 represented four SD from the mean. OD values below two SD or less than 0.52 were labeled nonsignificant. OD values above two SD but below three SD at OD values of 0.53–0.66 were categorized as 1+ reaction. OD values above three SD but less than four SD at OD values of 0.67–0.90 were categorized as 2+ reactions. OD values of 0.91–1.50 were categorized as 3+ reactions. OD values of 1.51–2.0 were categorized as 4+ reactions, and OD values >2.0 were categorized as 5+ reactions. The ODs of control wells coated only with BSA to which all other reagents were added were less than 0.15.

3.2. Immune Reactivity between Monoclonal Anti-Insulin and Anti-Insulin Receptor

3.2.1. Insulin. Our investigation found no specific immune reactivity with anti-insulin antibody and any of the 204 food antigens.

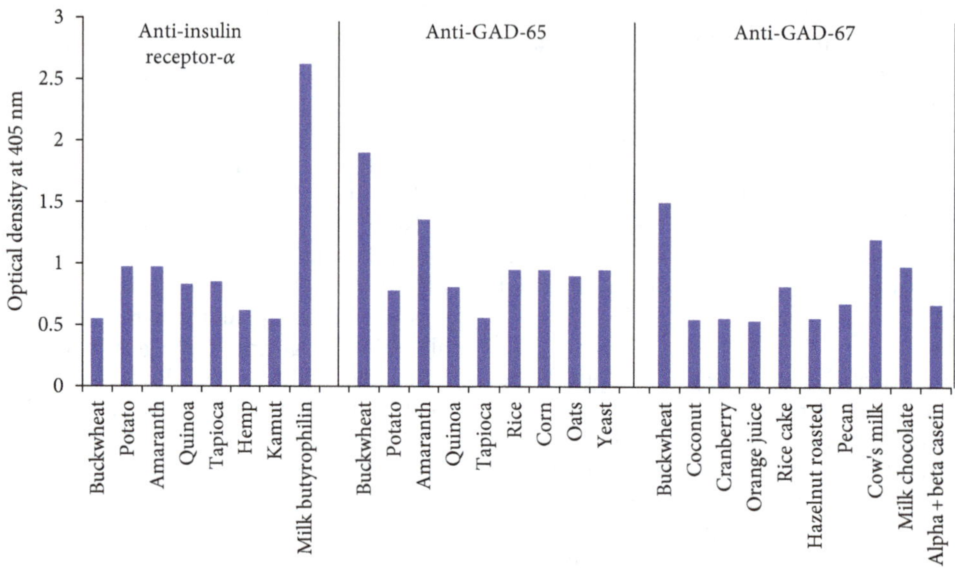

FIGURE 1: Reaction of polyclonal IR-A, GAD-65, and GAD-67 antibodies with different dietary proteins.

3.2.2. Insulin Receptors. Our investigation identified eight dietary proteins that exhibited immune reactivity with specific IR-A antibody: milk butyrophilin (5+), potato (3+), amaranth (3+), quinoa (2+), tapioca (2+), buckwheat (1+), hemp (1+), and kamut (1+) (see Figure 1). Our investigation identified no specific targeted immune reactivity by IR-B with any of the 204 dietary proteins (see Figure 1).

3.3. Immune Reactivity between Polyclonal GAD-65 and GAD-67 Antibodies and Dietary Proteins. Our investigation identified 9 dietary proteins that directly exhibited immune reactivity with specific targeted GAD-65 polyclonal antibody: of these, buckwheat (3+) was the most reactive, followed by amaranth (3+), rice (3+), corn (3+), and yeast (3+), potato (2+), quinoa (2+), and oats (2+), then tapioca (1+) (see Figure 1).

3.4. Immune Reactivity between Monoclonal IA2 Antibodies and Dietary Proteins. Our investigation found 27 dietary proteins that exhibited immune reactivity with specific target IA2 monoclonal antibody. Of these immune reactive proteins, seaweed (5+), guar gum (5+), and apricot (5+) were the most reactive, followed by pea lectin (3+), spinach (3+), cooked white and brown rice (3+), cooked garlic (3+), zucchini (3+), and mackerel (3+), egg yolk (2+), garbanzo bean (2+), carrageenan (2+), soy bean agglutinin (2+), bell pepper (2+), and mint (2+), then cooked lima bean (1+), gluten-free soy sauce (1+), tofu (1+), and mustard seed (1+). Rice apple, melon, watermelon, clam, cooked cod, cooked halibut, and cilantro had reactions that were insignificant (see Figure 2).

3.5. Immune Reactivity between Monoclonal ZnT8 Antibodies and Dietary Proteins. The ZnT8 antibody reacted with 30 dietary proteins. The most reactive were seaweed (5+), cooked lentil (5+), and pea protein (5+), followed by guar gum (4+), wheat (4+), peanut oleosin (4+), and cooked pea (4+), garbanzo bean (3+), soy bean oleosin (3+), roasted peanut (3+), and cooked tilapia (3+), egg yolk (2+), cooked lima bean (2+), mustard seed (2+), clam (2+), goat's milk (2+), roasted almond (2+), cashew vicilin (2+), tomato (2+), cooked yam and sweet potato (2+), banana (2+), and kiwi (2+), then gluten-free soy sauce (1+), tofu (1+), pea lectin (1+), spinach (1+), carrageenan (1+), macadamia nut (1+), cherry (1+), and salmon (1+) (see Figure 3).

In addition, 10 dietary proteins that directly exhibited immune reactivity with specific targeted GAD-67 polyclonal antibody: buckwheat (4+) was the most reactive, followed by cow's milk (3+); milk chocolate (3+) were the most reactive, followed by raw and roasted pecan (2+), alpha and beta casein (2+), and rice cake (2+), then coconut (1+), cranberry (1+), orange juice 1+), and roasted hazelnut (1+) (see Figure 1).

4. Discussion

There is some evidence showing that pancreatic beta islet cell antibodies in children are predictive for determining progression to diabetes using proportional hazards analysis [34]. Early identification of potential immunological reactive dietary protein triggers may aid clinicians in devising stratagems and protocols to reduce inflammatory sequelae and progression of the disease process in susceptible subgroups [35].

The focus of our laboratory research was to identify food proteins that have the potential to cross-react with pancreatic islet cells by evaluating immune reactivity between antibodies made against target tissue antigens involved in diabetes and various dietary proteins. The foods found to be immune reactive to pancreas target sites included the main food groups of gluten proteins, nongluten grains, and dairy proteins. Food groups tend to have homologous amino acid sequences. Reactivity to one food may also lead to immune

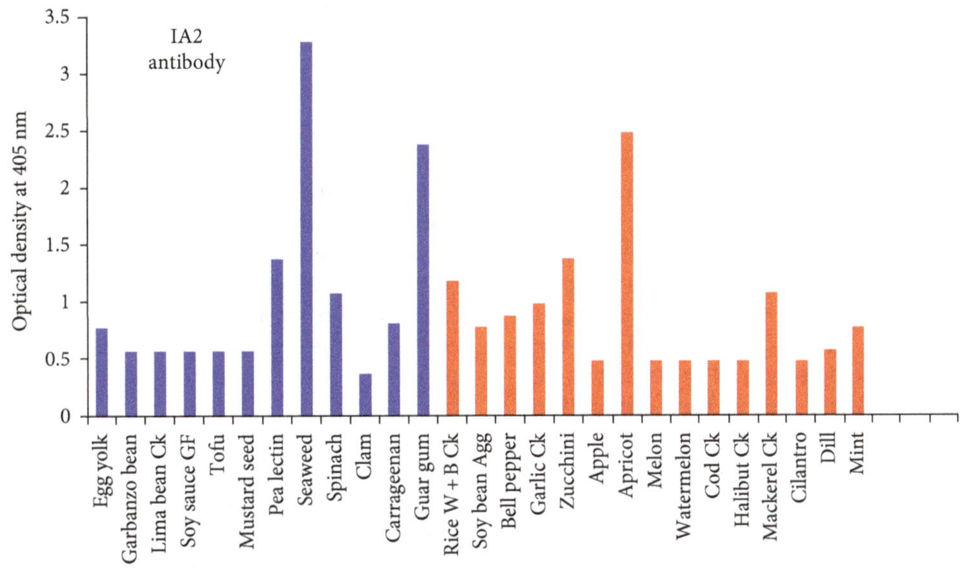

FIGURE 2: Reaction of monoclonal IA2 antibodies with different dietary proteins. The antigens in blue also reacted with ZnT8 antibodies.

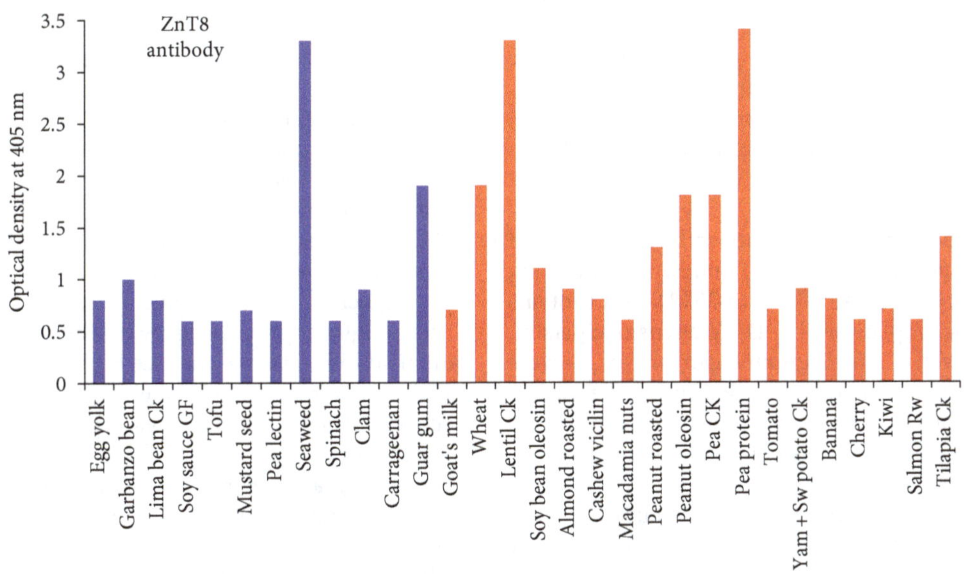

FIGURE 3: Reaction of monoclonal ZnT8 antibodies with different dietary proteins. The antigens in blue also reacted with IA2 antibodies.

reactivity with other dietary proteins in that food group. For example, several papers demonstrate that an isolated allergy to a single fish species leads to immune reactivity to other fish species due to amino acid structural similarity [36–39]. Coallergy reactions with legumes that share similar structural similarity were also identified by Bernhisel-Broadbent et al. [36], where they found that 37% of children immune reactive to one legume had reactions against all six major legumes, and 79% had binding to at least another legume [40]. Immune sensitivity with natural rubber latex allergens have also been reported to lead to cross-reactive sensitivity to foods that contain prohevein, such as banana, avocado, kiwi, chestnut, potato, and papaya, in what is called "latex-fruit syndrome" [41, 42].

In this current study, we examined possible cross-reactivity between islet cell antigens and different food proteins by measuring the reactivity of highly specific antibodies made against islet cell antigens with a variety of food antigens.

With IR-A, the strongest reaction was with milk butyrophilin, while with GAD-65, the strongest reactions were with buckwheat, amaranth, rice, corn, and yeast. With GAD-67, the strongest reactions were with buckwheat, cow's milk, and milk chocolate (see Figure 1).

With IA2 antibody, the strongest reactions were with seaweed, guar gum, and apricot, then pea lectin, spinach, cooked white, and brown rice, cooked garlic, zucchini, and mackerel (see Figure 2).

With ZnT8 antibody, the strongest reactions were with seaweed, cooked lentil, and pea protein, followed by guar gum, wheat, peanut oleosin, and cooked pea, then garbanzo bean, soy bean oleosin, roasted peanut, and cooked tilapia (see Figure 3).

Overall, we found that IA2 antibody reacted with 27 food proteins, ZnT8 antibody reacted with 30 food proteins, and GAD-65 reacted with 9 food proteins. Out of these foods, the same 12 foods reacted with both IA2 and ZnT8 antibodies. These 12 foods were egg yolk, garbanzo bean, cooked lima bean, gluten-free soy sauce, tofu, mustard seed, pea lectin, seaweed, spinach, clam, carrageenan, and guar gum. The detection of these dietary proteins cross-reactive with these major islet cell antigens, IA2, ZnT8, and GAD-65, especially the 12 foods that are dually reactive to both IA2 and ZnT8, warrants further investigation, because on the occasion of oral tolerance failure, if these foods manage to penetrate the epithelial barriers, the production of cross-reactive antibodies may contribute towards the destruction of islet cells.

Both IA2 and ZnT8 were also shown to be reactive to pea lectin (3+ and 1+, resp.). Lectins stimulate class II human leukocyte antigens (HLAs) of islet cells, which normally do not display them. Islet cells carry a very specific disaccharide determinant called N-acetyllactosamine, to which wheat, peanuts, soy, potato, and tomato lectins love to bind. This binding can result in islet cells expressing the class II HLAs and foreign antigens together, making the individual susceptible to autoimmune attack.

The ZnT8 antibody reacted not only with roasted peanut (3+) but also with peanut oleosin (4+) and soy bean oleosin (3+). Oleosins are relatively small (15 to 25 kDa) oil proteins that provide energy for plant seed cells. To a sensitive person, the ingestion of even a small amount can provoke severe reactions. Refined vegetable oils are used in a wide variety of food products, but oils from plants such as peanuts and soybeans have been recognized as potent antigens and allergens [43, 44].

Both IA2 and ZnT8 reacted very strongly to guar gum (5+ and 4+, resp.). Both also reacted to a lesser extent to carrageenan (2+ and 1+, resp.). Like oil, gums have an extremely broad range of commercial and industrial use, in not just food but including pharmaceuticals, printing, and other applications. Even though gums are generally recognized as safe by the FDA, gums do have a history of association with sensitivities or allergic reactions [45]. The fact that both of our tested islet cell antigens reacted strongly with gums raises concerns about the wide variety of commonly available products containing gums that may contribute to islet cell autoimmunity through the mechanism of this demonstrated cross-reactivity.

Aquaporin 4 (AQP4) is a class of water channels found in many cells of the body including the stomach, brain, lung, and skeletal muscle. Aquaporin is also found in many plants, and a recent study showed a significant similarity between the amino acid sequences of soy, spinach, corn, tomato, and tobacco with human aquaporin epitope 207–232 to elicit concerns about cross-reactivity. IA2 and ZnT8 had reactions in varying degrees with spinach, tomato, and different soy antigens (see Figure 2) [46].

Wheat has long been confirmed to be associated with a broad spectrum of autoimmune disorders, including T1D [44]. ZnT8 reacted strongly with wheat (4+). Considering the degree of cross-reactivity between wheat/gliadin/gluten and different neuronal antigens such as GAD-65, it should not be surprising that so many autoimmune reactivities can arise, and the significance of this reaction with wheat should be looked at closely. Animal models of autoimmune diabetes found that 6 months of a gluten-free diet had a beneficial effect on the preservation of islet cell function [47]. A population-based screening study of Danish children with autoimmune diabetes and celiac disease found improvements with a gluten-free diet in height and weight development during a 2-year follow-up [48].

The role of milk proteins and their involvement with autoimmune diabetes due to mimicry epitopes has previously been reported from epidemiological studies and from animal models that found that milk proteins play a diabetogenic role [21]. Our study showed that the islet cell antigens reacted with goat's milk, milk butyrophilin, cow's milk, milk chocolate, and $\alpha+\beta$ casein. Exposure to cow's milk proteins may prime the immune system to recognize and react to islet cell antigens that possess sequence homology to milk proteins, as reviewed by Vojdani [45].

Although many researchers have previously investigated the potential role of gluten and autoimmune diabetes, our largest immune reactive category was to nongluten grains, which has been less studied. These foods accounted for 4.4% of the screened dietary proteins and included rice, quinoa, hemp, yeast, oats, buckwheat, amaranth, and tapioca. This nongluten grain category was highly reactive to GAD-65 and insulin receptor alpha (see Figure 1, Table 2). The potential immune reactive role of gluten-free grains in susceptible subjects—such as celiac disease patients with autoimmune diabetes—is of concern, as those grains are often used as a substitute grain for individuals on a gluten-free diet. Many of these gluten-free grains demonstrated strong 3+ and even 4+ immunological reactions. Vojdani et al. previously published how these gluten-free grain proteins can also react with α-gliadin 33-mer antibody and explained why some individuals with gluten sensitivity do not respond to a gluten-free diet alone [49]. The results of our investigation show that many gluten-free grains that cross-react with gluten also have immune reactivity to pancreatic target sites. Immune reactivity to these grains may play a role in diabetes progression independent of gluten exposure or the high glycemic index of grain products.

The second largest reactive food category we identified was bean proteins. Beans (including black, white, navy, lima, pinto, garbanzo, soy, and kidney) are a winning combination of high-quality carbohydrates, lean protein, and soluble fiber that helps stabilize your body's blood-sugar levels and keeps hunger in check. Unfortunately, although they are generally considered a low glycemic index food, in our study, the islet cell antigens reacted with garbanzo bean, lima bean, gluten-free soy sauce, soy bean oleosin, soy bean agglutinin, tofu, pea lectin, pea protein, cooked pea, and cooked lentil.

Table 2: Reactivity of antibodies against pancreatic islet cell antigens with food proteins.

Food protein	Reactivity
Gluten	
Wheat	ZnT8 (4+)
Kamut	IR-A (1+)
Nongluten Grains	
Buckwheat	GAD-65 (4+), GAD-67 (3+), IR-A (1+)
Amaranth	GAD-65 (3+), IR-A (3+)
Quinoa	GAD-65 (2+), IR-A (2+)
Tapioca	IR-A (2+), GAD-65 (1+)
Oats	GAD-65 (2+)
Rice/rice cake	GAD-65 (3+), IA2 (3+), GAD-67 (2+)
Hemp	IR-A (1+)
Corn	GAD-65 (3+)
Beans & legumes	
Lentil	ZnT8 (5+)
Pea protein	ZnT8 (5+)
Pea cooked	ZnT8 (4+)
Pea lectin	IA2 (3+)
Garbanzo bean	ZnT8 (3+), IA2 (2+)
Lima bean	ZnT8 (2+), IA2 (1+)
Soy sauce gluten free	ZnT8 (1+), IA2 (1+)
Tofu	ZnT8 (1+), IA2 (1+)
Soy bean agglutinin	IA2 (2+)
Soy bean oleosin	ZnT8 (3+)
Seafood	
Clam	ZnT8 (2+)
Mackerel	IA2 (3+)
Salmon	ZnT8 (1+)
Tilapia	ZnT8 (3+)
Others	
Seaweed	ZnT8 (5+), IA2 (5+)
Egg yolk	ZnT8 (2+), IA2 (2+)
Yeast	GAD-65 (3+)
Mustard seed	ZnT8 (3+), IA2 (1+)
Milk proteins	
Goat's milk	ZnT8 (2+)
Cow's milk	GAD-67 (3+)
Milk chocolate	GAD-67 (3+)
Milk butyrophilin	IR-A (5+)
α+β casein	GAD-67 (2+)
Nuts	
Hazelnut	GAD-67 (1+)
Pecan	GAD-67 (2+)
Almond roasted	ZnT8 (2+)
Cashew vicilin	ZnT8 (2+)
Macadamia	ZnT8 (1+)
Peanut roasted	ZnT8 (3+)
Peanut oleosin	ZnT8 (4+)

Table 2: Continued.

Food protein	Reactivity
Gums	
Guar gum	IA2 (5+), ZnT8 (4+)
Carrageenan	IA2 (2+), ZnT8 (1+)
Fruit	
Apricot	IA2 (5+)
Banana	ZnT8 (2+)
Cherry	ZnT8 (1+)
Kiwi	ZnT8 (2+)
Coconut	GAD-67 (1+)
Cranberry	GAD-67 (1+)
Orange juice	GAD-67 (1+)
Vegetables	
Bell pepper	IA2 (2+)
Garlic Ck	IA2 (2+)
Tomato	ZnT8 (2+)
Potato	IR-A (3+), GAD-65 (2+)
Yam + Sw Potato	ZnT8 (2+)
Zucchini	IA2 (3+)
Herbs	
Dill	IA2 (1+)
Mint	IA2 (2+)

Our investigation identified 49 dietary proteins (24% of the 204 proteins) that are classified as low glycemic foods (glycemic index <55) to be reactive to antibodies made against pancreatic autoimmune target sites (see Table 3). Foods such as high-fiber grains, nuts, and dairy products that are encouraged for both type 1 and 2 diabetes patients were found to be highly reactive to antibodies against insulin receptors, islet cells, GAD-65, and GAD-67 (see Figures 1 and 2, Table 2). Current diabetes dietary management encourages the consumption of these foods [50]. Because the etiology of both juvenile type 1 diabetes and LADA is immunological, we suggest that future dietary management should include not only glycemic management but also the reduction or avoidance of immunoreactive dietary antigens shown to have a role in the etiology of autoimmune diabetes.

We must not forget that immune or sensitive reactions to food can also depend on whether the food is raw or cooked. A food in its natural state can be vastly different from the same food that has been cooked, processed, or modified. The food can react with sugar, lipids can be oxidized, peptide chains can be broken, and neoantigens can be formed. Thus, an individual that can eat a raw food safely may be highly reactive to the same food if cooked, or vice versa. It is not surprising then that in our tests, IA2 reacted strongly with cooked garlic (3+) but less with raw garlic (insignificant), strongly with pea lectin (4+) but not as much with pea protein (insignificant), and moderately with apple (2+) but less with apple cider (1+). In a similar fashion, ZnT8 reacted moderately with raw banana (2+) but less with cooked banana (insignificant), stronger against raw salmon (3+) but not as much

TABLE 3: Low glycemic index foods reactive with pancreatic islet cell antibodies.

Milk butyrophilin	Nuts	Corn
Cow's milk	Oats	Coconut
$\alpha+\beta$ casein	Quinoa	Cranberry
Goat's milk	Rice	Hazelnut
Milk chocolate	Hemp	Pecan
Guar gum	Seaweed	Vegetables
Carrageenan	Beans & Legumes	Seafood

Glycemic index <55.

with cooked salmon (1+), and very strongly with pea protein (5+) but less with pea lectin (3+).

It is important to note that cross-reactivity alone is not likely to initiate the pathogenesis of autoimmunity. However, the potential exists to upregulate subclinical or preexisting autoimmune conditions, and we suggest that immune reactivity is likely to promote the autoreactive process in susceptible subgroups if exposed to the specific antigens [51]. This susceptibility to dietary protein immune reactivity may occur if the gut immune system loses oral tolerance homeostasis and mucosal immune function, as found in autoimmunity [52, 53]. A cause for concern is that mechanisms of intestinal permeability, chronic intestinal inflammation, and impaired mucosal immune regulatory mechanisms have all been reported in children with type 1 diabetes [54].

These underlying mechanisms that may coexist with autoimmune diabetes and, in combination with immune reactive foods that share amino acid sequence homology, may lead to dietary proteins that can be diabetogenic in a subset of individuals. Further research to investigate the pathogenic role of these dietary proteins is necessary but must include confounding variables such as humoral and cellular immunity factors, intestinal permeability, mucosal regulatory mechanisms, and other factors that can determine whether exposure to dietary proteins is antigenic or immunologically benign; protein sequence similarity alone would not account for a pathogenic role. It is unlikely that the consumption of these dietary proteins alone would be diabetogenic in nonsusceptible populations. However, the immunoreactive dietary proteins we identified may act as cross-reactive food antigens for subsets of individuals who produce these antibodies due to loss of immunological tolerance.

5. Conclusion

The results of our study identified immune reactivity between antibodies to insulin, insulin receptors, islet cell antigens, and food antigens. Potential tissue antibody binding with various food antigens or food antibody binding to specific pancreatic sites can lead to the possibilities that some dietary proteins may play an antigenic role with autoimmune diabetes.

Even though many of the individual proteins in these groups may be considered safe or of low glycemic index, the consumption of these foods by a sensitive or predisposed individual may trigger immune reactions or autoimmunities.

Further research should be conducted to evaluate the specific epitope for each of the dietary proteins that react with these tissue-specific antibodies. It is necessary to determine the exact amino acid sequence homology, the immunological factors that convert dietary proteins from benign to pathogenic, and the clinical role that these dietary proteins play in autoimmune diabetes. However, the results of our research provide a first step in narrowing down a list of specific dietary proteins that, due to cross-reactivity, may potentially have an impact on autoimmune diabetes.

Disclosure

Dr. Aristo Vojdani is CEO of Immunosciences Lab, Inc. Dr. Datis Kharrazian and Dr. Martha Herbert have nothing to disclose.

Conflicts of Interest

The authors do not have any conflicts of interest.

References

[1] American Diabetes Association, *National Diabetes Fact Sheet*, http://www.diabetes.org/diabetes-basics/statistics/.

[2] Diabetes Control and Complications Trial Research Group, "The absence of a glycemic threshold for the development of long-term complications," *Diabetes*, vol. 45, pp. 1289–1298, 1996.

[3] WHO, "Diabetes Fact Sheet No. 312," October 2013. Archived from the original on 26 August 2013. Retrieved 25 March 2014.

[4] A. A. Elayat, M. M. el-Naggar, and M. Tahir, "An immunocyto-chemical and morphometric study of the rat pancreatic islets," *Journal of Anatomy*, vol. 186, Part 3, pp. 629–637, 1995.

[5] D. G. Gardner and D. Greenspan, Eds., *"Chapter 17". Greenspan's Basic & Clinical Endocrinology*, McGraw-Hill Medical, New York, NY, USA, 2011.

[6] E. Pipi, M. Marketou, and A. Tsirogianni, "Distinct clinical and laboratory characteristics of latent autoimmune diabetes in adults in relation to type 1 and type 2 diabetes mellitus," *World Journal of Diabetes*, vol. 5, no. 4, pp. 505–510, 2014.

[7] G. Schernthaner, S. Hink, H. P. Kopp, B. Muzyka, G. Streit, and A. Kroiss, "Progress in the characterization of slowly progressive autoimmune diabetes in adult patients (LADA or type 1.5 diabetes)," *Experimental and Clinical Endocrinology & Diabetes*, vol. 109, Supplement 2, pp. S94–S108, 2001.

[8] M. Landin-Olsson, "Latent autoimmune diabetes in adults," *Annals of the New York Academy of Sciences*, vol. 958, pp. 112–116, 2002.

[9] E. Laugesen, J. A. Østergaard, R. D. Leslie, and the Danish Diabetes Academy Workshop and Workshop Speakers, "Latent autoimmune diabetes of the adult: current knowledge and uncertainty," *Diabetic Medicine*, vol. 32, no. 7, pp. 843–852, 2015.

[10] S. Fourlanos, F. Dotta, C. J. Greenbaum et al., "Latent autoimmune diabetes in adults (LADA) should be less latent," *Diabetologia*, vol. 48, no. 11, pp. 2206–2212, 2005.

[11] D. B. Wilson, "Immunology: insulin auto-antigenicity in type 1 diabetes," *Nature*, vol. 438, no. 7067, article E5, 2005, discussion E5-6.

[12] K. T. Coppieters and M. von Herrath, "Antibody cross-reactivity and the viral aetiology of type 1 diabetes," *The Journal of Pathology*, vol. 230, no. 1, pp. 1–3, 2013.

[13] N. Lammi, M. Karvonen, and J. Tuomilehto, "Do microbes have a causal role in type 1 diabetes?," *Medical Science Monitor*, vol. 11, no. 3, pp. RA63–RA69, 2005.

[14] Y. Saeki and K. Ishihara, "Infection-immunity liaison: pathogen-driven autoimmune-mimicry (PDAIM)," *Autoimmunity Reviews*, vol. 13, no. 10, pp. 1064–1069, 2014.

[15] R. Root-Bernstein and D. Fairweather, "Complexities in the relationship between infection and autoimmunity," *Current Allergy and Asthma Reports*, vol. 14, no. 1, p. 407, 2014.

[16] J. Lis, A. Jarząb, and D. Witkowska, "Molecular mimicry in the etiology of autoimmune diseases," *Postępy Higieny I Medycyny Doświadczalnej (Online)*, vol. 66, pp. 475–491, 2012.

[17] L. Tuft and G. Blumstein, "Studies in food allergy II: sensitization to fresh fruits: clinical and experimental observations," *The Journal of Allergy*, vol. 13, no. 6, pp. 574–582, 1942.

[18] R. W. Weber, "Cross-reactivity of pollen allergens: impact on allergen immunotherapy," *Annals of Allergy, Asthma & Immunology*, vol. 99, no. 3, pp. 203–211, 2007.

[19] J. Karjalainen, J. M. Martin, M. Knip et al., "A bovine albumin peptide as a possible trigger of insulin-dependent diabetes mellitus," *The New England Journal of Medicine*, vol. 327, no. 5, pp. 302–307, 1992.

[20] C. Lévy-Marchal, J. Karjalainen, F. Dubois, W. Karges, P. Czernichow, and H. M. Dosch, "Antibodies against bovine albumin and other diabetes markers in French children," *Diabetes Care*, vol. 18, no. 8, pp. 1089–1094, 1995.

[21] H. E. Wasmuth and H. Kolb, "Cow's milk and immune-mediated diabetes," *The Proceedings of the Nutrition Society*, vol. 59, no. 4, pp. 573–579, 2000.

[22] I. Haladová, D. Cechurová, S. Lacigová, J. Gruberová, Z. Rušavý, and K. Balihar, "Celiac disease in adult patients with type 1 diabetes mellitus," *Vnitřní Lékařství*, vol. 60, no. 7-8, pp. 562–566, 2014, Czech.

[23] A. J. MacFarlane, K. M. Burghardt, J. Kelly et al., "A type 1 diabetes-related protein from wheat (*Triticum aestivum*). cDNA clone of a wheat storage globulin, Glb1, linked to islet damage," *The Journal of Biological Chemistry*, vol. 278, no. 1, pp. 54–63, 2003.

[24] J. C. Antvorskov, K. Josefsen, K. Engkilde, D. P. Funda, and K. Buschard, "Dietary gluten and the development of type 1 diabetes," *Diabetologia*, vol. 57, no. 9, pp. 1770–1780, 2014.

[25] K. Adler, D. B. Mueller, P. Achenbach et al., "Insulin autoantibodies with high affinity to the bovine milk protein alpha casein," *Clinical and Experimental Immunology*, vol. 164, no. 1, pp. 42–49, 2011.

[26] A. Belfiore, F. Frasca, G. Pandini, L. Sciacca, and R. Vigneri, "Insulin receptor isoforms and insulin receptor/insulin-like growth factor receptor hybrids in physiology and disease," *Endocrine Reviews*, vol. 30, no. 6, pp. 586–623, 2009.

[27] J. Giudice, F. C. Leskow, D. J. Arndt-Jovin, T. M. Jovin, and E. A. Jares-Erijman, "Differential endocytosis and signaling dynamics of insulin receptor variants IR-A and IR-B," *Journal of Cell Science*, vol. 124, Part 5, pp. 801–811, 2011.

[28] D. U. Rabin, S. M. Pleasic, J. A. Shapiro et al., "Islet cell antigen 512 is a diabetes-specific islet autoantigenrelated to protein tyrosine phosphatases," *Journal of Immunology*, vol. 152, no. 6, pp. 3183–3188, 1994.

[29] P. Arvan, M. Pietropaolo, D. Ostrov, and C. J. Rhodes, "Islet autoantigens: structure, function, localization, and regulation," *Cold Spring Harbor Perspectives in Medicine*, vol. 2, article a007658, 2012.

[30] J. M. Wenzlau, K. Juhl, L. Yu et al., "The cation efflux transporter ZnT8 (Slc30A8) is a major autoantigen in human type 1 diabetes," *Proceedings of the National Academy of Sciences*, vol. 104, pp. 17040–17045, 2007.

[31] Y. H. Kong, M. S. Kim, and D. Y. Lee, "Comparison of the prevalence of islet autoantibodies according to age and disease duration in patients with type 1 diabetes mellitus," *Annals of Pediatric Endocrinology & Metabolism*, vol. 18, no. 2, pp. 65–70, 2013.

[32] C. E. Taplin and J. M. Barker, "Autoantibodies in type 1 diabetes," *Autoimmunity*, vol. 41, no. 1, pp. 11–18, 2008.

[33] C. H. Thivolet, M. Tappaz, A. Durand et al., "Glutamic acid decarboxylase (GAD) autoantibodies are additional predictive markers of type 1 (insulin-dependent) diabetes mellitus in high risk individuals," *Diabetologia*, vol. 35, no. 6, pp. 570–576, 1992.

[34] J. M. Barker, K. J. Barriga, L. Yu et al., "Prediction of autoantibody positivity and progression to type 1 diabetes: diabetes autoimmunity study in the young (DAISY)," *The Journal of Clinical Endocrinology and Metabolism*, vol. 89, no. 8, pp. 3896–3902, 2004.

[35] J. M. Denham and I. D. Hill, "Celiac disease and autoimmunity: review and controversies," *Current Allergy and Asthma Reports*, vol. 13, no. 4, pp. 347–353, 2013.

[36] J. Bernhisel-Broadbent, S. M. Scanlon, and H. A. Sampson, "Fish hypersensitivity. I. In vitro and oral challenge results in fish-allergic patients," *The Journal of Allergy and Clinical Immunology*, vol. 89, no. 3, pp. 730–737, 1992.

[37] K. Aas, "Studies of hypersensitivity to fish. A clinical study," *International Archives of Allergy and Applied Immunology*, vol. 29, no. 4, pp. 346–363, 1966.

[38] C. Pascual, M. Martín Esteban, and J. F. Crespo, "Fish allergy: evaluation of the importance of cross-reactivity," *The Journal of Pediatrics*, vol. 121, no. 5, Part 2, pp. S29–S34, 1992.

[39] A. Helbling, R. Haydel Jr., M. L. McCants, J. J. Musmand, J. El-Dahr, and S. B. Lehrer, "Fish allergy: is cross-reactivity among fish species relevant? Double-blind placebo-controlled food challenge studies of fish allergic adults," *Annals of Allergy, Asthma & Immunology*, vol. 83, no. 6, Part 1, pp. 517–523, 1999.

[40] J. Bernhisel-Broadbent and H. A. Sampson, "Cross-allergenicity in the legume botanical family in children with food hypersensitivity," *The Journal of Allergy and Clinical Immunology*, vol. 83, pp. 435–440, 1989.

[41] A. Nel and C. Gujuluva, "Latex antigens: identification and use in clinical and experimental studies, including crossreactivity with food and pollen allergens," *Annals of Allergy, Asthma & Immunology*, vol. 81, pp. 388–396, 1998.

[42] Z. Chen, A. Posch, R. Cremer, M. Raulf-Heimsoth, and X. Baur, "Identification of hevein(Hev b 6.02) in Hevea latex as a major cross-reacting allergen with avocado fruitin patients with latex allergy," *Journal of Allergy and Clinical Immunology*, vol. 102, no. 3, pp. 476–481, 1998.

[43] C. Schwager, S. Kull, J. Behrends et al., "Peanut oleosins associated with severe peanut allergy-importance of lipophilic allergens for comprehensive allergy diagnostics," *The Journal of Allergy and Clinical Immunology*, 2017.

[44] L. Zuidmeer-Jongejan, M. Fernández-Rivas, M. G. Winter et al., "Oil body-associated hazelnut allergens including oleosins are underrepresented in diagnostic extracts but associated with severe symptoms," *Clinical and Translational Allergy*, vol. 4, no. 1, p. 4, 2014.

[45] A. Vojdani, "Molecular mimicry as a mechanism for food immune reactivity and autoimmunity," *Alternative Therapies in Health and Medicine*, vol. 21, Supplement 1, pp. 46–51, 2015.

[46] A. Vojdani, P. S. Mukherjee, J. Berookhim, and D. Kharrazian, "Detection of antibodies against human and plant aquaporins in patients with multiple sclerosis," *Autoimmune Diseases*, vol. 2015, Article ID 905208, 10 pages, 2015.

[47] M. R. Pastore, E. Bazzigaluppi, C. Belloni, C. Arcovio, E. Bonifacio, and E. Bosi, "Six months of gluten-free diet do not influence autoantibody titers, but improve insulin secretion in subjects at high risk for type 1 diabetes," *The Journal of Clinical Endocrinology and Metabolism*, vol. 88, no. 1, pp. 162–165, 2003.

[48] D. Hansen, B. Brock-Jacobsen, E. Lund et al., "Clinical benefit of a gluten-free diet in type 1 diabetic children with screening-detected celiac disease: a population-based screening study with 2 years' follow-up," *Diabetes Care*, vol. 29, no. 11, pp. 2452–2456, 2006.

[49] A. Vojdani and I. Tarash, "Cross-reaction between gliadin and different foods and tissue antigens," *Food and Nutrition Sciences*, vol. 4, pp. 20–32, 2013.

[50] http://www.ndei.org/ADA-diabetes-management-guidelines-diagnosis-A1C-testing.aspx.

[51] U. Christen and M. G. von Herrath, "Induction, acceleration or prevention of autoimmunity by molecular mimicry," *Molecular Immunology*, vol. 40, no. 14-15, pp. 1113–1120, 2004.

[52] O. Vaarala, "Is type 1 diabetes a disease of the gut immune system triggered by cow's milk insulin?," *Advances in Experimental Medicine and Biology*, vol. 569, pp. 151–156, 2005.

[53] L. C. Harrison and M. C. Honeyman, "Cow's milk and type 1 diabetes: the real debate is about mucosal immune function," *Diabetes*, vol. 48, no. 8, pp. 1501–1507, 1999.

[54] O. Vaarala, "Is the origin of type 1 diabetes in the gut?," *Immunology and Cell Biology*, vol. 90, no. 3, pp. 271–276, 2012.

17

Identification of Protein Kinase C Isoforms Involved in Type 1 Diabetic Encephalopathy in Mice

Jiayin Zheng,[1] Yue Wang,[2] Song Han,[1] Yanlin Luo,[1] Xiuli Sun,[1] Ning Zhu,[1] Li Zhao,[1] and Junfa Li[1]

[1]*Department of Neurobiology and Center of Stroke, Beijing Institute for Brain Disorders, Capital Medical University, Beijing 100069, China*
[2]*Department of Neurology, Beijing Chaoyang Hospital, Capital Medical University, Beijing, China*

Correspondence should be addressed to Li Zhao; zhaoli@ccmu.edu.cn and Junfa Li; junfali@ccmu.edu.cn

Academic Editor: Munmun Chattopadhyay

Diabetic encephalopathy is a complication of diabetes mellitus characterized by impaired cognitive functions. Protein kinase C (PKC) isoforms are rarely reported on diabetic encephalopathy, although they have been believed to play crucial roles in other diabetic complications. In this study, streptozotocin- (STZ-) induced diabetic mice were found to exhibit learning and memory deficits in the Morris water maze test. Meanwhile, the expression of cPKCβII, nPKCε, and cPKCγ did not change in the hippocampus, cortex, and striatum at 2 and 8 weeks after STZ injection. The nPKCε translocation to the membrane, where it is activated, was not altered in the above brain regions at 2 and 8 weeks after STZ injection. Nevertheless, cPKCβII translocation to the membrane was significantly decreased in the cortex and hippocampus at 8 weeks after STZ injection. The translocation of cPKCγ from the cytosol to the membrane was remarkably decreased in the hippocampus at 2 and 8 weeks and in the cortex and striatum at 8 weeks after STZ injection. In addition, deletion of cPKCγ aggravated the impairment of spatial learning and memory. In conclusion, our results suggest that the decrease in the activity of cPKCβII and cPKCγ, especially cPKCγ, may play key roles in the pathogenesis of diabetic encephalopathy.

1. Introduction

The prevalence rates of diabetes mellitus (DM) have increased rapidly over the past three decades in the world [1]. Some clinical studies have shown that high blood glucose increases the risk of Alzheimer's disease (AD) [2–4]. It has been manifested that type 1 diabetes mellitus (T1DM) has shown neurofibrillary and senile plaque, two major pathologic characteristics of AD, in the animal models [5, 6]. To describe cognitive impairment in diabetes, the term "diabetic encephalopathy" was introduced [7]. Now, diabetic encephalopathy is accepted as one of the most widespread diabetic complications in the central nervous system [8]. Because of a lack of effective treatment for diabetic encephalopathy, much interest now is focused on its molecular mechanism.

Constant hyperglycemia inside the cell increases the synthesis of diacylglycerol, which is one of the critical activating factors for protein kinase C (PKC) [9]. PKC, a family of Ser/Thr kinases that regulate a series of cellular processes, may play a key role in diabetes and its complications. According to the forms of activation, PKC isoforms are included in three groups: (1) conventional PKC isoforms (cPKCα, βI, βII, and γ) are activated by diacylglycerol, phosphatidylserine, and Ca^{2+} influx; (2) novel PKC isoforms (nPKCδ, ε, η, and θ) require diacylglycerol; and (3) atypical PKC isoforms (aPKCζ and ι/λ) do not bind either second messengers. It has been demonstrated that the cPKCβII, cPKCγ, and nPKCε, widely expressed in the nervous system, participate in many diabetic complications [10–14].

cPKCβII is the most studied isoform for diabetic complications. Deletion or inhibition of the cPKCβII can reduce glomerular, albuminuria, and mesangial expansion, which prevent the thickening of the glomerular basement membrane and the obliteration of glomerular capillaries in a diabetic kidney [15, 16]. The cPKCβII inhibitor can reverse acute blood glucose fluctuation-induced endothelial cell apoptosis increase, inflammatory cytokine level increase, and insulin signaling impairment, indicating that PKCβII may serve as a target for anticardiovascular diseases [11]. The cPKCβII inhibitor can also reduce the incidence of visual loss and prevent blood-retinal barrier breakdown in diabetic patients and animal models [17].

nPKCε is highly relative to insulin resistance. The key role of nPKCε for fat-induced hepatic insulin resistance is demonstrated with antisense oligonucleotide-mediated knockdown of nPKCε in high-fat feeding rats [18]. Several studies in type 2 diabetic patients have demonstrated that activation of nPKCε by hepatic accumulation of the diacylglycerol can result in hepatic insulin resistance and nonalcoholic fatty liver disease [19]. nPKCε deletion also enhances the amplifying pathways of glucose-stimulated insulin secretion and lipolysis in diabetic mouse beta-cells [20].

Compared to other PKC isoforms, cPKCγ is located only in the neurons of the central nervous system. Some studies have reported that the inhibitors of cPKCγ could reverse the DM-associated chronic impairment of neurovascular coupling [10]. The increase in cPKCγ expression in a trigeminal spinal nucleus is associated with orofacial thermal hyperalgesia in diabetic mice [21]. The increase in cPKCγ activity is also associated with diabetic embryonic dysmorphogenesis in rat [22]. However, few studies investigate the roles of the three specific PKC isoforms in the diabetic encephalopathy. In this study, we explored whether cPKCβII, cPKCγ, and nPKCε participated in the pathogenesis of type 1 diabetic encephalopathy induced by streptozocin (STZ) injection in mice.

2. Materials and Methods

2.1. Animals. C57BL/6 wild-type and cPKCγ knockout mice (male, 18–22 g) were purchased from Jackson Laboratory (Bar Harbor, Maine 04609, USA). Mice were housed, three per cage. The mice with free access to water and food were maintained in the Experimental Animal Center of Capital Medical University, the People's Republic of China. The experimental procedures were approved by the experimental animal ethics committee of Capital Medical University (permit number AEEI-2014-035) and conducted according to the recommendations in the Guide for the Care and Use of Laboratory Animals of the National Institutes of Health.

2.2. Induction of Type 1 Diabetes Mellitus in Mice. Animals were randomly divided into three groups, namely, the CON group (with citrate buffer treatment), T1DM group (with STZ treatment), and T1DM + cPKCγ group (cPKCγ knockout mice with STZ treatment). Following an overnight fast, T1DM mice were induced by low doses of freshly prepared STZ (50 mg/kg/day, i.p.), dissolved in a 0.1 M citrate buffer (pH 4.5), over five consecutive days. The control mice were only injected with citrate buffer (5 mL/kg/day, i.p.). The fasting blood glucose level was measured every week using a blood sample from the tail vein with the aid of a OneTouch® Ultra blood glucose meter (Milpitas, CA, USA). Mice with blood glucose levels over 11.1 mmol/L were considered diabetic and used for the study [23]. At 2 weeks and 8 weeks after STZ injection, the hippocampus, prefrontal cortex, and striatum of the mice in the CON and T1DM groups were prepared for the determination of PKC isoform expression levels and membrane translocation of PKC isoforms ($n = 6$ per group, resp.). At 8 weeks after STZ injection, the mice in the CON, T1DM, and T1DM + cPKCγ groups were tested in the Morris water maze ($n = 12$ per group, resp.).

2.3. Cytosolic and Membrane Fractions and Whole Tissue Homogenate Preparation. As previously reported [24], the dissected samples were first homogenized at 4°C in buffer A [50 mM Tris-Cl, pH 7.5, containing 1 mM DTT, 2 mM EDTA, 2 mM EGTA, 50 mM potassium fluoride (KF), 5 mM sodium pyrophosphate, and a protease inhibitor mixture]. Homogenates were centrifuged at 30,000*g* for 30 min, and the supernatant was collected as cytosolic fractions. The pellet fractions (membrane fractions) were resuspended in buffer A containing 2% SDS before being sonicated and centrifuged again. These two fractions were analyzed for membrane translocation of PKC isoforms. To analyze PKC isoform expression, the whole tissue was homogenized and sonicated in RIPA buffer. The concentration of protein was analyzed as previously reported [25].

2.4. Western Blot. As previously reported [26], the samples (30 μg) were subjected to 10% SDS-PAGE and transferred onto polyvinylidene difluoride membrane (GE Healthcare, UK); the membrane was blocked with 10% nonfat milk for 1 h and probed with anti-cPKCβII (number sc-210, Santa Cruz Biotechnology, Santa Cruz, USA), cPKCγ (number sc-211, Santa Cruz Biotechnology, Santa Cruz, USA), and nPKCε (number sc-214, Santa Cruz Biotechnology, Santa Cruz, USA). The horseradish peroxidase-conjugated goat anti-rabbit (number 31460, ThermoFisher Scientific, Rockford, USA) and anti-mouse IgG (number 31430, ThermoFisher Scientific, Rockford, USA) were used as second antibodies at a 1 : 4000 dilution for 1 h at room temperature. Signals were visualized via an enhanced chemiluminescent reagent solution (chemiluminescent HRP substrate, Millipore Corporation, USA). To verify the equal loading of protein, the blots were reprobed with primary monoclonal antibodies against β-actin (number 60008-1-lg, Proteintech, Rosemont, USA) or Na^+/K^+ ATPase (number 14418-1-AP, Proteintech, Rosemont, USA). The protein expression levels of PKC isoforms were calculated as 100% in the control group, and then the other groups were expressed as the percentage of the control group. Quantitative analysis for immunoblotting was done by Fusion Capt 16.15 software (Fusion FX6 XT, Vilber Lourmat, France).

2.5. Morris Water Maze. At 8 weeks after STZ injection, spatial learning and memory were tested by the Morris water maze. Briefly, a custom-built water tank (122 cm diameter, 50 cm height) with a white nonreflective interior surface was filled with opaque water (19–22°C) containing nontoxic titanium white-colored dye. The experiment was performed in a room with low-light indirect lighting. Four different extramaze cues were fixed at four quartiles of the tank periphery (Figure 1(e)). In the target quadrant (quadrant II), a platform was submerged 1 cm below the water surface. The mice were trained to find the hidden platform for 5 consecutive days, four trials of 90 seconds per day. In each trial, the mouse started from one of the four quadrants facing the wall of the pool and ended when the mouse climbed on the platform. If the mice did not find the platform in 90 s, they were guided to the platform. To test reference memory, the platform was removed on day 6 and the percentage of time that the mice spent in each quadrant was recorded. The visible platform tests (with the platform marked) were given on day 7 and day 8 to evaluate sensorimotor abilities and motivation of the animals. Swim paths were recorded on a CCD camera and analyzed using WaterMaze 3 Software. Average swimming speed was determined to exclude motor impairments.

2.6. Statistics Analysis. The values were presented as the mean ± SEM. Statistical analysis of Western blot was conducted by a one-way analysis of variance followed by all pairwise multiple comparison procedures using the Bonferroni test. The statistical analysis of the Morris water maze was conducted by a two-way analysis of variance followed by all pairwise multiple comparison procedures using the Bonferroni test. All results were regarded as at least $p < 0.05$ was considered statistically significant.

3. Results

3.1. Biochemical Characteristics of the Mice. At the beginning of the experiment, there was no significant difference among the groups in blood glucose and body weight. Following STZ injection, the mice developed DM rapidly with a mean blood glucose of 13.13 ± 4.74 mmol/L on day 3 after STZ injection, 18.87 ± 3.79 mmol/L at 2 weeks, and 26.7 ± 5.70 mmol/L at 8 weeks (Figure 1(a)). As shown in Figure 1(b), the body weight of the T1DM group increased (from 19.38 ± 2.03 g to 26.12 ± 2.36 g at 8 weeks after STZ injection) but much more slowly than the increase of the CON group (from 19.18 ± 1.54 g to 30.22 ± 1.43 g at 8 weeks after STZ injection). There was no significant difference in blood glucose and body weight between the cPKC$\gamma^{+/+}$ diabetic mice and the scPKC$\gamma^{-/-}$ diabetic mice (Figures 1(a) and 1(b)).

3.2. Expression of PKC Isoforms in the Hippocampus, Prefrontal Cortex, and Striatum of the T1DM Mice. In the next set of experiments, we observed whether diabetes mellitus affected the expression patterns of PKC isoforms in the hippocampus, prefrontal cortex, and striatum. As shown in Figures 2 and 3, we observed that the expression of cPKCβII, nPKCε, and cPKCγ did not change in the above brain regions at 2 or 8 weeks after STZ injection. These results indicated that chronic T1DM did not affect the expression of the three PKC isoforms in the hippocampus, prefrontal cortex, and striatum.

3.3. Membrane Translocation of PKC Isoforms in the Hippocampus, Prefrontal Cortex, and Striatum of the T1DM Mice. The activation of PKC relates to a transition from the cytosolic autoinhibited form to the membrane-associated active form [27]. To figure out whether PKC isoforms are involved in type 1 diabetic encephalopathy, we observed the membrane translocation of PKC isoforms in the hippocampus, prefrontal cortex, and striatum of the T1DM mice.

As shown in Figures 4(c) and 5(c), chronic T1DM did not affect the membrane translocation of nPKCε in the hippocampus, prefrontal cortex, and striatum at 2 weeks and 8 weeks after STZ injection. The ratio of membranal cPKCβII to cytosolic cPKCβII was not significantly altered in the three brain regions at 2 weeks (Figure 4(a)) but dramatically decreased in the prefrontal cortex and hippocampus at 8 weeks (Figure 5(a)). Moreover, chronic T1DM significantly reduced the ratio of membranal cPKCγ to cytosolic cPKCγ in the hippocampus at 2 weeks (Figure 4(b)) and in the prefrontal cortex, hippocampus, and striatum at 8 weeks (Figure 5(b)).

3.4. Effects of cPKCγ on Spatial Learning and Memory of Mice. To explore the role of cPKCγ in learning and memory, the Morris water maze test was used at 8 weeks after STZ injection. On day 5, the diabetic mice had a significantly increased latency to find the hidden platform compared to control mice (Figure 1(c)). Furthermore, the cPKCγ-deficient diabetic mice took more time to find the hidden platform than the wild-type diabetic mice (Figure 1(c)).

On day 6, swim patterns indicated that control mice swam immediately towards the target area, where the platform used was placed, tried to find the platform, and swam back and forth. In contrast, diabetic mice swam in random circles throughout the pool (Figure 1(e)). In addition, the cPKC$\gamma^{-/-}$ diabetic mice performed worse than the wild-type diabetic mice (Figure 1(e)).

The percentage of the time spent swimming in the target quadrant (quadrant II) was significantly lower for diabetic mice than for control mice (Figure 1(d)). Moreover, cPKC$\gamma^{-/-}$ diabetic mice spent less time in the target quadrant than cPKC$\gamma^{+/+}$ diabetic mice (Figure 1(d)), again indicating memory impairment in the cPKCγ knockout mice.

As both the vision and sensorimotor abilities of mice could affect the reliability of Morris water maze tests, the visible platform tests (with the platform marked) were given on day 7 and day 8. There were no significant differences in escape latency among groups (Figure 1(c)). As shown in Figure 1(f), no significant differences in average speed were observed among groups in 8 days. These results suggested that chronic T1DM could induce spatial learning and memory deficits of mice without affecting their visual and sensorimotor abilities and cPKCγ deficiency aggravated the spatial learning and memory impairment of T1DM mice.

4. Discussion

Several studies have reported that the expression of cPKCβII, cPKCγ, and nPKCε is altered by hyperglycemia. The expression of cPKCβII increases in the renal tissues of diabetic rats

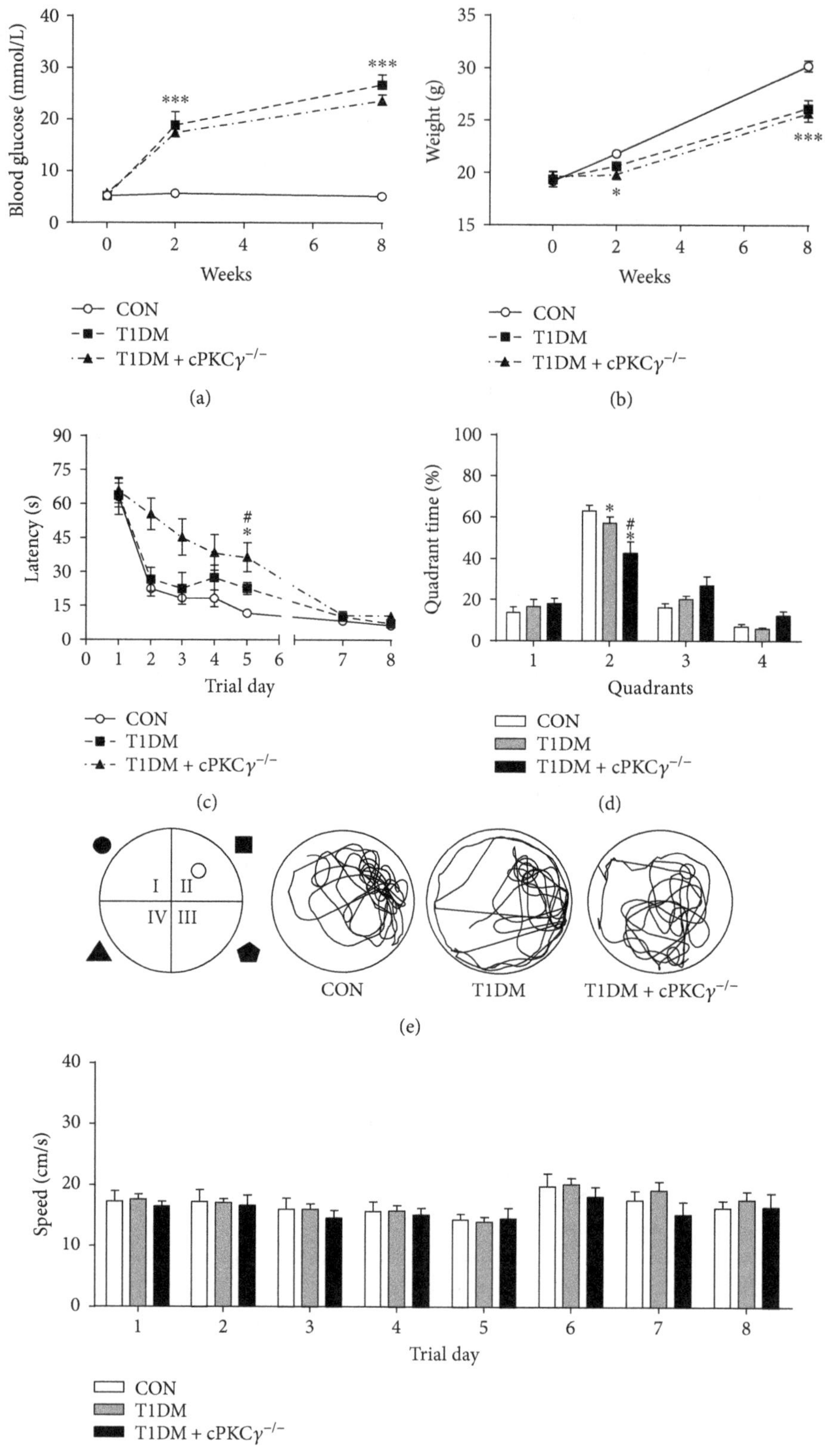

FIGURE 1: Changes of body weight, blood glucose, and spatial learning and memory deficits induced by STZ in mice. (a) Statistical results of blood glucose of each group. (b) Statistical results of body weight of each group. (c) The graph showed the escape latency of each group during 5 consecutive days of learning process and visible test (days 7 and 8). (d) Statistical results of the time spent in the target quadrant measured on day 6 by removing the platform. (e) The graph showed the swim path of each group on day 6. (f) Statistical results of speeds of each group every day. $^{*}p < 0.05$ compared with the CON group, $^{***}p < 0.001$ compared with the CON group, and $^{\#}p < 0.05$ compared with the T1DM group. $n = 12$ per group.

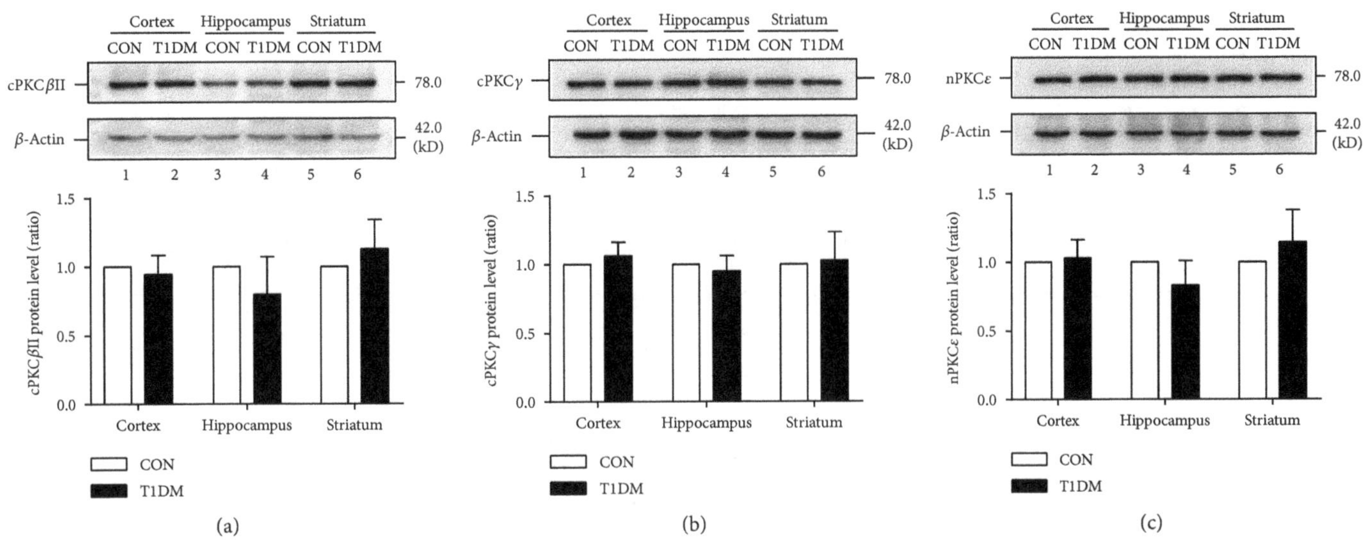

Figure 2: Expression of PKC isoforms in the cortex, hippocampus, and striatum at 2 weeks after STZ injection. (a) Representative and statistical results of Western blot analysis showed the levels of cPKCβII in the cortex, hippocampus, and striatum at 2 weeks after STZ injection. (b) Representative and statistical results of Western blot analysis showed the levels of cPKCγ in the cortex, hippocampus, and striatum at 2 weeks after STZ injection. (c) Representative and statistical results of Western blot analysis showed the levels of nPKCε in the cortex, hippocampus, and striatum at 2 weeks after STZ injection. $n = 6$ per group.

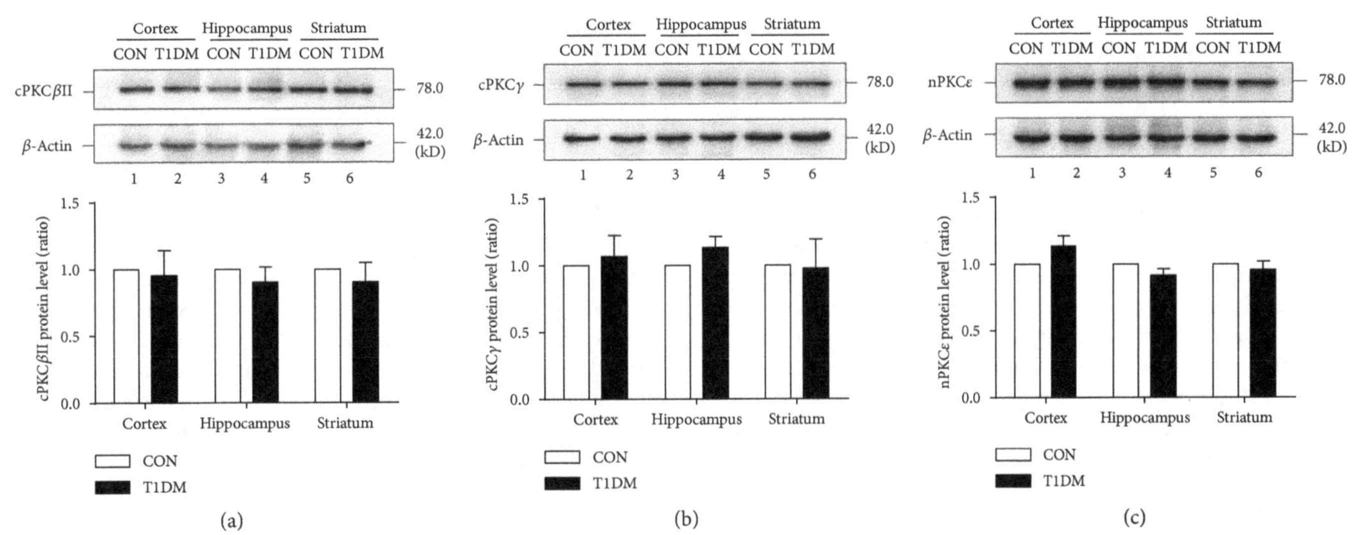

Figure 3: Expression of PKC isoforms in the cortex, hippocampus, and striatum at 8 weeks after STZ injection. (a) Representative and statistical results of Western blot analysis showed the levels of cPKCβII in the cortex, hippocampus, and striatum at 8 weeks after STZ injection. (b) Representative and statistical results of Western blot analysis showed the levels of cPKCγ in the cortex, hippocampus, and striatum at 8 weeks after STZ injection. (c) Representative and statistical results of Western blot analysis showed the levels of nPKCε in the cortex, hippocampus, and striatum at 8 weeks after STZ injection. $n = 6$ per group.

on 21 days after STZ injection [28]. The nPKCε level increases in the skeletal muscle of nutritionally induced diabetic rats in 3 weeks [29] and vessels of spontaneously diabetic rats [30]. And the expression of cPKCγ is also found to increase in the trigeminal spinal nucleus of T1DM mice on 14 days after STZ injection [21]. Interestingly, the expression of cPKCβII, cPKCγ, and nPKCε may not change in the cerebral cortex, but the levels of cPKCγ and nPKCε are decreased in the glio-pial tissue of T1DM rats at 16 weeks after STZ injection [31]. In this study, we explored the expression and activation of cPKCβII, cPKCγ, and nPKCε in the hippocampus, prefrontal cortex, and striatum, the regions important in the cognitive processes of learning, memory, and decision-making [32–34]. We observed that T1DM did not significantly change the protein expression of cPKCβII, cPKCγ, and nPKCε in the three brain regions at 2 weeks after STZ injection. Next, we prolonged the observation time. But we still did not find significant changes in the protein expression of cPKCβII, cPKCγ, and nPKCε at 8 weeks after STZ injection.

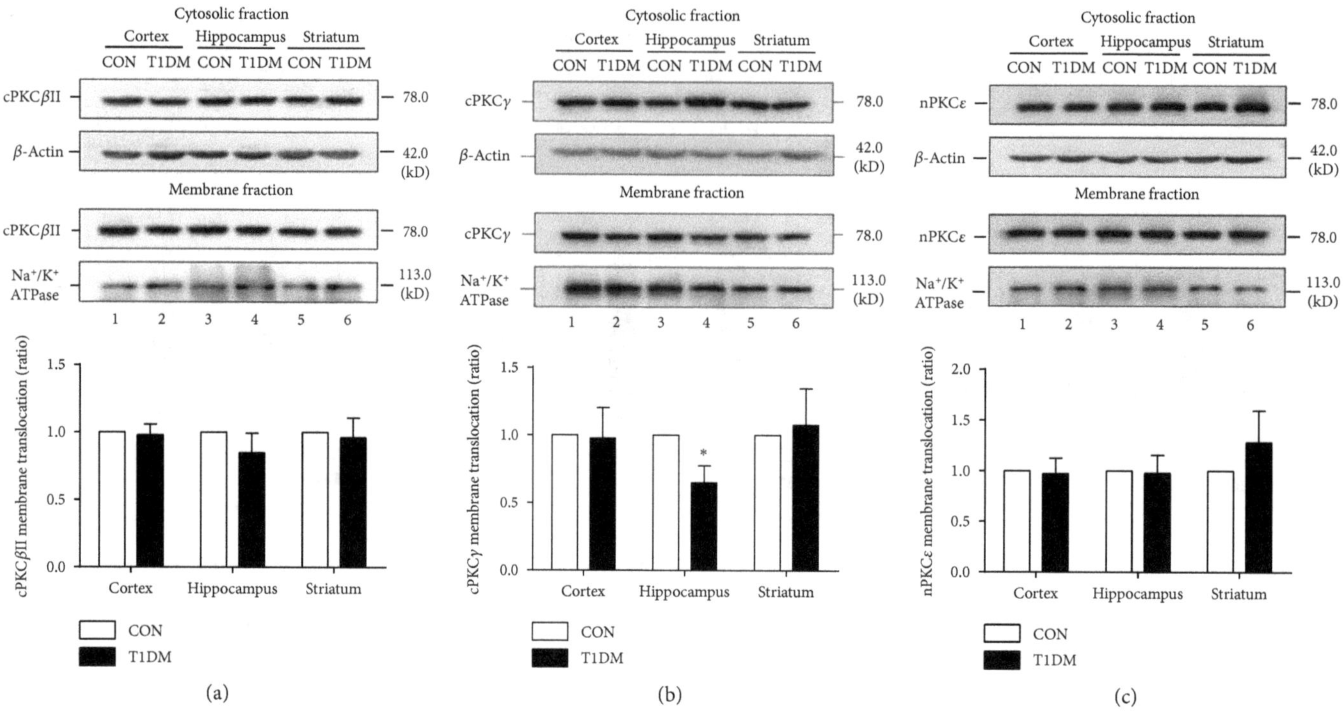

FIGURE 4: Membrane translocation of PKC isoforms in the cortex, hippocampus, and striatum at 2 weeks after STZ injection. (a) Representative and statistical results of Western blot analysis showed the membrane translocation of cPKCβII in the cortex, hippocampus, and striatum at 2 weeks after STZ injection. (b) Representative and statistical results of Western blot analysis showed the membrane translocation of cPKCγ in the cortex, hippocampus, and striatum at 2 weeks after STZ injection. (c) Representative and statistical results of Western blot analysis showed the membrane translocation of nPKCε in the cortex, hippocampus, and striatum at 2 weeks after STZ injection. $^*p < 0.05$ compared with the CON group. $n = 6$ per group.

Activation of PKC is associated with the translocation of enzymes from the cytosol to the membrane. The membrane translocation or activation of PKC isoforms is linked to the development of pathologies in diabetes. The acute blood glucose fluctuation significantly increased cPKCβII membrane translocation, which causes the apoptosis of vascular endothelial cell through increasing oxidative stress and induces impairment of insulin signaling in diabetic rats [11]. Activation of cPKCβII by hyperglycemia upregulates caspase 8-induced apoptosis in blood-brain barrier endothelial cells [35]. Activation of nPKCε, as a result of the accumulation of diacylglycerol, results in hepatic insulin resistance and nonalcoholic fatty liver disease in patients and type 2 diabetic mice [19, 36]. Activation of cPKCγ by early STZ-induced diabetes causes the inhibition of lens gap junction activity in rats [37]. In this study, we found that T1DM mice exhibited spatial learning and memory impairment in the Morris water maze at 8 weeks after STZ injection. Meanwhile, T1DM failed to affect nPKCε membrane translocation in the hippocampus, prefrontal cortex, and striatum at 8 weeks. However, the translocation of cPKCβII and cPKCγ from the cytosol to the membrane was significantly decreased in the brain of T1DM mice at 8 weeks, indicating that they might be involved in type 1 diabetic encephalopathy.

It is well accepted that cPKCβII is essential for learning and memory formation [38, 39]. The downregulation of cPKCβII in the hippocampus of offspring, especially in the CA3, CA1, and dentate gyrus, the regions important in the entorhinal-hippocampal trisynaptic circuit, is responsible for impaired learning and memory of prenatally stressed offspring [40]. The levels of cPKCβII decrease in the striatum and cortex of transgenic Huntington's disease mice, which is associated with impaired information storage and memory disorder [41]. The baseline asymmetry and lateralized changes of cPKCβII in the rat amygdale are associated with the cue and context in a classical fear conditioning paradigm [42]. And furthermore, the cPKCβII knockout mice also exhibit a loss of learning and suffer deficits in both cued and contextual fear conditioning [43].

cPKCγ is a neuron-specific isoform, and its activity is suggested to be related to spatial memory in aged rats [44, 45]. Activation of cPKCγ in the CA1 region participates in postsynaptic plasticity associated with spatial experiences and learning [46]. Young rats, those with the best spatial memory, are those with the highest concentrations of cPKCγ in the particulate fraction. Conversely, aged rats with poor spatial memory increase hippocampal cPKCγ concentrations in soluble fraction in comparison with young rats, which indicates that the decrease in cPKCγ activity is correlated with memory impairment [47]. In addition, cPKCγ is found to participate in the reversal of learning and memory deficits by intranasal insulin treatment in AD mice [48]. In this study, we found that the decrease in cPKCγ activity induced by T1DM came earlier and occurred in more brain regions than cPKCβII, suggesting that cPKCγ played a bigger role in the diabetic encephalopathy. Therefore, we deleted the

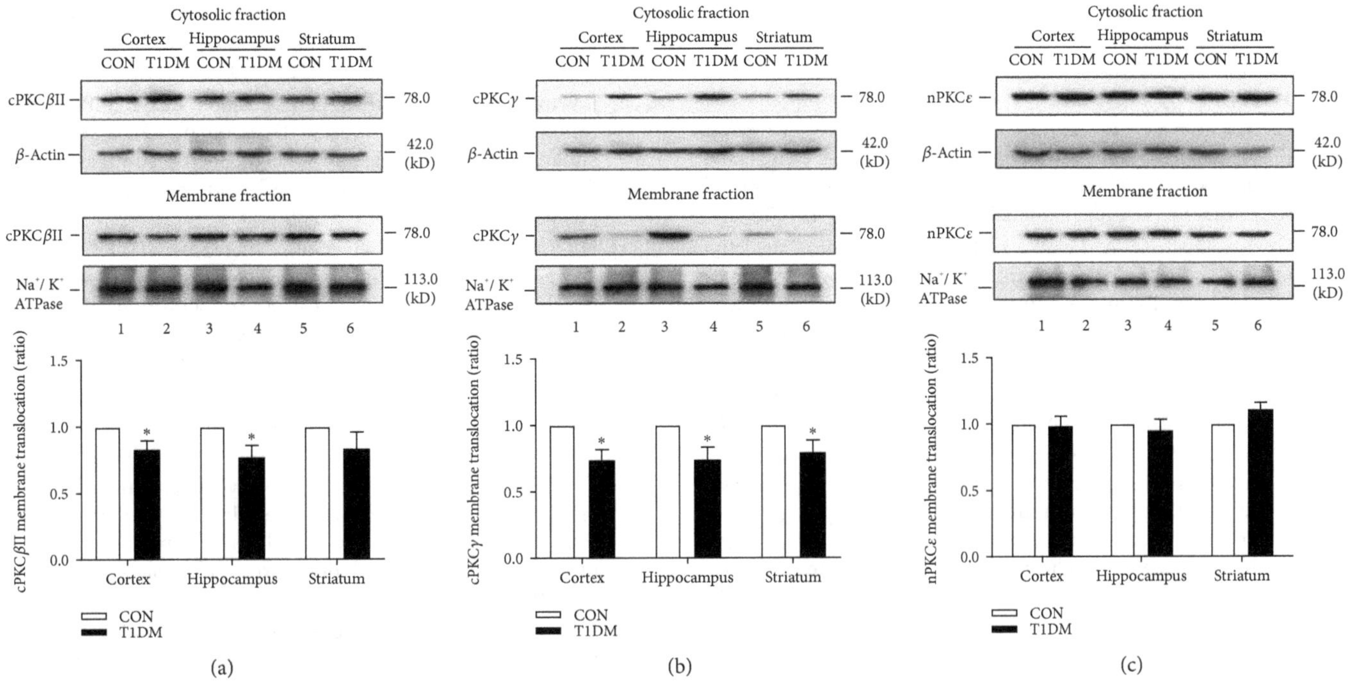

FIGURE 5: Membrane translocation of PKC isoforms in the cortex, hippocampus, and striatum at 8 weeks after STZ injection. (a) Representative and statistical results of Western blot analysis showed the membrane translocation of cPKCβII in the cortex, hippocampus, and striatum at 8 weeks after STZ injection. (b) Representative and statistical results of Western blot analysis showed the membrane translocation of cPKCγ in the cortex, hippocampus, and striatum at 8 weeks after STZ injection. (c) Representative and statistical results of Western blot analysis showed the membrane translocation of nPKCε in the cortex, hippocampus, and striatum at 8 weeks after STZ injection. $^*p < 0.05$ compared with the CON group. $n = 6$ per group.

cPKCγ gene in mice and then found that the spatial learning and memory of cPKC$\gamma^{-/-}$ diabetic mice are worse than those of wild diabetic mice.

Elevated glucose level and impaired glucose tolerance can affect the spatial learning and memory, which is associated with hippocampal apoptosis [49–52]. But in this study, we found that cPKCγ did not affect blood glucose level, demonstrating that the effect of cPKCγ on cognitive function is irrelevant to blood glucose. PKC activators have been reported to improve cognitive function by restoring PKC signaling and downstream activity, including stimulation of synaptic plasticity and development [53], reduction in accumulation of neurotoxic amyloid β, regulation of tau protein hyperphosphorylation [38], and support of antiapoptotic processes [54]. Further studies about the mechanism how cPKCγ can enhance spatial memory performance in T1DM mice are required.

5. Conclusion

Our results indicate that the activation of cPKCβII and cPKCγ, not nPKCε, may be involved in the development of the diabetic encephalopathy in mice. cPKCγ can dramatically improve learning and memory performances impaired by diabetes mellitus in mice.

Conflicts of Interest

The authors declare that there are no conflicts of interest.

Authors' Contributions

Li Zhao and Junfa Li designed the experiments. Jiayin Zheng, Yue Wang, Song Han, Xiuli Sun, and Ning Zhu performed the experiments. Jiayin Zheng and Yanlin Luo analyzed the data. Jiayin Zheng and Yue Wang wrote the paper. Li Zhao, Yue Wang, and Junfa Li revised the paper. Jiayin Zheng and Yue Wang contributed equally to this work.

Acknowledgments

The authors disclosed the receipt of the following financial support for the research, authorship, and/or publication of this article: National Natural Science Foundation of China (Grant nos. 81400948, 31671205, and 31471142) and Beijing Natural Science Foundation (Grant no. 7141001).

References

[1] World Health Organization, *Global Report on Diabetes*, World Health Organization, Geneva, 2016.

[2] B. Kim, C. Backus, S. Oh, and E. L. Feldman, "Hyperglycemia-induced tau cleavage in vitro and in vivo: a possible link between diabetes and Alzheimer's disease," *Journal of Alzheimer's Disease*, vol. 34, no. 3, pp. 727–739, 2013.

[3] N. Mukai, T. Ohara, J. Hata et al., "Alternative measures of hyperglycemia and risk of Alzheimer's disease in the community: the Hisayama study," *The Journal of Clinical Endocrinology and Metabolism*, vol. 102, no. 8, pp. 3002–3010, 2017.

[4] J. Q. Wang, J. Yin, Y. F. Song et al., "Brain aging and AD-like pathology in streptozotocin-induced diabetic rats," *Journal of Diabetes Research*, vol. 2014, Article ID 796840, 12 pages, 2014.

[5] C. G. Jolivalt, R. Hurford, C. A. Lee, W. Dumaop, E. Rockenstein, and E. Masliah, "Type 1 diabetes exaggerates features of Alzheimer's disease in APP transgenic mice," *Experimental Neurology*, vol. 223, no. 2, pp. 422–431, 2010.

[6] C. G. Jolivalt, C. A. Lee, K. K. Beiswenger et al., "Defective insulin signaling pathway and increased glycogen synthase kinase-3 activity in the brain of diabetic mice: parallels with Alzheimer's disease and correction by insulin," *Journal of Neuroscience Research*, vol. 86, no. 15, pp. 3265–3274, 2008.

[7] G. S. Mijnhout, P. Scheltens, M. Diamant et al., "Diabetic encephalopathy: a concept in need of a definition," *Diabetologia*, vol. 49, no. 6, pp. 1447-1448, 2006.

[8] S. Samarghandian, M. Azimi-Nezhad, and F. Samini, "Ameliorative effect of saffron aqueous extract on hyperglycemia, hyperlipidemia, and oxidative stress on diabetic encephalopathy in streptozotocin induced experimental diabetes mellitus," *BioMed Research International*, vol. 2014, Article ID 920857, 12 pages, 2014.

[9] M. Brownlee, "The pathobiology of diabetic complications: a unifying mechanism," *Diabetes*, vol. 54, no. 6, pp. 1615–1625, 2005.

[10] F. Vetri, M. Qi, H. Xu, J. Oberholzer, and C. Paisansathan, "Impairment of neurovascular coupling in type 1 diabetes mellitus in rats is prevented by pancreatic islet transplantation and reversed by a semi-selective PKC inhibitor," *Brain Research*, vol. 1655, pp. 48–54, 2017.

[11] N. Wu, H. Shen, Y. Wang et al., "Role of the PKCβII/JNK signaling pathway in acute glucose fluctuation-induced apoptosis of rat vascular endothelial cells," *Acta Diabetologica*, vol. 54, no. 8, pp. 727–736, 2017.

[12] B. Capuani, F. Pacifici, D. Pastore et al., "The role of epsilon PKC in acute and chronic diseases: possible pharmacological implications of its modulators," *Pharmacological Research*, vol. 111, pp. 659–667, 2016.

[13] A. M. Kay, C. L. Simpson, and J. A. Stewart Jr., "The Role of AGE/RAGE signaling in diabetes-mediated vascular calcification," *Journal of Diabetes Research*, vol. 2016, Article ID 6809703, 8 pages, 2016.

[14] M. C. Perez-Matos, M. C. Morales-Alvarez, and C. O. Mendivil, "Lipids: a suitable therapeutic target in diabetic neuropathy?," *Journal of Diabetes Research*, vol. 2017, Article ID 6943851, 9 pages, 2017.

[15] V. Thallas-Bonke and M. E. Cooper, "Tandem inhibition of PKC in diaβetic nephropathy: it takes two to tango?," *Diabetes*, vol. 62, no. 4, pp. 1010-1011, 2013.

[16] A. S. Al-Onazi, N. M. Al-Rasheed, H. A. Attia et al., "Ruboxistaurin attenuates diabetic nephropathy via modulation of TGF-β1/Smad and GRAP pathways," *The Journal of Pharmacy and Pharmacology*, vol. 68, no. 2, pp. 219–232, 2016.

[17] M. Amadio, C. Bucolo, G. M. Leggio, F. Drago, S. Govoni, and A. Pascale, "The PKCβ/HuR/VEGF pathway in diabetic retinopathy," *Biochemical Pharmacology*, vol. 80, no. 8, pp. 1230–1237, 2010.

[18] V. T. Samuel, Z. X. Liu, A. Wang et al., "Inhibition of protein kinase Cε prevents hepatic insulin resistance in nonalcoholic fatty liver disease," *The Journal of Clinical Investigation*, vol. 117, no. 3, pp. 739–745, 2007.

[19] A. L. Birkenfeld and G. I. Shulman, "Nonalcoholic fatty liver disease, hepatic insulin resistance, and type 2 diabetes," *Hepatology*, vol. 59, no. 2, pp. 713–723, 2014.

[20] J. Cantley, J. G. Burchfield, G. L. Pearson, C. Schmitz-Peiffer, M. Leitges, and T. J. Biden, "Deletion of PKCε selectively enhances the amplifying pathways of glucose-stimulated insulin secretion via increased lipolysis in mouse β-cells," *Diabetes*, vol. 58, no. 8, pp. 1826–1834, 2009.

[21] H. Y. Xie, F. Xu, Y. Li et al., "Increases in PKC gamma expression in trigeminal spinal nucleus is associated with orofacial thermal hyperalgesia in streptozotocin-induced diabetic mice," *Journal of Chemical Neuroanatomy*, vol. 63, pp. 13–19, 2015.

[22] M. Gareskog and P. Wentzel, "Altered protein kinase C activation associated with rat embryonic dysmorphogenesis," *Pediatric Research*, vol. 56, no. 6, pp. 849–857, 2004.

[23] X. Tian, Y. Liu, G. Ren et al., "Resveratrol limits diabetes-associated cognitive decline in rats by preventing oxidative stress and inflammation and modulating hippocampal structural synaptic plasticity," *Brain Research*, vol. 1650, pp. 1–9, 2016.

[24] J. Li, Y. Qu, P. Zu et al., "Increased isoform-specific membrane translocation of conventional and novel protein kinase C in human neuroblastoma SH-SY5Y cells following prolonged hypoxia," *Brain Research*, vol. 1093, no. 1, pp. 25–32, 2006.

[25] L. Zhao, X. Liu, J. Liang et al., "Phosphorylation of p38 MAPK mediates hypoxic preconditioning-induced neuroprotection against cerebral ischemic injury via mitochondria translocation of Bcl-xL in mice," *Brain Research*, vol. 1503, pp. 78–88, 2013.

[26] D. Zhang, S. Han, S. Wang, Y. Luo, L. Zhao, and J. Li, "cPKCγ-mediated down-regulation of UCHL1 alleviates ischaemic neuronal injuries by decreasing autophagy via ERK-mTOR pathway," *Journal of Cellular and Molecular Medicine*, vol. 21, no. 12, pp. 3641–3657, 2017.

[27] T. I. Igumenova, "Dynamics and membrane interactions of protein kinase C," *Biochemistry*, vol. 54, no. 32, pp. 4953–4968, 2015.

[28] E. Molina-Jijón, R. Rodríguez-Muñoz, M. del Carmen Namorado et al., "All-trans retinoic acid prevents oxidative stress-induced loss of renal tight junction proteins in type-1 diabetic model," *The Journal of Nutritional Biochemistry*, vol. 26, no. 5, pp. 441–454, 2015.

[29] Y. Ikeda, G. S. Olsen, E. Ziv et al., "Cellular mechanism of nutritionally induced insulin resistance in *Psammomys obesus*: overexpression of protein kinase Cε in skeletal muscle precedes the onset of hyperinsulinemia and hyperglycemia," *Diabetes*, vol. 50, no. 3, pp. 584–592, 2001.

[30] J. Radosinska, L. H. Kurahara, K. Hiraishi et al., "Modulation of cardiac connexin-43 by omega-3 fatty acid ethyl-ester supplementation demonstrated in spontaneously diabetic rats," *Physiological Research*, vol. 64, no. 6, pp. 795–806, 2015.

[31] F. Vetri, R. Chavez, H. L. Xu, C. Paisansathan, and D. A. Pelligrino, "Complex modulation of the expression of PKC isoforms in the rat brain during chronic type 1 diabetes mellitus," *Brain Research*, vol. 1490, pp. 202–209, 2013.

[32] J. D. Shin and S. P. Jadhav, "Multiple modes of hippocampal-prefrontal interactions in memory-guided behavior," *Current Opinion in Neurobiology*, vol. 40, pp. 161–169, 2016.

[33] O. Y. Chao, S. Nikolaus, M. Lira Brandao, J. P. Huston, and M. A. de Souza Silva, "Interaction between the medial

prefrontal cortex and hippocampal CA1 area is essential for episodic-like memory in rats," *Neurobiology of Learning and Memory*, vol. 141, pp. 72–77, 2017.

[34] M. Mendez-Couz, N. M. Conejo, H. Gonzalez-Pardo, and J. L. Arias, "Functional interactions between dentate gyrus, striatum and anterior thalamic nuclei on spatial memory retrieval," *Brain Research*, vol. 1605, pp. 59–69, 2015.

[35] Y. Cao, Z. Zhao, R. L. Eckert, and E. A. Reece, "Protein kinase Cβ2 inhibition reduces hyperglycemia-induced neural tube defects through suppression of a caspase 8-triggered apoptotic pathway," *American Journal of Obstetrics and Gynecology*, vol. 204, no. 3, pp. 226.e1–226.e5, 2011.

[36] M. C. Petersen, A. K. Madiraju, B. M. Gassaway et al., "Insulin receptor Thr1160 phosphorylation mediates lipid-induced hepatic insulin resistance," *The Journal of Clinical Investigation*, vol. 126, no. 11, pp. 4361–4371, 2016.

[37] D. Lin, R. Harris, R. Stutzman, G. A. Zampighi, H. Davidson, and D. J. Takemoto, "Protein kinase C-γ activation in the early streptozotocin diabetic rat lens," *Current Eye Research*, vol. 32, no. 6, pp. 523–532, 2007.

[38] B. P. Lucke-Wold, R. C. Turner, A. F. Logsdon et al., "Common mechanisms of Alzheimer's disease and ischemic stroke: the role of protein kinase C in the progression of age-related neurodegeneration," *Journal of Alzheimer's Disease*, vol. 43, no. 3, pp. 711–724, 2015.

[39] A. Olariu, K. Yamada, T. Mamiya, V. Hefco, and T. Nabeshima, "Memory impairment induced by chronic intracerebroventricular infusion of beta-amyloid (1-40) involves downregulation of protein kinase C," *Brain Research*, vol. 957, no. 2, pp. 278–286, 2002.

[40] J. Wu, T. B. Song, Y. J. Li, K. S. He, L. Ge, and L. R. Wang, "Prenatal restraint stress impairs learning and memory and hippocampal PKCbeta1 expression and translocation in offspring rats," *Brain Research*, vol. 1141, pp. 205–213, 2007.

[41] A. S. Harris, E. M. Denovan-Wright, L. C. Hamilton, and H. A. Robertson, "Protein kinase C beta II mRNA levels decrease in the striatum and cortex of transgenic Huntington's disease mice," *Journal of Psychiatry & Neuroscience*, vol. 26, no. 2, pp. 117–122, 2001.

[42] R. Orman and M. Stewart, "Hemispheric differences in protein kinase C βII levels in the rat amygdala: baseline asymmetry and lateralized changes associated with cue and context in a classical fear conditioning paradigm," *Neuroscience*, vol. 144, no. 3, pp. 797–807, 2007.

[43] E. J. Weeber, C. M. Atkins, J. C. Selcher et al., "A role for the β isoform of protein kinase C in fear conditioning," *The Journal of Neuroscience*, vol. 20, no. 16, pp. 5906–5914, 2000.

[44] M. A. Rossi, D. C. Mash, and L. deToledo-Morrell, "Spatial memory in aged rats is related to PKCγ-dependent G-protein coupling of the M1 receptor," *Neurobiology of Aging*, vol. 26, no. 1, pp. 53–68, 2005.

[45] L. Li, L. You, B. Sunyer et al., "Hippocampal protein kinase C family members in spatial memory retrieval in the mouse," *Behavioural Brain Research*, vol. 258, pp. 202–207, 2014.

[46] J. Nithianantharajah and M. Murphy, "Experience on the Barnes spatial maze influences PKCγ levels in the hippocampus," *The International Journal of Neuroscience*, vol. 119, no. 7, pp. 1014–1030, 2009.

[47] P. J. Colombo, W. C. Wetsel, and M. Gallagher, "Spatial memory is related to hippocampal subcellular concentrations of calcium-dependent protein kinase C isoforms in young and aged rats," *Proceedings of the National Academy of Sciences of the United States of America*, vol. 94, no. 25, pp. 14195–14199, 1997.

[48] T. S. Salameh, K. M. Bullock, I. A. Hujoel et al., "Central nervous system delivery of intranasal insulin: mechanisms of uptake and effects on cognition," *Journal of Alzheimer's Disease*, vol. 47, no. 3, pp. 715–728, 2015.

[49] H. Kuang, M. Sun, J. Lv et al., "Hippocampal apoptosis involved in learning deficits in the offspring exposed to maternal high sucrose diets," *The Journal of Nutritional Biochemistry*, vol. 25, no. 9, pp. 985–990, 2014.

[50] Y. Kohara, S. Kawaguchi, R. Kuwahara, Y. Uchida, Y. Oku, and K. Yamashita, "Genistein improves spatial learning and memory in male rats with elevated glucose level during memory consolidation," *Physiology & Behavior*, vol. 140, pp. 15–22, 2015.

[51] S. S. Patel, V. Mehta, H. Changotra, and M. Udayabanu, "Depression mediates impaired glucose tolerance and cognitive dysfunction: a neuromodulatory role of rosiglitazone," *Hormones and Behavior*, vol. 78, pp. 200–210, 2016.

[52] R. Codella, S. Benedini, S. Paini et al., "Effect of sugar versus mixed breakfast on metabolic and neurofunctional responses in healthy individuals," *Journal of Diabetes Research*, vol. 2017, Article ID 9634585, 10 pages, 2017.

[53] S. A. Patten and D. W. Ali, "PKCγ-induced trafficking of AMPA receptors in embryonic zebrafish depends on NSF and PICK1," *Proceedings of the National Academy of Sciences of the United States of America*, vol. 106, no. 16, pp. 6796–6801, 2009.

[54] M. K. Sun and D. L. Alkon, "Activation of protein kinase C isozymes for the treatment of dementias," *Advances in Pharmacology*, vol. 64, pp. 273–302, 2012.

18

Intralymphatic Glutamic Acid Decarboxylase-Alum Administration Induced Th2-Like-Specific Immunomodulation in Responder Patients: A Pilot Clinical Trial in Type 1 Diabetes

Beatriz Tavira,[1] Hugo Barcenilla,[1] Jeannette Wahlberg,[2] Peter Achenbach,[3] Johnny Ludvigsson,[1,4] and Rosaura Casas[1]

[1]*Division of Pediatrics, Department of Clinical and Experimental Medicine, Faculty of Medicine and Health Sciences, Linköping University, Linköping, Sweden*
[2]*Department of Endocrinology and Department of Medical and Health Sciences and Department of Clinical and Experimental Medicine, Linköping University, Linköping, Sweden*
[3]*Institute of Diabetes Research, Helmholtz Zentrum München, and Forschergruppe Diabetes, Klinikum Rechts der Isar, Technische Universität München, München, Germany*
[4]*Crown Princess Victoria Children's Hospital, Region Östergötland, Linköping, Sweden*

Correspondence should be addressed to Beatriz Tavira; beatriz.tavira@ki.se and Rosaura Casas; rosaura.casas@liu.se

Academic Editor: Toshiyasu Sasaoka

GAD-alum given into lymph nodes to type 1 diabetes patients participating in an open-label pilot trial resulted in preservation of C-peptide similar to promising results from other trials. Here, we compared the immunomodulatory effect of giving GAD-alum directly into lymph nodes versus that induced by subcutaneous administration. Samples from T1D patients ($n = 6$) who received 4 μg GAD-alum into lymph nodes (LNs), followed by two booster injections one month apart, and from patients ($n = 6$) who received two subcutaneous injections (SC) (20 μg) given one month apart were compared. GADA, IA-2A, GADA subclasses, IgE, GAD_{65}-induced cytokines, PBMC proliferation, and T cell markers were analyzed. Lower doses of GAD-alum into LN induced higher GADA levels than SC injections and reduced proliferation and IgG1 GADA subclass, while enhancing IgG2, IgG3, and IgG4. The cytokine profile was dominated by the Th2-associated cytokine IL-13, and GAD_{65} stimulation induced activated CD4 T cells. Patients responding clinically best account for most of the immunological changes. In contrast, SC treatment resulted in predominant IgG1, predominant IFN-γ, higher proliferation, and activated CD4 and CD8 cells. Patients from the LN group with best metabolic outcome seemed to have common immune correlates related to the treatment. This trial is registered with DIAGNODE (NCT02352974, clinicaltrials.gov) and DIABGAD (NCT01785108, clinicaltrials.gov).

1. Introduction

Type 1 diabetes (T1D) treatment consists of lifelong administration of insulin, a replacement therapy which does not satisfactorily prevent serious complications. Immune intervention trials in recent-onset T1D patients to delay or halt disease progression have shown no or limited efficacy [1–7], highlighting the complexity of translation from animal models to human T1D. Immunomodulation with autoantigens could potentially constitute the most specific and safe treatment for T1D. Subcutaneous administration of glutamic acid decarboxylase $(GAD)_{65}$ formulated with aluminum hydroxide (GAD-alum) showed efficacy in preserving residual insulin secretion in children and adolescents with recent-onset T1D [8], but subsequent phase II [9] and phase III [10] trials failed to reach their primary outcomes. However, significant efficacy was shown in prespecified subgroups in the phase III study [10], and we have recently shown that close administration of influenza vaccine might have influenced the study outcome [11]. Thus, it is plausible that treatment with GAD-alum is beneficial for some patients but has not been sufficiently effective [12].

Immunotherapy with allergens has been extensively used as treatment for allergic rhinitis and asthma [13, 14]. The most common forms of allergen immunotherapy have been through subcutaneous or sublingual allergen administration [15, 16], but even though they are quite safe and effective, recent studies have focused on further optimization of allergen vaccines to improve clinical efficacy. Intralymphatic administration of low doses of allergens has shown promising result, providing improved allergen exposure and triggering prompt immune changes [17–20]. The mechanism for this form of treatment remains unclear, although immune modulation of the immune responses and induction of tolerance has been suggested [21]. It is known that intralymphatic administration of antigens can maximize immunogenicity and hence efficacy and has shown to improve the efficacy of several vaccines [22, 23]. Thus, to render the presentation of GAD_{65} antigen to T cells in the lymph nodes more efficient than previously described [9, 10], GAD-alum was administrated into lymph nodes to six patients participating in an open-label clinical trial. Results from these patients showed that preservation of C-peptide appeared to be similar to promising results observed in patients from other immune intervention trials [24]. Here, we studied the immunomodulatory effect of giving low doses of GAD-alum directly into lymph glands versus that induced by subcutaneous administration of larger doses.

2. Methods

2.1. Participants. A group of recent-onset T1D patients ($n = 6$, <6 months from diagnosis) participating in a pilot trial (NCT02352974, clinicaltrials.gov) received a primary injection of 4 μg of GAD-alum (Diamyd Medical, Stockholm) into an inguinal lymph node, followed by two booster injections of 4 μg each with one-month interval [24, 25]. In parallel, they got vitamin D 2000 U/d per os. Another group of recent-onset T1D patients ($n = 6$, <4 months from diagnosis) participated in a double-blind, placebo-controlled pilot trial (NCT01785108, clinicaltrials.gov) (unpublished), where they received two subcutaneous injections (SC) of GAD-alum, 20 μg each, one month apart (Figure S1). They also in parallel got vitamin D 2000 U/d per os. These patients were selected under blind conditions, before code break according to availability of samples (Figure 1).

2.2. Laboratory Tests. Laboratory analyses were performed at Linköping University, Sweden. Blood and serum samples were collected at baseline and after 30, 60, 90, and 180 days in the LN group and after 15, 45, 90, and 180 days in the SC group. Samples were drawn during the morning hours, and PBMCs were isolated within 24 h using Leucosep (Greiner Bio-One) according to the manufacturer's instructions.

2.3. Serum Antibodies and IgG Subclasses. Serum GAD autoantibodies (GADA) and IA-2A were estimated in duplicate by means of a radio-binding assay, using ^{35}S-labeled recombinant human GAD_{65} as previously described [26]. Sepharose protein A was used to separate free from antibody-bound labeled GAD_{65}. A diabetes autoantibody standardization program (IASP) in which the laboratory participated in has shown that the GADA assay has a sensitivity of 70% and specificity of 100% and for IA-2A, 99% sensitivity and 100% specificity.

GADA IgG1, 2, 3, and 4 subclasses were measured by radio-binding assays [27] using IgG subclass-specific biotin-labeled mouse anti-human monoclonal antibodies bound on Streptavidin Sepharose High Performance beads (GE Healthcare Life Sciences, Freiburg, Germany). Mouse anti-human IgG1 (clone G17-1; BD Biosciences, Heidelberg, Germany), IgG2 (clone G18-21; BD Biosciences), IgG3 (clone HP6047; Invitrogen, Carlsbad, CA), and IgG4 (clone JDC-14; BD Biosciences) monoclonal antibodies were used. Nonspecific binding was determined for each serum using biotin-labeled mouse anti-rat IgM monoclonal antibody (clone G53-238; BD Biosciences) bound on Streptavidin Sepharose beads. Briefly, 2 μl of serum was incubated in duplicate with 25,000 cpm of ^{35}S-labeled recombinant human GAD_{65} in 25 μl of 50 mM Tris, 150 mM NaCl, and 1% Tween 20 (pH 7.4) (TBST) overnight at 4°C, before addition of 50 μl antibody-coated Streptavidin Sepharose bead suspension, incubation for 1 h at 4°C on a shaker, washing in cold TBST, and counting. Results were expressed as delta cpm (IgG subclass-specific cpm − anti-rat IgM cpm) and converted to arbitrary units (AU) proportional to the GADA IgG subclass-specific delta cpm of a local standard serum.

Total serum IgE was quantified using the ImmunoCap100E system (Phadia AB, Uppsala, Sweden). The measuring range for the assay was 2–50,000 kU/l, and calibrators were run in duplicate to obtain a full calibration curve. Levels of total IgE ≥ 85 kU/l were regarded as positive.

2.4. Lymphocyte Proliferation Assay. PBMCs were incubated in triplicate in round-bottom plates with 5 μg/ml rhGAD65 (Diamyd Medical, Stockholm, Sweden), CD3/CD28 beads (Gibco, Life Technologies AS, Oslo, Norway), and in the medium alone. After 3 days, cells were pulsed for 18 h with 0.2 μCi of [^{3}H] thymidine/well (Perkin Elmer) and harvested thereafter. Proliferation was recorded [28] and expressed as stimulation index (SI) and calculated as the mean of triplicates in the presence of stimulus divided by the mean of triplicates with the medium alone.

2.5. Cytokine Secretion Assay. For cytokine quantification, peripheral blood mononuclear cells (PBMCs) were cultured for 7 days in the presence of 5 μg/ml recombinant human GAD65 (Diamyd Medical, Stockholm, Sweden) or in the medium (AIM-V) alone at 37°C in 5% CO_2, as previously described [11, 28, 29]. The cytokines interleukin- (IL-) 2, IL-5, IL-10, IL-13, IL-17, tumor necrosis factor- (TNF-) α, and interferon- (IFN-) γ were measured in cell culture supernatants using Bio-Plex Pro Cytokine Panel (Bio-Rad, Hercules, CA, USA) according to the manufacturer's instructions. Data was collected using the Luminex 200™ (Luminex xMAP™ Corporation, Austin, TX, USA). The antigen-induced cytokine secretion level was calculated by subtracting the spontaneous secretion (i.e., secretion from

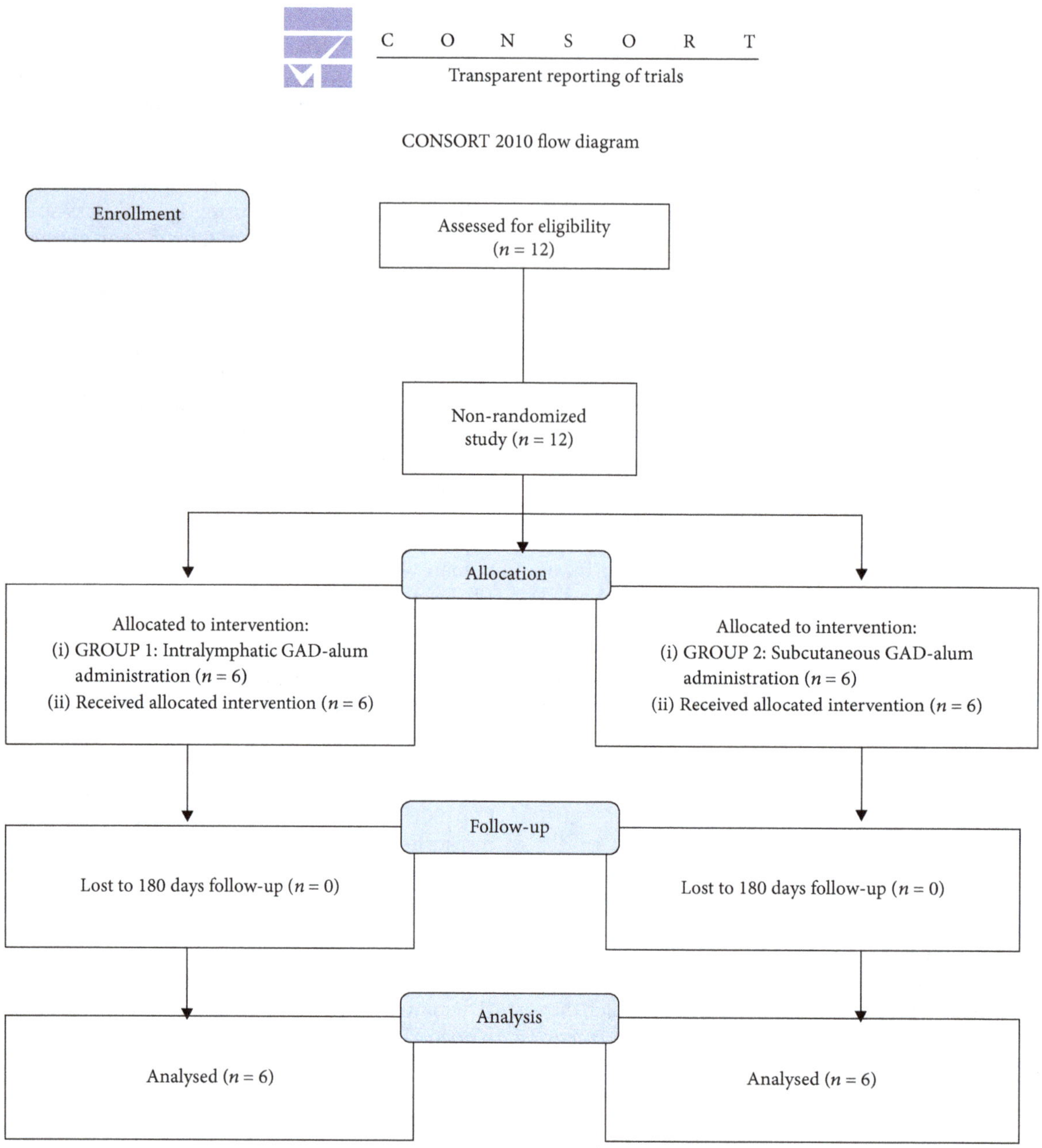

Figure 1: CONSORT flow diagram. A total of 12 patients were recruited in two different clinical studies ($n = 6$ each study) using different doses and administration of GAD-alum. None of the patients were excluded during these trials' follow-up.

PBMC cultured in the medium alone) from the one following stimulation with GAD65.

2.6. Flow Cytometry. PBMCs were incubated in the AIM-V medium with β-mercaptoethanol at 37°C, 5% CO_2 for 7 days, with or without 5 μg/ml recombinant GAD_{65}. Thereafter, cells were washed in PBS containing 0.1% BSA and subsequently stained with Alexa 700-conjugated anti-CD3 (clone UCHT1, BD Biosciences), Pacific Blue-conjugated anti-CD4 (clone RPA-T4, BD Biosciences), allophycocyanin- (APC-) H7-conjugated anti-CD8 (clone SK1, BD Biosciences), PerCP-Cy5.5-conjugated anti-CD45RA (clone HI100, BD Biosciences), phycoerythrin- (PE-) conjugated anti-CCR7 (clone G043H7, BioLegend), FITC-conjugated anti-CD127 (clone eBioRDR5, eBioscience), and PE-Cy7-conjugated anti-CD25 (clone BC96, eBioscience). Then, cells were fixed and permeabilized using the FOXP3-staining buffer set (eBioscience), according to the manufacturer's instructions. Cells were then stained with APC-conjugated anti-FOXP3 (clone PCH101, eBioscience) and acquired on a FACS Aria III (Becton Dickinson) running FACS Diva v8 software (Becton Dickinson). Data were analyzed using Kaluza v1.3 (Beckman Coulter).

2.7. Ethics. All patients and children's parents gave their oral and written informed consent. Both trials have been approved by the Research Ethics Committee, Linköping University, Sweden (DIAGNODE: Dnr 2014/153-31; DIABGAD-1: Dnr 2012/417-32), and by the Medical Product Agency, Uppsala, Sweden (DIAGNODE: Dnr 5.1-214-54385; DIABGAD-1: Dnr 2012-003251-11).

2.8. Statistical Analysis. Data distribution was tested using the Kolmogorov-Smirnov test. Variables that followed a normal distribution were presented as mean (i.e., age, insulin dose, HbA1c, and C-peptide), and differences within groups were calculated by a Student t-test. For nonnormally distributed variables, a nonparametric test was applied (Mann–Whitney test). A Wilcoxon test was used for related samples not normally distributed. Differences between categorical variables were calculated by a chi-square test (χ^2 test). A probability level of <0.05 was considered statistically significant. Calculations were performed using IBM SPSS Statistics version 23 (IBM SPSS, Armonk, NY, USA), and graphical illustrations were made in GraphPad Prism 5 for Windows (GraphPad Software, La Jolla, CA, USA). Due to the small sample size, the immunological and clinical data of the patients were individually represented.

3. Results

Patients were stratified into those who received lymph node (LN) or subcutaneous (SC) GAD-alum injections. Gender distribution was the same in both groups, while mean age was higher in LN patients (22 years) than in the SC group (14 years) ($p = 0.001$). Both groups had similar baseline mean C-peptide (fasting, max. stimulated, and AUC). Pretreatment HbA1c values tended to be higher in LN patients ($p = 0.054$), but there was no difference in the insulin dose/kg body weight, 24 hours between the groups. Baseline GADA and IA-2A autoantibody levels did not differ between the groups (Table S1). Follow-up of the patients showed that fasting and stimulated C-peptide (AUC) remained stable at 180 days in the LN group, while HbA1c levels and insulin dose/kg body weight, 24 hours decreased [24]. Patients in the SC group had a greater loss of stimulated C-peptide, as well as an increase in HbA1c and insulin requirement (Table S1).

3.1. GADA Titers and GADA Subclass Analysis. GADA levels and GADA subclass distribution at baseline did not differ between the two groups. Following the second injection of GAD-alum given in both SC and LN (Figure 2(a)), GADA levels were enhanced. However, LN administration of low GAD-alum doses induced median GADA 29 times higher than SC injection of higher doses (Figure 2(a)).

We looked next to the longitudinal GADA IgG1–4 subclass responses of the patients, and the distribution of IgG subclasses at each time point was calculated, as frequency of each subclass with respect to the combined sum of the AUs of all the subclasses in each sample. Baseline GADA subclass distribution was similar in the two groups, IgG1 being the most frequent, followed by IgG3 > IgG2 ≈ IgG4 (Figure 2(b), Figure S2). The proportion of IgG1 decreased from baseline to 90 days both in the LN and SC groups, while the proportion of the other subclasses increased. While GADA subclass distribution in the SC group at 180 days was similar to that observed at baseline, the proportion of IgG1 in the LN group was further reduced, with a marked increase of IgG2, IgG3, and IgG4 (Figure 2(c)).

To disregard a possible allergy-associated effect in response of GAD-alum, total IgE was measured at baseline and at 180 days. Baseline IgE levels were similar in patients receiving intralymphatic and subcutaneous injections and were not affected by the treatment but remained unchanged after 180 days (data not shown).

3.2. Cytokine Secretion and Relative Contribution. Baseline cytokine secretion in PBMC supernatants collected after 7 days culture was similar in the two groups. GAD_{65}-induced secretion of IL-5, IL-13, IFN-γ, and IL-17 was increased at 90 days, both after the second GAD-alum SC and LN doses, together with IL-2 in the SC group. The third GAD-alum injection into the LN resulted in a predominant secretion of IL-13 and low levels of IFN-γ at 180 days. Meanwhile, IFN-γ was the most secreted cytokine in the SC group at the same time point (Figure S3). We further assessed the relative contribution of each cytokine to the total GAD_{65}-induced cytokine secretion. In the LN group, a broad cytokine profile was observed at 90 days, following the second injection of GAD-alum, while cytokine secretion at 180 days, after the third injection, was dominated by the Th2-associated cytokine IL-13. In the SC group, cytokine profile was also characterized by a broad cytokine secretion at 90 days with a predominant secretion of Th2 cytokines, but cytokine distribution shifted in a dominant Th1-like response at 180 days (Figure 3).

3.3. In Vitro Stimulation with GAD65. GAD_{65}-induced proliferation was increased by the second injection of GAD-alum both into the LN and SC. The third injection to the LN group resulted in a reduction of proliferation at 180 days, while it remained stable in the SC group. Proliferation induced by stimulation with CD3/CD28 beads showed the same distribution as that induced by GAD_{65} (Figure S4).

3.4. T Cell Immunophenotype. We monitored the differentiation state and GAD_{65}-induced activation of T cells. A representative illustration of the gating strategy for the analysis of CD8, CD4, and regulatory T cells is shown (Figure S5). GAD_{65} stimulation induced activated $CD25^{+}CD127^{+}$ T cells in both groups after the second injection of GAD-alum. In the LN, higher frequency of activated CD4 T cells was detected in 3 patients, while activation of CD8 T cells was moderate or not detectable. In the SC group in contrast, the proportion of activated CD8 T cells was more predominant, with weaker expression of GAD_{65} activation of CD4 cells (Figures 4(a) and 4(b)).

The analysis of $CD4^{+}FOXP3^{+}CD25^{hi}CD127^{low/-}$ Tregs showed that resting Treg did not vary through the study, but antigen recall induced cells with regulatory phenotype at 180 days in both groups (Figures S6C and S6D). Further, addition of CD45RA revealed an increment in nonsuppressive $FOXP3^{lo}CD45RA^{-}$ T cells in both groups (Figures 4(e) and 4(f)).

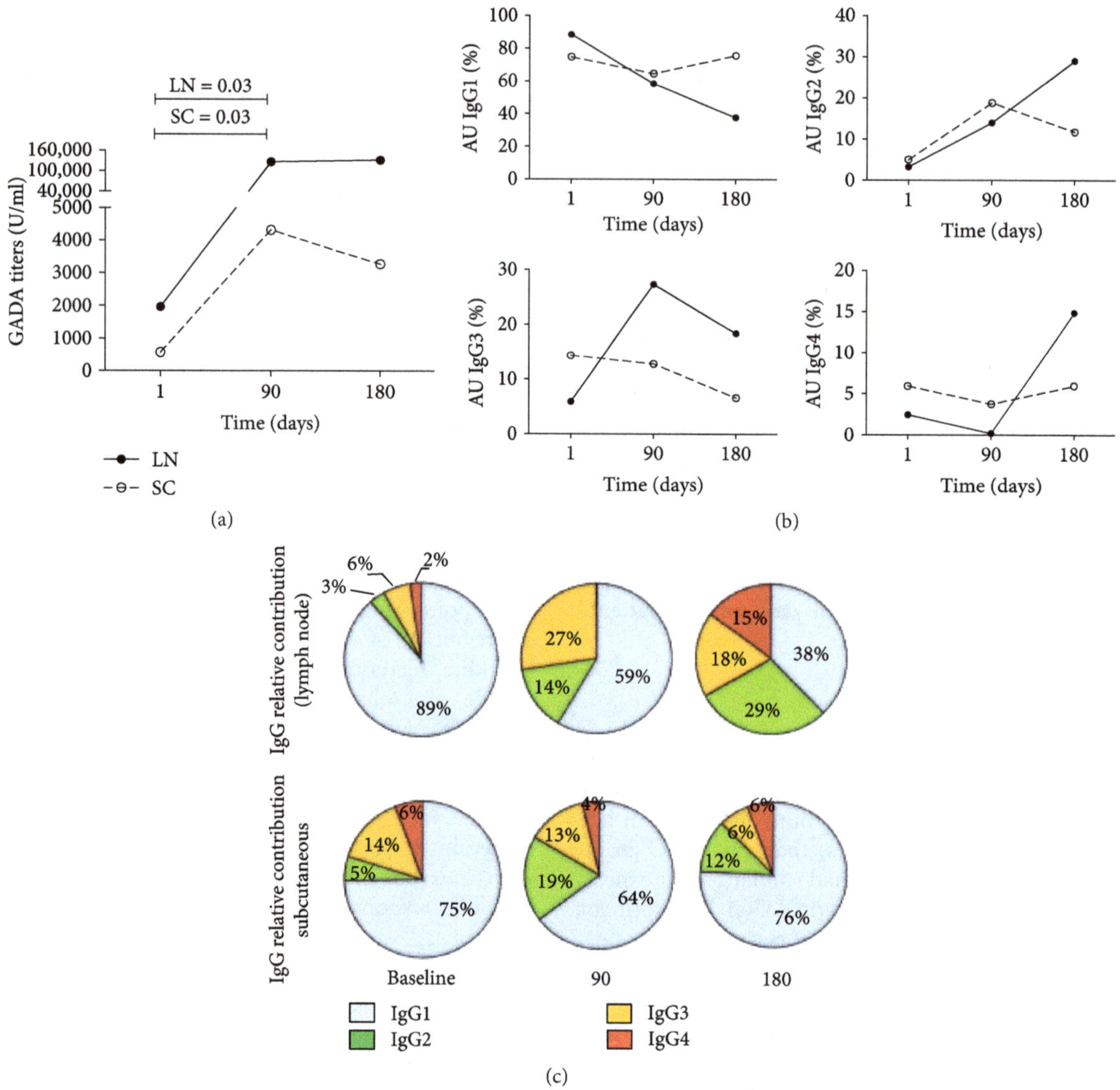

Figure 2: GADA titers and GADA subclass distribution in GAD-alum lymph node and subcutaneous treatment. (a) Median values of GADA titers in the lymph node (LN, $n = 6$) or subcutaneous vaccination (SC, $n = 6$). (b) Change of the frequency (%) of IgG1, IgG2, IgG3, and IgG4 GADA subclasses. Frequencies were calculated with respect to the combined sum of the AUs of the 4 subclasses in each sample. The median percentage with respect to the total IgG is shown for each respective subclass. (c) GADA subclass relative contribution at baseline, 90, and 180 days for LN and SC groups.

CD4 and CD8 T cells were further classified according to the expression of CD45RA and CCR7 as näive (T_N, $CD45RA^+CCR7^+$), central memory (T_{CM}, $CD45RA^-CCR7^+$), effector memory (T_{EM}, $CD45RA^-CCR7^-$), and terminally differentiated effector memory (T_{EMRA}, $CD45RA^+CCR7^-$) cells (Figure S6). Both groups showed a progressive reduction in the proportion of näive CD4 and CD8 T cells after 90 days, while the frequency of memory and effector cells increased in GAD65-stimulated PBMC (Figure S6).

3.5. Identifying Biomarkers of Clinical Outcome. Individual immunological changes induced by GAD-alum treatment were calculated as the ratio of GAD_{65}-induced immune responses at 90 and 180 days with respect to immune response pretreatment, and patients were stratified according to their metabolic and C-peptide preservation (Figure 5, Table S2).

Baseline immune response did not show any pretreatment feature that seemed to be related to the clinical outcome. Representation of induced changes of GAD_{65}-induced cytokine secretion posttreatment showed that Th1- and Th2-associated cytokines were enhanced after 90 days in most patients, independently of the administration route. However, changes in GAD_{65}-induced cytokines at 180 days were detectable in the LN patients with the best clinical response (patients 1, 2, and 3), with lower HbA1c, decreased insulin requirement, and best preservation of C-peptide secretion. Activated CD4 cells but no CD8 were observed in these three patients. Reduction of the proportion of IgG1

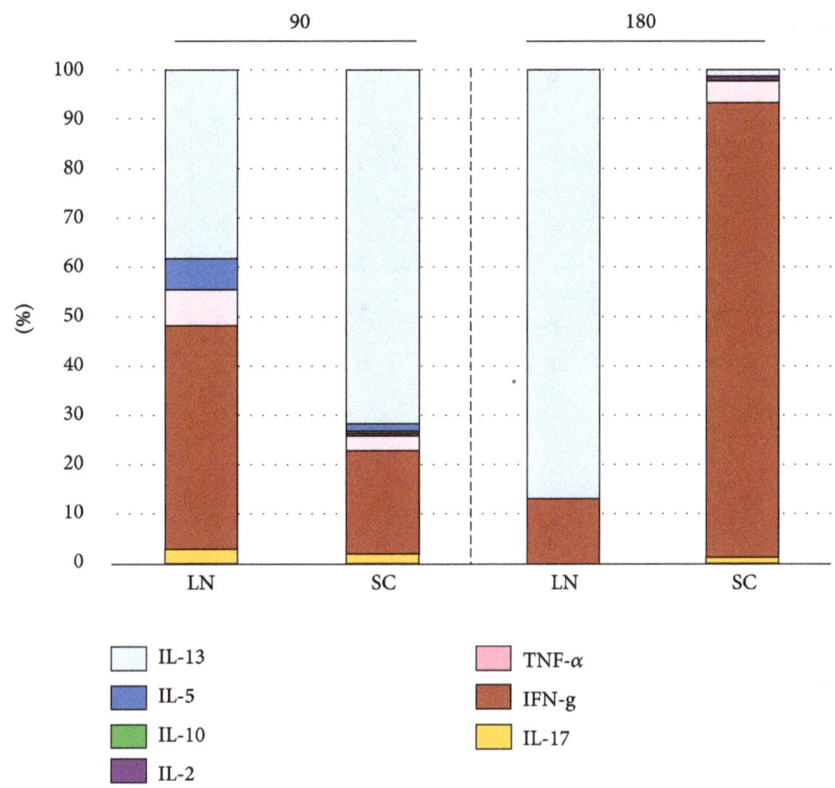

FIGURE 3: GAD65-induced cytokine secretion upon in vitro PMBC stimulation. Relative contribution (%) of the cytokines in LN patients and SC group at 90 and 180 days.

and enhancement of IgG2 and IgG4 were most pronounced in the patient with the best clinical response (patient 1), and this patient accounted for the observed increase of IgG4 in the LN group (Figure 5).

GAD_{65}-induced cytokine secretion in the patient with best clinical response in the SC group (patient 1) resembled that observed in the LN patients with best response, but in the SC-treated patient, IgG1 was the predominant GADA subclass, and both activated CD4 and CD8 cells were detected.

Calculation of the ratio of Th2 (IL-13 and IL-5)/Th1 (IFN-γ and TNF-α) cytokines at 180 days for the best responders in both groups ($n = 2$ in LN and $n = 1$ in SC) revealed that Th2 response was three times stronger in LN patients than in the SC group (ratio: 6.44 LN versus 2.24 SC).

4. Discussion

In this study, we assessed the influence of the administration route on the immunogenicity induced by GAD-alum treatment. Our results show that direct intralymphatic administration enhanced the immunogenicity of the treatment as compared with subcutaneous delivery. The intensity of the specific immune response induced by low doses of GAD-alum injected into the lymph nodes was comparable with that induced by higher doses given subcutaneously. No specific immune signatures before treatment were identified among the biomarkers included in this study. Although the patients in the SC group were slightly younger, the immunological profile at baseline was quite similar in both groups, supporting the idea that differences in the immune response observed at follow-up were due to the treatment. A common feature for both groups was that patients with better preservation of C-peptide secretion and improved metabolic outcome, that is, lower HbA1c and insulin needs, seemed to have some common immune correlates.

Modifications following therapy included a stepwise increment of GADA in the LN group, with titers peaking after the third injection. Boost of GADA was stronger following low doses given into the LN than by SC administration of larger doses. Intriguingly, GADA increase was associated with the reduction of GAD_{65}-induced proliferation after 180 days in the LN patients but not in the SC group. Increased antibody titers and lower proliferation against insulin have also been shown in a prevention trial using intranasal insulin given to at-risk individuals, suggesting induction of tolerance [30]. Reduction of proliferation in the LN group raises the question whether induction of tolerance was part of the immunological effect, but no Treg-associated cytokines or T cells with regulatory phenotype were detected. Instead, GAD_{65}-specific CD4 T cell responses were observed. The second injection, both into the LN and SC, induced a cytokine secretion profile dominated by Th2 cytokines. The third LN dose led to a cytokine distribution dominated by the Th2-associated cytokine IL-13 after 6 months, while TNF and IFN were the predominant cytokines in the SC group at the same time point. This is of particular interest, as a cytoprotective action of IL-13 has been shown

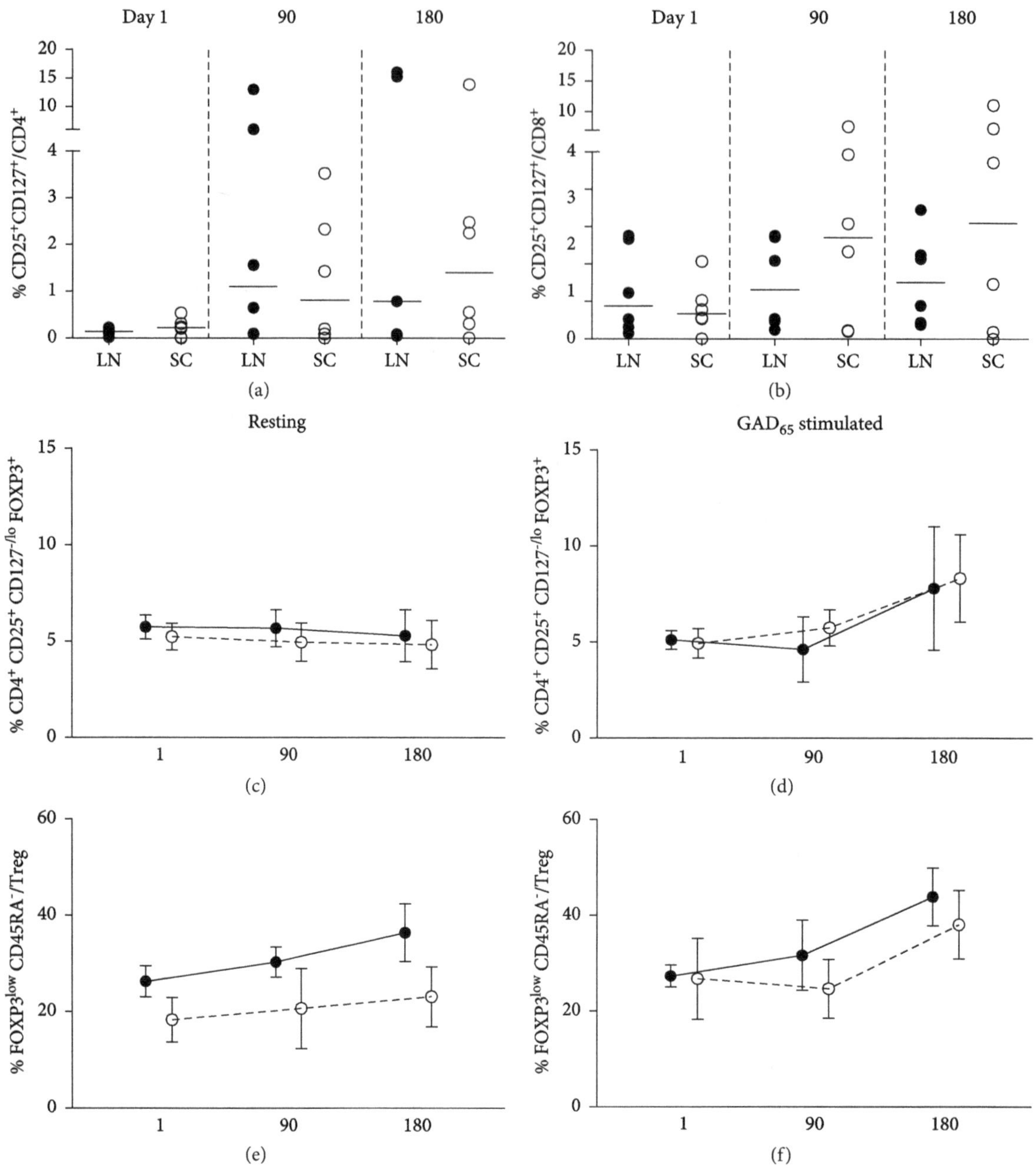

Figure 4: T cell activation induced by GAD65 in lymph node (LN, $n = 6$, black circles) and subcutaneous (SC, $n = 6$, white circles) GAD-alum patients. (a) Percentage of GAD65-activated $CD4^+CD25^+CD127^+$ T cells and (b) $CD8^+CD25^+CD127^+$ T cells. (c) Mean percentage of $CD4^+CD25^+CD127^{lo/-}FOXP3^+$ (Treg) in resting samples (medium alone) and (d) induced by GAD65 stimulation. (e) Mean percentage of $FOXP3^{lo}CD45RA^-$ nonsuppressor regulatory T cells in resting samples (medium alone) and (f) GAD65-stimulated samples.

in pancreatic β-cell viability [31], and IL-13 has been described as the main effector of suppression, reducing both Teff proliferation and IL-2 secretion [32]. IFN-γ was also detected in the same supernatants, and it could be argued that secretion of Th1-associated cytokines might not be desirable as part of GAD-alum-induced immune responses. However, cytokines can exert different effects depending on their concentrations and microenvironment [33], and IFN-γ has a wide-ranging effect on the innate and the adaptive immune system [34]. In that sense, the GAD-alum effect might not only be dependent on the induction of a predominant Th2 response but is also reliant upon a broader range of cytokines that may play a role in restoring the immune balance. T cells with regulatory phenotype were not part of the detected subpopulations, in agreement with results from previous studies [29, 35]. However, as the GAD-alum effect on the immune response is antigen specific [29, 36, 37], it cannot be excluded that the scarce number of GAD_{65}-specific cells precluded their identification.

As subclass frequencies can be associated with Th1/Th2 responses, we analyzed whether GAD-alum influenced GADA IgG subclass distribution. A relative reduction of IgG1, with a shift towards IgG2, IgG3, and IgG4 subclasses, was observed in the LN group. It was particularly interesting

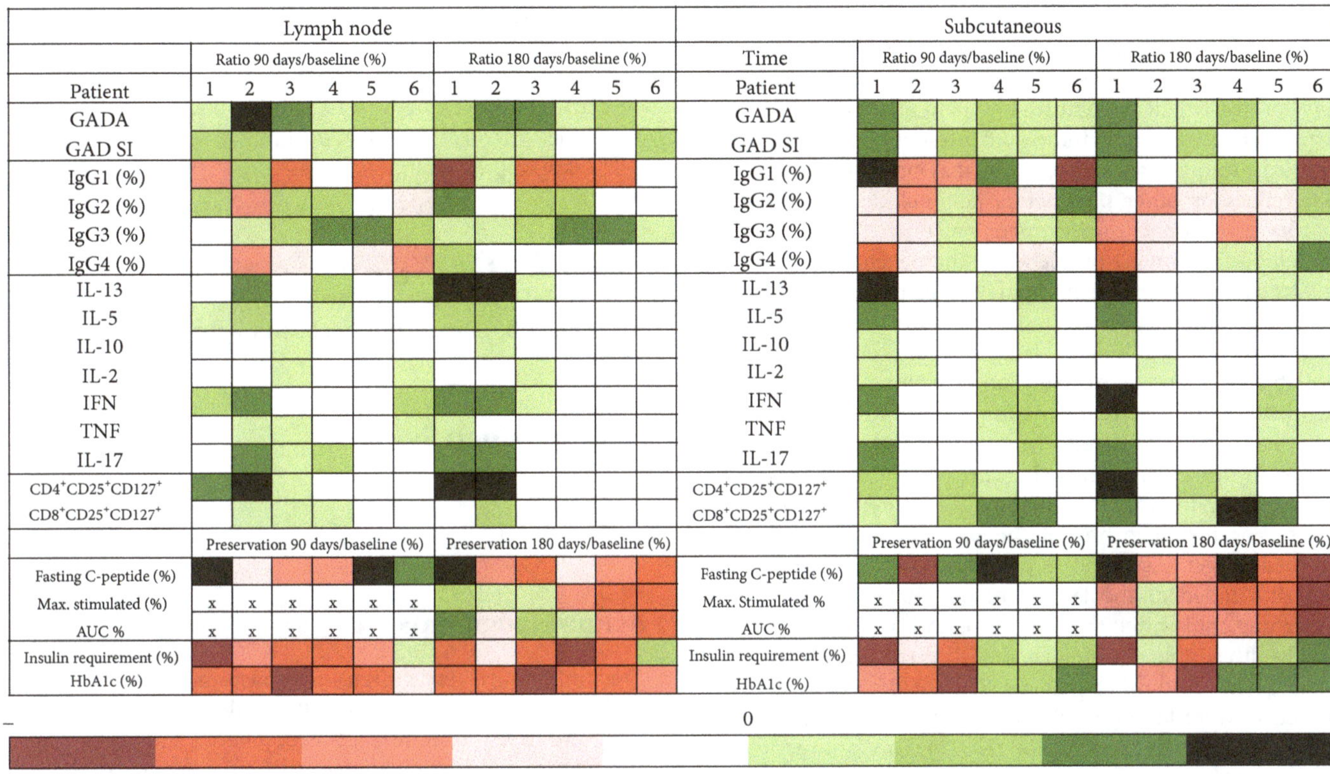

Figure 5: Heat map representing the immunological changes induced by GAD-alum treatment. Variations were calculated as the ratio of the values at 90 and 180 days with respect to the baseline. Patients received GAD-alum injections into the lymph nodes (LNs, $n = 6$) or subcutaneously (SC, $n = 6$), and they were stratified from left to right according to their clinical outcome at 180 days. Clinical variables are expressed as percentage of change from baseline (%). At 90 days, max. stimulated, and AUC C-peptide were not calculated, as meal tolerance tests were not performed, and are represented by "×". The color scales illustrate the posttreatment increase (green) or decrease (red) of variables in relation to baseline values.

to observe a high increase of IgG2 that has been described to correlate with IgG4 responses to tetanus vaccine in autoantibody negative children, and both subclasses correlated with IL-4 and IL-13 secretion [38]. The fact that both subclasses were not detectable or were very low in autoantibody-positive children in the same study was interpreted as a reduced capacity to mount Th2-associated responses in prediabetic children. The effect of SC administration of GAD-alum observed in the few patients included in this study is in line with the results from previous GAD-alum trials, where we observed only a transient increase of IgG3 and IgG4 and a reduction of IgG1 after SC administration of 2 doses of the same concentration [26, 28].

Based on the general consensus that T1D is due to the lack of tolerance and the involvement of autoreactive T cells, it has been expected that efficacy of immunotherapy with autoantigens should be accompanied by the induction of tolerance. Here, we observe that immune responses in individuals with better clinical outcome after LN injections were characterized by rise in the GADA levels, lower proliferation, and predominant Th2-like responses, supported by increase in IL-13 and shift of IgG subclasses. Although the direction of the immune responses to GAD_{65} was Th2 skewed in the LN group, there were however large interindividual differences. Strikingly, GAD_{65}-induced cytokines were detected in the LN group after 180 days solely in patients with the best clinical outcome. It could be argued that lack of T cell responses might be due to failure of injections into the lymph node. However, the GADA enhancement in those patients suggests that this explanation is less likely. It was particularly interesting that patients displaying a better clinical outcome were characterized by GAD-induced T cell responses deviated towards a Th2 cytokine profile, both after SC and LN treatments. We have shown that SC injection of 2 doses of GAD-alum induced a broad cytokine secretion that switched towards a more predominant Th2-associated profile over time [28]. Administration of further SC doses in the phase III study increased the secretion levels but did not affect the quality of the cytokine response, and cytokine profile was similar in patients receiving 2 or 4 doses of GAD-alum [28]. Thus, a different cytokine secretion profile after the third LN injection cannot be explained by an extra dose but rather by the administration route. Intralymphatic administration delivers more antigen to the site of immune response induction [39], and the difference in antigen dose available for stimulation of antigen-specific T cells may also lead to increased Th2 response. The adjuvant aluminum effect is associated with the induction of Th2 responses [40] and preferentially induces humoral rather than cellular immune responses. Therefore, alum has been the adjuvant of choice to minimize the possibility of promoting β-cell-mediated destruction together with GAD_{65}. We could not identify any pretreatment signature for patients who responded better. However, each individual presented unique clinical and immunological features, and it is possible that modest differences or other parameters not included in this study can have an impact on treatment outcome.

One of the main problems in the development of T1D treatment has been the extrapolation of results from animal models to humans, proven to be more difficult and less accurate than expected. Indeed, besides patient heterogeneity, the possible interference of many other factors as infections or medication during treatment might be more relevant than what has been considered when looking at the effect at group levels. In this open trial, we had the possibility to dissect the events along treatment and made some interesting observations. For instance, one of the patients in the LN group seemed to get a specific response to GAD_{65} after 90 days but that faded at the later control. That patient reported recurrent colds after the 90-day period and antihistaminic and health supplement intake, as well as the use of corticosteroid cream. Two other patients without detectable cytokine secretion were taking antihistaminic pills, and one of them even antidepressive medication. No concomitant medication of any type was reported for the patient responding clinically best and who displayed the strongest treatment-associated immunological changes. We have recently shown that H1N1 vaccination might have had an impact on the outcome of the phase III trial and that signs of possible vaccine interference were observed far beyond the time period during which concomitant vaccinations, excluding influenza, were forbidden in the trial [11]. Thus perhaps, it is reasonable to consider whether failure of reaching differences in placebo-controlled trials must immediately lead to treatments disregard. A beneficial effect in some patients might be good enough to support the use of the agent alone or in combination with other agents, in efforts to tailor treatment for each patient. Our results highlight the relevance of this kind of small pilot trials in treatment development, as they can give faster insight in many unsolved questions and help to speed experimental treatment modalities towards successful clinical use.

5. Conclusion

Intralymphatic administration of autoantigen in T1D might represent a promising therapeutic approach to increase the efficacy of autoantigen immunotherapy, although our observations are based on a small number of patients and have to be interpreted cautiously. Whether the immunological changes associated with clinical efficacy observed in the participants in this pilot trial might be regarded as a favorable immune outcome must be addressed in future larger double-blind studies. Nevertheless, results from small pilot trials are needed to test new approaches before the initiation of full-scale, randomized, controlled trials.

Disclosure

The current address of Johnny Ludvigsson is Division of Pediatrics, Department of Clinical and Experimental Medicine, Medical Faculty of Linköping University, 581 85 Linköping, Sweden.

Conflicts of Interest

No conflict of interest was declared by the authors.

Authors' Contributions

Johnny Ludvigsson and Rosaura Casas contributed equally to this work.

Acknowledgments

The authors are very grateful for Joachim Davidsson for his skillful performance of the needle-guided lymph node injections and to research nurses Sofia Sjöberg (Endocrine Clinic) and Anette Nilsson (Pediatric Clinic), University Hospital Linköping, for taking care of the patients. Ingela Johansson, Gosia Smolinska, and Claudia Matzke are thanked for their skillful laboratory work. The authors would like to address the technical support from the flow cytometry core facility unit of the Faculty of Medicine and Health Sciences. The study has been generously supported by Barndiabetesfonden (Swedish Child Diabetes Foundation), Diabetesfonden (Swedish Diabetes Foundation), and an unrestricted grant from Diamyd Medical.

Supplementary Materials

Table S1: baseline clinical and immunological parameters in the patients who received GAD-alum injections into the lymph nodes (LNs, $n = 6$) or subcutaneously (SC, $n = 6$). Table S2: clinical and immunological parameters at 90 and 180 days in the patients who received GAD-alum injections into the lymph nodes (LNs, $n = 6$) or subcutaneously (SC, $n = 6$). Figure S1: protocol of the GAD-alum treatment. Figure S2: GADA IgG1–4 subclasses expressed as arbitrary units (AU) in follow-up serum samples. (A) Lymph node patients and (B) subcutaneous vaccination. Figure S3: median levels of IL-13, IL-5, IL-10, IL-2, IL-17, TNF-α, and IFN-γ (pg/ml) at baseline, 90, and 180 days in lymph node (LN, black circles, $n = 6$) and subcutaneous (SC, white circles, $n = 6$) GAD-alum patients. Figure S4: median values of proliferative responses to GAD65 and CD3/CD28 beads in GAD-alum patients at baseline, 90, and 180 days. Figure S5: flow cytometry gating strategy. Figure S6: change of differentiation state (%) of $CD4^+$ and $CD8^+$ T cells in lymph node (LN, $n = 6$, black circles) and subcutaneous (SC, $n = 6$, white circles) GAD-alum patients. *(Supplementary Materials)*

References

[1] N. C. Schloot, G. Meierhoff, C. Lengyel et al., "Effect of heat shock protein peptide DiaPep277 on beta-cell function in paediatric and adult patients with recent-onset diabetes mellitus type 1: two prospective, randomized, double-blind phase II trials," *Diabetes/Metabolism Research and Reviews*, vol. 23, no. 4, pp. 276–285, 2007.

[2] B. Keymeulen, E. Vandemeulebroucke, A. G. Ziegler et al., "Insulin needs after CD3-antibody therapy in new-onset type 1 diabetes," *New England Journal of Medicine*, vol. 352, no. 25, pp. 2598–2608, 2005.

[3] K. C. Herold, W. Hagopian, J. A. Auger et al., "Anti-CD3 monoclonal antibody in new-onset type 1 diabetes mellitus," *New England Journal of Medicine*, vol. 346, no. 22, pp. 1692–1698, 2002.

[4] M. D. Pescovitz, C. J. Greenbaum, H. Krause-Steinrauf et al., "Rituximab, B-lymphocyte depletion, and preservation of beta-cell function," *New England Journal of Medicine*, vol. 361, no. 22, pp. 2143–2152, 2009.

[5] T. Orban, B. Bundy, D. J. Becker et al., "Co-stimulation modulation with abatacept in patients with recent-onset type 1 diabetes: a randomised, double-blind, placebo-controlled trial," *The Lancet*, vol. 378, no. 9789, pp. 412–419, 2011.

[6] P. Pozzilli, D. Pitocco, N. Visalli et al., "No effect of oral insulin on residual beta-cell function in recent-onset type I diabetes (the IMDIAB VII). IMDIAB group," *Diabetologia*, vol. 43, no. 8, pp. 1000–1004, 2000.

[7] M. Walter, A. Philotheou, F. Bonnici, A.-G. Ziegler, R. Jimenez, and on behalf of the NBI-6024 Study Group, "No effect of the altered peptide ligand NBI-6024 on beta-cell residual function and insulin needs in new-onset type 1 diabetes," *Diabetes Care*, vol. 32, no. 11, pp. 2036–2040, 2009.

[8] J. Ludvigsson, M. Faresjö, M. Hjorth et al., "GAD treatment and insulin secretion in recent-onset type 1 diabetes," *New England Journal of Medicine*, vol. 359, no. 18, pp. 1909–1920, 2008.

[9] D. K. Wherrett, B. Bundy, D. J. Becker et al., "Antigen-based therapy with glutamic acid decarboxylase (GAD) vaccine in patients with recent-onset type 1 diabetes: a randomised double-blind trial," *The Lancet*, vol. 378, no. 9788, pp. 319–327, 2011.

[10] J. Ludvigsson, D. Krisky, R. Casas et al., "GAD65 antigen therapy in recently diagnosed type 1 diabetes mellitus," *New England Journal of Medicine*, vol. 366, no. 5, pp. 433–442, 2012.

[11] B. Tavira, M. Cheramy, S. Axelsson, L. Akerman, J. Ludvigsson, and R. Casas, "Effect of simultaneous vaccination with H1N1 and GAD-alum on GAD65-induced immune response," *Diabetologia*, vol. 60, no. 7, pp. 1276–1283, 2017.

[12] C. A. Beam, the Type 1 Diabetes TrialNet Study Group, C. MacCallum et al., "GAD vaccine reduces insulin loss in recently diagnosed type 1 diabetes: findings from a Bayesian meta-analysis," *Diabetologia*, vol. 60, no. 1, pp. 43–49, 2017.

[13] O. Pfaar, C. Bachert, A. Bufe et al., "Guideline on allergen-specific immunotherapy in IgE-mediated allergic diseases," *Allergo Journal International*, vol. 23, no. 8, pp. 282–319, 2014.

[14] S. Dhami, U. Nurmatov, G. B. Pajno et al., "Allergen immunotherapy for IgE-mediated food allergy: protocol for a systematic review," *Clinical and Translational Allergy*, vol. 6, no. 1, p. 24, 2016.

[15] S. Tsabouri, A. Mavroudi, G. Feketea, and G. V. Guibas, "Subcutaneous and sublingual immunotherapy in allergic asthma in children," *Frontiers in Pediatrics*, vol. 5, p. 82, 2017.

[16] Y. Chelladurai, C. Suarez-Cuervo, N. Erekosima et al., "Effectiveness of subcutaneous versus sublingual immunotherapy for the treatment of allergic rhinoconjunctivitis and asthma: a systematic review," *The Journal of Allergy and Clinical Immunology: In Practice*, vol. 1, no. 4, pp. 361–369, 2013.

[17] K. J. Maloy, I. Erdmann, V. Basch et al., "Intralymphatic immunization enhances DNA vaccination," *Proceedings of the National Academy of Sciences*, vol. 98, no. 6, pp. 3299–3303, 2001.

[18] G. Senti, B. M. Prinz Vavricka, I. Erdmann et al., "Intralymphatic allergen administration renders specific immunotherapy faster and safer: a randomized controlled trial," *Proceedings of the National Academy of Sciences*, vol. 105, no. 46, pp. 17908–17912, 2008.

[19] A. M. Patterson, A. E. Bonny, W. E. Shiels II, and E. A. Erwin, "Three-injection intralymphatic immunotherapy in adolescents and young adults with grass pollen rhinoconjunctivitis," *Annals of Allergy, Asthma & Immunology*, vol. 116, no. 2, pp. 168–170, 2016.

[20] T. Hylander, O. Larsson, U. Petersson-Westin et al., "Intralymphatic immunotherapy of pollen-induced rhinoconjunctivitis: a double-blind placebo-controlled trial," *Respiratory Research*, vol. 17, no. 1, p. 10, 2016.

[21] G. Senti, R. Crameri, D. Kuster et al., "Intralymphatic immunotherapy for cat allergy induces tolerance after only 3 injections," *Journal of Allergy and Clinical Immunology*, vol. 129, no. 5, pp. 1290–1296, 2012.

[22] A. Mackensen, T. Krause, U. Blum, P. Uhrmeister, R. Mertelsmann, and A. Lindemann, "Homing of intravenously and intralymphatically injected human dendritic cells generated in vitro from $CD34^+$ hematopoietic progenitor cells," *Cancer Immunology, Immunotherapy*, vol. 48, no. 2-3, pp. 118–122, 1999.

[23] P. Johansen, A. . C. Häffner, F. Koch et al., "Direct intralymphatic injection of peptide vaccines enhances immunogenicity," *European Journal of Immunology*, vol. 35, no. 2, pp. 568–574, 2005.

[24] J. Ludvigsson, J. Wahlberg, and R. Casas, "Intralymphatic injection of autoantigen in type 1 diabetes," *New England Journal of Medicine*, vol. 376, no. 7, pp. 697–699, 2017.

[25] J. Ludvigsson, B. Tavira, and R. Casas, "More on intralymphatic injection of autoantigen in type 1 diabetes," *New England Journal of Medicine*, vol. 377, no. 4, pp. 403–405, 2017.

[26] M. Cheramy, C. Skoglund, I. Johansson, J. Ludvigsson, C. S. Hampe, and R. Casas, "GAD-alum treatment in patients with type 1 diabetes and the subsequent effect on GADA IgG subclass distribution, GAD65 enzyme activity and humoral response," *Clinical Immunology*, vol. 137, no. 1, pp. 31–40, 2010.

[27] E. Bonifacio, M. Scirpoli, K. Kredel, M. Füchtenbusch, and A. G. Ziegler, "Early autoantibody responses in prediabetes are IgG1 dominated and suggest antigen-specific regulation," *Journal of Immunology*, vol. 163, no. 1, pp. 525–532, 1999.

[28] S. Axelsson, M. Cheramy, L. Akerman, M. Pihl, J. Ludvigsson, and R. Casas, "Cellular and humoral immune responses in type 1 diabetic patients participating in a phase III GAD-alum intervention trial," *Diabetes Care*, vol. 36, no. 11, pp. 3418–3424, 2013.

[29] S. Axelsson, M. Chéramy, M. Hjorth et al., "Long-lasting immune responses 4 years after GAD-alum treatment in children with type 1 diabetes," *PLoS One*, vol. 6, no. 12, article e29008, 2011.

[30] L. C. Harrison, M. C. Honeyman, C. E. Steele et al., "Pancreatic beta-cell function and immune responses to insulin after administration of intranasal insulin to humans at risk for type 1 diabetes," *Diabetes Care*, vol. 27, no. 10, pp. 2348–2355, 2004.

[31] M. A. Russell, A. C. Cooper, S. Dhayal, and N. G. Morgan, "Differential effects of interleukin-13 and interleukin-6 on Jak/STAT signaling and cell viability in pancreatic β-cells," *Islets*, vol. 5, no. 2, pp. 95–105, 2013.

[32] L. Usero, A. Sánchez, E. Pizarro et al., "Interleukin-13 pathway alterations impair invariant natural killer T-cell-mediated regulation of effector T cells in type 1 diabetes," *Diabetes*, vol. 65, no. 8, pp. 2356–2366, 2016.

[33] K. J. Wood and B. Sawitzki, "Interferon gamma: a crucial role in the function of induced regulatory T cells in vivo," *Trends in Immunology*, vol. 27, no. 4, pp. 183–187, 2006.

[34] J. Fenimore and H. A. Young, "Regulation of IFN-γ expression," *Advances in Experimental Medicine and Biology*, vol. 941, pp. 1–19, 2016.

[35] M. Pihl, H. Barcenilla, S. Axelsson et al., "GAD-specific T cells are induced by GAD-alum treatment in type-1 diabetes patients," *Clinical Immunology*, vol. 176, pp. 114–121, 2017.

[36] M. Hjorth, S. Axelsson, A. Ryden, M. Faresjo, J. Ludvigsson, and R. Casas, "GAD-alum treatment induces GAD65-specific $CD4^{+}CD25^{high}FOXP3^{+}$ cells in type 1 diabetic patients," *Clinical Immunology*, vol. 138, no. 1, pp. 117–126, 2011.

[37] M. Pihl, L. Åkerman, S. Axelsson et al., "Regulatory T cell phenotype and function 4 years after GAD-alum treatment in children with type 1 diabetes," *Clinical & Experimental Immunology*, vol. 172, no. 3, pp. 394–402, 2013.

[38] S. Schmid, A. Molteni, M. Fuchtenbusch, H. E. Naserke, A. G. Ziegler, and E. Bonifacio, "Reduced IL-4 associated antibody responses to vaccine in early pre-diabetes," *Diabetologia*, vol. 45, no. 5, pp. 677–685, 2002.

[39] J. M. Martinez-Gomez, P. Johansen, I. Erdmann, G. Senti, R. Crameri, and T. M. Kundig, "Intralymphatic injections as a new administration route for allergen-specific immunotherapy," *International Archives of Allergy and Immunology*, vol. 150, no. 1, pp. 59–65, 2009.

[40] J. M. Brewer, M. Conacher, C. A. Hunter, M. Mohrs, F. Brombacher, and J. Alexander, "Aluminium hydroxide adjuvant initiates strong antigen-specific Th2 responses in the absence of IL-4- or IL-13-mediated signaling," *Journal of Immunology*, vol. 163, no. 12, pp. 6448–6454, 1999.

19

The Coincidence of Newly Diagnosed Type 1 Diabetes Mellitus with IgM Antibody Positivity to Enteroviruses and Respiratory Tract Viruses

Murat Karaoglan[1] and **Fahriye Eksi**[2]

[1]*Division of Pediatric Endocrinology, Gaziantep University Faculty of Medicine, Gaziantep, Turkey*
[2]*Department of Medical Microbiology, Gaziantep University Faculty of Medicine, Gaziantep, Turkey*

Correspondence should be addressed to Murat Karaoglan; muratkaraoglan@gantep.edu.tr

Academic Editor: Marco Songini

Objective. Viruses trigger and promote islet cell destruction and cause type 1 diabetes mellitus (T1DM). However, the existence of a cause-and-effect relationship is under debate. The aim of this study is to investigate the sero-epidemiological and molecular evidence on enteroviruses and respiratory viruses in patients with newly diagnosed T1DM during the cold season. *Design.* Forty children newly diagnosed with T1DM and 30 healthy children who presented to the clinic over the course of a year were included in the study. The IgM antibodies against enteroviruses and respiratory viruses were studied using the indirect immunofluorescence assay (IFA) test, and no CBV4-specific RNA was detected in the children. The onset times of T1DM were classified into fall-winter and spring-summer seasons and separated into cold, moderate, or warm months in terms of temperature. *Results.* The percentages of viral IgM antibodies against most common viruses were detected in the patients as follows: influenza B (IVB) (70%), echovirus 7 (ECHO7) (45%), parainfluenza virus 4 (PIV4) (40%), coxsackievirus A7 (CAV7) (27.5%), and H3N2 (22.5%). Compared with the control group, the above viruses had a significant association with T1DM ($p \leq 0.001$, $p \leq 0.001$, $p = 0.035$, $p = 0.003$, and $p = 0.023$, resp.). CBV4-specific RNA was not detected in any serum. A total of 75% and 95% patients were diagnosed with T1DM in the fall-winter seasons and cold-moderate months, respectively. *Conclusion.* Our study demonstrates the significant association between T1DM and the presence of IgM antibodies against IVB, ECHO7, PIV4, CAV7, and H3N2, and the majority of newly diagnosed T1DM appeared in the fall-winter season. It suggests that enteroviruses and respiratory viruses, in addition to seasonal variation, could play a role in the etiopathogenesis and clinical onset of T1DM.

1. Introduction

Many studies in recent decades have determined that enteroviruses (EV), in particular, and respiratory viruses play a role in the pathogenesis of type 1 diabetes (T1DM) [1–3]. Respiratory viruses share common clinical and pathological characteristics with enteroviruses. These viruses can grow in either the respiratory or intestinal tract. Most enteroviruses exhibit tropism to islet cells. In experimental and epidemiologic studies, it has been shown that influenza viruses can affect islet cells [4, 5]. Moreover, viruses lead to beta cell destruction through indirect or direct pathways [6, 7]. These patterns are known as T1a (autoimmune) and T1b (nonimmune or cytopathic).

The onset time of T1DM exhibits seasonal variations [8]. The seasonal pattern coincides with the typical influenza season seen during the fall and winter season [4, 9]. In addition, the incidence of T1DM has been demonstrated to increase during the aftermath of outbreaks of influenza and mumps [10]. Likewise, many viruses, including respiratory viruses and enteroviruses, lead to beta cell destruction after recurrent, cumulative, and prolonged chronic inflammation with a "multiple hit" of viruses. The onset of T1DM appears by means of a "final hit" of viruses after a long unapparent process [11]. Moreover, mixed viruses trigger and potentiate each other during the process of target tissue damage [12].

T1DM is one of the most chronic and dysmetabolic childhood disorders, resulting from an interaction between the host immune system and heterogeneous environmental factors in the polygenic background [7]. Numerous longitudinal, epidemiological, animal, and human modeling studies have been conducted using sero-epidemiological, molecular, and pathological evidence, indicating that viruses are strongly linked with T1DM [6, 7].

Gut microbiota is actively involved in the interplay between the host immune system and islet destruction [13]. In support of this idea, many studies have been documented in recent decades that have related the alteration in gut microbiota to a pathological process, leading to autoimmune diabetes [14]. In addition, a prospective study showed that a sibling of a child newly diagnosed with T1DM who was EV-seropositive developed T1DM after intrafamilial transmission of EV [15].

The present study, the first to include seasonal variations in Turkey, has been designed to investigate the association between T1DM and multiple EV and respiratory tract viruses, which are postulated to be diabetogenic viruses.

2. Materials and Methods

The study was carried out retrospectively. The medical records of children who were newly diagnosed with T1DM between September 2013 and October 2014 in Gaziantep Province, Southeast Turkey, were collected. We included 40 children aged 1–16 years (mean age = ±3.85 years) who were newly diagnosed with T1DM and 30 healthy children who had presented to pediatric policlinics during the same period. The one-year period was classified into two groups to determine time variations in the spread of a virus: group 1 = fall/winter (September to February) and spring/summer (March to August) and group 2 = cold months (November, December, January, and February), moderate months (September, October, March, and April), and warm months (May, June, July, and August). In respect of temperature and climate, seasons and months were classified according to the Köppen-Geiger climate classification for Gaziantep Province [16]. The DMS latitude and longitude coordinates for Gaziantep are 37°03′33.98″N and 37°22′57.00″E, respectively. Type C climate is dominant in Gaziantep.

T1DM was diagnosed using the following criteria: history of polyuria and/or polydipsia, blood glucose above 200 mg/dL, low insulin and C-peptide level, glycated hemoglobin A1C (HbA1C) above 6.5%, and insulin dependency. Blood was drawn from patients with newly diagnosed T1DM for the following assays: glutamic acid decarboxylase antibodies (GADA), islet cell antibodies (ICA), and insulin autoantibodies (IAA), routinely. GADA and ICA levels were classified into three groups: (1) the low group included GADA levels of 0–19 U/mL and ICA levels of 1 : 10 titer, (2) the moderate group included GADA levels of 20–199 U/mL and ICA levels of 1 : 32 titer, and (3) the high group included GADA levels of 100 U/mL or higher and ICA levels of 1 : 100 titer. The control group consisted of nonobese and nonoverweight healthy children whose viral IgM antibodies had been studied. We recorded the dates when the blood samples were drawn. One healthy child was chosen for every patient in the same month. If more than five patients were included in the same month, a maximum of five children were chosen for the control group.

The following viruses were studied in every child in the study and control groups: influenza virus A (H1N1, H3N2), with respect to the Köppen-Geiger climate classification for Gaziantep Province [16]. Influenza virus B (IVB); parainfluenza viruses 1, 2, 3, and 4 (PIV1, PIV2, PIV3, and PIV4); adenovirus 3 (AdV3); respiratory syncytial virus (RSV); echovirus 7 (ECHO7), coxsackievirus A7 (CAV7); and coxsackievirus B1 IgM antibodies and coxsackievirus B4 RNA were investigated using PCR. Serum samples were drawn within 1–19 days of admission (mean 6.04 ± 4.32) and stored at −80°C until analysis. Virus IgM antibodies were analyzed with respiratory tract profile 1 kits (Euroimmun, Germany) using the indirect immunofluorescence assay (IFA) test.

We used the composition of the Euroimmun IF kit (FI 2821-1001-1 G "respiratory tract profile 1" IgG field A: verification BIOCHIP). IgM antibodies were studied against the following viruses in the respiratory tract profile kit: RSV, adenovirus type 3, influenza virus type A (H1N1 and H3N2), influenza virus type B, parainfluenza virus types [1–4], echo virus type 7, and coxsackievirus types B1 and A7.

The test procedure was as follows: the fluorescence uptake of the infected cells used as a substrate is observed in all parts of the cell in the case of being positive in pathogen substrates. Positive cytoplasmic fluorescence is seen in viral substrates. The results are reported as "positive" or "negative" according to the fluorescence composition of the infected cells seen in the fluorescence microscope. The dilution ratios that are positive for each viral IgM antibody are given in Table 1. We did not study the IgG antibody against viruses. As this study is limited to viruses, the bacterial IgM antibody results were not given. The RNA extraction process was shown as follows: RNA was extracted using the RNA Purification Kit (Thermo Scientific, Vilnius, Lithuania). RNA templates were mixed in a 50 μL multiplex reaction consisting of 1x buffer, 1.5 mM magnesium chloride (MgCl), 0.2 M deoxynucleotide triphosphate (dNTP) (Thermo Scientific, Lithuania), and 0.4 pmol and 1.25 U Taq polymerase of each primer (Thermo Scientific, Lithuania). The primers and probes of the viral protein (VP1) and VP2 genes of enterovirus were used for enterovirus PCR. As we did not detect any CBV4-specific RNA, RNA sequence analysis was not conducted for CVB4.

This study was approved by the Gaziantep University Clinical Research Ethics Committee (reference number: 387/2017; date: 27 November 2017) for three months. Written informed consent was obtained from the parents/legal guardian of the eligible children before recruitment.

3. Statistics

Descriptive statistics, such as mean, standard deviation, and frequency distributions, were used to compare the two groups. A chi-square test was used to compare the presence

TABLE 1: Serum titer, if positivity is considered for each virus.

Respiratory tract profile 1	Dilution rates (IgM)
Respiratory syncytial virus	
Adenovirus type 3	
Influenza virus type A (H1N1)	1:10
Influenza virus type A (H3N2)	
Influenza virus type B	
Parainfluenza type 1	
Parainfluenza type 2	1:10
Parainfluenza type 3	
Parainfluenza type 4	1:100
Coxsackievirus type B1	
Coxsackievirus type A7	1:10
ECHO 7	

of viral agents in the patient and control groups. The results were evaluated at a 95% significance level ($p < 0.05$). Statistical analyses were calculated using the Statistical Package for the Social Sciences (SPSS) for Windows version 22.0 pocket program (IBM Corp., Armonk, NY).

4. Results

The characteristics of all the participating children at the onset of the newly diagnosed T1DM are shown in Table 2. The study group consisted of 23 boys (57.5%) and 17 girls (42.5%). Six children were Syrian refugees. Seven patients (17%) were younger than three years old. A total of 55% of patients had clinical signs of diabetic ketoacidosis at the onset of T1DM. Two of the patients with newly diagnosed T1DM were classmates who were diagnosed with T1DM in the same month. Both classmates were from the city of Kilis on the border of Gaziantep Province. They were eight years old. The second case presented to our clinic two weeks after the first case. The two children had been admitted with signs of diabetic ketoacidosis in December 2013, and they had also IgM positivity against the same virus profiles (Table 3). Both of the classmates had antiviral IgM antibodies against CAV7, ECHO7, and IVB. In addition, two siblings were admitted to the hospital with diagnosed diabetic ketoacidosis in the same month. Two siblings were admitted with newly diagnosed T1DM in November 2014. One of them was 2 years old, and the other was 10 years old. The boy who was 2 years old was diagnosed with T1DM three weeks after his brother. They had also the same viral IgM antibody (Table 3). The two siblings had antiviral IgM antibodies against IVB, PIV4, and CAV7.

The distribution of patients according to season and month is shown in Figures 1 and 2. Thirty patients (75%) were diagnosed in the fall-winter season. The distribution of patients according to month of admission was as follows: October = 7, November = 9, December = 9, January = 3, February = 2, March = 4, April = 4, and May = 2. No patients with newly diagnosed T1DM were admitted in June, July, August, or September. While there was a significant association between high GADA levels and CBV4-seropositive

TABLE 2: Characteristics of the children in the study and control groups.

	T1DM ($n = 40$)	Control group ($n = 30$)
Onset age[&] (years), mean ± SD	8.17 ± 3.85	7.50 ± 4.28
Boys/girls (n)	23/17	19/11
History of T1DM in the classmate or family of the proband (n)	2	
Glucose (mg/dL), mean ± SD	472.63 ± 194.16	87.45 ± 17.34
HbA1c (%)	10.59 ± 2.52	4.7 ± 0.78
Day of admission**	6.04 ± 4.32	
C-peptide	0.32 ± 0.21	
Ketoacidosis, n/%	22/55	
Thyroid antibodies (n) at onset	3 cases	
Celiac antibodies (n) at onset	1 case	
Patients (n) in year		
2013	15	10
2014	25	20
Patients (n) in season		
Fall-winter	30	21
Spring-summer	10	9
Patients (n) in months		
Cold	23	19
Moderate	15	10
Warm	2	1
Islet antibodies, n/%		
GADA	35/87.5	—
ICA	28/70	—
IAA	19/47.5	—
Number of islet antibodies, n/%		
Any	3/7.5	1/3.3
One	7/17.5	
Two	15/37.5	
Three	15/37.5	

[&]At the same time. n: number of cases—both classmates and siblings. **Blood samples drawn.

patients ($p = 0.019$), high ICA levels were found, significantly more often in IVB- and ECHO7-seropositive patients ($p = 0.006$ and $p = 0.007$, resp.).

The distribution (n) of IgM seropositivity for each virus is shown in Table 3. In terms of comparing the control group with the study group, the most common virus seropositivity and percentages were as follows: IVB (70%), ECHO7 (45%), PIV4 (40%), CAV7 (27.5%), and influenza virus A H3N2 (22.5%). We found that there was a significant association between the IgM seropositivity of these viruses and T1DM, with respect to the control group. Whereas only three patients (10%) had a dual mixed viral IgM antibody in the control group, 24 patients (60%) in the study group had multiple (two or more) viral IgM seropositivity, concurrently.

The incidence of viral IgM seropositivity according to season and month is shown in Figures 1 and 2. In the

Table 3: Distribution of positive antiviral IgM antibodies in the study and control groups.

	Study group ($n = 40$)		Control group ($n = 30$)		
	Positive n (%)	Negative n (%)	Positive n (%)	Negative n (%)	p
Influenza A					
H1N1	0	40 (100)	0	30 (100)	
H3N2	9 (22.5)	31 (77.5)	1 (3.3)	29 (96.7)	0.023*
Influenza B	28 (70)	12 (30)	8 (26.7)	22 (73.3)	≤0.001*
Parainfluenza					
PIV1	No	40 (100)	No	30 (100)	
PIV2	1 (2.5)	39 (97.5)	1 (3.3)	29 (96.7)	0.836
PIV3	No	40 (100)	No	30 (100)	
PIV4	16 (40)	24 (60)	5 (16.7)	25 (83.3)	0.035*
Coxsackievirus					
CVB1	3 (7.5)	37 (92.5)	No	30 (100)	
CAV7	11 (27.5)	29 (72.5)	No	30 (100)	0.003*
ECHO7	18 (45)	22 (55)	1 (3.3)	29 (96.7)	≤0.001*
AdV3	3 (7.5)	37 (92.5)	No	30 (100)	0.125
RSV	2 (5)	38 (95)	1 (3.3)	39 (96.7)	0.733
Any IgM Ab	—	3 (7.5)	—	20 (66.6)	0.002*
One IgM Ab	13 (32.5)	—	7 (23.3)	—	
Mix IgM Ab					
Two	11 (27.5)	—	3 (10)	—	
Three*	6 (15)	—	No	—	
Four	4 (10)	—	No	—	
Five	3 (7.5)	—	No	—	

PIV: parainfluenza; CVB: coxsackievirus B; CAV7: coxsackievirus A7; AdV3: adenovirus 3. *Classmates had the same viral IgM antibodies against viruses: CAV7, ECHO7, and IVB, and siblings had the same viral IgM antibodies against viruses: IVB, PIV4, and CAV7.

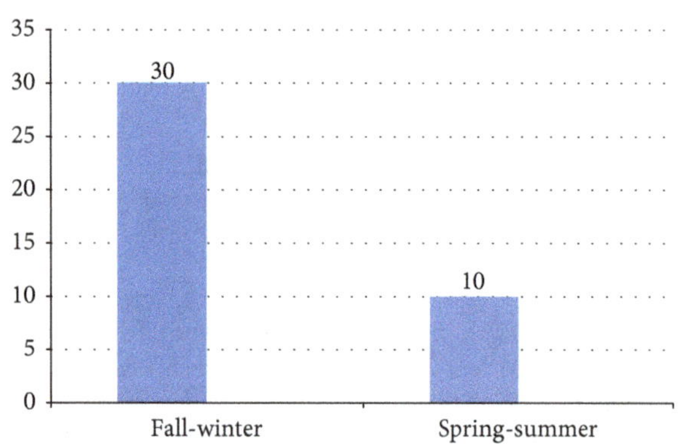

Figure 1: The distribution of patients newly diagnosed with T1DM (n) in each season.

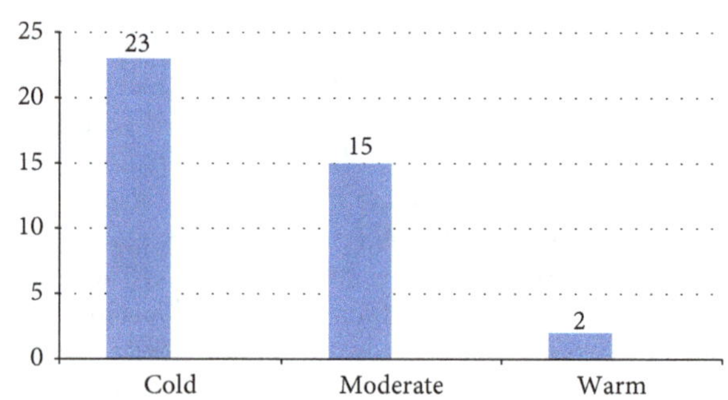

Figure 2: The distribution patients newly diagnosed with T1DM (n) in each month group.

study group, 75.5% of IgM viral seropositivity was detected in the fall-winter season. In addition to this, 90.1% of viruses were detected in the cold or moderate months. No child in the study group or control group had CBV4 RNA in their serum. In patients with IgM seropositivity of two or more, the mean GADA level (540 ± 718.34) was higher than that in patients with IgM seropositivity of one (mean 63.1 ± 73.39) ($p = 0.02$).

5. Discussion

The present study demonstrates that the time of the onset of newly diagnosed T1DM coincided with the fall-winter season, which is the typical season for respiratory tract viruses, and T1DM patients had an association with respiratory viruses and enteroviruses including IVB, ECHO7, PIV4, CAV7, and H3N2 at the clinical onset. These results indicate that enteroviruses and respiratory tract viruses, in addition to seasonal variation, could play a role in the etiopathogenesis and clinical onset of T1DM.

The incidence of T1DM, as well as of other autoimmune diseases, has been steadily increasing around the world. The largest increase has been seen in developed Northern European countries, such as Finland. However, the worldwide increase is occurring too rapidly, which is explained simply by changes in the genetic pool of populations [17]. From an evolutionary perspective, the increasing incidence of T1DM in wealthy countries arises from rapid changes in environmental forces [18]. A strong immune system has developed in human species to ward off many infectious agents. This has simultaneously made it more susceptible to autoimmune diseases in highly hygienic environments [19]. The defective immune response activates the bystander autoreactive cytotoxic T lymphocyte, leading to inhibited immune tolerance. This defective immune reaction skews the T helper 2 response to T helper 1 [20, 21], thus triggering an autoimmune disorder, resulting in islet cell damage. In line with the present data, the cause of the increased incidence of T1DM suggests that it is a trade-off in protection against life-threatening viruses, including respiratory viruses and enteroviruses.

The clinical onset of T1DM exhibits seasonal variations [9]. T1DM usually appears in the fall-winter season, which is seen as the typical season for respiratory infections. Moreover, it has been shown that T1DM incidence increases in the aftermath of outbreaks of influenza, mumps, and rubella. As previously documented in epidemiological reports, our study similarly demonstrated that the majority of newly diagnosed cases of T1DM occurred in the fall-winter season (75%) and during the cold or moderate months (90.1%). In a study involving influenza data from the last 12 years in Turkey, it was reported that influenza viruses A and B repeated every year during the fall-winter season [22]. In the 2013-2014 seasons, while influenza virus A H3N2 (73.6%) and IVB (26.4%) were predominant, H1N1 was detected in only 2% of cases in Turkey [22]. Similarly, in our study, while IVB (70%) and H3N2 (22.5%) were more common, IgM antibodies against H1N1 were not found in the same season.

According to the data obtained from Gaziantep Children's Hospital during 2013-2014, 142 children were newly diagnosed with T1DM. Gaziantep Children's Hospital and Gaziantep University Medical Hospital have a high density of cases with T1DM and are located in the seventh biggest city in Turkey. Gaziantep has a population of 2 million. The study population consisted of patients not only from our own province but also from the surrounding area. This high frequency of patients newly diagnosed with T1DM is due largely to the number of Syrian pediatric patients in our region. According to the Turkish Statistical Institute (TSI), in 2014, the total population of Gaziantep was 1,889,466 and the total population in the 0–14 age bracket was 644,872. The calculated T1DM incidence based on this data was 28.2/105/year for Gaziantep City. In comparison, the incidence of T1DM for Diyarbakir, another large city in the same region, was 7.2/105/year in 2010. Approximately 46.3% of newly diagnosed patients are refugee children. Therefore, we suspect that this is the reason why our province's annual prevalence and incidence of T1DM are significantly higher than those of other provinces [17]. The majority of new T1DM cases diagnosed at Regional Children's Hospital also arose during the fall-winter season. In total, 84.6% of cases were diagnosed in the cold or moderate months during 2013-2014.

Compared with the control group, the IgM positivity to IVB, ECHO7, PIV4, CAV7, and H3N2 viruses in T1DM patients was statistically significant. There have been many studies investigating the relationship between enteroviruses, in particular CVB4 and T1DM [3]. In the present study, CBV4-specific RNA was not found in any blood sample in the patient or control groups. However, the number and type of viruses that cause infections can vary in each region. For example, in a previous study conducted in our country, CBV4 RNA was not detected in either the control or the study group [17].

The sibling of a proband patient and the classmate of another proband patient had the same seropositivity as their probands in the same months, strongly supporting the relationship between T1DM and viral etiology. In a prospective study investigating the intrafamilial spread of enteroviruses, siblings of seropositive patients newly diagnosed with T1DM were also studied at the time of the clinical onset in the proband. The same enterovirus seropositivity was then determined in those same siblings. Subsequently, one sibling was found to have islet antibody positivity, followed by T1DM [15].

It has been reported that multiple viruses, especially enteroviruses, can cause diabetes [23]. Enteroviruses and respiratory viruses growing via replicative cycles lead to progressive and persistent chronic inflammation in target tissues. We serologically detected IgM antibodies against a single virus in 32% ($n = 23$) and mixed viruses in 60% ($n = 24$) of the patients. Each patient had a mean virus seropositivity of 2.34. Correspondingly, it has been reported that mixed viruses can cause fulminant T1DM [4]. Mixed viruses that activate and impact each other can also aggravate the existing damage in target tissue. Likewise, replicative cycles that result in "multiple hits" lead to recurrent and cumulative inflammation in target tissues [1, 11]. When compared with patients with single seropositivity, we found a higher mean GADA in mixed seropositive patients. This finding indicates that multiple viruses may contribute to the exacerbation of damage to tissue. While respiratory viruses and enteroviruses accelerate pancreatic islet disruption by means of multiple hits, on the other hand, they also give rise to the clinical onset of T1DM.

This study is one of the few in Turkey to have investigated the association between T1DM and a large number of enteroviruses and respiratory viruses. At the same time, the diabetogenic effect of viruses on the etiopathogenesis of T1DM is still debated. Therefore, viral evidence indicating the potential for T1DM may be found during seasons when enteroviruses and respiratory viruses are prevalent. When the presence of a causative relationship between T1DM and respiratory viruses is proven, it could provide opportunities for new approaches to predicting, preventing, and treating T1DM.

6. Conclusion

In conclusion, this study demonstrated that newly diagnosed T1DM appears during the fall/winter season and during months when the temperature is cold or moderate and coincides with seropositivity for both respiratory viruses and enteroviruses including IVB, ECHO7, PIV4, CAV7, and H3N2 at the time of T1DM diagnosis. These results suggest that respiratory viruses and enteroviruses may play a diabetogenic role in addition to the seasonality of the onset of clinical manifestation of T1DM.

Consent

Written informed consent was obtained from the parents/legal guardian of the eligible children before recruitment.

Conflicts of Interest

The authors declare that they have no competing interests.

Authors' Contributions

Murat Karaoglan participated in the design of the study. Fahriye Eksi carried out the indirect immunofluorescence assay (IFA) test, investigated CBV RNA using PCR, and also performed the statistical analysis.

References

[1] M. Hiltunen, H. Hyöty, M. Knip et al., "Islet cell antibody seroconversion in children is temporally associated with enterovirus infections," *The Journal of Infectious Diseases*, vol. 175, no. 3, pp. 554–560, 1997.

[2] D. Hober, F. Sane, H. Jaïdane, K. Riedweg, A. Goffard, and R. Desailloud, "Immunology in the clinic review series; focus on type 1 diabetes and viruses: role of antibodies enhancing the infection with coxsackievirus-B in the pathogenesis of type 1 diabetes," *Clinical & Experimental Immunology*, vol. 168, no. 1, pp. 47–51, 2012.

[3] L. C. Stene and M. Rewers, "Immunology in the clinic review series; focus on type 1 diabetes and viruses: the enterovirus link to type 1 diabetes: critical review of human studies," *Clinical & Experimental Immunology*, vol. 168, no. 1, pp. 12–23, 2012.

[4] C. Valdés, N. Unanue, M. Hernández et al., "Is there a link between influenza and type I diabetes? Increased incidence of TID during the pandemic H1N1 influenza of 2009 in Chile," *Pediatric endocrinology reviews*, vol. 11, no. 2, pp. 161–166, 2013.

[5] I. Capua, A. Mercalli, M. S. Pizzuto et al., "Influenza A viruses grow in human pancreatic cells and cause pancreatitis and " diabetes in an animal model, *Journal of Virology*, vol. 87, no. 1, pp. 597–610, 2013.

[6] F. A. Grieco, G. Sebastiani, I. Spagnuolo, A. Patti, and F. Dotta, "Immunology in the clinic review series; focus on type 1diabetes and viruses: how viral infections modulate beta cell function," *Clinical & Experimental Immunology*, vol. 168, no. 1, pp. 24–29, 2012.

[7] R. S. Eringsmark and A. Lernmark, "The environment and the origins of islet autoimmunity and Type 1 diabetes," *Diabetic Medicine*, vol. 30, no. 2, pp. 155–160, 2013.

[8] C. C. Patterson, E. Gyürüs, and J. Rosenbaueretal, "Seasonal variation in month of diagnosis in children with type 1 diabetes registered in 23 European centers during 1989-2008: little short-term influence of sunshine hours or average temperature," *Pediatric Diabetes*, vol. 16, no. 8, pp. 573–580, 2015.

[9] M. I. Kalliora, A. Vazeou, D. Delis, E. Bozas, I. Thymelli, and C. S. Bartsocas, "Seasonal variation of type 1 diabetes mellitus diagnosis in Greek children," *Hormones*, vol. 10, no. 1, pp. 67–71, 2011.

[10] B. Piccini, S. Toni, L. Lenzi, M. Guasti, F. Barni, and M. De Martino, "Type 1 diabetes onset and pandemic influenza A (H1N1)," *International Journal of Immunopathology and Pharmacology*, vol. 25, no. 2, pp. 547–549, 2012.

[11] D. A. Schneider and M. G. von Herrath, "Viruses and type 1 diabetes: a dynamic labile equilibrium," *Diabetes Management*, vol. 3, no. 3, pp. 217–223, 2013.

[12] J. L. Waner, "Mixed viral infections: detection and management," *Clinical Microbiology Reviews*, vol. 7, no. 2, pp. 143–151, 1994.

[13] M. OutiVaarala, A. Atkinson, and J. Neu, "The "perfect storm" for type 1 diabetes: the complex interplay between intestinal microbiota, gut permeability, and mucosal immunity," *Diabetes*, vol. 57, no. 10, pp. 2555–2562, 2008.

[14] O. Vaarala, "Gut microbiota and type 1 diabetes," *The Review of Diabetic Studies*, vol. 9, no. 4, pp. 251–259, 2012.

[15] A. Salvatoni, A. Baj, G. Bianchi, G. Federico, M. Colombo, and A. Toniolo, "Intrafamilial spread of enterovirus infections at the clinical onset of type 1 diabetes," *Pediatric Diabetes*, vol. 14, no. 6, pp. 407–416, 2013.

[16] M. Z. Öztürk, G. Çetinkaya, and S. Aydın, "Climate types of Turkey according to Köppen-Geiger climate classification," *Journal of Geography*, vol. 35, pp. 17–27, 2017.

[17] Y. Çekin, E. Özkaya, H. Gülkesen, S. Akçurin, and D. Çolak, "Investigation of enterovirus infections, autoimmune factors and HLA genotypes in patients with T1DM," *Minerva Endocrinol*, vol. 39, no. 1, pp. 67–74, 2014.

[18] C. A. Canas and F. Canas, "The biological significance of evolution in autoimmune phenomena," *Autoimmune Diseases*, vol. 2012, Article ID 784315, 12 pages, 2012.

[19] D. W. Dunne and A. Cooke, "A worm's eye view of the immune system: consequences for evolution of human autoimmune disease," *Nature Reviews Immunology*, vol. 5, no. 5, pp. 420–426, 2005.

[20] K. Lind, M. H. Hühn, and M. Flodström-Tullberg, "Immunology in the clinic review series; focus on type 1 diabetes and viruses: the innate immune response to enteroviruses and its possible role in regulating type 1 diabetes," *Clinical & Experimental Immunology*, vol. 168, no. 1, pp. 30–38, 2012.

[21] Y. Simoni, J. Diana, L. Ghazarian, L. Beaudoin, and A. Lehuen, "Therapeutic manipulation of natural killer (NK) T cells in autoimmunity: are we close to reality?," *Clinical & Experimental Immunology*, vol. 171, no. 1, pp. 8–19, 2013.

[22] D. Zipris, "Epidemiology of type 1 diabetes and what animal models teach us about the role of viruses in disease mechanisms," *Clinical Immunology*, vol. 131, no. 1, pp. 11–23, 2009.

[23] M. A. Atkinson and G. S. Eisenbarth, "Type 1 diabetes: new perspectives on disease pathogenesis and treatment," *The Lancet*, vol. 358, no. 9277, pp. 221–229, 2001.

Exercise Training Induced Cardioprotection with Moderate Hyperglycemia versus Sedentary Intensive Glycemic Control in Type 1 Diabetic Rats

Matthew W. McDonald,[1] Michelle S. Dotzert,[1] Mao Jiang,[1] Michael R. Murray,[1] Earl G. Noble,[1,2] and C. W. James Melling[1]

[1]*Exercise Biochemistry Laboratory, School of Kinesiology, Western University, London, ON, Canada*
[2]*Lawson Health Research Institute, London, ON, Canada*

Correspondence should be addressed to C. W. James Melling; jmelling@uwo.ca

Academic Editor: Markus Wallner

Intensive insulin therapy (IIT; 4–7 mmol/L) is the preferred treatment for type 1 diabetes mellitus (T1DM) patients to reduce the risk of cardiovascular disease (CVD). However, this treatment strategy has been questioned as it is accompanied with a sedentary lifestyle leading to weight gain and insulin resistance. T1DM patients who partake in high-intensity aerobic training (AT_{high}) to reduce CVD often utilize conventional insulin therapy (CIT; 9–15 mmol/L) to offset the risk of hypoglycemia. Moreover, exercise modalities incorporating resistance training (RT) have been shown to further reduce this risk. The purpose of this investigation was twofold: (1) to determine if CIT paired with AT_{high} results in larger cardioprotection from an ischemia-reperfusion (I-R) injury than IIT and (2) to establish if the integration of RT with AT_{high} (ART) results in similar cardioprotection as AT_{high}. Diabetic (D) male Sprague-Dawley rats were divided into D-IIT ($n = 12$), D-CIT ($n = 12$), D-AT_{high} ($n = 8$), D-RT ($n = 8$), and D-ART ($n = 8$). T1DM was induced with streptozotocin, and blood glucose was adjusted with insulin. D-AT_{high} occurred on a treadmill (27 m/min; 1 hr), D-RT performed weighted ladder climbs, and D-ART alternated daily between AT_{high} and RT. Exercise occurred 5 days/wk for 12 wks. This investigation demonstrates that cardioprotection following an I-R injury was similar between D-AT_{high} and D-IIT. This cardioprotection is not exercise-specific, and each provides unique advantages. D-AT_{high} leads to improved glycemia while insulin sensitivity was enhanced following resistance exercises. Thus, exercise is an effective means to elicit cardioprotection in T1DM. However, in addition to glycemia, other factors should be considered when tailoring an exercise program for T1DM patients.

1. Introduction

Individuals with type 1 diabetes mellitus (T1DM) exhibit a heightened risk for cardiovascular disease (CVD) not entirely accounted for by traditional risk factors (hyperglycemia, obesity, hypertension, dyslipidemia, and smoking) [1]. To date, the most characterized strategies to limit CVD development have been intensive insulin therapy (IIT) [2] and regular exercise [3–5]. However, both IIT and exercise potentiate the risk of hypoglycemia, especially when attempted collectively [2, 6]. To counteract hypoglycemia risk, individuals with T1DM often intentionally elevate their blood glucose concentrations prior to exercise through changes in insulin dosing and/or carbohydrate ingestion [7]. As such, individuals with T1DM who are more physically active typically prescribe to a more conventional insulin therapy (CIT) and have higher HbA1c values with reduced focus on glycemic control [8].

Additional work is needed to better evaluate the cardiovascular benefits and risks associated with regular exercise in physically active individuals with T1DM that often prescribe to less stringent glycemic control, since elevations in glycemia (HbA_{1c}) are known to increase the risk of cardiovascular complications [2]. Our group has demonstrated that the combination of less stringent blood glucose control and high-intensity aerobic exercise training (AT_{high}) in experimental T1DM rats not only decreases the risk of exercise-induced hypoglycemia [4] but also has numerous cardiovascular benefits such as increased recovery from an ischemic insult [4], reduction in cardiovascular autonomic dysfunction [9], improvement in systolic and diastolic heart function [5], and improved vascular reactivity [10, 11]. It is unknown how these cardiovascular benefits would compare to stringent blood glucose control alone (i.e., IIT), the predominant treatment option for individuals with T1DM [2, 12]. This is a significant question that needs to be answered since IIT is associated with cardiovascular risk factors such as increased sedentary behaviour, weight gain, and insulin resistance [8, 13, 14].

Additionally, it has been established both experimentally [15] and clinically [16] that poor glycemic control leads to hepatic glycogen deficiencies. Restoration of hepatic glycogen content could represent a mechanism for combatting hypoglycemia, as hepatic glycogen is the predominant source of blood glucose during exercise [17] and insulin overcorrection [18]. Our laboratory has recently shown that ten weeks of AT_{high} fails to normalize hepatic glycogen in T1DM rats despite significantly elevated levels of hepatic glycogenic storage enzymes [15]. In contrast, resistance training (RT) has been shown to increase hepatic glycogen content in rats [19], while also alleviating the risk of exercise-induced hypoglycemia in T1DM [4, 20]. While still allowing for the cardiovascular benefits associated with regular aerobic exercise, the integration of RT with aerobic exercise may allow individuals with T1DM to exercise safely by reducing the risk of hypoglycemia development. Indeed, the Canadian Diabetes Association recommends that RT be incorporated into aerobic exercise regimes at least twice a week [21].

The objective of the present study was to examine whether moderate blood glucose control and AT_{high} result in greater levels of cardioprotection than more stringent blood glucose control. Secondly, it was determined whether combining RT with AT_{high} resulted in similar cardioprotection and less exercise-induced blood glucose fluctuations. Additionally, the potential relationship between glycemic status and cardioprotection was explored.

2. Methods

This study was approved by the Research Ethics Board of the University of Western Ontario which is in compliance with the guidelines of the Canadian Council on Animal Care. Eight-week-old male Sprague-Dawley rats were obtained from Charles River Laboratories, provided standard rat chow ad libitum, and housed in pairs at a standard temperature and humidity (21.5°C and 50% humidity).

2.1. Experimental Protocol. Sprague-Dawley rats were randomly divided into one of five diabetic groups (D): conventional insulin therapy (D-CIT; $n = 12$), intensive insulin therapy (D-IIT; $n = 12$), high-intensity aerobic exercise training (D-AT_{high}; $n = 8$), resistance exercise training (D-RT; $n = 8$), and combination aerobic/resistance exercise training (D-ART; $n = 8$). During experimental week one, T1DM was induced after five consecutive daily injections of streptozotocin (Sigma-Aldrich; 20 mg/kg; dissolved in 0.1 M citrate buffer, pH 4.5) and T1DM was confirmed after two nonfasting blood glucose concentrations greater than 18 mmol/L. After diabetes confirmation, subcutaneous insulin pellets (Linshin, Toronto, Canada) were implanted in the abdomen (experimental week two). Through insulin pellet adjustments, it was intended to maintain blood glucose concentrations in D-CIT, D-AT_{high}, D-RT, and D-ART between 9 and 15 mmol/L and D-IIT between 4 and 9 mmol/L. Exercise training occurred five times a week over a twelve-week period (experimental week 3 to 14). D-AT_{high} rats exercised on a motorized treadmill at 27 m/min (six percent grade) for one hour. Continuous running was encouraged by small blasts of compressed air at the rear of the treadmill. In D-RT rats, resistance training consisted of climbing a vertical ladder with weights secured to the proximal portion of the tail, as previously described [4]. Familiarization occurred the week prior to training (experimental week 2) and consisted of 10 climbs a day with varying weights attached (5%, 15%, 20%, and 35% of each rat's body mass). Regular resistance training sessions (experimental week 3 to 14) consisted of incremental increases in weight (50%, 75%, and 90% of maximal lifting capacity) followed by 100% of their maximal lifting capacity until exhaustion (unable to finish climb despite tactile stimulation to haunches). Maximum lifting capacity was calculated every fourth exercise session and was determined by sequentially adding 30 grams of weight to the rat's tail until exhaustion (starting at 75% of their body mass). In D-ART rats, exercise training consisted of alternating daily between the aerobic and resistance exercises.

2.2. Blood Analysis. Blood samples were taken over two consecutive days from the saphenous vein during the last week of exercise training (experimental week 14; pre/postexercise) to determine if antecedent AT_{high} or RT altered the blood glucose response to a subsequent exercise bout [22]. In D-ART, this measure was conducted at week 11 and week 12 of training (experimental week 13 and 14, resp.) to determine if performing AT_{high} (or RT) first had an effect on glucoregulation following a subsequent bout of RT (or AT_{high}). Blood glucose concentrations were detected using a OneTouch Ultra 2 Blood Glucose Monitoring System (Lifescan Canada Ltd., Burnaby, BC, Canada) and OneTouch test strips (Lifescan Canada Ltd.). Epinephrine concentrations prior to and after exercise were determined via ELISA (Cusabio, catalog number CSB-E08678r). Fructosamine concentrations were determined using the procedure outlined by Oppel et al. [23]. Briefly, serum samples taken at the completion of the study were added to a carbonate buffer (pH 10.8) containing 0.25 mM nitroblue tetrazolium (NBT) at 37°C. Following a 20-minute incubation at 37°C, the reaction was read at 530 nm and compared to standards of 1-deoxy,1-morpholinofructose (DMF; Sigma-Aldrich) and albumin (40 g/L).

2.3. Langendorf Heart Preparation. Three days following the last exercise bout, all rats were anaesthetized with isoflurane and hearts were extracted and placed in cold

TABLE 1: General animal characteristics at the completion of the study.

	D-CIT	D-IIT	D-AT_{high}	D-RT	D-ART
Body mass (g)	567 ± 20	598 ± 21[3,4,5]	510 ± 15	520 ± 21	534 ± 19
Blood glucose conc. (mmol/L)	15.0 ± 1.2	10.9 ± 1.2[1,3,5]	15.6 ± 0.5	12.4 ± 1.9[5]	16.7 ± 1.4
Fructosamine conc. (mmol/L)	3.0 ± 0.5	1.0 ± 0.2[1,5]	1.3 ± 0.3[1,5]	2.0 ± 0.1	2.6 ± 0.7
Exogenous insulin (IU)	27.3 ± 5.4	35.8 ± 7.8	19.0 ± 7.7	11.1 ± 7.1[2]	4.1 ± 2.0[1,2]
Insulin resistance (AU)	10,665 ± 2078[5]	16,055 ± 4558[3,4,5]	4722 ± 1988	1438 ± 62[3]	1260 ± 601[3]

Data are means ± SE. [1]Different from D-CIT; [2]different from D-IIT; [3]different from D-AT_{high}; [4]different from D-RT; [5]different from D-ART.

Krebs-Henseleit buffer (KHB; 120 mM NaCl, 4.63 mM KCl, 1.17 mM KH_2PO_4, 1.25 mM $CaCl_2$, 1.2 mM $MgCl_2$, 20 mM $NaHCO_3$, and 8 mmol/L glucose). Hearts were rapidly cannulated for unpaced retrograde perfusion of KHB (37°C; gassed with 95% O_2 and 5% CO_2) at 15 mL/min. A small water-filled latex balloon was inserted through the mitral valve and into the left ventricle. Hearts were equilibrated to the preparation for 30 minutes (preischemia) followed by the termination of flow for 50 minutes. Subsequently, reperfusion occurred for a total of 30 minutes at 15 m/min. Left ventricle pressures (LVDP, left ventricle developed pressure; LVEDP, left ventricle end-diastolic pressure) were measured with a pressure transducer (Statham Gould P23ID), and the rate of pressure development (+dp/dt) and relaxation (−dp/dt) were obtained using a PowerLab 8/30 data acquisition system and analyzed by LabChart 7.0 Pro software (ADInstruments, Colorado Springs, Colorado, USA). Area under the curve (AUC) was determined for the pressure curves of each rat in the study in order to correlate measures to glycemic control and insulin resistance.

2.4. Glucose Tolerance Test. Intravenous glucose tolerance tests (IVGTT) were conducted following training (experimental week 14) after an 8–12-hour fast and consisted of a sterile injection (1 g/kg) of dextrose solution (50% dextrose, 50% ddH_2O) into the lateral tail vein. Blood glucose concentrations were measured at 5, 10, 20, 30, and 40 minutes post-injection, and area under the curves (AUC) were determined for each individual rat. Prior to the IVGTT, blood samples were taken from the saphenous vein and exogenous insulin concentrations were measured via ELISA (Alpco, Salem, NH: catalog number 80-INSHU-E01.1). The measure of insulin resistance was considered the AUC of the IVGTT multiplied by exogenous insulin concentration. We have previously reported that when using this T1DM model, sedentary rats can become insulin resistant and require substantial more exogenous insulin in order to maintain the desired blood glucose concentrations [15, 24]. Accordingly, when determining the insulin resistance measure, the amount of circulating insulin present in the rat during the IVGTT was factored into the calculation.

2.5. Western Blotting. Liver (extracted during sacrifice at end of study) and left ventricles were homogenized in buffer (100 mM NaCl, 50 mM Tris base, 0.1 mM EDTA, and 0.1 EGTA, pH ~7.5) using a polytron, and total protein concentrations were determined by the Bradford protein assay. Homogenates (40–80 μg of protein) were mixed with equal volumes of sample buffer (0.125 M Tris, 20% glycerol, 4% SDS, 10% β-mercaptoethanol, 0.015% bromophenol blue, pH ~6.8), separated by SDS-PAGE (4% stacking, 10% separating) and transferred to nitrocellulose membranes. Membranes were blocked in 5% nonfat dairy milk in TTBS (10 mM Tris, 100 mM NaCl, and 0.1% Tween-20, pH 7.5) for 1 hour and incubated overnight at 4°C with primary antibodies (Cell Signaling: Hsp70 1:4000, glycogen synthase 1:1000; Abcam: glycogen phosphorylase 1:2000, SERCA2 1:1000; Santa Cruz: glucose-6-phosphotase 1:200) diluted in TTBS with 2% nonfat dairy milk. Following washes in TTBS, membranes were exposed to corresponding secondary antibodies (IgG-HRP conjugated, Bio-Rad) in TTBS with 2% nonfat dairy milk for 1 hour at room temperature. After successive washes in TTBS, protein bands were visualized with a luminol-based chemiluminescent substrate (Western C Enhanced Chemiluminescent Kit; Bio-Rad), imaged with the Chemidoc XRS System (Bio-rad), and analyzed with Quantity One Software (Bio-Rad). Optical densities were normalized to a consistent non-T1DM control sample and subsequently β-actin.

2.6. Statistical Analysis. Body mass, blood glucose, fructosamine, exogenous insulin, insulin resistance, and Western blot data were compared using a one-way analysis of variance (ANOVA). Langendorf measures were compared using a two-way repeated measure ANOVA. Blood glucose concentrations and epinephrine concentrations in response to exercise, and over consecutive days, were compared using a two-way repeated measures ANOVA. When a significant difference was found, a least squares difference post hoc test was performed and significance was set at $p < 0.05$. Relationships between left ventricular mechanical performance and fructosamine or insulin resistance were determined via Pearson correlation. All data are presented as a mean ± standard error. All statistical analyses were completed using GraphPad Prism 6.

3. Results

3.1. Animal Characteristics. Blood glucose concentrations were lower in D-IIT compared to D-CIT (p=0.03), D-AT_{high} ($p = 0.02$), and D-ART ($p = 0.007$), and lower in D-RT compared to D-ART ($p = 0.04$) (Table 1). Body mass was higher in D-IIT compared to D-AT_{high} ($p = 0.003$), D-RT ($p = 0.01$), and D-ART ($p < 0.04$). Fructosamine concentrations were lower in D-IIT compared to D-CIT ($p < 0.001$) and D-ART ($p = 0.01$). Further, fructosamine concentrations

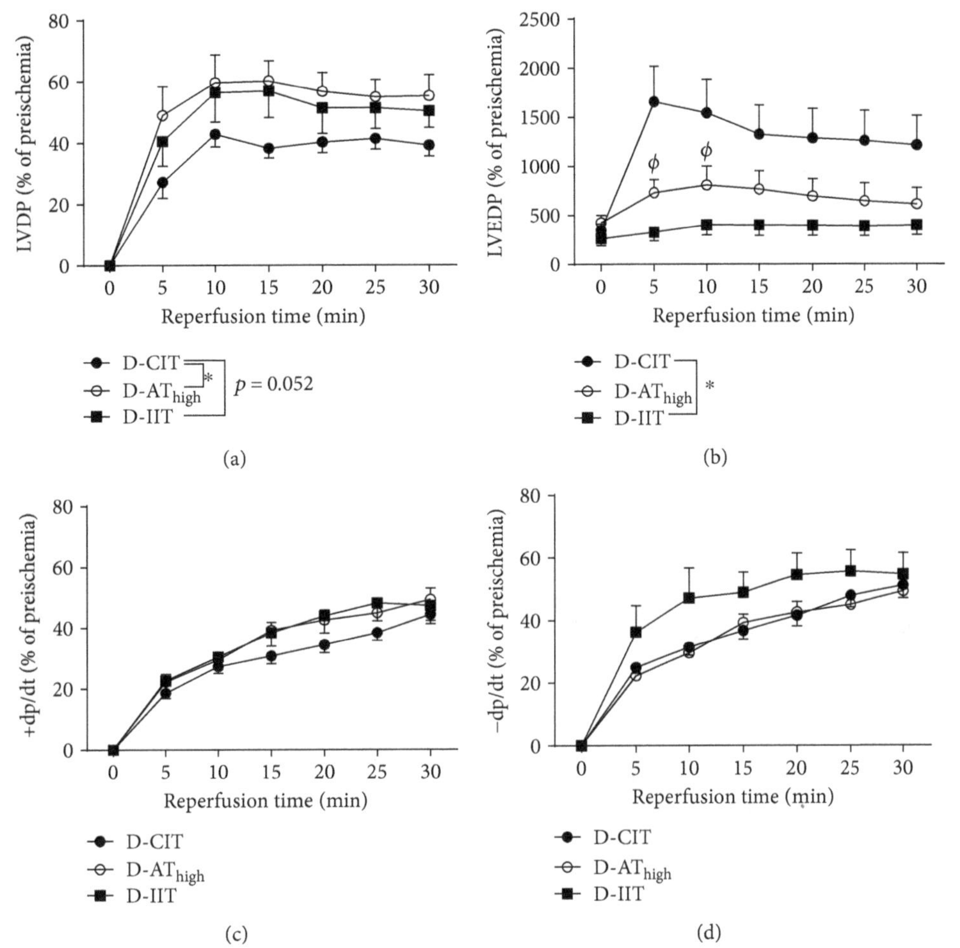

FIGURE 1: Left ventricle mechanical performance during ischemia-reperfusion. The data are presented in time course format. LVDP (a), LVEDP (b), +dP/dt (c), −dP/dt (d). *Significant main effect ($p < 0.05$); (φ) different from D-CIT ($p < 0.05$). Data are presented as a mean ± SE.

were lower in D-AT_{high} compared to D-CIT ($p = 0.003$) and D-ART ($p = 0.04$). Exogenous insulin concentrations were lower in D-RT compared to D-IIT ($p = 0.01$), and lower in D-ART compared to D-CIT ($p = 0.02$) and D-IIT ($p < 0.001$). The insulin resistance measure was higher in D-IIT compared to D-AT_{high} ($p = 0.02$), D-RT ($p = 0.008$), and D-ART ($p = 0.003$). Further, D-CIT displayed higher insulin resistance compared to D-ART ($p = 0.04$).

3.2. Left Ventricular Mechanical Performance. For the first objective of the study, we compared left ventricular mechanical performance following ischemia in D-CIT, D-AT_{high}, and D-IIT. There was a significant increase in LVDP in D-AT_{high} compared to D-CIT (Figure 1(a); $p = 0.03$). No difference in LVDP was observed between D-AT_{high} and D-IIT ($p = 0.5$), and LVDP between D-CIT and D-IIT did not reach significance ($p = 0.052$). LVEDP was lower in D-IIT compared to D-CIT (Figure 4.1B; $p = 0.004$), while D-AT_{high} was lower than D-CIT at 5 ($p < 0.0001$) and 10 minutes ($p = 0.03$) during reperfusion. There was no difference in +dp/dt ($p = 0.4$) or −dp/dt ($p = 0.2$) across any of the groups (Figures 1(c) and 1(d)).

For the second objective of the study, we compared left ventricle mechanical performance following ischemia in D-AT_{high}, D-RT, and D-ART. There were no differences in LVDP ($p = 0.6$) or LVEDP ($p = 0.9$) among D-AT_{high}, D-RT, and D-ART (Figures 2(a) and 2(b)). Compared to D-AT_{high}, D-ART had a higher +dp/dt at 25 ($p = 0.01$) and 30 minutes ($p = 0.005$) during reperfusion (Figure 2(c)). Compared to D-RT, D-ART had a higher +dp/dt at 25 ($p = 0.009$) and 30 minutes ($p = 0.002$) during reperfusion. D-AT_{high} had a slower −dp/dt than D-RT at 20 ($p = 0.04$), 25 ($p = 0.001$), and 30 minutes ($p < 0.0001$) (Figure 2(d)). Further, D-AT_{high} had a slower −dp/dt than D-ART at 20 ($p = 0.04$), 25 ($p = 0.002$), and 30 minutes ($p < 0.0001$).

3.3. Correlations of Left Ventricular Mechanical Performance. There was a significant correlation between the AUC of LVDP and fructosamine concentration (Table 2; $p = 0.01$; $r = -0.4$), while no correlation was evident between the AUC of LVEDP ($p = 0.8$), +dp/dt ($p = 0.7$), −dp/dt ($p = 0.8$), and fructosamine concentration. There was a significant correlation between the AUC of +dp/dt and insulin resistance ($p = 0.03$; $r = -0.4$), but no correlation between insulin resistance and the AUC of LVDP ($p = 0.7$), LVEDP ($p = 0.65$), or −dp/dt ($p = 0.5$).

3.4. Molecular Analysis. An elevation in left ventricle Hsp70 content was evident in D-AT_{high} compared to both D-CIT

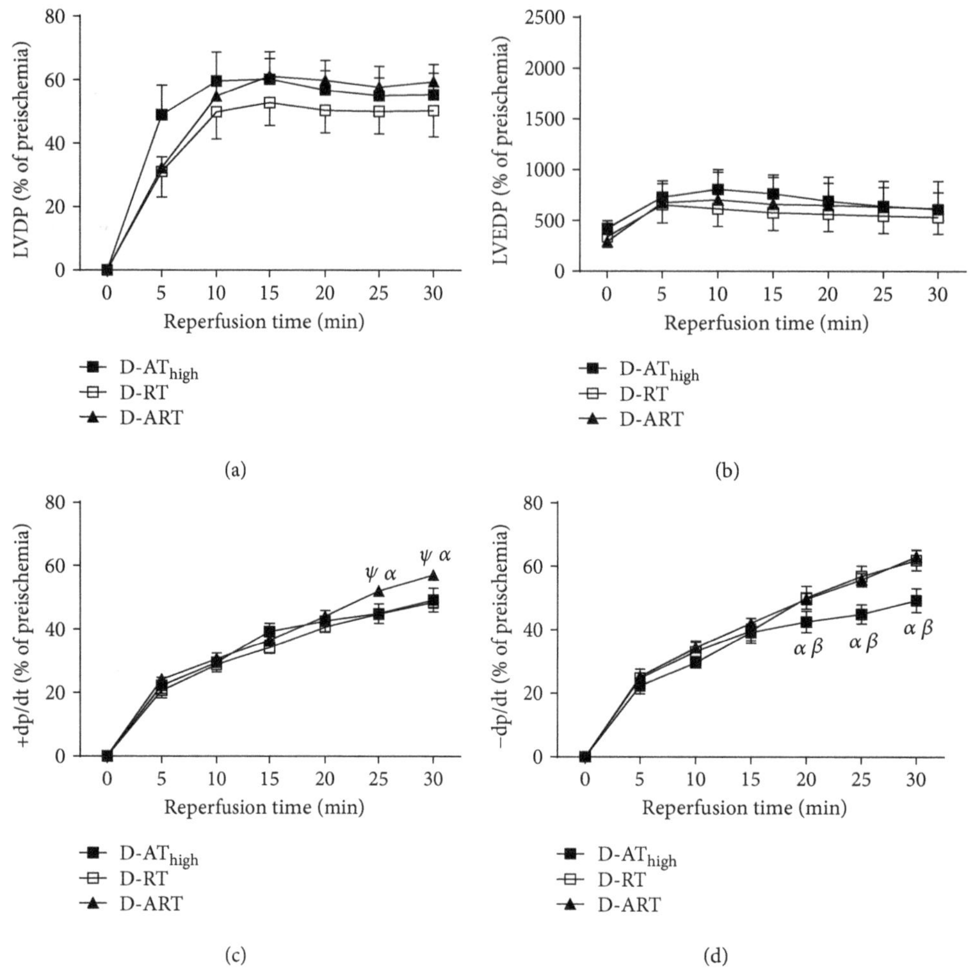

FIGURE 2: Left ventricle mechanical performance during ischemia-reperfusion and following different modalities of exercise training. The data are presented in time course format. LVDP (a), LVEDP (b), +dP/dt (c), −dP/dt (d). ψ: different from D-AT$_{high}$ ($p < 0.05$); α: different from D-RT ($p < 0.05$); β: different from D-ART ($p < 0.05$). Data are presented as a mean ± SE.

TABLE 2: Correlation of left ventricle mechanical performance on glycemia and insulin resistance.

	Versus fructosamine (mmol/L)		Versus insulin resistance (AU)	
	p value	r	p value	r
LVDP (AUC)	*0.01**	−0.4	0.7	—
LVEDP (AUC)	0.8	—	0.7	—
+dp/dt (AUC)	0.7	—	*0.03**	−0.4
−dp/dt (AUC)	0.8	—	0.5	—

*Significant ($p < 0.05$).

($p = 0.003$) and D-IIT ($p = 0.009$) (Figure 3(a)), while no differences were evident in SERCA2 among D-CIT, D-IIT, and D-AT$_{high}$ (Figure 3(b); $p = 0.8$). Differences existed between exercise regimes in that D-AT$_{high}$ resulted in higher left ventricle Hsp70 compared to D-RT ($p = 0.02$), but did not differ significantly from D-ART (Figure 3(a); $p = 0.1$). No differences in SERCA2 expression were evident among exercise regimes (Figure 4.3B; $p = 0.4$).

3.5. Hepatic Glycogen Content and Regulatory Enzymes. Hepatic glycogen content was higher in D-CIT compared to D-AT$_{high}$ ($p = 0.05$), D-RT ($p = 0.01$), and D-ART ($p = 0.004$) (Figure 4(a)). Hepatic glycogen was also higher in D-IIT compared to D-AT$_{high}$ ($p = 0.04$), D-RT ($p = 0.01$), and D-ART ($p = 0.004$). No differences in glycogen synthase ($p = 0.9$), glycogen phosphorylase ($p = 0.9$), and glycogen-6-phosphatase ($p = 0.7$) were apparent between experimental groups (Figures 4(b)–4(d)).

3.6. Exercise-Mediated Changes in Blood Glucose. Significant declines in blood glucose concentrations following exercise were apparent in D-AT$_{high}$ at day 1 and day 2 of exercise (week 12 of training; Table 3; $p < 0.0001$). No change in blood glucose concentrations was apparent following RT at day 1 or day 2 (week 12 of training; $p = 0.5$). In D-ART, significant declines in blood glucose concentrations were apparent only on AT$_{high}$ days at both week 11 ($p = 0.0003$) and week 12 ($p < 0.0001$) of training. In D-AT$_{high}$, no change in epinephrine concentrations was evident from pre to postexercise (week 12 of training; $p = 0.4$; Table 4), and epinephrine concentrations were similar between day 1 and day 2 (week 12 of training; $p = 0.2$). In D-RT, no change in

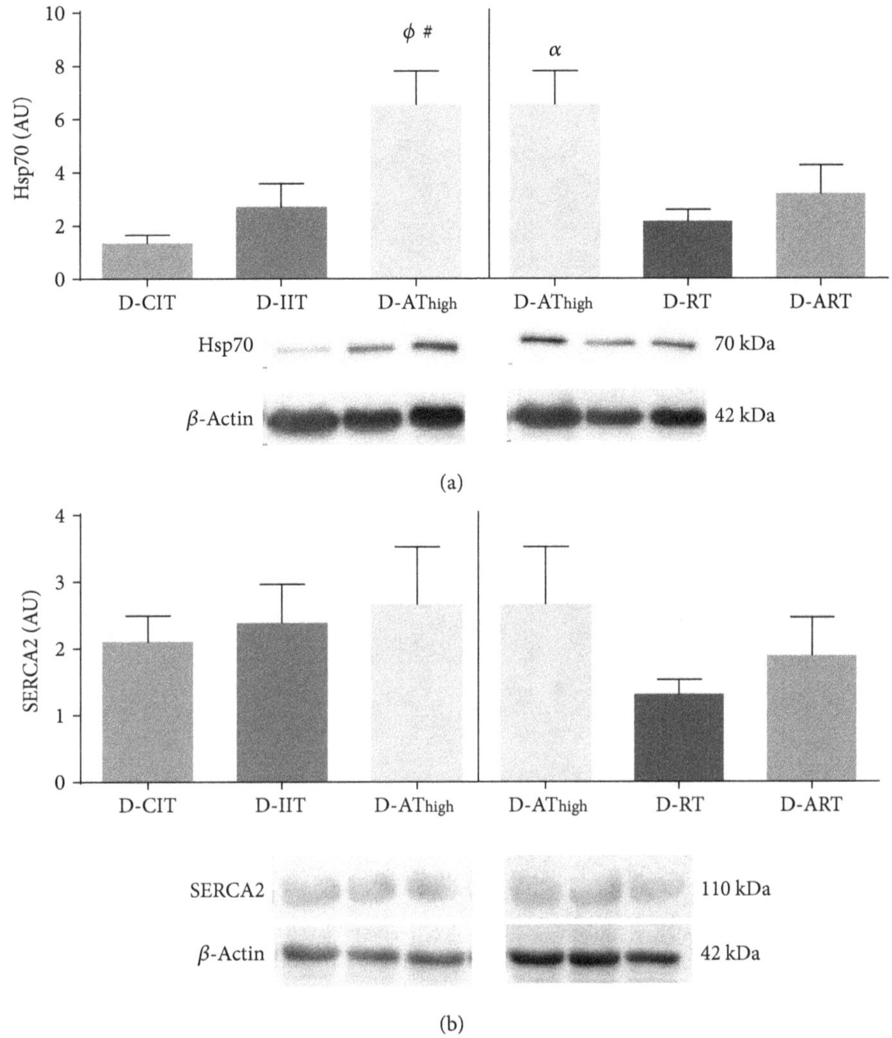

FIGURE 3: Left ventricle Hsp70 (a) and SERCA2 (b) protein content. ϕ: different from D-CIT; #: different from D-IIT; α: different from D-RT. Significance $p < 0.05$. Data are presented as a mean ± SE.

epinephrine concentrations was evident from pre to postexercise (week 12 of training; $p = 0.7$); however, epinephrine concentrations were lower overall on day 2 compared to day 1 (week 12 of training; $p = 0.02$). In D-ART, when RT occurred the day before AT_{high} (week 11 of training), epinephrine concentrations were reduced overall during AT_{high} ($p = 0.007$). In D-ART, no change in epinephrine occurred from pre to postexercise at both week 11 ($p = 0.5$) and week 12 ($p = 0.2$) of training.

4. Discussion

Stringent management of blood glucose concentrations through intensive insulin therapy is the primary treatment strategy in order to limit the progression of CVD in patients with T1DM [2]. Indeed, D-IIT resulted in greater recovery from an I-R injury than D-CIT, supporting the deleterious effects of chronic hyperglycemia on the macrovasculature in individuals with T1DM [12, 25]. In a previous study, we reported that six weeks of high-intensity aerobic exercise led to significant improvements in I-R functional recovery [4]. Here, we demonstrate that this modality of exercise when combined with CIT can lead to comparable recovery from an I-R injury as IIT alone. It is important to note that while exercised animals were maintained in a chronic hyperglycemic state, AT_{high} exhibited similar serum fructosamine concentrations as IIT. It is likely that glycemic control played a significant role in contributing to the increased cardioprotection of IIT and AT_{high}, since both exhibited similar serum fructosamine concentrations. Indeed, the negative correlation between serum fructosamine, indicative of glycemic control, and LVDP would support this finding.

While it is well-recognized that regular exercise can improve glycemic control (lowered HbA_{1C}) in type 2 diabetes, results in T1DM have generally failed to show this glycemic benefit [3]. A number of factors may contribute to this lack of evidence in previous studies, including the predominant use of adolescent subjects, the use of questionnaires to estimate activity levels, or the increased food consumption that is typically associated with the initiation of an exercise program [3]. Although comparable to HbA_{1c}, the measure of glycosylated hemoglobin, fructosamine is a measure of

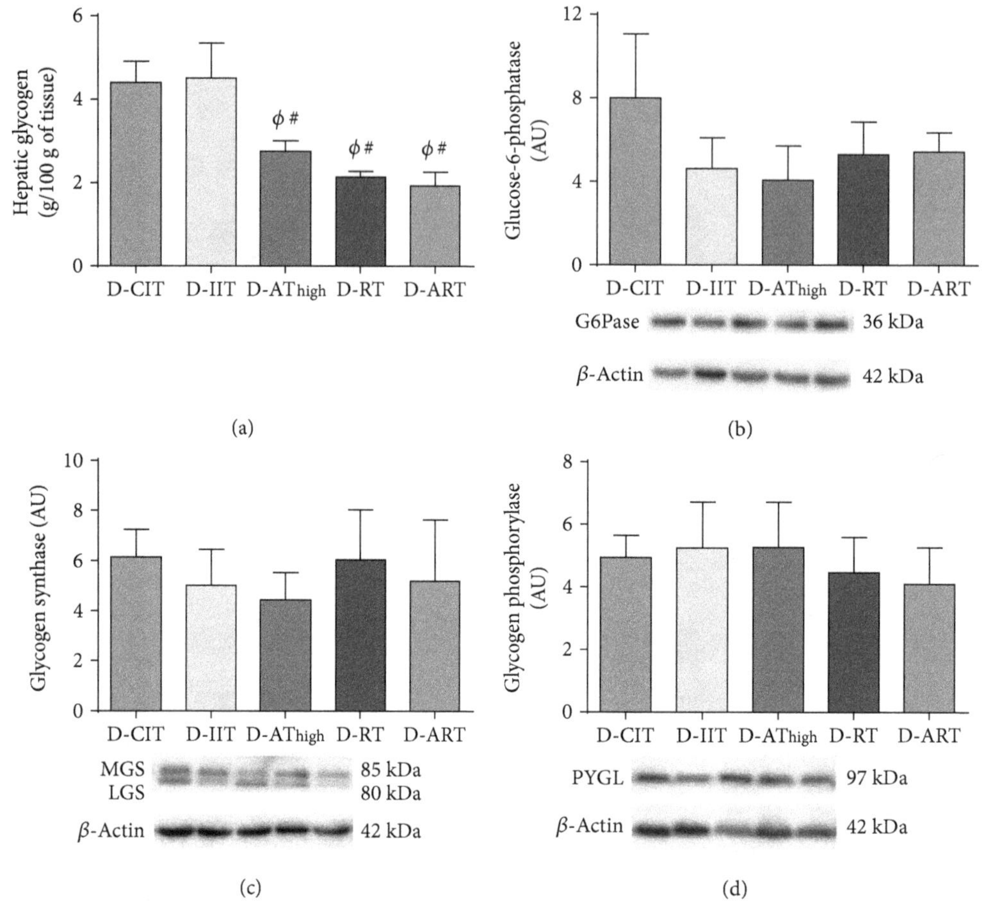

FIGURE 4: Hepatic glycogen content (a), glycogen-6-phosphatase (b), glycogen synthase (MGS: muscle glycogen synthase; LGS: liver glycogen synthase) (c), and glycogen phosphorylase (d). ϕ: different from D-CIT ($p < 0.05$); #: different from D-IIT ($p < 0.05$). Data are presented as a mean ± SE.

TABLE 3: Blood glucose concentrations in response to exercise at week 11 or week 12 of training.

	Day 1		Day 2	
	Preexercise (mmol/L)	Postexercise (mmol/L)	Preexercise (mmol/L)	Postexercise (mmol/L)
D-AT_{high}	15.0 ± 0.4	8.0 ± 1.1*	14.6 ± 0.5	6.9 ± 1.0*
D-RT	12.2 ± 1.6	12.0 ± 0.9	13.6 ± 2.2	15.1 ± 1.6
D-ART (week 11; RT then AT_{high})	14.9 ± 1.6	15.6 ± 1.2	15.4 ± 1.7	8.0 ± 1.8*
D-ART (week 12; AT_{high} then RT)	16.7 ± 1.4	8.8 ± 1.4*	15.2 ± 2.0	15.6 ± 1.2

Data are means ± SE. *Significantly lower than preexercise ($p < 0.05$).

TABLE 4: Epinephrine concentrations in response to exercise at week 11 or week 12 of training.

	Day 1		Day 2	
	Preexercise (pg/mL)	Postexercise (pg/mL)	Preexercise (pg/mL)	Postexercise (pg/mL)
D-AT_{high}	254.3 ± 44.6	93.1 ± 24.9	237.0 ± 43.8	298.0 ± 109.1
D-RT	320.8 ± 72.2	238.3 ± 58.2	110.0 ± 46.1*	136.3 ± 66.3*
D-ART (week 11; RT then AT_{high})	254.3 ± 107.2	150.8 ± 98.0	38.7 ± 9.3*	57.8 ± 15.1*
D-ART (week 12; AT_{high} then RT)	331.0 ± 169.8	112.6 ± 45.7	202.2 ± 33.0	184.6 ± 41.8

Data are means ± SE. *Significantly lower than day 1 ($p < 0.05$).

the amount of serum proteins that have undergone glycation and is thus a better marker for shorter-term glycemic control (approximately two weeks). While there is a shortage of evidence supporting increased glycemic control in T1DM following aerobic exercise [3], exercise intensity appears to play a significant role as to whether glycemic benefits are obtained [3, 26]. In the present study, the aerobic exercise training program was intensive, representing approximately 70–80% of the rats VO_{2max} [27]. The potential ability of RT to improve glycemic control (determined by HbA_{1C}) in populations with T1DM is inconclusive [28], and the present results would support work citing that it has no benefit on long-term glycemia [29]. There was no improvement in fructosamine levels in D-ART, despite supplementing RT with AT_{high}, suggesting that the frequency of AT_{high} may be an important factor to experience glycemic benefits. However, since food consumption was not directly measured in the current study, it cannot be completely discounted that the diets of experimental groups may not have been isocaloric.

In a previous report, we demonstrated that six weeks of RT provided little protection against an I-R injury in T1DM rats [4]. The current study demonstrated that longer term RT, conducted alone or paired with AT_{high} (D-ART), is necessary in order to provide similar levels of cardioprotection as performing strictly AT_{high}. Indeed, it has been demonstrated in non-T1DM rats that short-term RT provides little cardioprotection [30]; however, if the RT is prolonged, the cardioprotective effects of this form of exercise become evident, as demonstrated by reduced infarct size following an I-R injury [31]. Again, it is of importance to note that we see unique advantages associated with RT that were not evident in other modalities of exercise. The maximal rate of pressure development (+dp/dt) and relaxation (−dp/dt) in T1DM rats were significantly improved in experimental groups utilizing RT that were not evident in D-AT_{high}. It has been reported that just a single bout of RT can improve the rate of left ventricular systolic pressure in hypertensive rats undergoing Langendorf perfusion [32]. Further, Melo et al. [33] reported faster cardiomyocyte contraction and relaxation in rats following eight weeks of RT, believed to be due to increased sarcoplasmic reticulum Ca^{2+}-ATPase (SERCA2a) expression. While neither +dp/dt nor −dp/dt were altered in D-AT_{high}, these results may not be surprising as little change in Ca^{2+} regulatory mechanisms is reported elsewhere in rat hearts following 12 weeks of treadmill training [34]. Thus, these findings may support the incorporation of RT into the treatment of T1DM, since slowed Ca^{2+} clearing and abnormal cardiomyocyte excitation-contraction coupling are prominent in T1DM [35].

The finding that rates of pressure development and relaxation were increased in D-RT and D-ART despite no improvement in glycemia (fructosamine) indicates that other factors may contribute to changes in rates of pressure development. For example, cardiomyocytes from insulin-resistant rats have demonstrated mechanical defects and impaired Ca^{2+} handling [36, 37]. In the present investigation, we report a negative correlation between the degree of insulin resistance and the rate of developed pressure. Indeed, the experimental groups that demonstrated the greatest insulin sensitivity, D-RT and D-ART, also displayed the quickest rates of pressure development and relaxation. In the insulin-resistant state, impaired SERCA activity is well documented to contribute to cardiomyocyte dysfunction [38], and RT itself has been shown to increase SERCA expression [33]. In the present study, SERCA2 expression was not changed as a result of RT or ART. This lack of change may not reflect changes in the activity levels of this enzyme, as impaired SERCA activity has been reported in insulin-resistant animals despite normal protein content [38]. Nonetheless, the implications of insulin resistance in the recovery from an I-R injury are significant and require further investigation, given the emerging evidence of "double diabetes," a separate classification of patients with T1DM that exhibit both insulin deficiency and resistance [39].

In seeking to explain the mechanistic means by which a specific exercise training regime may prove to be more beneficial for the functional recovery of the heart during an I-R injury, we examined cardiac Hsp70 protein expression in each of the groups [40, 41]. We observed an increase in left ventricular Hsp70 content in D-AT_{high} compared to both sedentary T1DM groups (D-CIT and D-IIT). Our laboratory, as well as others, has established the importance of exercise-induced Hsp70 expression in recovery from an I-R injury [40, 41]. This finding is in line with previous work from our laboratory that demonstrated both short- and long-term aerobic exercise can result in increased Hsp70 in the hearts of insulin-treated T1DM rats [4, 5]. Further, we showed that D-AT_{high} had higher Hsp70 expression than D-RT which supports an earlier finding by our laboratory [4]. While it is not clear why differences in the expression of Hsp70 exist between exercise modalities, it may be reflective of frequency, duration, and/or intensity of the exercise. We have previously shown that antioxidant enzymes are elevated in the myocardium following AT_{high}, but not following RT [4]. Increases in myocardial antioxidant defenses have been shown to be dependent on the duration and frequency of training [42], while exercise-induced elevations in Hsp70 are known to be intensity-dependent [43]. It is plausible that D-RT did not undergo the same quantity or intensity of exercise as was achieved in D-AT_{high}.

The largest barrier to exercise prescription for individuals with T1DM is exercise-induced hypoglycemia [6]. Thus, independent of which exercise provides the largest cardiovascular benefit, the risk of exercise-induced hypoglycemia must also be considered. Similar to past findings [4], D-AT_{high} resulted in a significant drop in blood glucose immediately following exercise, while D-RT did not. Interestingly, the integration of RT and AT_{high} (D-ART) did not alter the abrupt drop in blood glucose in response to AT_{high}. Recently, our group has demonstrated that both sedentary and aerobically trained T1DM rats using CIT demonstrate hepatic glycogen deficiencies [15], similar to what has been reported using clinical populations [16]. Despite increased glycemic control in IIT, there was no difference in hepatic glycogen content between D-IIT and D-CIT. Further, exercise-trained T1DM rats, regardless of training modality, demonstrated significantly lower liver glycogen content. It is expected that the amount of insulin in circulation in the treatment groups contributed to different hepatic glycogen levels. Both D-CIT and D-IIT had similar exogenous insulin concentrations, which would in turn regulate glycogen storage by increasing the activity of glycogen synthase [44].

Moreover, independent of exercise modality, trained T1DM rats displayed the smallest amounts of hepatic glycogen, concurrent with the lowest exogenous insulin requirements. Despite the apparent cardiovascular benefits associated with regular exercise, the decreased hepatic glycogen content in trained T1DM rats could have implications for combatting hypoglycemia, since hepatic glycogen is a prominent source of blood glucose during glucose-demanding states [17, 18]. However, it is important to note that T1DM rats in each of the different training modalities failed to reach hypoglycemic blood glucose concentrations (less than 3 mmol/L).

In conclusion, the first objective of the present investigation was to determine if AT_{high} coupled with CIT resulted in larger cardioprotective benefits than IIT alone. Findings presented here demonstrate that when CIT was paired with AT_{high}, the increase in cardioprotection from an I-R injury was similar to that of D-IIT. In fact, the current findings may suggest that CIT with AT_{high} may lead to a larger cardiac improvement in T1DM rats than IIT alone, given the potential role of elevated expression of left ventricular Hsp70 with this form of exercise. For the second objective, we determined that following long-term exercise training, both D-ART and D-RT resulted in similar levels of overall cardioprotection as D-AT_{high}; although each exercise training modality did appear to provide unique benefits. For example, improved glycemic control was only evident in D-AT_{high}, while the largest improvements in insulin sensitivity measures were evident in exercises that utilize resistance exercise (D-ART, D-RT). This study underlines the need to consider other factors besides glycemic control (i.e., insulin resistance) when tailoring an exercise treatment program for the patient with T1DM to reduce the risk of developing CVD.

Conflicts of Interest

The authors declare that they have no conflicts of interest.

Acknowledgments

This study was supported by Natural Sciences and Engineering Council Discovery Grant (RGPGP-2015-00059).

References

[1] J. K. Snell-Bergeon and K. Nadeau, "Cardiovascular disease risk in young people with type 1 diabetes," *Journal of Cardiovascular Translational Research*, vol. 5, no. 4, pp. 446–462, 2012.

[2] D. M. Nathan and for the DCCT/EDIC Research Group, "The diabetes control and complications trial/epidemiology of diabetes interventions and complications study at 30 years: overview," *Diabetes Care*, vol. 37, no. 1, pp. 9–16, 2014.

[3] M. Chimen, A. Kennedy, K. Nirantharakumar, T. T. Pang, R. Andrews, and P. Narendran, "What are the health benefits of physical activity in type 1 diabetes mellitus? A literature review," *Diabetologia*, vol. 55, no. 3, pp. 542–551, 2012.

[4] M. W. McDonald, K. E. Hall, M. Jiang, E. G. Noble, and C. W. J. Melling, "Ischemia-reperfusion injury and hypoglycemia risk in insulin-treated T1DM rats following different modalities of regular exercise," *Physiological Reports*, vol. 2, no. 11, pp. e12201–e12212, 2014.

[5] C. W. J. Melling, K. N. Grisé, C. P. Hasilo et al., "A model of poorly controlled type 1 diabetes mellitus and its treatment with aerobic exercise training," *Diabetes & Metabolism*, vol. 39, no. 3, pp. 226–235, 2013.

[6] A.-S. Brazeau, R. Rabasa-Lhoret, I. Strychar, and H. Mircescu, "Barriers to physical activity among patients with type 1 diabetes," *Diabetes Care*, vol. 31, no. 11, pp. 2108-2109, 2008.

[7] D. P. Zaharieva and M. C. Riddell, "Prevention of exercise-associated dysglycemia: a case study–based approach," *Diabetes Spectrum: A Publication of the American Diabetes Association*, vol. 28, no. 1, pp. 55–62, 2015.

[8] Diabetes Control and Complications Trial/Epidemiology of Diabetes Interventions and Complications, L. M. Delahanty, D. M. Nathan et al., "Association of diet with glycated hemoglobin during intensive treatment of type 1 diabetes in the diabetes control and complications trial," *The American Journal of Clinical Nutrition*, vol. 89, no. 2, pp. 518–524, 2009.

[9] K. N. Grisé, T. D. Olver, M. W. McDonald et al., "High intensity aerobic exercise training improves deficits of cardiovascular autonomic function in a rat model of type 1 diabetes mellitus with moderate hyperglycemia," *Journal of Diabetes Research*, vol. 2016, Article ID 8164518, 13 pages, 2016.

[10] J. M. Murias, A. Dey, O. A. Campos et al., "High-intensity endurance training results in faster vessel-specific rate of vasorelaxation in type 1 diabetic rats," *PLoS One*, vol. 8, no. 3, article e59678, 2013.

[11] T. D. Olver, M. W. McDonald, K. N. Grisé et al., "Exercise training enhances insulin-stimulated nerve arterial vasodilation in rats with insulin-treated experimental diabetes," *American Journal of Physiology, Regulatory, Integrative and Comparative Physiology*, vol. 306, no. 12, pp. R941–R950, 2014.

[12] The Diabetes Control and Complications Trial Research Group, "The effect of intensive treatment of diabetes on the development and progression of long-term complications in insulin-dependent diabetes mellitus," *The New England Journal of Medicine*, vol. 14, no. 3, pp. 286-287, 1994.

[13] S. J. Cleland, "Cardiovascular risk in double diabetes mellitus—when two worlds collide," *Nature Reviews Endocrinology*, vol. 8, no. 8, pp. 476–485, 2012.

[14] R. Schechter and S. Reutrakul, "Management of severe insulin resistance in patients with type 1 diabetes," *Current Diabetes Reports*, vol. 15, no. 10, pp. 77–88, 2015.

[15] M. W. McDonald, M. R. Murray, K. N. Grise et al., "The glucoregulatory response to high-intensity aerobic exercise following training in rats with insulin-treated type 1 diabetes mellitus," *Applied Physiology, Nutrition, and Metabolism*, vol. 41, no. 6, pp. 631–639, 2016.

[16] M. G. Bischof, M. Krssak, M. Krebs et al., "Effects of short-term improvement of insulin treatment and glycemia on hepatic glycogen metabolism in type 1 diabetes," *Diabetes*, vol. 50, no. 2, pp. 392–398, 2001.

[17] J. Vissing, J. L. Wallace, and H. Galbo, "Effect of liver glycogen content on glucose production in running rats," *Journal of Applied Physiology*, vol. 66, no. 1, pp. 318–322, 1989.

[18] P. Kishore, I. Gabriely, M. H. Cui et al., "Role of hepatic glycogen breakdown in defective counterregulation of hypoglycemia in intensively treated type 1 diabetes," *Diabetes*, vol. 55, no. 3, pp. 659–666, 2006.

[19] J. Prestes, R. Leite, G. Pereira et al., "Resistance training and glycogen content in ovariectomized rats," *International Journal of Sports Medicine*, vol. 33, no. 7, pp. 550–554, 2012.

[20] J. E. Yardley, G. P. Kenny, B. A. Perkins et al., "Resistance versus aerobic exercise acute effects on glycemia in type 1 diabetes," *Diabetes Care*, vol. 36, no. 3, pp. 537–542, 2013.

[21] M. J. Armstrong and R. J. Sigal, "Physical activity clinical practice guidelines: what's new in 2013?," *Canadian Journal of Diabetes*, vol. 37, no. 6, pp. 363–366, 2013.

[22] D. A. Sandoval, D. L. A. Guy, M. A. Richardson, A. C. Ertl, and S. N. Davis, "Effects of low and moderate antecedent exercise on counterregulatory responses to subsequent hypoglycemia in type 1 diabetes," *Diabetes*, vol. 53, no. 7, pp. 1798–1806, 2004.

[23] K. Oppel, L. Bárdos, A. Ferencz et al., "A new, modern, cost-saving micro/macro method for the determination of serum fructosamine," *Acta Veterinaria Hungarica*, vol. 48, no. 3, pp. 285–291, 2000.

[24] K. E. Hall, M. W. McDonald, K. N. Grisé, O. A. Campos, E. G. Noble, and C. W. J. Melling, "The role of resistance and aerobic exercise training on insulin sensitivity measures in STZ-induced type 1 diabetic rodents," *Metabolism*, vol. 62, no. 10, pp. 1485–1494, 2013.

[25] The Diabetes Control and Complications Trial (DCCT)/Epidemiology of Diabetes Interventions and Complications (EDIC) Study Research Group, "Intensive diabetes treatment and cardiovascular outcomes in type 1 diabetes: the DCCT/EDIC study 30-year follow-up," *Diabetes Care*, vol. 39, no. 5, pp. 686–693, 2016.

[26] M. A. Salem, M. A. Aboelasrar, N. S. Elbarbary, R. A. Elhilaly, and Y. M. Refaat, "Is exercise a therapeutic tool for improvement of cardiovascular risk factors in adolescents with type 1 diabetes mellitus? A randomised controlled trial," *Diabetology and Metabolic Syndrome*, vol. 2, no. 1, p. 47, 2010.

[27] T. G. Bedford, C. M. Tipton, N. C. Wilson, R. A. Oppliger, and C. V. Gisolfi, "Maximum oxygen consumption of rats and its changes with various experimental procedures," *Journal of Applied Physiology*, vol. 47, no. 6, pp. 1278–1283, 1979.

[28] J. E. Yardley, R. J. Sigal, B. A. Perkins, M. C. Riddell, and G. P. Kenny, "Resistance exercise in type 1 diabetes," *Canadian Journal of Diabetes*, vol. 37, no. 6, pp. 420–426, 2013.

[29] A. C. Ramalho, M. de Lourdes Lima, F. Nunes et al., "The effect of resistance versus aerobic training on metabolic control in patients with type-1 diabetes mellitus," *Diabetes Research and Clinical Practice*, vol. 72, no. 3, pp. 271–276, 2006.

[30] Y. Doustar, F. G. Soufi, A. Jafary, M. M. Saber, and R. Ghiassie, "Role of four-week resistance exercise in preserving the heart against ischaemia-reperfusion-induced injury," *Cardiovascular Journal of Africa*, vol. 23, no. 8, pp. 451–455, 2012.

[31] F. G. Soufi, M. M. Saber, R. Ghiassie, and M. Alipour, "Role of 12-week resistance training in preserving the heart against ischemia-reperfusion-induced injury," *Cardiology Journal*, vol. 18, no. 2, pp. 140–145, 2011.

[32] A. A. Fernandes, T. O. Faria, R. F. Ribeiro Júnior et al., "A single resistance exercise session improves myocardial contractility in spontaneously hypertensive rats," *Brazilian Journal of Medical and Biological Research*, vol. 48, no. 9, pp. 813–821, 2015.

[33] S. Melo, V. Barauna, M. Júnior et al., "Resistance training regulates cardiac function through modulation of miRNA-214," *International Journal of Molecular Sciences*, vol. 16, no. 12, pp. 6855–6867, 2015.

[34] J. Delgado, A. Saborido, M. Morán, and A. Megías, "Chronic and acute exercise do not alter Ca2 + regulatory systems and ectonucleotidase activities in rat heart," *Journal of Applied Physiology*, vol. 87, no. 1, pp. 152–160, 1999.

[35] J. Ren and A. J. Davidoff, "Diabetes rapidly induces contractile dysfunctions in isolated ventricular myocytes," *American Journal of Physiology-Heart and Circulatory Physiology*, vol. 272, no. 1, pp. H148–H158, 1997.

[36] K. Dutta, D. A. Podolin, M. B. Davidson, and A. J. Davidoff, "Cardiomyocyte dysfunction in sucrose-fed rats is associated with insulin resistance," *Diabetes*, vol. 50, no. 5, pp. 1186–1192, 2001.

[37] M. L. Schwanke, K. Dutta, D. A. Podolin, and A. J. Davidoff, "Cardiomyocyte dysfunction in insulin-resistant rats: a female advantage," *Diabetologia*, vol. 49, no. 5, pp. 1097–1105, 2006.

[38] L. Wold, K. Dutta, M. Mason et al., "Impaired SERCA function contributes to cardiomyocyte dysfunction in insulin resistant rats," *Journal of Molecular and Cellular Cardiology*, vol. 39, no. 2, pp. 297–307, 2005.

[39] S. J. Cleland, B. M. Fisher, H. M. Colhoun, N. Sattar, and J. R. Petrie, "Insulin resistance in type 1 diabetes: what is "double diabetes" and what are the risks?," *Diabetologia*, vol. 56, no. 7, pp. 1462–1470, 2013.

[40] J. J. Hutter, R. Mestril, E. K. W. Tam, R. E. Sievers, W. H. Dillmann, and C. L. Wolfe, "Overexpression of heat shock protein 72 in transgenic mice decreases infarct size in vivo," *Circulation*, vol. 94, no. 6, pp. 1408–1411, 1996.

[41] Z. Paroo, J. V. Haist, M. Karmazyn, and E. G. Noble, "Exercise improves postischemic cardiac function in males but not females," *Circulation Research*, vol. 90, no. 8, pp. 911–917, 2002.

[42] S. K. Powers, D. Criswell, J. Lawler et al., "Rigorous exercise training increases superoxide dismutase activity in ventricular myocardium," *The American Journal of Physiology*, vol. 265, no. 6, pp. H2094–H2098, 1993.

[43] K. J. Milne and E. G. Noble, "Exercise-induced elevation of HSP70 is intensity dependent," *Journal of Applied Physiology*, vol. 93, no. 2, pp. 561–568, 2002.

[44] A. R. Saltiel and C. R. Kahn, "Insulin signalling and the regulation of glucose and lipid metabolism," *Nature*, vol. 414, no. 6865, pp. 799–806, 2001.

21

Meprin Metalloprotease Deficiency Associated with Higher Mortality Rates and More Severe Diabetic Kidney Injury in Mice with STZ-Induced Type 1 Diabetes

John E. Bylander,[1] Faihaa Ahmed,[2] Sabena M. Conley,[2] Jean-Marie Mwiza,[2] and Elimelda Moige Ongeri[2]

[1]*Department of Environmental Sciences, Pennsylvania State University, Harrisburg, Middletown, PA 17057, USA*
[2]*Department of Biology, North Carolina A&T State University, Greensboro, NC 27411, USA*

Correspondence should be addressed to Elimelda Moige Ongeri; eongeri@ncat.edu

Academic Editor: Konstantinos Papatheodorou

Meprins are membrane-bound and secreted metalloproteinases consisting of α and/or β subunits that are highly expressed in kidney epithelial cells and are differentially expressed in podocytes and leukocytes (macrophages and monocytes). Several studies have implicated meprins in the progression of diabetic nephropathy (DN) and fibrosis-associated kidney disease. However, the mechanisms by which meprins modulate DN are not understood. To delineate the role of meprins in DN, we subjected meprin $\alpha\beta$ knockout ($\alpha\beta$KO) mice and their wild-type (WT) counterparts to streptozotocin-induced type 1 diabetes. The 18-week survival rates were significantly lower for diabetic meprin $\alpha\beta$KO mice when compared to those for their WT counterparts. There were significant decreases in mRNA and protein levels for both meprin α and β in diabetic WT kidneys. Furthermore, the blood urea nitrogen levels and urine albumin/creatinine ratios increased in diabetic meprin $\alpha\beta$KO but not in diabetic WT mice, indicating that meprins may be protective against diabetic kidney injury. The brush border membrane levels of villin, a meprin target, significantly decreased in diabetic WT but not in diabetic meprin $\alpha\beta$KO kidneys. In contrast, isoform-specific increases in cytosolic levels of the catalytic subunit of PKA, another meprin target, were demonstrated for both WT and meprin $\alpha\beta$KO kidneys.

1. Introduction

Meprins are zinc metalloproteases of the astacin family that are abundantly expressed in the brush border membranes (BBM) of kidney proximal tubules and small intestines [1, 2]. Other locations with documented meprin expression include the skin [3], podocytes [4], and leukocytes (macrophages and monocytes) [5]. Meprins are composed of two subunits, alpha (α) and beta (β), that are encoded by distinct genes on chromosomes 6 and 18, respectively, in humans, and chromosomes 17 and 18, respectively, in mice [6–8]. These result in two protein isoforms, meprin A and meprin B. Meprin A is a homooligomer of α subunits or a heterooligomer of α and β subunits, while meprin B is a homooligomer of β subunits [9, 10]. Meprins have been implicated in the pathology of acute and chronic kidney injury. The levels of expression and localization of meprins have been associated with acute kidney injury induced by ischemia/reperfusion (IR) [11, 12]. While meprin localization is restricted to the BBM in healthy kidneys, both meprin A and meprin B get redistributed to the cytoplasm and basolateral membranes in IR [11, 12]. Pretreatment of rats with the meprin inhibitor, actinonin, and disruption of the meprin β gene both protected mice from IR-induced renal injury [11, 13], suggesting that meprins enhance kidney injury in IR.

A role for meprin β in the progression of diabetic nephropathy (DN) and fibrosis-associated kidney disease has been demonstrated by several studies in both rodents and humans [14–16]. Db/db mice, a common mouse model of type 2 diabetes, manifested decreased meprin α and meprin β gene and protein expression before the development of clinical kidney disease [15]. Furthermore, meprin A enzymatic activity was lower in the diabetic db/db mice when compared to that in the control nonobese mice. Rats with streptozotocin- (STZ-) induced type 1 diabetes were also shown to have significant increases in urinary meprin A excretion. Additionally, their kidney proximal tubule BBM protein levels and meprin A activity were both decreased [15]. In humans, meprin β gene polymorphisms were associated with DN in the Pima Indians, a United States Native American ethnic group with an extremely high incidence of type 2 diabetes, and a prevalence of end stage renal disease (ESRD) that is 23 times that of the general population [16]. A study involving 154 diabetic individuals revealed 19 single-nucleotide polymorphisms (SNPs) of the meprin β gene. Nine of the SNPs had significant within-family associations, suggesting a role for meprin β in DN. However, the mechanisms by which meprins modulate the progression of DN are not known. Several extracellular (ECM) proteins (e.g., collagen IV, fibronectin, laminin, and nidogen-1) and modulators of inflammation (e.g., IL-1β, IL-6, IL-18, and MCP-1) are proteolytically processed by meprins, suggesting that meprins could impact inflammation and the fibrosis observed in DN. The objective of the present study was to evaluate how meprin deficiency impacts the pathology of kidney injury in mice with STZ-induced type 1 diabetes.

2. Materials and Methods

2.1. Experimental Animals. Eight-week-old male mice on a congenic C57BL/6 background were used for these studies. We compared wild-type (WT) and meprin $\alpha\beta$ knockout ($\alpha\beta$KO) mice in which the genes for both meprin α and meprin β were disrupted. The mice were housed at the Pennsylvania State University, College of Medicine, Hershey, Pennsylvania. All the mice were kept under a 12 : 12 light: dark cycle and provided rodent chow and fresh deionized water ad libitum. The animal procedures used were approved by the Institutional Animal Care and Use Committees (IACUC).

2.2. Induction of Diabetes. Type 1 diabetes was induced in male mice at age 8 weeks ($n = 7$ for each group) by intraperitoneal injection of STZ. We first used high-dose STZ (100 mg/kg body weight for 2 days) to determine whether diabetes affects meprin expression. The WT mice for this experiment were sacrificed at 12 weeks post-STZ injection and real-time PCR was used to evaluate the expression of meprin α and meprin β. After confirming a decrease in meprin mRNA levels, we sought to find out how meprin expression impacts the progression of DN. To this end, we induced type 1 diabetes in both WT and meprin $\alpha\beta$KO mice. However, because of the side effects associated with high-dose STZ, we used low-dose STZ and planned to keep the mice for 24 weeks, a time point that has been used for C57BL/6 mice in previous studies. The mice were injected with low-dose STZ, (55 mg/kg daily for 5 consecutive days) following the protocol described by Tesch and Allen [17] and recommended by the Animal Models of Diabetic Complications Consortium (AMDCC; http://amdcc.org/). The mice were fasted for 6 hours before STZ injection. The STZ was dissolved in sodium citrate solution (pH 4.5) and injected within 15 minutes using insulin syringes. Control mice ($n = 4$ for each group) were injected with equivalent volumes of the sodium-citrate vehicle solution. Biochemical assessments of diabetes were done by measuring blood glucose levels at 10 days post-STZ injection. STZ-injected mice with a nonfasting glucose of >15 mmol/L (>280 mg/DL) were considered diabetic and used for the study. Body weights were monitored on a weekly basis. Blood and urine samples were collected at 4-week intervals. Blood was sampled into heparin tubes by tail nicking and by cardiac puncture or aspiration from the abdominal aorta at the time the mice were sacrificed. Spot urine samples were collected by bladder massage onto sterile petri dishes, and metabolic cages were used for collecting 24 h urine samples. The high mortality rate associated with meprin deficiency was unexpected, leading us to sacrifice the mice at 18 weeks post-STZ injection so we could analyze the kidney tissue and avoid losing all the meprin $\alpha\beta$ KO mice.

2.3. Biochemical Assays for Kidney Function. Kidney function was evaluated by assays for blood urea nitrogen (BUN), serum creatinine, and urine albumin to creatinine ratio. Measurement of BUN was performed with Vitros DT60II chemistry slides (Ortho Clinical Diagnostics, Rochester, NY). Serum and urine creatinine were assayed by ELISA (Diazyme Laboratories, San Diego, CA). Urinary albumin excretion was also determined by ELISA (Exocell, Philadelphia PA).

2.4. Processing of Kidney Tissue. The mice were weighed and sacrificed by isoflurane asyphyxiation followed by cervical dislocation. The kidneys were excised, decapsulated, and individually weighed. One longitudinal half of the right kidney tissue was fixed in methyl Carnoy's fixative (6 : 3 : 1 methanol-chloroform-acetic acid), transferred to 70% ethanol, and subsequently paraffin embedded for histological analysis. The other half was combined with the left kidney and snap frozen in liquid nitrogen for protein extraction. The left kidneys from mice subjected to the high-dose STZ treatment were homogenized immediately in TRIzol and processed for RNA extraction.

2.5. RNA Extraction. Total RNA was extracted from the left kidneys of the mice injected with high-dose STZ using TRIzol (Invitrogen, Carlsbad, CA). The quantity and integrity of total RNA were determined using an absorption ratio at 260 and 280 nm and agarose-formaldehyde gel electrophoresis, respectively.

2.6. Real-Time PCR. Synthesis of cDNA was performed with 2 μg of each RNA preparation, SuperScript III reverse transcriptase (Invitrogen), and hexanucleotide random primers (Roche, Indianapolis, IN). A reaction without reverse transcriptase was run in parallel for each RNA sample to control for DNA amplification. PCR primers were designed with

Primer Express 1.5 software (Applied Biosystems), and the Spidey data-mining tool (National Center for Biotechnology Information) was used to minimize DNA amplification. Primers were as follows: meprin α forward, CGCCTCAAGT CTTGTGTGGATT; reverse, ATTTCATGTTCAATGGTGG CCTT (product size, 164 bp); meprin β forward, AGGATTC AGCCAGGCAAGGA; reverse, CGTGACGATGGTAGACT CTGTCC (product size, 144 bp); and β-actin forward, TGA CGTTGACATCCGTAAAGACC; reverse, CTCAGGAGGA GCAATGATCTTGA (product size, 148 bp). Quantitative fluorescent real-time PCR analysis was performed in an ABI 7700 sequence detector (Applied Biosystems) using the QuantiTect SYBR green PCR kit and 300 nM gene-specific primers. The cycle profile was 15 min at 95°C followed by 40 cycles of 15 s at 94°C, 30 s at 55°C, and 30 s at 71°C. Analyses of 40 ng of cDNA for meprin β and 16 ng for meprin α and β-actin were performed in triplicate, and reverse transcriptase negative control reactions were performed in duplicate. For determination of standard curves and PCR efficiencies, standards were prepared using dilutions of C57Bl/6 mouse kidney total RNA. Differences between slopes were <0.1, and PCR efficiencies were >1.97 for all primer pairs. Data were normalized to β-actin and analyzed using the comparative threshold cycle method. The results are presented as fold expression relative to nondiabetic (sodium citrate-injected) control mice.

2.7. Kidney Protein Extraction. The frozen kidney tissues were thawed on ice and homogenized in 9 volumes of homogenization buffer (2 mM Tris-HCl and 10 mM Mannitol; pH 7.0) with protease inhibitors and fractionated into BBM- and cytosolic-enriched protein fractions as previously described [12, 18]. In addition, RIPA buffer was used to obtain nonfractionated total protein lysates from each kidney. The protein levels were quantified using a Bradford protein assay and Bio-Rad's protein reagent and subsequently stored in aliquots at −80°C until analyzed by Western blot.

2.8. Western Blot Analysis. Western blot analysis coupled with optic densitometry were used to quantify the protein levels for meprin A, meprin B, villin, the catalytic subunit of protein kinase A (PKA C), and phosphor-PKA C in kidney tissue. To this end, 20 μg of BBM-enriched proteins or 60 μg of cytosolic-enriched protein samples were electrophoretically separated using 10% acrylamide gels and transferred onto nitrocellulose membranes. Nonspecific binding sites on the membranes were blocked in 5% fat-free milk made in tris-buffered saline with 0.5% Tween 20 (TBS-T) for 1 h at room temperature (RT). The membranes were then probed using primary antibodies against each of the proteins and incubated at RT for 1 h or at 4°C overnight. The antibodies used were rabbit polyclonal antimeprin α (HMC14, gift from Dr. Judith Bond, Pennsylvania State University, College of Medicine, Hershey, Pennsylvania) diluted 1 : 3000, rabbit polyclonal antimeprin β (HMC77, gift from Dr. Judith Bond, Pennsylvania State University, College of Medicine, Hershey, Pennsylvania) diluted 1 : 5000, rabbit polyclonal antivillin (Santa Cruz Biotechnology, Santa Cruz CA) diluted 1 : 1000, mouse monoclonal anti-PKA C (BD Biosciences, San Jose, CA) diluted 1 : 1000, and phosphor-PKA C (Cell Signaling, Danvers, MA) diluted 1 : 1000. The nitrocellulose membranes were washed three times for 10 min in TBS-T and incubated with HRP-conjugated secondary antibodies (Bio-Rad, Hercules, CA) diluted 1 : 15,000 in TBS-T at RT for 1 h or at 4°C overnight. The membranes were then washed in TBS-T for 15 min, three times, and exposed to Chemiluminiscence substrate, and protein bands developed by exposure to X-ray film. The membranes were stripped and probed for tubulin as a loading control. The intensities of the protein bands were quantified using Bio-Rad's GS800 calibrated densitometer coupled with QuantityOne software. The relative OD were calculated as a ratio of the OD for each protein and the OD for the tubulin loading control. The relative OD data were subjected to statistical analysis using 2-way ANOVA (GraphPad Prism software).

2.9. Immunohistochemical Analysis and Microscopic Imaging. Kidney tissues were paraffin embedded at the Pennsylvania State University, College of Medicine, Histology Core Facility, Hershey, PA. Serial kidney sections (4 μm) were cut onto Superfrost® slides and deparaffinized by sequential exposure to xylenes (3 × 5 minutes), 100% ethanol (2 × 10 minutes), 95% ethanol (3 × 5 minutes), and distilled water (2 × 5 minutes). The kidney tissue sections were stained in periodic acid-Schiff and hematoxylin-eosin staining to evaluate tubular dilation. Analysis for localization of meprins was performed using standard immunohistochemical protocols previously described [12, 19]. The sections were imaged using light microscopy and ImageJ was used to evaluate tubular dilation.

2.10. Statistical Analysis. The ELISA assays were performed in triplicate and analyzed by two-way ANOVA. The intensity of protein bands for Western blot were quantified using Bio-Rad's GS800 calibrated densitometer and QuantityOne software (Bio-Rad, Hercules, CA). The densitometric data for Western blots for individual mouse samples were normalized to tubulin levels and analyzed by two-way ANOVA with pairwise comparisons for all treatment groups using GraphPad Prism software. The data are presented as mean ± SEM. p values ≤0.05 were considered statistically significant. Comparison of survival curves utilized chi-square and the Gehan-Breslow-Wilcoxon test.

3. Results

3.1. Severe Diabetes Caused a Significant Decrease in Kidney Meprin mRNA and Protein Levels. We first determined the impact of severe diabetes on renal meprin expression levels. Wild-type mice treated with high-dose STZ were sacrificed at 12 weeks post-STZ injection, and real-time PCR was used to determine the kidney meprin α and meprin β mRNA levels. The diabetic mice had a significant decrease in kidney mRNA levels of 43% for meprin α ($p \leq 0.05$) and 61% for meprin β ($p \leq 0.01$) (Figure 1(a)). Western blot analysis with BBM-enriched kidney protein fractions also demonstrated an 18% decrease in BBM meprin α protein levels ($p \leq 0.05$) and a 53% decrease in meprin β protein levels ($p \leq 0.01$) in

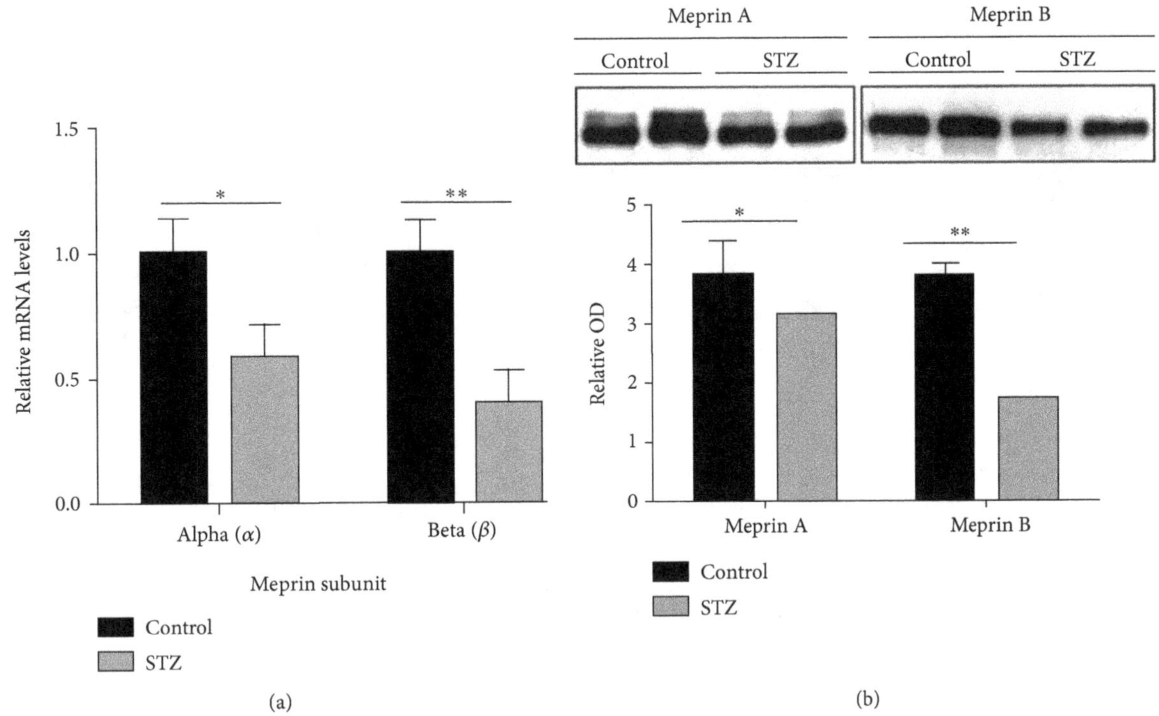

FIGURE 1: (a) Messenger RNA levels for meprin α and meprin β. Kidneys from WT mice injected with high-dose STZ were harvested at 12 weeks post-STZ injection and Trizol was used to extract RNA. Real-time PCR was used to amplify meprin α and meprin β mRNA. Data were normalized to β-actin and analyzed using the comparative threshold cycle method. The results are presented as fold expression ± SEM ($n = 7$) relative to nondiabetic (sodium citrate-injected) control mice. $^*p < 0.05$, $^{**}p < 0.01$. (b) Protein levels for meprin A and meprin B in the brush border membrane (BBM) of kidneys from wild-type (WT) mice with STZ-induced type 1 diabetes. Proteins were extracted from WT mice injected with low-dose STZ at 18 weeks post STZ injection, and Western blot analysis used to evaluate meprin protein levels in the BBM-enriched fraction. Diabetic kidneys had a significant decrease in the levels of both meprin A and meprin B proteins ($p \leq 0.05$). However, the fold change in protein levels was greater for meprin B (53%) than for meprin A (18%). $^*p < 0.05$, $^{**}p < 0.01$.

mice injected with low-dose STZ at 18 weeks post-STZ (Figure 1(b)).

3.2. Meprin Deficiency Was Associated with Higher Mortality Rates in Diabetic Mice. We initially sought to evaluate the impact of meprin deficiency on the pathology of DN over a 24-week period. To this end, we used low-dose STZ to induce type 1 diabetes. The meprin $\alpha\beta$KO mice (with disruption of both meprin α and meprin β genes) with STZ-induced type 1 diabetes had significantly lower relative survival rates at 18 weeks compared to wild-type mice ($p \leq 0.02$) (Figure 2). The 18-week survival rate for the meprin $\alpha\beta$KO mice was only 40%, leading us to terminate the experiment at 18 weeks post-STZ injection. The relative survival rates for each group were determined as a ratio of the survival of the diabetic mice to that of the nondiabetic control mice in the same genotype.

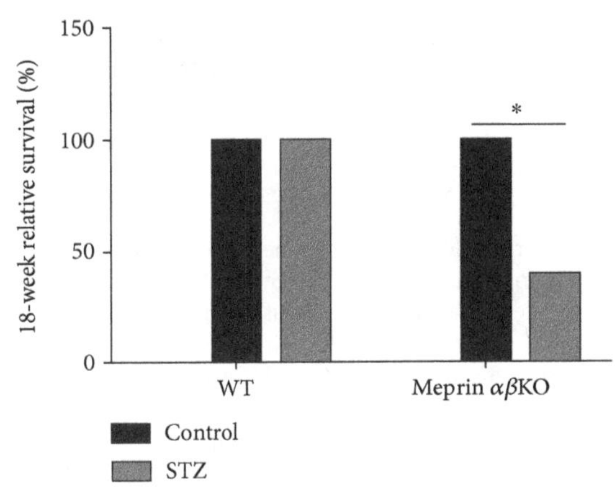

FIGURE 2: Survival rates for mice with STZ-induced type 1 diabetes. Low-dose STZ was used to induce type 1 diabetes in 8-week-old male mice. The relative survival rates at 18 weeks post-STZ were normalized to those of nondiabetic control mice in each group. Meprin $\alpha\beta$ double-KO mice had a significantly lower 18-week survival rate (40%) when compared to wild-type mice (100%) ($p \leq 0.02$). $^*p \leq 0.05$.

3.3. Meprin Deficiency Resulted in Greater Impairment of Kidney Function. Kidney phenotyping data showed greater loss of kidney function in meprin-deficient mice. The meprin $\alpha\beta$KO mice with low-dose STZ-induced type 1diabetes had progressively higher BUN levels at 4 and 8 weeks post-STZ injection. At 12 weeks post-STZ, the BUN levels were significantly higher ($p \leq 0.05$) in diabetic meprin $\alpha\beta$KO mice when compared to those in their WT counterparts (Figure 3). Another important finding was a significantly higher albumin/creatinine ratio in diabetic meprin $\alpha\beta$KO mice when compared to that in their diabetic WT counterparts at 8 weeks post-STZ (Figure 4). While renal hypertrophy was significantly higher in diabetic kidneys, there was no

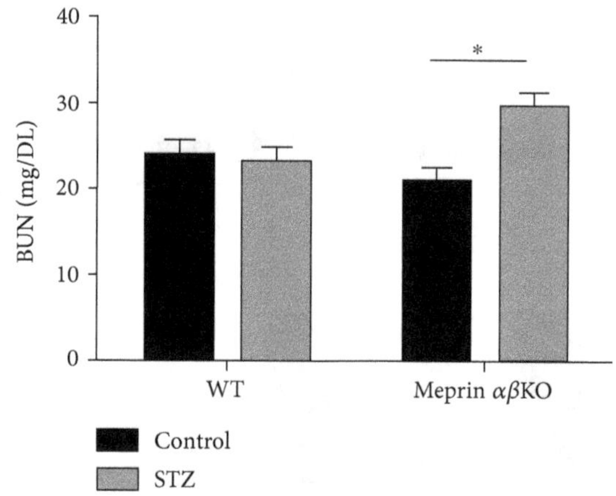

FIGURE 3: Blood urea nitrogen (BUN) levels at 12 weeks post-STZ injection. Blood was collected by tail nicking and plasma BUN levels were determined by use of BUN slides that were read on a Vitros DT6011 analyzer (Ortho Clinical Diagnostics, Rochester, NY). BUN levels were significantly higher ($p \leq 0.05$) in diabetic meprin $\alpha\beta$ double-KO mice when compared to those in nondiabetic controls at 12 weeks post-STZ injection. This difference was not significant in the wild-type mice. $^{*}p \leq 0.05$.

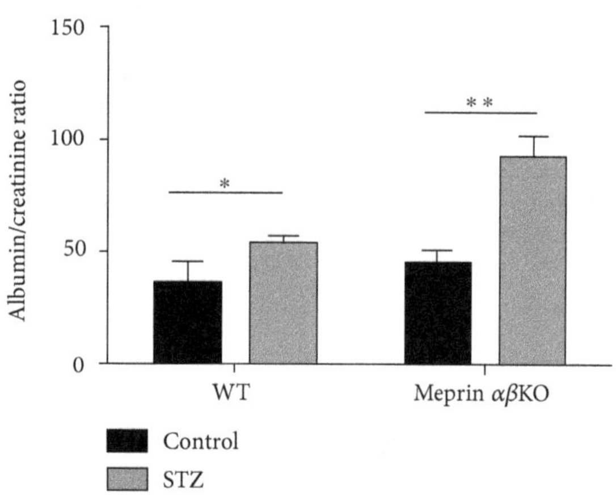

FIGURE 4: Urine albumin/creatinine ratio. Urine samples were collected onto sterile petri dishes by bladder massage. Albumin levels were determined by ELISA using murine Albuwell ELISA kits (Exocell, Philadelphia, PA). Creatinine levels in the same samples were determined by use of ELISA (Diazyme Laboratories). The 8-week albumin/creatinine ratios were significantly higher in diabetic meprin $\alpha\beta$KO mice when compared to those in their diabetic WT counterparts ($p \leq 0.05$). $^{*}p \leq 0.05$, $^{**}p \leq 0.01$.

significant association with meprin expression or deficiency (Figure 5).

3.4. Levels and Phosphorylation Status of the Catalytic Subunit of Protein Kinase A (PKA C) Correlated with Meprin Expression in Diabetic Kidneys. The PKA pathway has previously been shown to play a role in extracellular matrix (ECM) protein metabolism and the fibrosis associated with DN. Previous in vitro studies by our group had shown that the catalytic subunit of PKA (PKA C) is a meprin substrate and that meprin A is expressed in the glomeruli of diabetic mouse

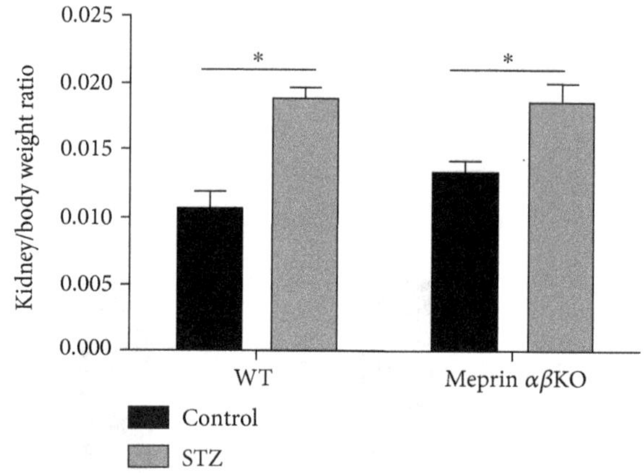

FIGURE 5: The kidney/body weight ratio at 18 weeks post-STZ injection. Kidneys were decapsulated and individually weighed. There was a significant renal hypertrophy in diabetic mice when compared to that in nondiabetic control mice in both genotypes. However, there was no significant difference between meprin $\alpha\beta$KO mice and WT mice. $^{*}p \leq 0.05$.

kidneys [19–21]. We therefore sought to evaluate the levels of phospho-PKA C in the kidneys of wild-type and meprin $\alpha\beta$KO mice with STZ-induced type 1 diabetes and compare them to those of nondiabetic controls for each genotype. Western blot analysis showed that the levels of the 42 kDa PKA C protein isoform in cytosolic-enriched kidney proteins were significantly higher in the kidneys from diabetic mice for both genotypes (Figure 6(a)). This increase was not observed for the 57 kDa PKA C isoform. We then determined the levels of phosphor-PKA C (p-PKA C) in the kidneys of diabetic mice. Western blot with phosphospecific anti-PKA C antibodies showed that the levels of the 42 kDa phospho-PKA increased in the kidneys of both WT and meprin $\alpha\beta$KO mice with STZ-induced diabetes when compared to those of their control counterparts. In contrast, the levels of the 57 kDa p-PKA C isoform decreased in both genotypes.

3.5. Diabetic Nephropathy Associated with a Decrease in Brush Border Villin Levels in Meprin Expressing Kidneys. Histological analysis showed loss of brush border microvilli and dilation of proximal tubules from the kidneys of diabetic wild-type mice (Figures 7(a) and 7(b)). This was especially apparent in stained sections probed with antimeprin antibodies (Figure 7(a)). To determine whether the tubular dilation is associated with loss of cytoskeletal proteins that constitute the structure of the brush border microvilli, we used Western blot analysis to compare the levels of villin, a meprin B target and a major component of the kidney proximal tubule BBM [12], in the BBM-enriched kidney proteins. Our data showed a significant decrease ($p \leq 0.05$) in BBM villin levels in diabetic WT mice when compared to those in their meprin $\alpha\beta$KO counterparts (Figure 7(c)).

4. Discussion

Meprin metalloproteases have been implicated in the pathology of diabetic nephropathy (DN), the major single cause of end-stage renal disease (ESRD). Diabetic nephropathy is

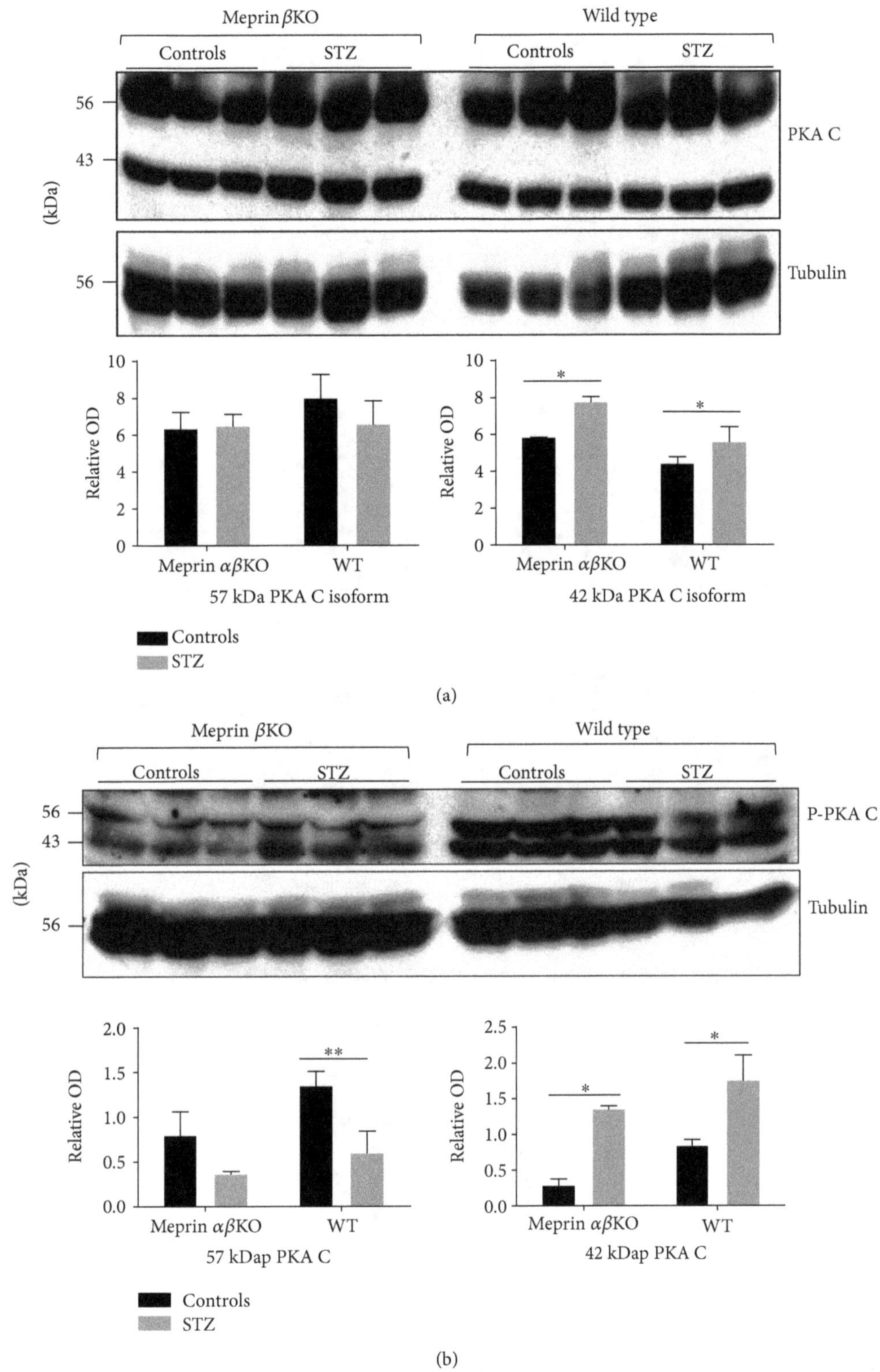

Figure 6: (a) Representative immunoblot for the catalytic subunit of protein kinase A (PKA C) in cytosolic kidney protein fraction; (b) representative immunoblot for p-PKA C in cytosolic-enriched kidney proteins. Proteins were extracted from kidney tissue at 18 weeks post-STZ injection and fractionated into cytosolic- and BBM-enriched fractions using differential centrifugation. Western blot analysis using anti-PKA C and p-PKA C-specific antibodies coupled with optic densitometry were used to quantify the PKA C protein levels. The levels of the 42 kDa PKA C protein isoform (a) were significantly higher in kidneys from diabetic mice, but there were no significant changes in the levels of the 57 kDa isoform. The levels of the 42 kDa p-PKA C increased while the levels of the 57 p-KCA isoform decreased for both genotypes. $^{*}p \leq 0.05$, $^{**}p \leq 0.01$.

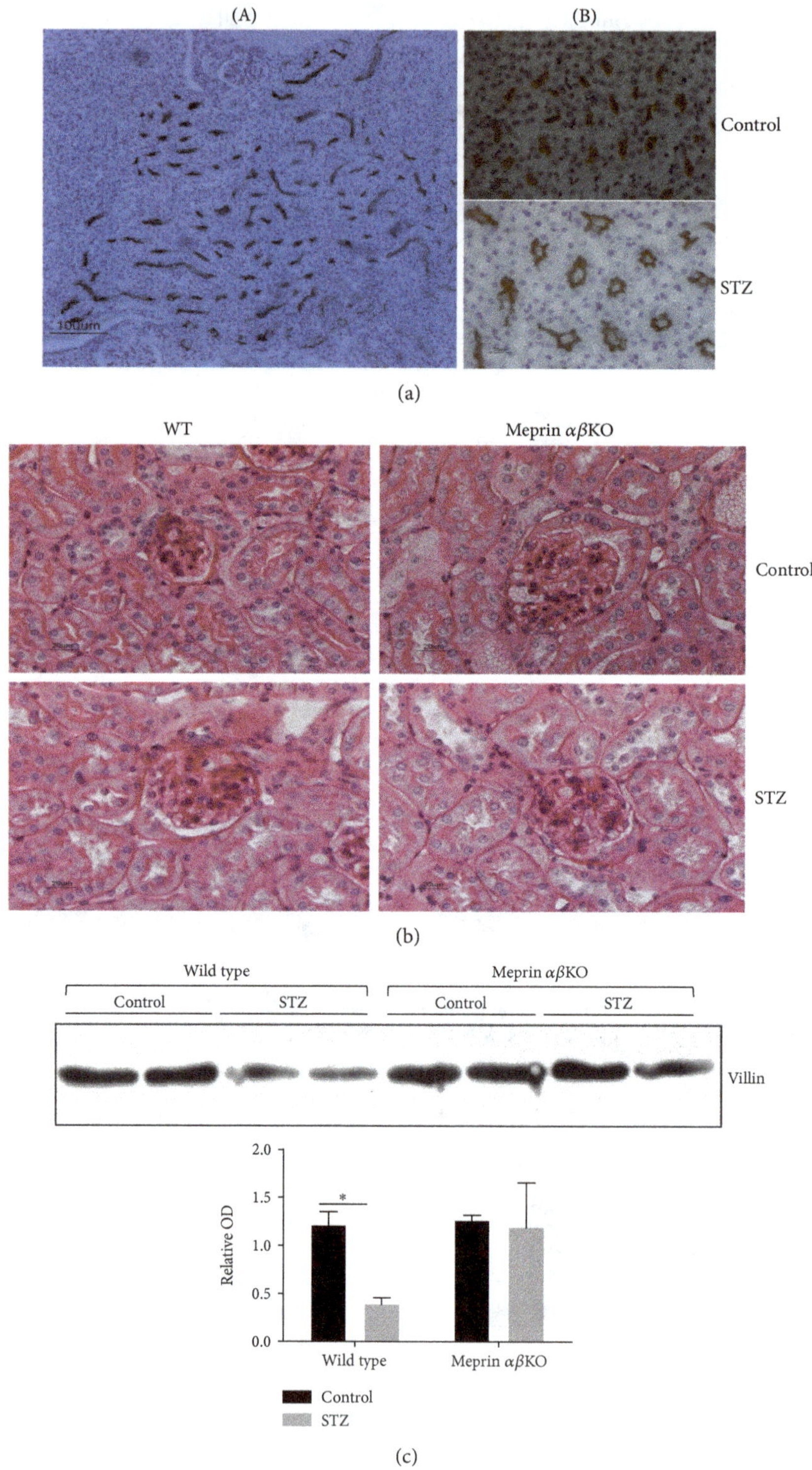

FIGURE 7: Localization of meprin B in the juxtamedullary region of the kidney (a), acid Schiff-stained kidney sections (b), and representative immunoblot for villin in BBM-enriched kidney protein fractions from wild-type and meprin $\alpha\beta$KO mice at 18 weeks post-STZ (c). There was no noticeable redistribution of meprins from the BBMs to other cell compartments. Significant tubular dilation was evident in the kidneys from diabetic mice when compared to that from nondiabetic controls. There was more tubular dilation in STZ-treated mice when compared to that in nondiabetic vehicle-treated controls. The levels of villin were significantly lower in diabetic WT mice when compared to those in nondiabetic controls ($p \leq 0.05$). This decrease was not observed in meprin $\alpha\beta$KO mice. $^*p \leq 0.05$.

characterized by albuminuria [22], renal hypertrophy [23], and excess accumulation of extracellular matrix (ECM) within the glomerulus and interstitium [24–28]. In humans, polymorphisms in the meprin β gene were associated with DN in the Pima Indians of Arizona, a US ethnic group with an extremely high incidence of type 2 diabetes and ESRD

[16]. Several studies have also demonstrated an association between meprin expression and the development of renal fibrosis, but the underlying mechanisms are not understood. Gene and protein expression levels for both meprin α and meprin β were downregulated in the kidneys of diabetic rats and in db/db mice before the development of overt kidney disease [15]. Data from the present study show a significant downregulation of gene and protein expression levels for both meprin α and meprin β in a mouse model of type I diabetes. By comparing congenic wild-type and meprin $\alpha\beta$ knockout mice, we have shown more severe diabetic kidney damage in meprin-deficient mice as evidenced by significantly higher blood urea nitrogen (BUN) levels and higher albumin/creatinine ratios. Mice with disruption of the meprin α and meprin β genes also had higher mortality rates associated with STZ-induced type 1 diabetes.

Two key pathological changes in DN, thickening of the glomerular basement membrane (GBM) and tubular interstitial fibrosis, are directly related to excessive ECM protein buildup. Identified meprin targets in the kidney include ECM proteins and proteins involved in ECM metabolism and thus linked to the renal fibrosis associated with DN [12, 19, 29–32]. In vitro and in vivo studies showed that meprins proteolytically process several ECM proteins (e.g., type IV collagen, type VI collagen, nidogen-1, laminin, and fibronectin) [33–37] and could thus directly impact the levels of ECM proteins via degradation. Other meprin substrates involved in ECM metabolism include proinflammatory cytokines and chemokines (e.g., interleukin 1β (IL-1β) [31, 32], interleukin 6 (IL-6) [38], and prointerleukin-18 (pro-IL-18) [30] and chemoattractant protein-1 (MCP-1), the catalytic subunit of protein kinase A (PKA) [19, 39], and protein kinase C (PKC) [40]). Meprins were previously implicated in inflammation and fibrosis in other pathologies, for example, meprin β expression is downregulated in collagen IVA3 knockout mice that develop Alport's syndrome [41] and meprin α was identified as a susceptibility gene for inflammatory bowel disease (IBD) [42, 43]. The PKA signaling pathway has been shown to interact with TGF β1 signaling to regulate ECM metabolism. We recently demonstrated isoform-specific proteolytic processing of the catalytic subunit of PKA (PKAC) by meprins which resulted in reduced kinase activity [19]. We further showed meprin expression in the glomerular of mice with STZ-induced type 1 diabetes. The protein kinase A (PKA) signaling pathway has been shown to play a role in ECM metabolism. Meprins could thus modulate the progression of DN via modulation of ECM metabolism through interactions with the PKA signaling pathway. In the present study, we demonstrated modest increases in the cytosolic levels of the 42 kDa (corresponding to the size of PKA Cα and Cβ1 splice variants) and 57 KDa PKA C (corresponding to the size of PKA Cβ4 splice variant) isoforms in diabetic nephropathy in both wild-type and meprin knockout mice. More importantly, we show a correlation between meprin expression and the phosphorylation status of PKA C isoforms. Since proteolytic processing by meprins reduces the kinase activity of PKA C, this could impact downstream mediators of the PKA signaling pathway in the kidney. The data suggest that in addition to directly cleaving ECM proteins, meprins could play an indirect role in ECM metabolism via proteolysis of signaling molecules such as PKA C, which are involved in ECM metabolism and the inflammatory response. Previous studies had shown that high blood glucose, the hallmark of diabetes, causes oxidative stress which induces synthesis of ECM proteins such as laminin and fibronectin in mesangial cells [44–46]. The glucose-mediated oxidative stress could be mimicked by the PKA agonist, forskolin, and inhibited by the PKA inhibitor, H89 [47]. Additionally, high glucose levels were shown to activate PKA, leading to phosphorylation and inhibition of G6PD in renal cortical extracts from diabetic rats [48]. Phosphorylation of the cAMP response-binding protein (CREB) also increased fibronectin production in rats with STZ-induced DN [45, 49]. The PKA signaling pathway further regulates TGF-β1 induction of epithelial-to-mesenchymal transition (EMT), an event that is related to the pathology of fibrotic kidney disease [50–52]. It is probable that the loss of kinase activity could impact downstream targets of the PKA signaling pathway, including TGF-β1-mediated regulation of the metabolism and catabolism of ECM, as well as the production of inflammatory response mediators. The downstream modulators of the PKA-TGF-β1-induced response are known to be cell type specific and depend on the cellular environment, and further studies are needed to delineate the impact of meprins on these pathways.

Meprins also cleave two cytoskeletal proteins, villin and actin, which would cause injury to the brush border membranes of proximal kidney tubules [12]. Data from the current study shows a significant reduction in the levels of villin in the kidneys from WT but not from meprin $\alpha\beta$KO mice. Villin is a critical part of the proximal tubule brush border membrane and degradation of villin could contribute to the appearance of dilation of the tubular lumen as observed in DN. While expression of meprins is most abundant in the BBM of proximal kidney tubules, meprins are redistributed from the BBM to the cytosol and basolateral membranes under pathological conditions such as ischemia reperfusion-(IR-) induced renal injury [11, 12]. Recent studies have documented the expression of meprins in rat podocytes [4] and in human and mouse leukocytes [5]. Our group recently demonstrated glomerular expression of meprins in the kidneys of diabetic mice but not in nondiabetic controls [19], suggesting that meprins could play a role in both tubular and glomerular renal pathology. Data from the present study indicate that meprin deficiency contributes to a more severe pathology observed in DN. Taken together, the data suggest that meprins play a protective role in kidney injury induced by diabetes. This could be via modulation of inflammation, an underlying cause of fibrosis, or through proteolytic processing of ECM proteins. Proteolytic processing by meprin B was shown to inactivate IL-6 [38]. In contrast, cleavage of IL-1β and pro-IL-18 by meprin B caused their activation [30, 31]. Meprin A was also shown to play a role in the release of the anti-inflammatory peptide, Ac-SDKP, from thymosin β4 [53]. Compared to human diabetic patients, rodent models of DN develop modest elevations in albuminuria and serum creatinine, and kidney histological lesions associated with DN in mice are also modest. This resistance to renal damage makes most strains of mice unsuitable as models for human DN. Because expression of meprins is much higher in the mouse kidneys when compared to that in humans [54], these data suggest that meprin expression may in part explain the modest DN observed in many mouse models of DN. Meprin-deficient mice could thus be a good model for studies on DN.

Disclosure

The content is solely the responsibility of the authors and does not necessarily represent the official views of the NIH.

Conflicts of Interest

The authors declare that there is no conflict of interest regarding the publication of this paper.

Acknowledgments

The authors wish to thank Dr. Judith Bond, Pennsylvania State University, College of Medicine, Hershey, Pennsylvania, for the meprin knockout mice and antimeprin α and antimeprin β antibodies used in this study and support for the experiments. The research in this publication was supported by the National Institutes of Health (NIH)/National Institute of General Medical Sciences (NIGMS) under Award no. SC3GM102049 to Elimelda Moige Ongeri. John E. Bylander was supported by the National Institutes of Diabetes and Digestive and Kidney Diseases (NIDDK) under Award no. DK19691 to Judith S. Bond. Faihaa Ahmed and Jean-Marie Mwiza were supported by the RISE Program under NIH/NIGMS Grant no. R25GM076162 to Goldie Byrd.

References

[1] G. P. Kaushal, P. D. Walker, and S. V. Shah, "An old enzyme with a new function: purification and characterization of a distinct matrix-degrading metalloproteinase in rat kidney cortex and its identification as meprin," *The Journal of Cell Biology*, vol. 126, no. 5, pp. 1319–1327, 1994.

[2] R. J. Beynon and J. S. Bond, "Expression of the Mep-1 gene regulating meprin, a kidney brush border proteinase," *Progress in Clinical and Biological Research*, vol. 180, pp. 185–194, 1985.

[3] C. Becker-Pauly, M. Howel, T. Walker et al., "The alpha and beta subunits of the metalloprotease meprin are expressed in separate layers of human epidermis, revealing different functions in keratinocyte proliferation and differentiation," *The Journal of Investigative Dermatology*, vol. 127, no. 5, pp. 1115–1125, 2007.

[4] B. Oneda, N. Lods, D. Lottaz et al., "Metalloprotease meprin beta in rat kidney: glomerular localization and differential expression in glomerulonephritis," *PLoS One*, vol. 3, no. 5, article e2278, 2008.

[5] Q. Sun, H. J. Jin, and J. S. Bond, "Disruption of the meprin alpha and beta genes in mice alters homeostasis of monocytes and natural killer cells," *Experimental Hematology*, vol. 37, no. 3, pp. 346–356, 2009.

[6] J. S. Bond, K. Rojas, J. Overhauser, H. Y. Zoghbi, and W. Jiang, "The structural genes, MEP1A and MEP1B, for the alpha and beta subunits of the metalloendopeptidase meprin map to human chromosomes 6p and 18q, respectively," *Genomics*, vol. 25, no. 1, pp. 300–303, 1995.

[7] W. Jiang, G. Dewald, E. Brundage et al., "Fine mapping of MEP1A, the gene encoding the alpha subunit of the metalloendopeptidase meprin, to human chromosome 6P21," *Biochemical and Biophysical Research Communications*, vol. 216, no. 2, pp. 630–635, 1995.

[8] J. F. Reckelhoff, P. E. Butler, J. S. Bond, R. J. Beynon, and H. C. Passmore, "Mep-1, the gene regulating meprin activity, maps between Pgk-2 and Ce-2 on mouse chromosome 17," *Immunogenetics*, vol. 27, no. 4, pp. 298–300, 1988.

[9] C. M. Gorbea, P. Marchand, W. Jiang et al., "Cloning, expression, and chromosomal localization of the mouse meprin beta subunit," *The Journal of Biological Chemistry*, vol. 268, no. 28, pp. 21035–21043, 1993.

[10] C. M. Gorbea, A. V. Flannery, and J. S. Bond, "Homo- and heterotetrameric forms of the membrane-bound metalloendopeptidases meprin A and B," *Archives of Biochemistry and Biophysics*, vol. 290, no. 2, pp. 549–553, 1991.

[11] J. Bylander, Q. Li, G. Ramesh, B. Zhang, W. B. Reeves, and J. S. Bond, "Targeted disruption of the meprin metalloproteinase beta gene protects against renal ischemia-reperfusion injury in mice," *American Journal of Physiology. Renal Physiology*, vol. 294, no. 3, pp. F480–F490, 2008.

[12] E. M. Ongeri, O. Anyanwu, W. B. Reeves, and J. S. Bond, "Villin and actin in the mouse kidney brush-border membrane bind to and are degraded by meprins, an interaction that contributes to injury in ischemia-reperfusion," *American Journal of Physiology. Renal Physiology*, vol. 301, no. 4, pp. F871–F882, 2011.

[13] S. Carmago, S. V. Shah, and P. D. Walker, "Meprin, a brush-border enzyme, plays an important role in hypoxic/ischemic acute renal tubular injury in rats," *Kidney International*, vol. 61, no. 3, pp. 959–966, 2002.

[14] D. M. Sadlier, S. B. Connolly, N. E. Kieran et al., "Sequential extracellular matrix-focused and baited-global cluster analysis of serial transcriptomic profiles identifies candidate modulators of renal tubulointerstitial fibrosis in murine Adriamycin-induced nephropathy," *The Journal of Biological Chemistry*, vol. 279, no. 28, pp. 29670–29680, 2004.

[15] R. Mathew, S. Futterweit, E. Valderrama et al., "Meprin-alpha in chronic diabetic nephropathy: interaction with the renin-angiotensin axis," *American Journal of Physiology. Renal Physiology*, vol. 289, no. 4, pp. F911–F921, 2005.

[16] A. R. Red Eagle, R. L. Hanson, W. Jiang et al., "Meprin beta metalloprotease gene polymorphisms associated with diabetic nephropathy in the Pima Indians," *Human Genetics*, vol. 118, no. 1, pp. 12–22, 2005.

[17] G. H. Tesch and T. J. Allen, "Rodent models of streptozotocin-induced diabetic nephropathy," *Nephrology*, vol. 12, no. 3, pp. 261–266, 2007.

[18] A. J. Kenny and J. Ingram, "Proteins of the kidney microvillar membrane. Purification and properties of the phosphoramidon-insensitive endopeptidase ('endopeptidase-2') from rat kidney," *The Biochemical Journal*, vol. 245, no. 2, pp. 515–524, 1987.

[19] J. M. Niyitegeka, A. C. Bastidas, R. H. Newman, S. S. Taylor, and E. M. Ongeri, "Isoform-specific interactions between meprin metalloproteases and the catalytic subunit of protein kinase A: significance in acute and chronic kidney injury,"

American Journal of Physiology. Renal Physiology, vol. 308, no. 1, pp. F56–F68, 2015.

[20] E. Alhanaty, J. Patinkin, M. Tauber-Finkelstein, and S. Shaltiel, "Degradative inactivation of cyclic AMP-dependent protein kinase by a membranal proteinase is restricted to the free catalytic subunit in its native conformation," *Proceedings of the National Academy of Sciences of the United States of America*, vol. 78, no. 6, pp. 3492–3495, 1981.

[21] E. Alhanaty and S. Shaltiel, "Limited proteolysis of the catalytic subunit of cAMP-dependent protein kinase—a membranal regulatory device?" *Biochemical and Biophysical Research Communications*, vol. 89, no. 2, pp. 323–332, 1979.

[22] P. Fioretto, M. L. Caramori, M. Dalla Vestra, and M. Mauer, "Risk predictors in patients with diabetic nephropathy," *Current Diabetes Reports*, vol. 1, no. 3, pp. 245–250, 2001.

[23] P. G. Duffy, S. R. Johnston, and R. A. Donaldson, "Idiopathic retroperitoneal fibrosis in twins," *The Journal of Urology*, vol. 131, no. 4, p. 746, 1984.

[24] R. Osterby, "Kidney structural abnormalities in early diabetes," *Advances in Metabolic Disorders*, vol. 2, Supplement 2, pp. 323–340, 1973.

[25] S. M. Mauer, M. W. Steffes, E. N. Ellis, D. E. Sutherland, D. M. Brown, and F. C. Goetz, "Structural-functional relationships in diabetic nephropathy," *The Journal of Clinical Investigation*, vol. 74, no. 4, pp. 1143–1155, 1984.

[26] M. W. Steffes, R. Osterby, B. Chavers, and S. M. Mauer, "Mesangial expansion as a central mechanism for loss of kidney function in diabetic patients," *Diabetes*, vol. 38, no. 9, pp. 1077–1081, 1989.

[27] M. W. Steffes, R. W. Bilous, D. E. Sutherland, and S. M. Mauer, "Cell and matrix components of the glomerular mesangium in type I diabetes," *Diabetes*, vol. 41, no. 6, pp. 679–684, 1992.

[28] P. H. Lane, M. W. Steffes, P. Fioretto, and S. M. Mauer, "Renal interstitial expansion in insulin-dependent diabetes mellitus," *Kidney International*, vol. 43, no. 3, pp. 661–667, 1993.

[29] T. Jefferson, U. Auf dem Keller, C. Bellac et al., "The substrate degradome of meprin metalloproteases reveals an unexpected proteolytic link between meprin beta and ADAM10," *Cellular and Molecular Life Sciences: CMLS*, vol. 70, no. 2, pp. 309–333, 2013.

[30] S. Banerjee and J. S. Bond, "Prointerleukin-18 is activated by meprin beta in vitro and in vivo in intestinal inflammation," *The Journal of Biological Chemistry*, vol. 283, no. 46, pp. 31371–31377, 2008.

[31] C. Herzog, G. P. Kaushal, and R. S. Haun, "Generation of biologically active interleukin-1beta by meprin B," *Cytokine*, vol. 31, no. 5, pp. 394–403, 2005.

[32] C. Herzog, R. S. Haun, V. Kaushal, P. R. Mayeux, S. V. Shah, and G. P. Kaushal, "Meprin A and meprin alpha generate biologically functional IL-1beta from pro-IL-1beta," *Biochemical and Biophysical Research Communications*, vol. 379, no. 4, pp. 904–908, 2009.

[33] D. Kohler, M. Kruse, W. Stocker, and E. E. Sterchi, "Heterologously overexpressed, affinity-purified human meprin alpha is functionally active and cleaves components of the basement membrane in vitro," *FEBS Letters*, vol. 465, no. 1, pp. 2–7, 2000.

[34] M. N. Kruse, C. Becker, D. Lottaz et al., "Human meprin alpha and beta homo-oligomers: cleavage of basement membrane proteins and sensitivity to metalloprotease inhibitors," *The Biochemical Journal*, vol. 378, Part 2, pp. 383–389, 2004.

[35] C. Herzog, R. Marisiddaiah, R. S. Haun, and G. P. Kaushal, "Basement membrane protein nidogen-1 is a target of meprin beta in cisplatin nephrotoxicity," *Toxicology Letters*, vol. 236, no. 2, pp. 110–116, 2015.

[36] P. D. Walker, G. P. Kaushal, and S. V. Shah, "Meprin A, the major matrix degrading enzyme in renal tubules, produces a novel nidogen fragment in vitro and in vivo," *Kidney International*, vol. 53, no. 6, pp. 1673–1680, 1998.

[37] D. Kronenberg, B. C. Bruns, C. Moali et al., "Processing of procollagen III by meprins: new players in extracellular matrix assembly?" *The Journal of Investigative Dermatology*, vol. 130, no. 12, pp. 2727–2735, 2010.

[38] T. R. Keiffer and J. S. Bond, "Meprin metalloproteases inactivate interleukin 6," *The Journal of Biological Chemistry*, vol. 289, no. 11, pp. 7580–7588, 2014.

[39] A. Chestukhin, K. Muradov, L. Litovchick, and S. Shaltiel, "The cleavage of protein kinase A by the kinase-splitting membranal proteinase is reproduced by meprin beta," *The Journal of Biological Chemistry*, vol. 271, no. 47, pp. 30272–30280, 1996.

[40] S. Boyd, R. Newman, and E. Ongeri, "Protein kinase C alpha is a target for the meprin B metalloproteinase (690.14)," *The FASEB Journal*, vol. 28, Supplement 1, article 690.14, 2014.

[41] N. S. Sampson, S. T. Ryan, D. A. Enke, D. Cosgrove, V. Koteliansky, and P. Gotwals, "Global gene expression analysis reveals a role for the alpha 1 integrin in renal pathogenesis," *The Journal of Biological Chemistry*, vol. 276, no. 36, pp. 34182–34188, 2001.

[42] S. Banerjee, B. Oneda, L. M. Yap et al., "MEP1A allele for meprin A metalloprotease is a susceptibility gene for inflammatory bowel disease," *Mucosal Immunology*, vol. 2, no. 3, pp. 220–231, 2009.

[43] S. Banerjee, G. Jin, S. G. Bradley et al., "Balance of meprin A and B in mice affects the progression of experimental inflammatory bowel disease," *American Journal of Physiology. Gastrointestinal and Liver Physiology*, vol. 300, no. 2, pp. G273–G282, 2011.

[44] L. P. Singh and E. D. Crook, "Hexosamine regulation of glucose-mediated laminin synthesis in mesangial cells involves protein kinases A and C," *American Journal of Physiology. Renal Physiology*, vol. 279, no. 4, pp. F646–F654, 2000.

[45] L. P. Singh, J. Andy, V. Anyamale, K. Greene, M. Alexander, and E. D. Crook, "Hexosamine-induced fibronectin protein synthesis in mesangial cells is associated with increases in cAMP responsive element binding (CREB) phosphorylation and nuclear CREB: the involvement of protein kinases A and C," *Diabetes*, vol. 50, no. 10, pp. 2355–2362, 2001.

[46] J. I. Kreisberg and S. H. Kreisberg, "High glucose activates protein kinase C and stimulates fibronectin gene expression by enhancing a cAMP response element," *Kidney International. Supplement*, vol. 51, pp. S3–S11, 1995.

[47] L. Hui, Y. Hong, Z. Jingjing, H. Yuan, C. Qi, and Z. Nong, "HGF suppresses high glucose-mediated oxidative stress in mesangial cells by activation of PKG and inhibition of PKA," *Free Radical Biology & Medicine*, vol. 49, no. 3, pp. 467–473, 2010.

[48] Y. Xu, B. W. Osborne, and R. C. Stanton, "Diabetes causes inhibition of glucose-6-phosphate dehydrogenase via activation of PKA, which contributes to oxidative stress in rat kidney cortex," *American Journal of Physiology. Renal Physiology*, vol. 289, no. 5, pp. F1040–F1047, 2005.

[49] J. Wang, H. Huang, P. Liu et al., "Inhibition of phosphorylation of p38 MAPK involved in the protection of nephropathy by emodin in diabetic rats," *European Journal of Pharmacology*, vol. 553, no. 1–3, pp. 297–303, 2006.

[50] L. Wang, Y. Zhu, and K. Sharma, "Transforming growth factor-beta1 stimulates protein kinase A in mesangial cells," *The Journal of Biological Chemistry*, vol. 273, no. 14, pp. 8522–8527, 1998.

[51] Y. Yang, X. Pan, W. Lei et al., "Regulation of transforming growth factor-beta 1-induced apoptosis and epithelial-to-mesenchymal transition by protein kinase A and signal transducers and activators of transcription 3," *Cancer Research*, vol. 66, no. 17, pp. 8617–8624, 2006.

[52] L. Bu, S. Qu, X. Gao et al., "Enhanced angiotensin-converting enzyme 2 attenuates angiotensin II-induced collagen production via AT1 receptor-phosphoinositide 3-kinase-Akt pathway," *Endocrine*, vol. 39, no. 2, pp. 139–147, 2011.

[53] N. Kumar, P. Nakagawa, B. Janic et al., "The anti-inflammatory peptide Ac-SDKP is released from thymosin-beta4 by renal meprin-alpha and prolyl oligopeptidase," *American Journal of Physiology. Renal Physiology*, vol. 310, no. 10, pp. F1026–F1034, 2016.

[54] R. E. Yura, S. G. Bradley, G. Ramesh, W. B. Reeves, and J. S. Bond, "Meprin A metalloproteases enhance renal damage and bladder inflammation after LPS challenge," *American Journal of Physiology. Renal Physiology*, vol. 296, no. 1, pp. F135–F144, 2009.

22

Incidence and Mortality Rates and Clinical Characteristics of Type 1 Diabetes among Children and Young Adults in Cochabamba, Bolivia

Elizabeth Duarte Gómez,[1] Gabriel Andrew Gregory,[2,3] Miriam Castrati Nostas,[1] Angela Christine Middlehurst,[2,4] Alicia Josephine Jenkins,[3] and Graham David Ogle[2,3,4]

[1]*Centro Vivir con Diabetes, Av. Simón López, No. 375, Cochabamba, Bolivia*
[2]*International Diabetes Federation Life for a Child Program, Glebe, NSW 2037, Australia*
[3]*NHMRC Clinical Trials Centre, University of Sydney, Sydney, NSW 2006, Australia*
[4]*Diabetes NSW, Glebe, NSW 2037, Australia*

Correspondence should be addressed to Graham David Ogle; grahamo@diabetesnsw.com.au

Academic Editor: Konstantinos Papatheodorou

Objectives. To determine incidence, mortality, and clinical status of youth with diabetes at the Centro Vivir con Diabetes, Cochabamba, Bolivia, with support from International Diabetes Federation Life for a Child Program. *Methods.* Incidence/mortality data analysis of all cases (<25 year (y)) diagnosed January 2005–February 2017 and cross-sectional data (December 2015). *Results.* Over 12.2 years, 144 cases with type 1 diabetes (T1D) were diagnosed; 43.1% were male. Diagnosis age was 0.3–22.2 y; peak was 11-12 y. 11.1% were <5 y; 29.2%, 5–<10 y; 43.1%, 10–<15 y; 13.2%, 15–<20 y; and 3.5%, 20–<25 y. The youngest is being investigated for monogenic diabetes. Measured incidence in Cercado Province (Cochabamba Department) was 2.2/100,000 children < 15 y/y, with ≈80% ascertainment, giving total incidence of 2.7/100,000 children < 15 y/y. Two had died. Crude mortality rate was 2.3/1000 patient years. Clinical data on 141 cases <35 y: mean/median HbA1c was 8.5/8.2% (69/62 mmol/mol), levels higher in adolescents. Three were on renal replacement therapy; four others had substantial renal impairment. Elevated BMI, triglycerides, and cholesterol were common: 19.1%, 18.3%, and 39.1%, respectively. *Conclusions.* Bolivia has low T1D incidence. Reasonable glycemic control is being achieved despite limited resources; however, some have serious complications and adverse cardiovascular risk factor profiles. Further attention is needed for complications.

1. Introduction

For any nation, understanding the epidemiology and clinical status of young people with diabetes is essential for training health professionals and also for conducting advocacy with the respective government to plan and improve the appropriate clinical services.

Very little published material is available on diabetes in youth in Bolivia. The International Diabetes Federation (IDF) Atlas estimates of children < 15 years with type 1 diabetes in Bolivia [1] are extrapolated from the data from Peru that is over two decades old [2, 3], a time during which the incidence of type 1 diabetes has been increasing at 2-3% or more per annum in many countries [1].

In 2005, the IDF Life for a Child (LFAC) Program [4], with the assistance of Rotary International, commenced support for the Centro Vivir con Diabetes (CVcD), a multidisciplinary clinic in Cochabamba. Satellite networks were established in five other cities. LFAC Program commenced professional mentoring and provision of insulin (initially with support of Insulin for Life Australia [5]). Later, blood glucose meters and test strips (three tests/day), HbA1c testing, and educational materials were provided.

This study presents epidemiological data on all young people with diabetes known to CVcD from January 2005 to February 2017 and the clinical features of the cohort receiving care at the end of 2015 and documents the initial impact of the LFAC Program.

2. Materials and Methods

The study was approved by the Board of Centro Vivir con Diabetes.

2.1. Epidemiology Data. Data (age, gender, and diabetes type) were compiled on all people diagnosed with diabetes at age < 25 years (y) and seen by CVcD and its five satellite clinics from January 2005 to February 2017. Diabetes was diagnosed according to the standard World Health Organization (WHO) criteria [6], and the diabetes type was determined by the local investigators based on clinical features. It is not possible to determine the exact national incidence as other diabetes care providers exist in Bolivia and no secondary ascertainment sources are available. However, in Cochabamba Province—comprising Cochabamba city and its immediate environs—where 63 (43.8%) of cases were living at diagnosis, CVcD is well-known and the ascertainment rate is estimated at 80%. A minimum incidence for Cercado Province was calculated according to census data [7], with population interpolated or extrapolated according to the annual growth rate of 1.6% [8].

The crude mortality rate was calculated as the total number of deaths in the cohort of 144 subjects divided by the total number of years from diagnosis until the last follow-up (February 2017) or, if they had died, date of death. Results are expressed as mortality per 1000 patient years.

2.2. Clinical Status. Clinical information was collated on all 141 subjects being followed from September to December 2015, who aged <25 y at diabetes diagnosis and ≤35 y at the time of this assessment. These 141 subjects included some cases diagnosed before January 2005 and excluded some cases included in the incidence study who were now being seen by other centres. The data were collected via LFAC Annual Clinical Data Sheets. Data included sex, date of birth, diabetes diagnosis date, details of diabetes treatment regimen, and physical and biochemistry measures. Also, social parameters as to whether diabetes was limiting school attendance, if subjects were in the age-appropriate grade, and how well overall the young person was, in their doctor's opinion, psychologically coping with their diabetes (rated as good, with some problems, or poor) were also recorded. Body weight and height were measured by electronic scales and a stadiometer, respectively, with subjects wearing light-weight clothing and without shoes. Body mass index (BMI) was then calculated. BMI SD scores were calculated using the WHO standards for <5 years [9], >5 years, and <19 years [10]. Blood pressure SD score was calculated from published data from the United States [11].

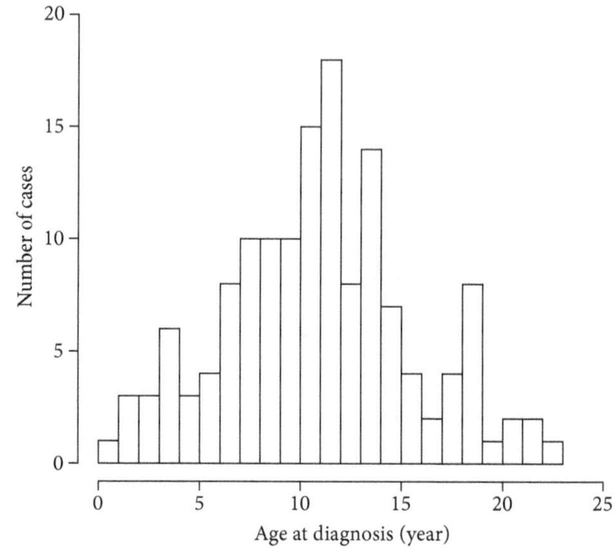

Figure 1: Age at diagnosis of type 1 diabetes in Bolivia, 2005–2017.

The presence of cataracts, retinopathy, and peripheral neuropathy was recorded. However, the methodology was not prescribed and therefore could have varied across centres and physicians.

2.3. Biochemistry. Glycosylated haemoglobin (HbA1c), serum creatinine, total cholesterol, triglycerides, and HDL cholesterol were measured in local biochemistry laboratories, with the exception of HbA1c at Cochabamba where it was measured with a Siemens DCA Vantage machine (Erlangen, Germany). Lipid tests were done on fasting samples. LDL cholesterol was calculated using the Friedewald equation and hence is only available on the subset of patients who had HDL cholesterol levels [12].

Estimated glomerular filtration rate (eGFR) was calculated for subjects ≥ 14 y by the CKD-EPI (Chronic Kidney Disease Epidemiology Collaboration) formula [13], adjusted for individual surface area.

Initial impact of Life for a Child Program was measured by assessing all HbA1c levels of all subjects having data at baseline (program commencement in 2004) and then at either six- or 12-month follow-up.

2.4. Statistics. Data and descriptive statistics were managed in Excel and analysed in R 3.3.1 (R Core Team, Vienna, Austria) with RStudio integrated development environment (RStudio Team, Boston, USA).

3. Results

3.1. Epidemiological Data

3.1.1. Sex Distribution and Age of Onset. Of the 144 subjects diagnosed at age < 25 y between January 2005 and February 2017, 62 (43.1%) were males. Age of onset ranged from 0.3–22.2 y, with a peak at 11 years (see Figure 1 histogram). Sixteen subjects (11.1%) were diagnosed at age 0–4 y, 42 (29.2%) were diagnosed at age 5–9 y, 62 (43.1%) were

Table 1: Clinical and biochemical characteristics.

Parameter	n	Mean (SD)	Range
Age at diagnosis (years)	141	9.9 (4.4)	0.3–22.2
Diabetes duration (years)	141	8.1 (5.7)	0.1–26.9
BMI SD score	137	0.9 (1.1)	−2.2–3.7
Systolic SD score	21	0.7 (0.8)	−1.4–2.0
Diastolic SD score	21	1.1 (0.7)	−0.1–2.6
HbA1c (%)*	135	8.5 (1.9) %	5.4–14.0%
HbA1c (mmol/mol)*	135	69 (21) mmol/mol	36–130 mmol/mol
Serum creatinine (mg/dL)	130	0.92 (0.69)	0.5–6.2
Total cholesterol (mg/dL)	122	167 (43.2)	81–334
Triglycerides (mg/dL)	121	112 (63)	42–497
HDL cholesterol (mg/dL)	27	43 (14.2)	7.9–59
LDL cholesterol (mg/dL, calculated)	27	124 (38)	43–191
Non-HDL cholesterol (mg/dL, calculated)	27	149 (44)	58–216

*HbA1c not included on six subjects assessed within six months of diagnosis.

diagnosed at age 10–14 y, 19 (13.2%) were diagnosed at age 15–19 y, and 5 (3.5%) were diagnosed at age 20–24 y.

Genetic studies are being arranged for the child diagnosed at 3 months to check for a monogenic form of diabetes. This child has no other medical problems.

3.1.2. Minimum Incidence. Sixty-three cases of diabetes (diagnosed at <25 years of age) occurred in the Cercado Province of Cochabamba Department in the 12.2 y study period from January 2005 to February 2017. Forty-nine were <15 y at diagnosis and 14 were 15–24 y. This is a measured incidence of 2.2 per 100,000 children < 15 y/y. Ascertainment is estimated as 80%, resulting in an estimated total incidence of 2.7 per 100,000 children < 15 y/y.

3.1.3. Mortality Rate. Of the 144 subjects followed up for 0.1–12.2 y (mean ± SD 5.9 ± 3.4 y), two had died, a male aged 22.8 y from gastric ulcer haemorrhage and a female aged 13.4 y from ketoacidosis (who had been abandoned by her family). The crude mortality rate was 2.3/1000 patient years.

3.2. Clinical Status

3.2.1. Demographics. One hundred and forty-one T1D subjects diagnosed at <25 years of age and ≤35 y were being followed up by CvCD at the end of 2015. Sixty-four (45%) patients were male. Sixty (43%) were from Cochabamba Department; 31 (22%), Santa Cruz; 27 (19%), La Paz; 12 (8.5%), Sucre; 6 (4.3%), Tarija; and 5 (3.5%), Potosi. One child also had cerebral palsy, one had Down syndrome, and one child also had epilepsy. Age at diagnosis and diabetes duration are shown in Table 1.

3.2.2. Diabetes Care. Ninety-four subjects (67%) were adjusting their insulin dose (data available on 141 subjects), with the remainder giving a fixed insulin dose set in agreement with their treating clinicians. Regarding insulin types ($n = 138$), 99 (72%) were on short- and long-acting human insulin only. Twenty-five (18%) were using analogue insulin, of which nine (7%) were using analogue only. Thirteen (9%) were on premixed insulin, and one patient was receiving long-acting human insulin only.

For the number of insulin injections per day ($n = 122$), 18 subjects (158%) were taking two injections per day; 70 (57%), three injections; 24 (20%), four injections; and the remaining 10 (8%), five injections. Insulin usage ranged 0.35–1.76 units/kg/day (mean ± SD 0.99 ± 0.29) ($n = 136$).

The frequency of self-blood glucose tests per week ($n = 139$) was 14–28 (mean ± SD 21.3 ± 1.4). The frequency of clinic visits in the last year ($n = 131$) was 1–8 (mean ± SD 3.5 ± 1.3).

3.2.3. Social Parameters. School/college attendance was regular in 93 (96%) of the 97 patients for whom this information was available, and the year of schooling was age-appropriate in 94%. Out of 105 patients for whom a response was recorded on the question of how well they thought their patients were coping with their diabetes, 62 (59%) of the responses were "good," 38 (37%) were with "some problems," and four (4%) were "poor."

3.2.4. Physical Measurements. Height and weight information was available for 137 patients, and 81 of these were under 19 years, permitting BMI SD score calculation (shown in Table 1).

Blood pressure was measured on 21 subjects < 20 years, with systolic and diastolic SD scores shown in Table 1. Both systolic and diastolic mean SD scores were above zero ($p < 0.001$ for both, by one-sided t-test). None of the patients for whom SD scores were available were noted to have hypertension (as defined by local clinical standards) or be on antihypertensive medications.

3.2.5. HbA1c. HbA1c was measured in the 135 subjects with duration of diabetes > 6 months. Mean and median HbA1c levels were 8.5% (69 mmol/mol) and 8.2% (66 mmol/mol), respectively (see also Table 1). Forty-four subjects (33%)

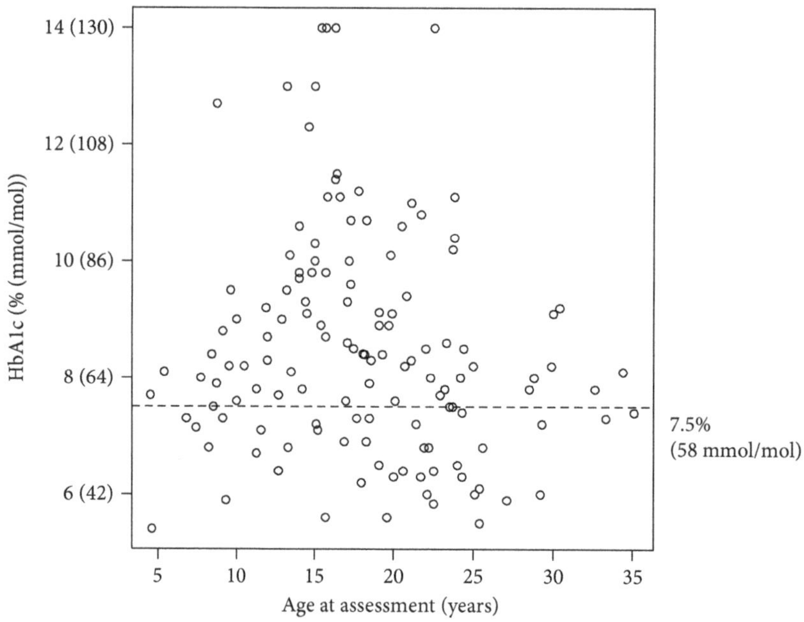

FIGURE 2: Relationship of age to HbA1c.

had HbA1c levels in the recommended target range of <7.5% (58 mmol/mol); 35 (25%), 7.5%–8.49% (58–69 mmol/mol); 48 (36%), 8.5%–12% (69–108 mmol/mol); and the remaining eight subjects (5.8%), >12% (108 mmol/mol). Twenty-six percent of those aged <15 y and 30% of those aged 15–24 y had target HbA1c < 7.5% (58 mmol/mol). A series of one-way ANOVAs on log-transformed HbA1c levels were performed, finding trends towards relationships between HbA1c levels, the number of insulin injections per day ($p = 0.07$), and the use of analogue insulin ($p = 0.06$), but not for gender ($p = 0.38$).

A pattern of increased HbA1c levels and variance during adolescence was observed from a plot of HbA1c by age (Figure 2). For those aged 0–13 y, the HbA1c mean ± SD was 7.9% (63 mmol/mol) ± 1.3% (14 mmol/mol); for those aged 13–20 y, the HbA1c mean ± SD was 9.4% (78 mmol/mol) ± 2.0% and for those aged >20 y, the HbA1c mean ± SD was 7.9% (63 mmol/mol) ± 1.7% (18 mmol/mol). This indicates a significant difference in HbA1c levels between age groups ($p = 0.0002$ by one-way ANOVA on log-transformed values). However, Levene's test for heterogeneity of variance was not statistically significant ($p = 0.24$).

Mean/median HbA1c levels by a diabetes clinic site were 9.0%/8.4% (75/68 mmol/mol) in Cochabamba, 7.9%/7.6% (63/60 mmol/mol) in La Paz, 8.0%/7.4% (64/57 mmol/mol) in Potosi, 8.5%/8.4% (69/68 mmol/mol) in Santa Cruz, 8.5%/8.3% (69/67 mmol/mol) in Sucre, and 7.1%/6.8% (54/51 mmol/mol) in Tarija, with no statistical difference between clinics on ANOVA.

3.2.6. Lipids. Lipid levels are shown in Table 1. No subjects were on lipid-lowering agents. For total cholesterol, 97 patients (80%) had <200 mg/dL (5.2 mmol/L), 16 patients (13%) had 200–239 mg/dL (5.2–6.2 mmol/L), and nine (7.3%) had ≥240 mg/dL (≥6.2 mmol/L). Total cholesterol levels were not correlated with concurrent HbA1c levels ($p = 0.14$ by Pearson's correlation).

Triglyceride levels ($n = 121$) were <1.7 mmol/L (150 mg/dL) in 99 patients (82%), 1.7–2.2 mmol/L (150–199 mg/dL) in 11 (9%) patients, and 2.3–5.6 mmol/L (200–499 mg/dL) in 11 (9%) patients (all subjects had <4.5 mmol/L (450 mg/dL). Log-transformed triglyceride levels were correlated with concurrent HbA1c levels ($p = 0.03$ by Pearson's correlation).

HDL cholesterol was measured in 27 patients from the Department of La Paz (see Table 1). None of these patients were on renal replacement therapy. Fifteen patients (56%) had HDL < 1.0 mmol/L (40 mg/dL) for men or 1.3 mmol/L (50 mg/dL) for women. There were no significant correlations between HDL cholesterol and either HbA1c or log-transformed triglyceride levels.

Seven patients (26%) had calculated LDL cholesterol levels < 100 mg/dL (<2.6 mmol/L), 10 patients (37%) had 100–129 mg/dL (2.6–3.3 mmol/L), and 10 patients (37%) had ≥130 mg/dL (3.3 mmol/L).

Table 2 shows the percentage of subjects meeting target levels for cardiovascular risk factors (BMI, triglycerides, total cholesterol, and HbA1c), for the 115 subjects that had values for all four measurements.

3.2.7. Renal Function. Serum creatinine values are shown in Table 1. Five patients (4%) had serum creatinine levels above the recommended level of 1.3 mg/dL (115 μmol/L) for males or 1.1 mg/dL (97 μmol/L) for females. eGFR for the 115 subjects ≥ 14 y ranged from 10.4–178.9 mL/min/1.73m^2 (mean ± SD 104.9 ± 31.0 mL/min/1.73m^2). Three patients on renal replacement therapy (see below) were excluded from this analysis.

Two subjects were receiving haemodialysis (age 28.5 and 28.8 y) (duration of diabetes to start of haemodialysis 16.5 and 1.25 y), one had received a renal transplant after 0.3 y

TABLE 2: Risk factors for cardiovascular disease.

Risk factor	Definition	n	%
High BMI	For <19 years, SD score ≥ 2.0; if ≥19 years, BMI ≥ 25	22	19.1
Elevated fasting triglycerides	≥150 mg/dL (≥1.7 mmol/L)	21	18.3
Elevated fasting total cholesterol	≥175 mg/dL (≥4.5 mmol/L)	45	39.1
HbA1c above target range	≥7.5% (58 mmol/mol)	74	64.3
One risk factor	—	44	38.3
Two risk factors	—	34	29.6
Three risk factors	—	14	12.2
Four risk factors	—	2	1.7

($n = 115$).

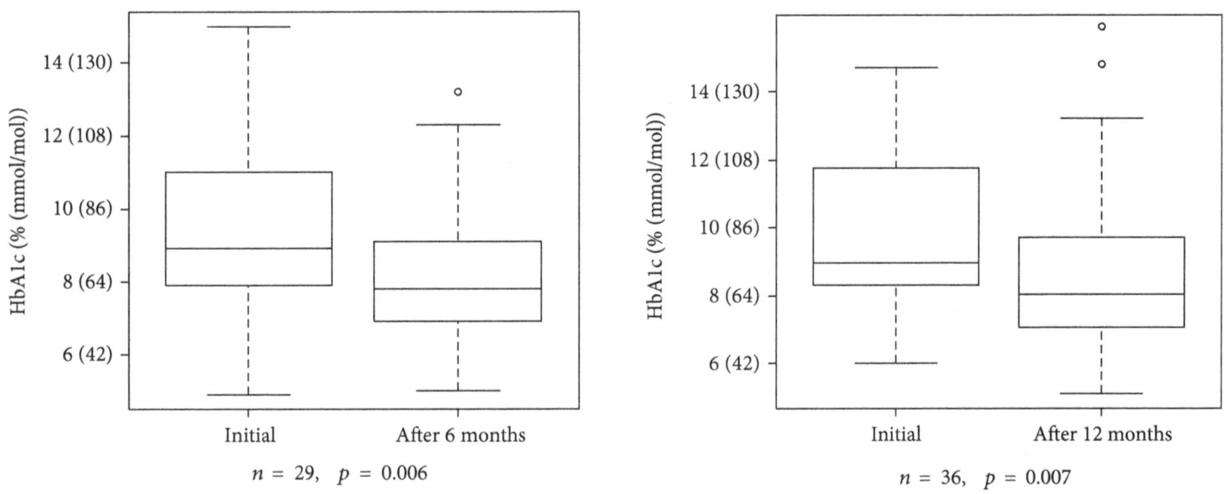

FIGURE 3: Initial impact at commencement of Life for a Child support.

on haemodialysis (age 30.4 y, duration of diabetes to time of haemodialysis 17.3 y) and the other was noted as having chronic renal failure (24.4 y, duration 20.5 y, eGFR 12.8 mL/min/1.73m^2). Three other subjects had eGFR < 50 mL/min/1.73m^2, all with diabetes duration of at least 16 years. Two of these three were receiving treatment for hypertension, and one was also treated with erythropoietin injections for associated anaemia.

Seventeen subjects ≥ 14 y had an eGFR of ≥140 mL/min/1.73m^2, suggestive of hyperfiltration.

3.2.8. Other Complications. One subject had hypothyroidism which was being treated. One subject had experienced a severe hypoglycemia episode in the past resulting in severe cognitive and motor impairment. Three patients were recorded as having diabetic retinopathy, and five subjects had cataracts (two of whom also had retinopathy). Neuropathy (loss of vibration and light touch) was recorded in one subject.

3.3. Initial Impact of Life for a Child Program. HbA1c results at the start of the LFAC Program in 2004-2005 were available for 57 subjects. Values ranged from 4.9–15% (30–140 mmol/mol), with mean ± SD 9.6 ± 2.2% (81 ± 24 mmol/mol). For six-month paired data, mean ± SD HbA1c at baseline was 9.4 ± 2.3% (79 ± 25 mmol/mol), and mean ± SD HbA1c at six months was 8.1 ± 1.8% (65 ± 20 mmol/mol) ($n = 29$, $p = 0.006$ by one-sided paired t-test). For 12-month paired data, mean ± SD HbA1c at baseline was 9.7 ± 2.1% (83 ± 23 mmol/mol), and mean ± SD HbA1c at twelve months was 8.7 ± 2.5% (72 ± 27 mmol/mol) ($n = 36$, $p = 0.007$ by one-sided paired t-test) (see Figure 3).

4. Discussion

Globally, the incidence rates of type 1 diabetes in children vary widely due to differences in genetic susceptibility, combined with inadequately understood but powerful and evolving environmental factors [1–3].

There have been no previous studies on type 1 diabetes incidence in Bolivia. Rates vary substantially in Central/South American and other Hispanic populations. Estimates for Bolivia in the IDF Atlas [1] are extrapolated from a 1990–1991 study in Lima, Peru, which found an incidence of 0.5 per 100,000 children < 15 y/y [2]. Other studies in South America in the early 1990s (all <15 y) showed rates per 100,000 ranging from 0.1 in Caracas, Venezuela, to 8.3 in Montevideo [2, 3]. Countries with both recent and older data are seeing sharp rises in type 1 diabetes incidence—in

Mexico, from 3.4 (per 100,000) in 2000 to 6.2 in 2012 for young people < 20 y in the Instituto Mexicano del Seguro Social (IMSS) health insurance service [14]; in Chile, from 5.7 in 2006 to 12.1 in 2012 for those aged <20 y [15], with the sharpest increase in the <5 y age group; and in Brazil, a trend for increased incidence in those aged <15 y from 1986 to 2006 [16].

Further afield for Hispanic populations, rates (<15 y) are 20.6 in Spain (<15 y, 1995–2001) [1], 13.2 in Portugal (<15 y, 1994–1998) [1], and 14.1 in Hispanic Whites in the USA (<15 y, 2002–2003) [17], with a recent study showing an increase of 4.2% per year in 2003–2012 on numbers < 20 y [18].

Some of the variance in South American populations is thought to be due to lower rates of type 1 diabetes in Central/South American indigenous peoples as compared to those of Hispanic White/mixed descent [2, 19]. Larenas et al. [20] found 3.8 times higher rates in Caucasian Chileans than in Mapuche (native Chileans). Bolivia has, by a substantial margin, the highest proportion of indigenous peoples in Central/South America [21]. This lower rate in indigenous populations is likely largely genetic in origin due to differences in HLA haplotypes [19, 22, 23]. However, differing exposure to environmental factors may also be potent influencers: rates of type 1 diabetes have increased in many countries as standards of living have increased. Incidence rates were found to be higher in high socioeconomic communes in Santiago de Chile [24].

The observed type 1 diabetes rate in Cercado in this study—2.2 per 100,000 children < 15 y/y with an estimated ascertainment of 80%, giving an estimated incidence of 2.7 per 100,000—is five times higher than the figure previously used for Bolivia (based on the Peruvian data from 1990–1991 [2]. It is likely that type 1 incidence is increasing in Bolivia; however, further studies will be needed to confirm this. This is still a low incidence rate compared to global figures. The female preponderance seen in Bolivia is common in low incidence studies [25] and is believed to be due to fathers with type 1 susceptibility genes being more likely to survive and pass on diabetogenic genes than mothers, with fathers' genes more likely to cause type 1 diabetes in female offspring and mothers' genes to cause diabetes in male offspring. In addition, it is thought that fathers' genes may be more diabetogenic than similar genes in mothers [26, 27].

Monogenic diabetes has been reported from various countries, and it is likely that the child diagnosed at 3 months of age has this form of diabetes—genetic testing is being arranged. If there is a gene defect, alternate noninsulin therapy may be possible depending on the specific gene [28].

Like various other less-resourced countries [29], the Bolivian government health service does not cover the cost of care for people with diabetes at any age. Most families cannot afford the cost of care, which can be prohibitive in such countries for families with lower incomes [30], and this can translate into the premature death of the child or young adult with diabetes, as occurred once in this Bolivian cohort. Furthermore, in Bolivia, there are very few paediatric endocrinologists and, due to its relative rarity, limited knowledge of type 1 among general paediatricians. Therefore, the support from a centre such as CvCD ± LFAC is crucial for families with limited resources. CvCD provides a multidisciplinary service of not just health professionals in diabetology but also health professionals in ophthalmology, nutrition, psychology, social work, foot care and podiatry, physiotherapy and rehabilitation, laboratory services, and pharmacy. There is also a young group or people with type 1 diabetes which encourage and support each other through meetings and the use of the social media platform "WhatsApp." The IDF Life for a Child Program provides insulin and, since 2009, also provides blood glucose test strips, educational materials, and point-of-care HbA1c testing in Cochabamba.

The initial impact seen in the LFAC follow-up data from 2004–2005 has been sustained. Mortality is low at 2.3 per 1000 patient years, and the mean/median HbA1c of 8.5/8.2% (69/62 mmol/mol) is surprisingly good, considering the substantial challenges faced in caring for these young people. Twenty-seven percent of those aged <15 y and 28% of those aged 15–24 y were achieving the recommended HbA1c target of <7.5% (58 mmol/mol). This is not substantially different from the mean of 29/30% (male/female) for subjects aged <15 y and from the mean of 24/20% (male/female) for those aged 15–24 y in a large international study in which 15 of 16 countries were high-income nations [31].

The higher HbA1c values seen in adolescents/emerging adults are similar to those of other reports [32] and likely reflect lifestyle and behavioural factors and growth spurt-related insulin resistance. As in other countries, thoughtful medical attention and support are warranted during this period, along with provision of insulin supply security.

It is of great concern that three young people with diabetes required renal replacement therapy and four others have substantial renal impairment (eGFR <50 mL/1.73m^2). Furthermore, 17 had hyperfiltration, which may be a risk factor for diabetic nephropathy, although recent evidence suggests this may not be the case [33, 34]. The presence of ESRD at a young age suggests that blood glucose control must have been poor for some years, and we note that for most of the Bolivian subjects evaluated herein, regular self-blood glucose monitoring has only been possible since 2009. Anderzén et al. [35] has shown the importance of a good early start in terms of blood glucose control, if later complications are to be reduced.

Further assessment should be done for early signs of nephropathy such as microalbuminuria and hypertension, with management (with ACE inhibitors or LDL-lowering "statin" drugs) being informed by the forthcoming results of the Adolescent Type 1 Diabetes Cardio-Renal Intervention Trial (ADDIT) [36]. Given the number with renal complications, it is likely that a thorough systematic assessment would lead to more subjects being found with other microvascular complications such as neuropathy and retinopathy, for whom early intervention with risk factor control and increased screening rates is appropriate.

The common cause of death of people with type 1 diabetes is cardiovascular disease, for which dyslipidaemia is a major risk factor and is treatable, with significant LDL-C, cardiovascular event, and mortality reduction with statins [37]. The substantial numbers with one or more lipid risk factors such as high triglycerides and total cholesterol and low HDL cholesterol levels, combined with the suggestion of blood pressure elevation, raise the possibility that some patients have features of the metabolic syndrome, which is recognised in type 1 diabetes and associated with higher rates of diabetes vascular complications [38, 39]. This "double diabetes" may benefit from the addition of metformin to insulin and risk factor control [40], though clinical trials with vascular end-points are still awaited.

The study has three other limitations. It is possible that with further study (autoantibodies and C-peptide, unfortunately not available in this clinical context), some of the subjects diagnosed with type 1 diabetes may be recategorised as having type 2 diabetes. Secondly, HbA1c measurements were not standardised across clinics, and so it is possible that results could be affected by the different methods used. Finally, the 80% ascertainment is an estimated figure, and Cercado Province may not be fully representative of Bolivia—incidence may vary in other parts of the country due to ethnic or socioeconomic factors.

5. Conclusion

This study has estimated the incidence of type 1 diabetes in Bolivia, confirming that incidence is relatively low compared to that in many other countries. The results demonstrate that reasonable blood glucose control and low mortality can be achieved in many subjects in a low-resourced setting with international support. However, there is a significant risk of early long-term complications in some subjects, as evidenced by renal impairment and substantial levels of cardiovascular risk factors.

Conflicts of Interest

None of the authors have any conflicts of interest in regard to this study.

Authors' Contributions

Elizabeth Duarte Gómez collected the data and contributed to the manuscript, Gabriel Andrew Gregory analysed the data and wrote the manuscript, Miriam Castrati Nostas collected the data and contributed to the manuscript, Angela Christine Middlehurst assisted in the data analysis and contributed to the manuscript, Alicia Josephine Jenkins helped with interpretation of the data and contributed to the manuscript, and Graham David Ogle designed the study and cowrote the manuscript.

Acknowledgments

The authors acknowledge the dedicated efforts of all at Centro Vivir con Diabetes and the determination of all these young people with diabetes and their families. They also thank the supporters of the IDF Life for a Child and Insulin for Life Programs and Rotary International (Rotary Club of Cochabamba, Quillacollo, District 6940, and the Rotary Foundation). Finally, they thank Sarah Garnett for helping with the SD scores. This work was supported by the Leona M. and Harry B. Helmsley Charitable Trust. Gabriel Andrew Gregory was partly funded by the University of Sydney Summer Research Scholarship. Alicia Josephine Jenkins is funded by the NHMRC (Australia) Practitioner Fellowship and the Sydney Medical School Foundation Fellowship.

References

[1] C. Patterson, L. Guariguata, G. Dahlquist, G. Soltész, G. Ogle, and M. Silink, "Diabetes in the young – a global view and worldwide estimates of numbers of children with type 1 diabetes," *Diabetes Research and Clinical Practice*, vol. 103, pp. 161–175, 2014.

[2] M. Karvonen, M. Viik-Kajander, E. Moltchanova, I. Libman, R. LaPorte, and J. Tuomilehto, "Incidence of childhood type 1 diabetes worldwide. Diabetes Mondiale (DiaMond) Project Group," *Diabetes Care*, vol. 23, pp. 1516–1526, 2000.

[3] DIAMOND Project Group, "Incidence and trends of childhood type 1 diabetes worldwide 1990-1999," *Diabetic Medicine*, vol. 23, pp. 857–866, 2006.

[4] International Diabetes Federation, "International Diabetes Federation Life for a Child Program," February 2017, http://www.lifeforachild.org.

[5] Insulin for Life, "Insulin for life," April 2017, http://www.insulinforlife.org.

[6] World Health Organization, *Definition and Diagnosis of Diabetes Mellitus and Intermediate Hyperglycemia. Report of a WHO/IDF Consultation*, WHO, Geneva, 2006, December 2016, http://apps.who.int/iris/bitstream/10665/43588/1/9241594934_eng.pdf.

[7] Instituto Nacional de Estadística, "Resultado Censo de Población y Vivienda 2012," April 2017, http://datos.ine.gob.bo/binbol/RpWebEngine.exe/Portal?BASE=CPV2012COM&lang=esp.

[8] The World Bank, "World development indicators, Bolivia," April 2017, http://databank.worldbank.org/data/reports.aspx?source=2&series=SP.POP.GROW&country=BOL.

[9] World Health Organization, *WHO Child Growth Standards: Length/Height-for-age, Weight-for-age, Weight-for-Length, Weight-for-Height and Body Mass Index-for-age: Methods and Development*, WHO, Geneva, 2006.

[10] M. De Onis, A. W. Onyango, E. Borghi, A. Siyam, C. Nishida, and J. Siekmann, "Development of a WHO growth reference for school-aged children and adolescents," *Bulletin of the World Health Organization*, vol. 85, pp. 660–667, 2007.

[11] National High Blood Pressure Education Program Working Group on High Blood Pressure in Children and Adolescents, "The fourth report on the diagnosis, evaluation, and treatment of high blood pressure in children and adolescents," *Pediatrics*, vol. 114, Supplement 2, pp. 555–576, 2004.

[12] W. T. Friedewald, R. I. Levy, and D. S. Fredrickson, "Estimation of the concentration of low-density cholesterol in plasma without use of the preparative ultracentrifuge," *Clinical Chemistry*, vol. 18, pp. 499–502, 1972.

[13] A. S. Levey, L. A. Stevens, C. H. Schmid et al., "A new equation to estimate glomerular filtration rate," *Annals of Internal Medicine*, vol. 150, pp. 604–612, 2009.

[14] R. A. Gómez-Díaz, G. Pérez-Pérez, I. T. Hernández-Cuesta et al., "Incidence of type 1 diabetes in Mexico: data from an institutional register 2000-2010," *Diabetes Care*, vol. 35, article e77, 2012.

[15] C. Garfias, A. Borzutzky, J. Cerda et al., "Dramatic increase in type 1 diabetes in Chilean children between 2006 and 2012," *Pediatric Diabetes*, vol. 15, Supplement 19, p. 121, 2014.

[16] C. A. Negrato, J. P. Dias, M. F. Teixeira et al., "Temporal trends in incidence of type 1 diabetes between 1986 and 2006 in Brazil," *Journal of Endocrinological Investigation*, vol. 33, pp. 373–377, 2010.

[17] The Writing Group for the SEARCH Study for Diabetes in Youth Study Group, D. Dabelea, R. A. Bell et al., "Incidence of diabetes in youth in the United States," *JAMA*, vol. 297, pp. 2716–2724, 2007.

[18] E. J. Mayer-Davis, J. M. Lawrence, D. Dabelea et al., "Incidence trends of type 1 and type 2 diabetes among youths, 2002-2012," *The New England Journal of Medicine*, vol. 376, pp. 1419–1429, 2017.

[19] F. C. Collado-Mesa, A. Barceló, K. L. Arheart, and S. E. Messiah, "An ecological analysis of childhood-onset type 1 diabetes incidence and prevalence in Latin America," *Pan American Journal of Public Health*, vol. 15, pp. 388–394, 2004.

[20] G. Larenas, A. Montecinos, M. Manosalva, M. Barthou, and T. Vidal, "Incidence of insulin-dependent diabetes mellitus in the IX region of Chile: ethnic differences," *Diabetes Research and Clinical Practice*, vol. 34, Supplement 34, pp. S147–S151, 1996.

[21] Center for Latin American Studies, Georgetown University, "Indigenous peoples, democracy and political participation," April 2017, http://pdba.georgetown.edu/IndigenousPeoples/demographics.html.

[22] C. Gorodezky, A. Alaez, A. Murguía et al., "HLA and autoimmune diseases: type 1 diabetes (T1D) as an example," *Autoimmunity Reviews*, vol. 5, pp. 187–194, 2006.

[23] F. S. Giraudo Abarca, E. Carrasco, E. Codner, and F. Pérez-Bravo, "Genetic of type 1 diabetes (T1D) in South America," *Pediatric Diabetes*, vol. 15, Supplement 19, p. 88, 2014.

[24] F. Torres-Avilés, E. Carrasco, G. Icaza, and F. Pérez-Bravo, "Clustering of cases of type 1 diabetes in high socioeconomic communes in Santiago de Chile: spatio-temporal and geographical analysis," *Acta Diabetologica*, vol. 47, pp. 251–257, 2010.

[25] M. Karvonen, M. Pitkäniemi, J. Pitkäniemi et al., "Sex-difference in the incidence of insulin-dependent diabetes mellitus: an analysis of the recent epidemiological data. World Health Organization DIAMOND Project Group," *Diabetes/Metabolism Reviews*, vol. 13, pp. 275–291, 1997.

[26] J. Tuomilehto, T. Podar, E. Tuomilehto-Wolf, and E. Virtala, "Evidence for importance of gender and birth cohort for risk of IDDM in offspring of IDDM parents," *Diabetologia*, vol. 38, pp. 975–982, 1995.

[27] T. Waldhör, E. Schober, B. Rami, J. Tuomilehto, and the Austrian Diabetes Incidence Study Group, "The prevalence of IDDM in the first degree relatives of children newly diagnosed with IDDM in Austria-a population-based study," *Experimental and Clinical Endocrinology & Diabetes*, vol. 107, pp. 323–327, 1999.

[28] O. Rubio-Cabezas, A. T. Hattersley, P. R. Njølstad et al., "The diagnosis and management of monogenic diabetes in children and adolescents," *Pediatric Diabetes*, vol. 15, Supplement 20, pp. 47–64, 2014.

[29] G. D. Ogle, A. C. Middlehurst, and M. Silink, "The IDF Life for a Child Program index of diabetes care for children and youth," *Pediatric Diabetes*, vol. 17, pp. 374–384, 2016.

[30] G. D. Ogle, H. Kim, A. C. Middlehurst, M. Silink, and A. J. Jenkins, "Financial costs for families of children with type 1 diabetes in lower-income countries," *Diabetic Medicine*, vol. 33, pp. 820–826, 2016.

[31] J. A. McKnight, S. H. Wild, M. J. E. Lamb et al., "Glycaemic control of type 1 diabetes in clinical practice early in the 21st century: an international comparison," *Diabetic Medicine*, vol. 32, pp. 1036–1050, 2015.

[32] M. A. Clements, N. C. Foster, D. M. Maahs et al., "Hemoglobin A1c (HbA1c) changes over time among adolescent and young adult participants in the T1D exchange clinic registry," *Pediatric Diabetes*, vol. 17, pp. 327–336, 2016.

[33] M. C. Thomas, J. L. Moran, V. Harjutsalo et al., "Hyperfiltration in type 1 diabetes: does it exist and does it matter for nephropathy," *Diabetologia*, vol. 55, pp. 1505–1513, 2012.

[34] C. Chatzikyrkou and H. Haller, "Hyperfiltration - a risk factor for nephropathy in T1DM?," *Nature Reviews. Endocrinology*, vol. 8, pp. 385-386, 2012.

[35] J. Anderzén, U. Samuelsson, S. Gudbjörnsdottir, L. Hanberger, and K. Åkesson, "Teenagers with poor metabolic control already have a higher risk of microvascular complications as young adults," *Journal of Diabetes and its Complications*, vol. 30, no. 3, pp. 533–536, 2016.

[36] The Adolescent type 1 Diabetes cardio-renal Interventional Trial Research Group, "Adolescent type 1 diabetes cardio-renal intervention trial (AdDIT)," *BMC Pediatrics*, vol. 9, p. 79, 2009.

[37] Cholesterol Treatment Trialists' (CTT) Collaborators, P. M. Kearney, L. Blackwell et al., "Efficacy of cholesterol-lowering therapy in 18,686 people with diabetes in 14 randomised trials of statins: a meta-analysis," *Lancet*, vol. 371, pp. 117–125, 2008.

[38] M. McGill, L. Molyneaux, S. M. Twigg, and D. K. Yue, "The metabolic syndrome in type 1 diabetes: does it exist and does it matter?," *Journal of Diabetes and its Complications*, vol. 22, pp. 18–23, 2008.

[39] S. D. Sibley, I. H. de Boer, M. W. Steffes, J. D. Brunzell, and Diabetes Control and Complications Trial/Epidemiology of Diabetes Interventions and Complications (DCCT/EDIC) Research Study Group, "Intra-abdominal fat and elevated urine albumin excretion in men with type 1 diabetes," *Diabetes Care*, vol. 30, pp. 1898–1900, 2007.

[40] S. Vella, L. Buetow, P. Royle, S. Livingstone, H. M. Colhoun, and J. R. Petrie, "The use of metformin in type 1 diabetes: a systematic review of efficacy," *Diabetologia*, vol. 53, pp. 809–820, 2010.

23

Association between Early Neuroretinal Dysfunction and Peripheral Motor Unit Loss in Patients with Type 1 Diabetes Mellitus

Fabiana Picconi,[1] Giorgia Mataluni,[2] Lucia Ziccardi,[3] Mariacristina Parravano,[3] Antonio Di Renzo,[3] Dorina Ylli,[4] Patrizio Pasqualetti,[5] Valeria Studer,[2,6] Laura Chioma,[1] Girolama Alessandra Marfia,[2] and Simona Frontoni[1]

[1]*Unit of Endocrinology, Diabetes and Metabolism, S. Giovanni Calibita Fatebenefratelli Hospital, Department of Systems Medicine, University of Rome Tor Vergata, Rome, Italy*
[2]*Unit of Disimmune Neuropathies, Department of Systems Medicine, University of Rome Tor Vergata, Rome, Italy*
[3]*IRCCS-G.B. Bietti Foundation, Rome, Italy*
[4]*Division of Endocrinology MedStar Washington Hospital Center, MedStar Health Research Institute, Washington, DC, USA*
[5]*Fatebenefratelli Foundation for Health Research and Education, AFaR Division, Rome, Italy*
[6]*Neuroimmunology and Neuromuscolar Diseases Unit, Foundation IRCCS Neurological Institute Carlo Besta, Milan, Italy*

Correspondence should be addressed to Simona Frontoni; frontoni@uniroma2.it

Academic Editor: Mark Yorek

Objectives. It has been already confirmed that retinal neurodegeneration has a predictive value in the development of microvascular alterations in diabetic retinopathy. However, no data are available on the association between neuroretinal dysfunction and peripheral motor unit loss. Our study, therefore, was aimed at investigating the hypothesis that retinal neurodegeneration could be considered an early marker of diabetic peripheral neuropathy (DPN). *Methods.* 20 T1DM patients with no symptoms/signs of peripheral polyneuropathy, without DR or with very mild nonproliferative DR, and 14 healthy controls (C) age- and gender-matched were enrolled. The following electrophysiological tests were performed: standard nerve conduction studies (NCS) and incremental motor unit number estimation (MUNE) from the abductor hallux (AH) and abductor digiti minimi (ADM). Neuroretinal function was studied by multifocal electroretinogram (MfERG) recordings, measuring response amplitude density (RAD) and implicit time (IT) from rings and sectors of superior (S)/inferior (I)/temporal (T)/nasal (N) macular sectors up to 10 degrees of foveal eccentricity. *Results.* MfERG RADs from rings and sectors were significantly reduced in T1DM ($p < 0.05$) vs. C. ADM MUNE and AH MUNE were significantly decreased in T1DM ($p = 0.039$ and $p < 0.0001$, respectively) vs. C. A positive correlation between mean MfERG RADs from the central 5 degrees of the four (S, I, T, and N) macular sectors and lower limb motor unit number ($r = 0.50$, $p = 0.041$; $r = 0.64$, $p = 0.005$; $r = 0.64$, $p = 0.006$; and $r = 0.61$, $p = 0.010$, respectively) was observed in T1DM patients. No abnormalities of NCS were found in any subject. *Conclusions.* The motor unit loss on the one hand and neuroretinal dysfunction on the other hand are already present in T1DM patients without DPN. The relationship between neuroretinal dysfunction and motor unit decline supports the hypothesis that neuroretina may represent a potential "window" to track the early neurogenic damage in diabetes.

1. Introduction

Diabetic peripheral neuropathy (DPN) is one of the most debilitating complications of diabetes mellitus (DM), determining sensory loss and neuropathic pain and late weakness [1]. The diagnosis of diabetic neuropathy is also based on the use of neurophysiologic techniques and the evaluation of advanced signs and symptoms. Moreover, the ability of standard electrophysiological techniques (nerve conduction studies and electromyographic evaluation) to identify neuronal dysfunction is confined to overt neuropathic damage. On the other hand, the new procedures, such as skin biopsy, showed to be helpful in detecting neuropathy in the early and subclinical stages but they are still demanding because they are invasive, require expensive laboratory equipment and trained personnel, and still have limited reproducibility [2]. A painless, noninvasive, cost-effective, and clinically available tool is therefore necessary, for the early detection, staging, and monitoring of peripheral diabetic neuropathy [3].

Recently, emerging evidence shows that the neuropathic process, contrary to the conventional view, is not only confined to the peripheral sensory nerves but also involved the whole nervous system, thus suggesting the possible identification of new observational "windows" of the neurodegenerative process [4]. Particularly, in few studies on animal models and in humans, an early impairment of the motor nerves has also been demonstrated [5, 6]. These alterations are likely associated to a "dying back" of motor nerve terminals, similar to the death process that occurs in sensory epidermal nerve fibers [6].

On the other hand, the process of retinal neurodegeneration is known to precede vascular damage, representing so far an early marker of diabetic retinopathy (DR) [7–9]. However, despite its prominence at clinical examination, vasculature makes up less than 5% of the retinal mass, so that the retina can be more appropriately considered as a vascularized neuronal tissue [10, 11]. Therefore, since hyperglycemia adversely affects the entire neurosensory retina, by accelerating neuronal apoptosis or altering metabolism of neuroretinal supporting cells [11, 12], some authors suggest to consider diabetic retinopathy, as a neuropathy that affects the retinal parenchyma, similar to peripheral diabetic neuropathy [13]. The aim of this observational study is to explore neuronal damage in type 1 diabetes mellitus through new clinically accessible "windows" as the retinal nerve tissue and peripheral motor units and to analyze if their dysfunctions are potential early markers of neurodegeneration in patients without peripheral diabetic neuropathy.

2. Materials and Methods

We followed the methods of Picconi et al. [14]. From the Unit of Endocrinology, Diabetes and Metabolism, S. Giovanni Calibita Fatebenefratelli Hospital of Rome, we recruited 20 patients with type 1 DM (T1DM). 14 healthy participants, without history of ocular disease and no family history of glaucoma or any relevant systemic disease, were enrolled as control group (C), from the medical staff of the Medical Retina Unit, G.B. Bietti Eye Foundation-IRCCS, Rome. Inclusion criteria for the type 1 DM patients were (1) documented diagnosis of type 1 DM, according to ADA criteria [15]; (2) age between 18 and 75 years; (3) treated with continuous subcutaneous insulin infusion or with multiple daily insulin injections; and (4) no signs of retinal vasculopathy (noDR) or very mild nonproliferative diabetic retinopathy (NPDR). Exclusion criteria were (1) symptomatic diabetic polyneuropathy not even with positive sensory symptoms such as pain, burning, paresthesia, or prickling; (2) history of possible confounding diseases (alcohol abuse, vitamin deficiency, malignancy treated with chemotherapy agents, central nervous system diseases, entrapment mononeuropathies, and cervical or lumbosacral radiculopathies); (3) a Michigan Neuropathy Screening Instrument [16] score equal to or greater than 2 points; (4) microalbuminuria (urinary albumin/creatinine ratio > 30 mg/g); (5) spherical refractive error > ±3 diopters, astigmatism (cyl) > ±2 diopters, active or past retinal pathologies, diagnosis of glaucoma or ocular hypertension, and opacities of optical media that could influence functional and structural retinal testing; and (6) history of ocular surgery. This study complied with the principles of the Declaration of Helsinki. All subjects gave their written informed consent.

All subjects underwent a general medical examination and anthropometric parameters. After an overnight fast, blood and urine samples were obtained for the determination of laboratory measurements. Each person underwent a complete ophthalmological examination, with determination of best-corrected visual acuity, anterior segment examination, fundus photography, and multifocal electroretinogram (MfERG) recordings. Neurological evaluation was performed at Disimmune Neuropathies Unit, Policlinico Tor Vergata of Rome. All patients underwent electrophysiological examination including bilateral standard sensory motor nerve conduction studies (NCS) and motor unit number estimation (MUNE). Extensive clinical neurological evaluation was performed; strength was assessed by means of Medical Research Council (MRC) sum score (with a maximum score of 60/60 indicating full strength) [17]. The MRC score of the muscles from which MUNE was derived (abductor digiti minimi (ADM) and abductor hallux (AH)) was also calculated.

2.1. MUNE Evaluation. MUNE is an electrophysiological method that can be used to determine the approximate functioning number of motor neuron units or axons innervating a single muscle. In addition, MUNE methods provide a means of measuring motor unit size, enabling tracking of both loss of motor units and the compensatory phenomenon of collateral reinnervation, and have the advantage of measuring the severity of nerve injury in neuropathy with retained CMAP amplitude; MUNE is already used in neuromuscular disorders such as amyotrophic lateral sclerosis, spinal muscular atrophy, and neuropathies to monitor neuronal loss [18, 19].

Recordings are performed using Medtronic Keypoint EMG equipment (Skovlunde Denmark). Limb temperature is maintained between 32 and 34°C by a heating lamp. Filter settings are 2 Hz/10 kHz. The maximal compound motor action potential (CMAP) is obtained by supramaximal stimulation of the peroneal nerve at the lower limbs and of the ulnar nerve at the upper limbs, with constant current square waves at the fibular head site and from the wrist site, respectively. Measurement of the CMAP negative peak area (from the onset of the first negative peak to the first crossing of the baseline) is preferred to peak-to-peak amplitude or negative peak amplitude measurements, as it minimizes the cancellation error [20] and better considers collateral reinnervation phenomena. Recordings are made from the abductor digiti minimi (ADM) for the ulnar nerve and from the abductor hallux (AH) for the tibial posterior nerve, with a single active surface electrode over the belly of the muscle, an inactive electrode over the tendon, and a ground surface electrode positioned between the recording site and stimulating site, similar to the arrangement for routine NCS. In this study, we determined the MUNE of ADM and AH using the manual incremental method [21], in which the assumption is made that each small, stepwise increase in CMAP amplitude with slight increments of stimulus intensity represented the addition of another single motor unit potential (SMUP) to the growing waveform [22]. A series of consecutive stimuli of progressively higher intensity are therefore applied at the stimulation site to obtain 10 distinct SMUP, elicited in an all-or-nothing manner. The area of each increment is measured and averaged to get the average SMUP area for that nerve and muscle. As the maximal CMAP area represents the total motor unit population firing together, dividing the maximal CMAP area by the average SMUP area yields an estimate of the number of motor units within that nerve. MUNE value is therefore expressed as maximal CMAP area/average SMUP area. In addition to an estimate of motor unit number, the average SMUP size obtained with these methods is also calculated, in order to quantify the extent of collateral reinnervation.

2.2. MfERG Recordings. VERIS Clinic™ 4.9 (Electro-Diagnostic Imaging, San Mateo, California, USA) was used for MfERG assessment using our previously published method [23–25]. The multifocal stimulus, consisting of 61 scaled hexagons, was displayed on a high-resolution, black-and-white monitor (size: 30 cm width and 30 cm height) with a frame rate of 75 Hz. The array of hexagons subtended 20 degrees of visual field. Each hexagon was independently alternated between black (1 cd/m^2) and white (200 cd/m^2) according to a binary *m*-sequence. This resulted in a contrast of 99%. In all eyes, MfERGs were binocularly recorded in the presence of pupils that were maximally pharmacologically dilated with 1% tropicamide to a diameter of 7–8 mm. Pupil diameter was measured by an observer (LZ) by means of a ruler and a magnifying lens and stored for each tested eye. The cornea was anesthetized with 1% Dicaine. MfERGs were recorded bipolarly between an active electrode (Dawson Trick Litzkow (DTL) bipolar contact electrode) and a reference electrode (Ag/AgCl electrode placed on the correspondent temporal side of the frontal lobe). A small Ag/AgCl skin ground electrode was placed at the center of the forehead. Interelectrode resistance was less than 3 KOhms. Binocular MfERG recording was preferred for helping subjects to have a stable target fixation. Eyes that did exhaustively meet the inclusion criteria were selected from each patient. The signal was amplified (gain 100.000) and filtered (band pass 1–100 Hz) by BM 6000 (Biomedica Mangoni, Pisa, Italy). After automatic rejection of artifacts (by VERIS Clinic™ 4.9 software), the first-order kernel response, K1, was examined.

2.2.1. Ring Analysis. MfERG ring analysis was selected to differentiate changes of the bioelectrical responses of the central foveal regions with respect to the more eccentric retinal areas in the macular region. We analyzed the averaged response obtained from three concentric annular retinal regions (rings) centered on the fovea: 0 to 2.5° (ring 1, R1), from 2.5 to 5° (ring 2, R2), from 5 to 10° (ring 3, R3). We also analyzed the responses from unified rings enclosing responses derived from the total area from 0–5° (R1 + R2) and from the fovea up to 10°(R1 + R2 + R3). For each obtained averaged response, we evaluated the amplitude densities (RAD, expressed in nanovolt/degree^2) between the first negative peak, N1, and the first positive peak, P1, and the implicit time (IT) of the first positive peak (P1).

2.2.2. Sector Analysis. MfERG sector analysis was selected to differentiate changes of the bioelectrical responses of the central macular region in 4 quadrants: inferior (I), nasal (N), superior (S), and temporal (T). We considered isolated and combined responses from the foveal center to external areas (sector 1, S1: 0–2.5°; sector 2, S2: 0–5°; and sector 3, S3: 0–10°) and S1 + S2 and S1 + S2 + S3, respectively. A similar analysis was recently adopted to study retinal functional changes in a hereditary ocular pathology [26].

2.3. Laboratory Measurements. Plasma glucose concentrations were measured by the hexokinase method (Modular P Analyzer, Roche). The intra-assay coefficient of variation (CV) was 1.1%, and interassay CV was 1.9%. The sensitivity of the method was 2 mg/dl (0.11 mmol/l). HbA1c was analyzed by high-performance liquid chromatography (VARIANT 2; BioRad Laboratories, Munich, Germany), with intra- and interassay CV of 0.46–0.77 and 0.69–0.91%, respectively. Plasma total cholesterol, high-density lipoprotein cholesterol (HDL chol), and low-density lipoprotein cholesterol (LDL chol) were analyzed with a colorimetric enzymatic method (CHOD-PAP, Roche Diagnostics). The intra-assay CV was 1%, and the interassay CV was 2.7%. The sensitivity of the method was 0.08 mmol/l. Plasma triglycerides were analyzed with a colorimetric enzymatic method (GPO-PAP, Roche Diagnostics). The intra-assay CV was 1.5%, and the interassay CV was 2.4%. The sensitivity of the method was 0.05 mmol/l. Urinary albumin was determined by the Tina-quant immunoturbidimetric assay (Cobas, Roche Diagnostic, Indianapolis, IN) and urinary creatinine by an enzymatic colorimetric test (Beckmann Coulter, California, USA). C underwent an oral glucose tolerance test, to exclude diabetes and impaired glucose tolerance.

3. Statistical Analysis

The main statistical analysis aimed at assessing the difference among T1DM and C groups in terms of MfERG RADs and MUNE. Thus, a general linear model was applied, allowing to adjust for eventual demographic, anthropometric, and metabolic differences.

Correlations among interval variables were measured through Pearson's index, after appropriate log-transformation when necessary. In order to verify the robustness of correlations, influence statistics (standardized DfBetas) were

Table 1: Clinical and laboratory characteristics of controls (C) and subjects with diabetes (T1DM), mean (SD).

	C $n = 14$	T1DM $n = 20$	p value
Gender (M/W)	5/9	9/11	$p = 0.588$
Age (yrs)	39.07 (14.4)	42.3 (12.4)	$p = 0.721$
Diabetes duration (yrs)	—	17.9 (9.5)	—
BMI (kg/m^2)	22.5 (±2)	24.9 (± 2.5)	$p < 0.001$
Glycemia (mmol/l)	4.9 (0.6)	8.9 (1.4)	$p < 0.0.001$
HbA1c (%) (mmol/mol)	—	7.5 (0.8) 58 (15)	—
Tot chol (mmol/l)	4.0 (0.6)	4.3 (0.44)	$p = 0.089$
HDL chol (mmol/l)	1.7 (0.2)	1.5 (0.2)	$p = 0.002$
Trigl (mmol/l)	0.8 (0.1)	0.75 (0.1)	$p = 0.08$
Microalb/creat (mg/gr)	—	7.2 (5.2)	—
Sural nerve (lateral malleolus)	—	Distal SNAP amp (μV) 13.4 (±4.3)	—
		SCV (ms) 56.4 (±6.9)	—
Tibial nerve (AH)*	—	Distal CMAP latency (ms) 3.2 (±0.4)	—
		Distal cMAP amplitude (μV) 11.9 (±4.6)	—
		MCV (ms) 47.3 (±4.5)	—
Ulnar nerve (ADM)*	—	Distal CMAP latency (ms) 2.2 (±1.7)	—
		Distal cMAP amplitude (μV) 9.8 (±1.7)	—
		MCV (ms) 59.7 (±5.3)	—

*No patient showed abnormalities (temporal dispersion or conduction block) in intermediate and proximal nerve segments. M: men; W: women; BMI: body mass index; HbA1c: hemoglobin glycated; Tot chol: total cholesterol; HDL chol: high-density lipoprotein cholesterol; Trigl: triglycerides; Microalb/creat: microalbuminuria/creatininuria; AH: abductor hallux; ADM: abductor digiti minimi; SNAP: sensory nerve action potential; MCV: motor conduction velocity; SCV: sensory conduction velocity; t-test. Statistical significance $p < 0.05$.

computed and, in case of outliers, correlations were computed after their elimination.

4. Results and Discussion

Clinical and laboratory characteristics of the diabetic patients and of the C group are reported in Table 1. Seven out of 20 patients had mild NPDR. The T1DM and C groups were not different, except for body mass index (BMI), fasting glucose, and HDL cholesterol levels. All patients had an MRC score of 60/60 at neurological examination indicating full strength. From the MfERG analysis, the mean MfERG RADs of R1 (0–2.5°), R2 (2.5–5°), and R3 (5–10°) differed significantly between the C and diabetic groups ($p < 0.01$). Combined sector analysis of mean MfERG RADs from S1 + S2 (0–5°) and S1 + S2 + S3 (0–10°) in superior, temporal and nasal sectors showed significantly reduced values in T1DM subjects vs. C ($p < 0.05$). There was also a reduced, but not statistically significant, RAD value from the inferior sector (0.055). In addition, significant sector X group interaction was found ($F(3,81) = 6.07$; $p = 0.001$), since the difference between DM and C was larger in the temporal and nasal sectors with respect to the superior and inferior sectors (consistently, $p < 0.005$) (Figure 1). For the IT parameter, no significant differences were found between the C and diabetic groups. No significant differences were found between noDR and NPDR patients for both RADs and ITs.

No abnormalities of conventional NCS were found in any subject. The number of motor units was significantly decreased in both the lower and upper limbs in T1DM vs. C (ADM MUNE: 82.55 ± 54.37 vs. 126.96 ± 65.85, $p = 0.039$; AH MUNE 101.87 ± 41.09 vs. 199.90 ± 69.81, $p < 0.001$), while AH SMUP was significantly increased in T1DM vs. C (0.55 ± 0.17 vs. 0.35 ± 0.13 μV/msec, $p = 0.001$) (Figures 2 and 3).

Since BMI and HDL chol were significantly different among the two groups, we added these variables as covariates in the previous analyses and the patterns remained stable.

A positive correlation between the mean MfERG RADs of S1 + S2 of the four sectors (S, I, T, and N) and AH MUNE ($r = 0.50$, $p = 0.041$; $r = 0.64$, $p = 0.005$; $r = 0.64$, $p = 0.006$; and $r = 0.61$, $p = 0.010$, respectively) was observed in

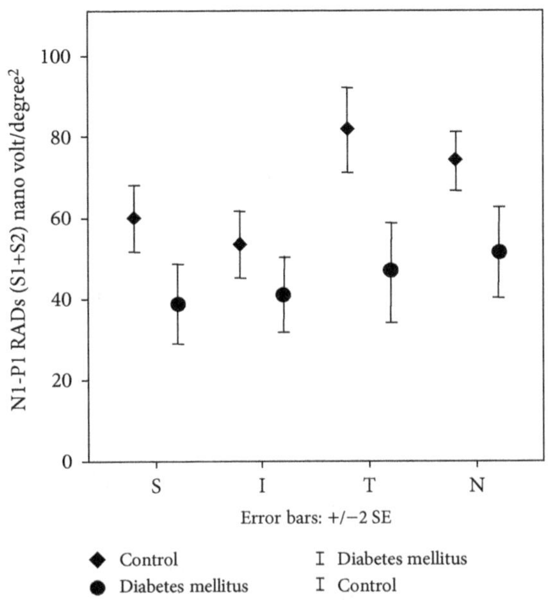

FIGURE 1: Combined sector analysis of mean MfERG RADs from S1 + S2 (0–5°) in the superior, temporal, and nasal sectors showed significantly reduced values in T1DM subjects vs. C ($p < 0.05$). There was also a reduced but not statistically significant RAD value from the inferior sector (0.055). In addition, significant sector X group interaction was found ($F(3,81) = 6.07$; $p = 0.001$), since the difference between DM and C was larger in the temporal and nasal sectors with respect to the superior and inferior sectors (consistently, $p < 0.005$) N1-P1 RADs are defined as amplitude densities between the first negative peak, N1, and the first positive peak, P1. S: superior; I: inferior; T: temporal; N: nasal macular quadrants.

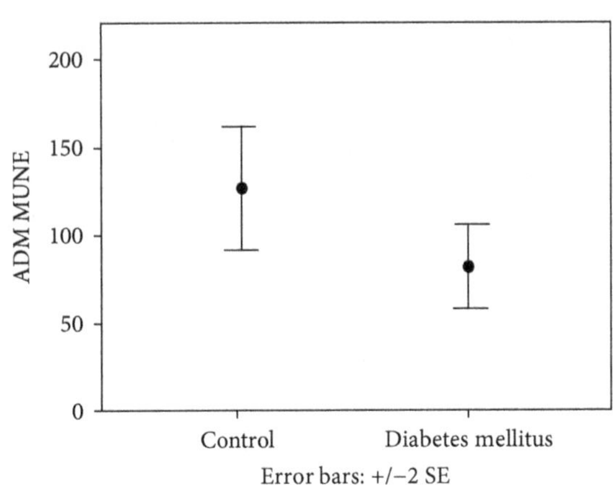

FIGURE 2: Motor unit number estimation (MUNE) (mean ± SEM) of abductor digiti minimi (ADM) in the diabetic groups and controls. ADM MUNE was significantly decreased in T1DM vs. C ($p < 0.05$).

T1DM patients (Figure 4). Since such correlations could be significantly affected by outliers, influence statistics (standardized DfBetas) were computed. After eliminating cases with values higher than the cutoff (2/sqrt(n)), r correlations resulted similar ($r = 0.49$, $p = 0.065$; $r = 0.64$, $p = 0.015$; $r = 0.64$, $p = 0.013$; and $r = 0.52$, $p = 0.048$, respectively).

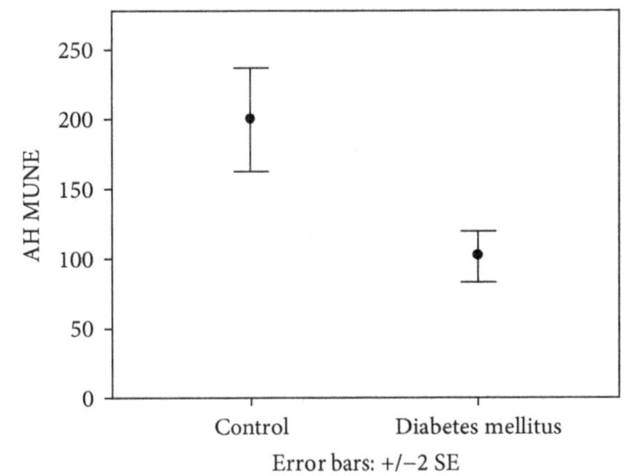

FIGURE 3: Motor unit number estimation (MUNE) (mean ± SEM) of abductor hallux (AH) in the diabetic groups and controls. AH MUNE was significantly decreased in T1DM vs. C ($p < 0.001$).

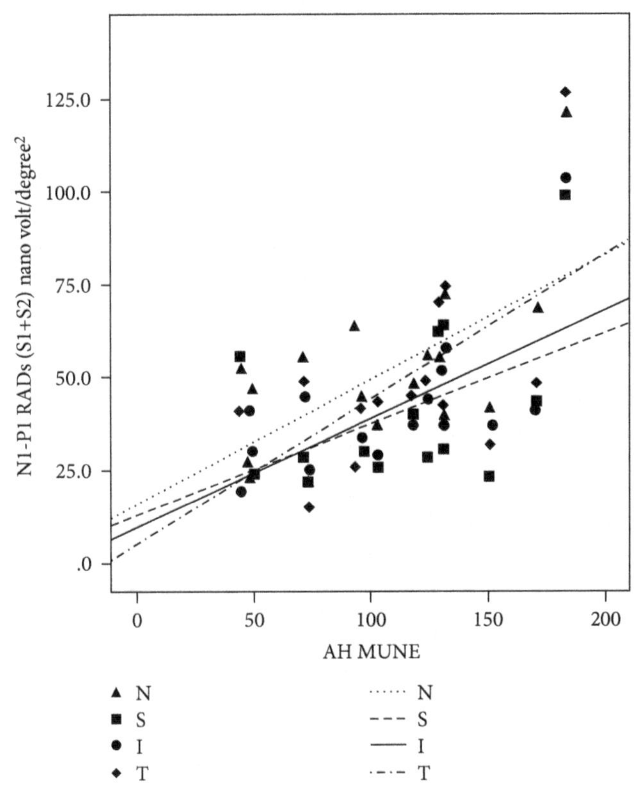

FIGURE 4: Scatter plot between MfERG RADS of S1 + S2 of the N (nasal), S (superior), I (inferior), and T (temporal) sectors and motor unit number estimation of the abductor hallux (AH MUNE) in type 1 DM patients. A positive correlation between the mean MfERG RADs of the four quadrants (S, I, T, and N) and AH MUNE ($r = 0.50$, $p = 0.041$; $r = 0.64$, $p = 0.005$; $r = 0.64$, $p = 0.006$; and $r = 0.61$, $p = 0.010$, respectively) was observed in T1DM patients. Since such correlations could be significantly affected by outliers, influence statistics (standardized DfBetas) were computed. After eliminating cases with values higher than the cutoff (2/sqrt(n)), r correlations resulted similar ($r = 0.49$, $p = 0.065$; $r = 0.64$, $p = 0.015$; $r = 0.64$, $p = 0.013$; and $r = 0.52$, $p = 0.048$, respectively).

We did not observe a significant correlation between the HbA1c and metabolic parameters and retinal macular function or MUNE (consistently, $p > 0.2$).

In this study, the diabetic subjects were highly selected without DPN, both clinically and after routine electrophysiological examination. Moreover, the good glycemic control and the absence of other microvascular complications and comorbidities allowed to perform these evaluations in the absence of confounding factors. Despite this, we observed a significant reduction in the number of motor units of both the ADM muscle (upper limb) and, more pronounced, the AH muscle (lower limb), consistent with length-dependent neurodegeneration expected in diabetes. The MUNE technique is increasingly used in studies on amyotrophic lateral sclerosis, but it is more rarely used in other peripheral nerve disorders, including diabetic neuropathy [6, 27–30].

Our findings imply that loss of motor units occurs early in the neurodegenerative process in diabetic patients and MUNE can detect motor unit abnormalities, even in the absence of signs of diabetic neuropathy at clinical exam and conventional NCS. Similarly to what is observed for epidermal nerve fiber densities, the dying back of motor nerve terminals occurs early and in the absence of clinical sensory-motor symptoms and signs in DM [31]. We also observed an increase in AH SMUP in the diabetic subjects compared to the control group. In diabetic peripheral neuropathy, a process of chronic denervation, the germination of small intact motor units can lead to larger SMUPs. We know that a motor unit includes a single motor neuron and the group of muscle fibers that it innervates. The increase in the average size of motor units suggests a preferential loss of smaller motor units or the enlargement of these units by compensatory germination [32]. The size of the motor units can also increase with axonal sprouting, which reinnervates the denervated muscle fibers to compensate for the loss of adjacent functional motor units [32–34]. The findings of concurrent AH SMUP enlargement can account for the existence of a similar process already ongoing in these asymptomatic diabetic patients. The only electrophysiological parameter currently used to describe the neuronal loss in neuropathies is the amplitude of distal cMAP, but this parameter remains into normal range until the reinnervation process is effective. Only when a marked loss of the motor units is reached, the force production will decrease in parallel, resulting in the reduction of cMAP amplitude in conventional NSC studies and muscle weakness as described in diabetic patients with more advanced peripheral neuropathy. Then, MUNE may represent an early noninvasive marker of a subclinical DNP. Such a marker has potential therapeutic implications, allowing an early treatment approach for DPN, when the probability of regeneration of sensorimotor fibers is still good [6].

We also showed that multifocal electroretinogram is a valuable tool in order to examine local neuroretinal dysfunction in T1DM with or without diabetic retinopathy. Therefore, it is able to detect functionally the most vulnerable areas, even in the absence of ophthalmoscopic early signs of retinal abnormalities. MfERG allows for the simultaneous recording of the activity of bipolar cells with small contributions from photoreceptors from different areas of the retina [35]. In diabetic population studies, the use of MfERG [36–39] identified significant abnormalities in retinal function, characterized by increased peak latencies and/or reduced amplitudes, suggesting a compromised inner retinal function, secondary to neuronal transmission alterations [40]. The topographic mapping of neuroretinal dysfunction by MfERG has been shown to be predictive of the onset of DR [36] and is able to detect these abnormalities earlier than morphological studies [41, 42]. Recently, in adolescents with T1DM and noDR, an early alteration of the inner retina, confirmed also by a delay of IT in MfERG recordings, has been observed [43]. The nasal retina had abnormal IT compared with the temporal retina, whereas alteration of the amplitude parameter was more evident in the temporal retina in T1DM adolescents [44]. Moreover, Holm and Adrian [45] described that the nasal area of the macula, where there is a higher density of cones and ganglion cells, was more vulnerable to neurodegenerative processes than the temporal region, showing a lower amplitude and longer implicit time in this specific area with the MfERG analysis. The innovative MfERG sector analysis allowed to identify the specific retinal areas of neuroretinal damage that in our group of patients are mainly represented by the nasal and temporal sectors, anatomically crucial regions for the function of collector cells to the small axons of the optic nerve forming the papillomacular bundle. The neurodegenerative theory, for which the photoreceptors are involved early in the course of diabetes in patients, has been also supported by recent *in vivo* studies using adaptive optics ophthalmoscopy [46]. The authors have shown that early pathological disruption of the parafoveal cone mosaic in patients with type 1 diabetes, even before any sign of diabetic retinopathy, was found on fundoscopy. Furthermore, through the use of spectral domain optical coherence tomography (SD-OCT) analysis, we recently observed an increased macular thickness of the inner nuclear layer (INL) and a decrease in the retinal nerve fiber layer (RNFL) thickness in the nasal quadrant of the macular area in T1DM persons with noDR and NPDR, compared to healthy groups. In order to analyze the role of glycemic control on the neuroretina, we also found that only glycemic variability was associated with abnormalities of these specific retinal layers, while no association was observed with HbA1c [14]. Finally, we studied the relationship between functional changes in the neuroretina and early signs of peripheral neuropathic damage. We have found that motor unit loss was associated with the amplitude densities' reduction in all four macular sectors, from the foveal center up to the 5° external areas. At the moment, the available evidence on the link between retinal neurodegeneration and diabetic neuropathy is scanty; it is related exclusively to morphological evidence and identifiable especially in DM1 or DM2 patients already affected by peripheral neuropathic damage diagnosed with standard examinations [47–51]. Recently, in a prospective study, defining longitudinal alterations to the RNFL thickness of the optic nerve head in individuals with DM1, with and without DPN, patients with DPN showed a progressive global RNFL thinning, especially in the superior quadrant. Therefore, it is possible to hypothesize common pathways for retinal and peripheral neurodegeneration that are independent of DPN risk factors [51]. Polyol pathway activation, hexosamine pathway and protein kinase C (PKC) isoform activation, and accumulation of advanced glycation end products (AGEs) resulting in imbalance of the mitochondrial redox state and in excess formation reactive oxygen species may represent common mechanisms to neuroretinal and peripheral neurodegeneration. Furthermore, a key role of the glial component has been described in the early stages of both neuronal and neuroretinal damages [14, 52, 53]. Despite promising evidence linking morphological alterations of the neuroretina to the overt presence of diabetic neuropathy, a functional analytical approach is required to identify and characterize initial stages of neuropathic damage. Very few studies have investigated the role of early outer retinal deficit at the base of retinal neurodegeneration [46], and, to our knowledge, this is the first work that allowed to observe a relationship between this dysfunction at the early peripheral neuropathic damage. In light of this, our result of an association between neuroretinal (photoreceptors and bipolar cells) dysfunction and subclinical damage of the peripheral nerve in asymptomatic diabetic subjects seems particularly interesting. MfERG recording could represent an accessible, noninvasive, and well-tolerated tool in the detection also of neuronal damage in diabetic patients. However, our study has some limitations: small sample size and the presence in the diabetic population of subjects with diabetic vascular retinopathy, although not proliferating and of a very mild degree, the lack of an association with standardized methods of early DN diagnosis, such as skin biopsy. The inclusion of a cohort of patients with overt DN or a longitudinal observation could allow to understand the associative link between the two neurodegeneration processes. Nevertheless, we believe that the identification of these potential markers of very early neuropathic damage in diabetes (retinal neurodegeneration and morphofunctional alterations of the motor unit) is an important point of strength of our study. Our findings, therefore, strongly support a new vision of the neuropathic damage in diabetes, as an overall neuronal damage.

5. Conclusions

In conclusion, motor unit loss and neuroretinal dysfunction are already present in T1DM patients without DPN. The relationship between neuroretinal dysfunction and early peripheral motor unit decline supports the hypothesis that the neuroretina is a potential "window" onto the early neurogenic process, in diabetes.

Disclosure

Parts of this study were presented in abstract form during a poster presentation at the 27th Annual Scientific Meeting of Neurodiab, Coimbra, Portugal, 9–11 September 2017, and as a poster presentation of the 53rd European Association for the Study of Diabetes meeting, 11–15 September 2017, Lisbon, Portugal.

Conflicts of Interest

The authors declare that there is no conflict of interest regarding the publication of this paper.

Authors' Contributions

Fabiana Picconi and Giorgia Mataluni have equally contributed.

Acknowledgments

Research for this study (for LZ, ADR, and MP) was financially supported by the Ministry of Health and by Rome Foundation. This work was partially supported by Fatebenefratelli Foundation for Health Research and Education, AFaR Division of Rome.

References

[1] S. Tesfaye, A. J. M. Boulton, P. J. Dyck et al., "Diabetic neuropathies: update on definitions, diagnostic criteria, estimation of severity, and treatments," *Diabetes Care*, vol. 33, no. 10, pp. 2285–2293, 2010.

[2] P. J. Dyck, B. Argyros, J. W. Russell et al., "Multicenter trial of the proficiency of smart quantitative sensation tests," *Muscle & Nerve*, vol. 49, no. 5, pp. 645–653, 2014.

[3] S. Srinivasan, N. Pritchard, G. P. Sampson et al., "Diagnostic capability of retinal thickness measures in diabetic peripheral neuropathy," *Journal of Optometry*, vol. 10, no. 4, pp. 215–225, 2017.

[4] D. Selvarajah, I. D. Wilkinson, M. Maxwell et al., "Magnetic resonance neuroimaging study of brain structural differences in diabetic peripheral neuropathy," *Diabetes Care*, vol. 37, no. 6, pp. 1681–1688, 2014.

[5] G. J. Francis, J. A. Martinez, W. Q. Liu et al., "Motor end plate innervation loss in diabetes and the role of insulin," *Journal of Neuropathology and Experimental Neurology*, vol. 70, no. 5, pp. 323–339, 2011.

[6] C. Toth, V. Hebert, C. Gougeon, H. Virtanen, J. K. Mah, and D. Pacaud, "Motor unit number estimations are smaller in children with type 1 diabetes mellitus: a case-cohort study," *Muscle & Nerve*, vol. 50, no. 4, pp. 593–598, 2014.

[7] N. G. Congdon, D. S. Friedman, and T. Lietman, "Important causes of visual impairment in the world today," *JAMA*, vol. 290, no. 15, pp. 2057–2060, 2003.

[8] E. Midena and E. Pilotto, "Emerging insights into pathogenesis," *Developments in Ophthalmology*, vol. 60, pp. 16–27, 2017.

[9] A. J. Barber and B. Baccouche, "Neurodegeneration in diabetic retinopathy: potential for novel therapies," *Vision Research*, vol. 139, pp. 82–92, 2017.

[10] D. A. Antonetti, R. Klein, and T. W. Gardner, "Diabetic retinopathy," *New England Journal of Medicine*, vol. 366, no. 13, pp. 1227–1239, 2012.

[11] D. A. Antonetti, A. J. Barber, S. K. Bronson et al., "Diabetic retinopathy: seeing beyond glucose-induced microvascular disease," *Diabetes*, vol. 55, no. 9, pp. 2401–2411, 2006.

[12] Y. Jiang, J. Pagadala, D. Miller, and J. J. Steinle, "Reduced insulin receptor signaling in retinal Müller cells cultured in high glucose," *Molecular Vision*, vol. 19, p. 804, 2013.

[13] N. Cheung, P. Mitchell, and T. Y. Wong, "Diabetic retinopathy," *The Lancet*, vol. 376, no. 9735, pp. 124–136, 2010.

[14] F. Picconi, M. Parravano, D. Ylli et al., "Retinal neurodegeneration in patients with type 1 diabetes mellitus: the role of glycemic variability," *Acta Diabetologica*, vol. 54, no. 5, pp. 489–497, 2017.

[15] American Diabetes Association, "Diagnosis and classification of diabetes mellitus," *Diabetes Care*, vol. 35, pp. S64–S71, 2012, Supplement_1.

[16] G. Bax, C. Fagherazzi, F. Piarulli, A. Nicolucci, and D. Fedele, "Reproducibility of Michigan Neuropathy Screening Instrument (MNSI). A comparison with tests using the vibratory and thermal perception thresholds," *Diabetes Care*, vol. 19, no. 8, pp. 904-905, 1996.

[17] R. P. Kleyweg, F. G. A. Van Der Meché, and P. I. M. Schmitz, "Interobserver agreement in the assessment of muscle strength and functional abilities in Guillain–Barré syndrome," *Muscle & Nerve*, vol. 14, no. 11, pp. 1103–1109, 1991.

[18] F. Sartucci, P. Maritato, G. Moscato et al., "Motor unit number estimation (MUNE) as a quantitative measure of disease progression and motor unit reorganization in amyotrophic lateral sclerosis," *International Journal of Neuroscience*, vol. 117, no. 9, pp. 1229–1236, 2009.

[19] V. H. Lawson, A. Gordon Smith, and M. B. Bromberg, "Assessment of axonal loss in Charcot-Marie-Tooth neuropathies," *Experimental Neurology*, vol. 184, no. 2, pp. 753–757, 2003.

[20] M. B. Bromberg, "Updating motor unit number estimation (MUNE)," *Clinical Neurophysiology*, vol. 118, no. 1, pp. 1–8, 2007, Epub 2006 Sep 25.

[21] A. J. McComas, "Invited review: motor unit estimation: methods, results, and present status," *Muscle & Nerve*, vol. 14, no. 7, pp. 585–597, 1991.

[22] C. L. Gooch, T. J. Doherty, K. M. Chan et al., "Motor unit number estimation: a technology and literature review," *Muscle & Nerve*, vol. 50, no. 6, pp. 884–893, 2014.

[23] V. Parisi, L. Ziccardi, G. Stifano, L. Montrone, G. Gallinaro, and B. Falsini, "Impact of regional retinal responses on cortical visually evoked responses: multifocal ERGs and VEPs in the retinitis pigmentosa model," *Clinical Neurophysiology*, vol. 121, no. 3, pp. 380–385, 2010.

[24] V. Parisi, L. Perillo, M. Tedeschi et al., "Macular function in eyes with early age-related macular degeneration with or without contralateral late age-related macular degeneration," *Retina*, vol. 27, no. 7, pp. 879–890, 2007.

[25] V. Parisi, L. Ziccardi, M. Centofanti et al., "Macular function in eyes with open-angle glaucoma evaluated by multifocal electroretinogram," *Investigative Opthalmology & Visual Science*, vol. 53, no. 11, p. 6973, 2012.

[26] M. L. Cascavilla, V. Parisi, G. Triolo et al., "Retinal dysfunction characterizes subtypes of dominant optic atrophy," *Acta Ophthalmologica*, vol. 96, no. 2, pp. e156–e163, 2018.

[27] I. K. Bayrak, A. O. Bayrak, H. E. Tilki, M. S. Nural, and T. Sunter, "Ultrasonography in carpal tunnel syndrome: comparison with electrophysiological stage and motor unit number estimate," *Muscle & Nerve*, vol. 35, no. 3, pp. 344–348, 2007.

[28] S. Hansen and J. P. Ballantyne, "Axonal dysfunction in the neuropathy of diabetes mellitus: a quantitative electrophysiological study," *Journal of Neurology, Neurosurgery, and Psychiatry*, vol. 40, no. 6, pp. 555–564, 1977.

[29] R. A. Lewis, J. Li, D. R. Fuerst, M. E. Shy, and K. Krajewski, "Motor unit number estimate of distal and proximal muscles in Charcot-Marie-Tooth disease," *Muscle & Nerve*, vol. 28, no. 2, pp. 161–167, 2003.

[30] K. L. Peterson, M. Graves, G. S. Berke et al., "Role of motor unit number estimate electromyography in experimental canine laryngeal reinnervation," *Otolaryngology and Head and Neck Surgery*, vol. 121, no. 3, pp. 180–184, 1999.

[31] T. Umapathi, W. L. Tan, S. C. Loke, P. C. Soon, S. Tavintharan, and Y. H. Chan, "Intraepidermal nerve fiber density as a marker of early diabetic neuropathy," *Muscle & Nerve*, vol. 35, no. 5, pp. 591–598, 2007.

[32] N. Ramji, C. Toth, J. Kennedy, and D. W. Zochodne, "Does diabetes mellitus target motor neurons?," *Neurobiology of Disease*, vol. 26, no. 2, pp. 301–311, 2007.

[33] G. Grimby, G. Einarsson, M. Hedberg, and A. Aniansson, "Muscle adaptive changes in post-polio subjects," *Scandinavian Journal of Rehabilitation Medicine*, vol. 21, no. 1, pp. 19–26, 1989.

[34] S. L. Tam and T. Gordon, "Mechanisms controlling axonal sprouting at the neuromuscular junction," *Journal of Neurocytology*, vol. 32, no. 5-8, pp. 961–974, 2003.

[35] D. C. Hood, J. G. Odel, C. S. Chen, and B. J. Winn, "The multifocal electroretinogram," *Journal of Neuro-Ophthalmology*, vol. 23, no. 3, pp. 225–235, 2003.

[36] K. P. Dhamdhere, M. A. Bearse Jr, W. Harrison, S. Barez, M. E. Schneck, and A. J. Adams, "Associations between local retinal thickness and function in early diabetes," *Investigative Ophthalmology & Visual Science*, vol. 53, no. 10, pp. 6122–6128, 2012.

[37] M. A. Bearse Jr, A. J. Adams, Y. Han et al., "A multifocal electroretinogram model predicting the development of diabetic retinopathy," *Progress in Retinal and Eye Research*, vol. 25, no. 5, pp. 425–448, 2006.

[38] W. W. Harrison, M. A. Bearse Jr, J. S. Ng et al., "Multifocal electroretinograms predict onset of diabetic retinopathy in adult patients with diabetes," *Investigative Ophthalmology & Visual Science*, vol. 52, no. 2, pp. 772–777, 2011.

[39] W. W. Harrison, M. A. Bearse Jr, M. E. Schneck et al., "Prediction, by retinal location, of the onset of diabetic edema in patients with nonproliferative diabetic retinopathy," *Investigative Ophthalmology & Visual Science*, vol. 52, no. 9, pp. 6825–6831, 2011.

[40] T. S. Kern and A. J. Barber, "Retinal ganglion cells in diabetes," *The Journal of Physiology*, vol. 586, no. 18, pp. 4401–4408, 2008.

[41] E. Midena, T. Segato, M. Giuliano, and M. Zucchetto, "Macular recovery function (nyctometry) in diabetics without and with early retinopathy," *British Journal of Ophthalmology*, vol. 74, no. 2, pp. 106–108, 1990.

[42] E. Midena and S. Vujosevic, "Visual psychophysics in diabetic retinopathy," in *Visual Disfunction in Diabetes*, J. T. Tink, C. J. Barnstable, and T. W. Gardner, Eds., pp. 69–105, Springer, New York, NY, USA, 2012.

[43] W. Tan, T. Wright, A. Dupuis, E. Lakhani, and C. Westall, "Localizing functional damage in the neural retina of adolescents and young adults with type 1 diabetes," *Investigative Ophthalmology & Visual Science*, vol. 55, no. 4, pp. 2432–2441, 2014.

[44] M. Laron, M. A. Bearse Jr, K. Bronson-Castain et al., "Association between local neuroretinal function and control of adolescent type 1 diabetes," *Investigative Ophthalmology & Visual Science*, vol. 53, no. 11, pp. 7071–7076, 2012.

[45] K. Holm and M. L. Adrian, "In diabetic eyes, multifocal ERG reflects differences in function between the nasal part and the temporal part of the macula," *Graefe's Archive for Clinical and Experimental Ophthalmology*, vol. 250, no. 8, pp. 1143–1148, 2012.

[46] M. Lombardo, M. Parravano, S. Serrao, L. Ziccardi, D. Giannini, and G. Lombardo, "Investigation of adaptive optics imaging biomarkers for detecting pathological changes of the cone mosaic in patients with type 1 diabetes mellitus," *PLoS One*, vol. 11, no. 3, article e0151380, 2016.

[47] A. M. Shahidi, G. P. Sampson, N. Pritchard et al., "Retinal nerve fibre layer thinning associated with diabetic peripheral neuropathy," *Diabetic Medicine*, vol. 29, no. 7, pp. e106–e111, 2012.

[48] S. Srinivasan, N. Pritchard, G. P. Sampson et al., "Focal loss volume of ganglion cell complex in diabetic neuropathy," *Clinical & Experimental Optometry*, vol. 99, no. 6, pp. 526–534, 2016.

[49] S. Srinivasan, N. Pritchard, D. Vagenas et al., "Retinal tissue thickness is reduced in diabetic peripheral neuropathy," *Current Eye Research*, vol. 41, no. 10, pp. 1359–1366, 2016.

[50] L. Salvi, P. Plateroti, S. Balducci et al., "Abnormalities of retinal ganglion cell complex at optical coherence tomography in patients with type 2 diabetes: a sign of diabetic polyneuropathy, not retinopathy," *Journal of Diabetes and its Complications*, vol. 30, no. 3, pp. 469–476, 2016.

[51] C. Dehghani, S. Srinivasan, K. Edwards et al., "Presence of peripheral neuropathy is associated with progressive thinning of retinal nerve fiber layer in type 1 diabetes," *Investigative Ophthalmology & Visual Science*, vol. 58, no. 6, article BIO234, 2017.

[52] E. L. Feldman, K. A. Nave, T. S. Jensen, and D. L. H. Bennett, "New horizons in diabetic neuropathy: mechanisms, bioenergetics, and pain," *Neuron*, vol. 93, no. 6, pp. 1296–1313, 2017.

[53] R. Simó and C. Hernández, "Neurodegeneration in the diabetic eye: new insights and therapeutic perspectives," *Trends in Endocrinology and Metabolism*, vol. 25, no. 1, pp. 23–33, 2014.

24

Interaction of Pubertal Development and Metabolic Control in Adolescents with Type 1 Diabetes Mellitus

M. Plamper,[1] B. Gohlke,[1] J. Woelfle,[1] K. Konrad,[2,3] T. Rohrer,[4] S. Hofer,[5] W. Bonfig,[6,7] K. Fink,[8] and R. W. Holl[8]

[1]*Pediatric Endocrinology Division, Children's Hospital, University of Bonn, Bonn, Germany*
[2]*Department of Pediatrics and Adolescent Medicine, University of Cologne, Cologne, Germany*
[3]*Department of Pediatric and Adolescent Medicine, Elisabeth Hospital Essen, Essen, Germany*
[4]*Department of Pediatrics, University of Saarland, Homburg, Germany*
[5]*Department of Pediatrics, University of Innsbruck, Innsbruck, Austria*
[6]*Department of Pediatrics, Technical University Munich, Munich, Germany*
[7]*Department of Pediatrics, Klinikum Wels-Grieskirchen, Wels, Austria*
[8]*Institute for Epidemiology and Medical Biometry, ZIBMT University of Ulm and German Center for Diabetes Research (DZD), Neuherberg, München, Germany*

Correspondence should be addressed to M. Plamper; Michaela.Hamm@ukb.uni-bonn.de and J. Woelfle; joachim.woelfle@ukb.uni-bonn.de

Academic Editor: Andrea Scaramuzza

Background. In T1DM, delayed pubertal development and reduced final height are associated with inadequate metabolic control. *Objective.* To assess whether T1DM affects pubertal growth spurt and whether metabolic control during puberty is gender-related. *Methods.* Using a large multicentre database, longitudinal data from 1294 patients were analysed. Inclusion criteria: complete records of height and HbA1c from the age of seven to 16 years. Exclusion criteria: other significant chronic diseases and medications, T1DM duration less than three months, and initial BMI < 3rd or >97th percentile. *Results.* Growth velocity (GV) was impaired with a significant reduction of peak GV by 1.2 cm in boys. HbA1c increase during male puberty was lower except for a period of 1.5 years. The highest HbA1c increase in boys coincided with maximum growth spurt. In girls, the highest HbA1c increase was observed during late puberty. Even though there is impaired GV, both sexes reach a height at 16 years of age which corresponds to the background population height. *Conclusion.* Worsening of metabolic control is sex-discordant and associated with gender-specific alterations of GV. However, the vast majority of boys and girls with T1DM seems to reach normal height at the age of 16 years.

1. Introduction

Type 1 diabetes mellitus (T1DM) is a chronic disease frequently manifesting in childhood or adolescence. Like other chronic diseases, T1DM can have a negative impact on growth and pubertal development. Several studies describe a delayed onset of puberty in both sexes and a delay of menarche in girls with diabetes [1–4].

Although the therapeutic regimen in children and adolescents has changed over the years towards a diversified arsenal of differently acting insulin types and a larger fraction of patients treated with CSII, adult height remains still reduced in patients with T1DM in the 21st century [5, 6].

Metabolic control in T1DM frequently worsens during puberty [7–9]. In this context, puberty-related insulin resistance may play an important role; in addition, inadequate adherence to diabetes management seems to be involved [9].

In this study, we analysed the relationship between pubertal growth spurt and HbA1c deterioration. Furthermore, we analysed whether differences in metabolic control are sex-specific. Since adult height is impaired in children with T1DM, we speculated that an impaired pubertal growth

Table 1: Clinical characteristics of 1294 type 1 diabetic patients, depending on sex and metabolic control (data expressed as median and interquartile range).

	All	Female	Male	HbA1c < 7.5%	HbA1c > 7.5%
n	1294	630	664	647	647
Age at study start (yr)	7.25 (7.21; 7.29)	7.25 (7.22; 7.29)	7.25 (7.21; 7.29)	7.25 (7.21; 7.29)	7.25 (7.22; 7.29)
Age at end of study (yr)	15.75 (15.7; 15.79)	15.74 (15.69; 15.79)	15.75 (15.7; 15.79)	15.75 (15.7; 15.78)	15.74 (15.69; 15.79)
Diabetes duration at study start (yr)	2.56 (1.23; 4.09)	2.46 (1.15; 4.08)	2.63 (1.30; 4.15)	2.40 (1.22; 3.91)	2.84 (1.26; 4.29)
Diabetes duration at study end (yr)	11.07 (9.7; 12.58)	10.94 (9.66; 12.57)	11.13 (9.78; 12.61)	10.9 (9.67; 12.37)	11.3 (9.71; 12.79)
Height SDS at study start	0.17 (−0.45; 0.85)	0.17 (−0.43; 0.84)	0.17 (−0.45; 0.85)	0.25 (−0.32; 0.92)	0.12 (−0.51; 0.75)
Height SDS at study end	0.01 (−0.64; 0.65)	0.04 (−0.65; 0.69)	−0.02 (−0.64; 0.62)	0.19 (−0.44; 0.80)	−0.18 (−0.79; 0.48)
BMI-SDS at study start	0.37 (−0.18; 0.82)	0.38 (−0.15; 0.84)	0.35 (−0.21; 0.78)	0.36 (−0.20; 0.82)	0.39 (−0.17; 0.82)
BMI-SDS at study end	0.39 (−0.16; 0.89)	0.61 (0.12; 1.06)	0.18 (−0.40; 0.68)	0.30 (−0.24; 0.86)	0.46 (−0.07; 0.92)
HbA1c at study start (%)	7.17 (6.51; 7.89)	7.17 (6.51; 7.92)	7.15 (6.51; 7.88)	6.77 (6.22; 7.20)	7.72 (7.13; 8.32)
HbA1c at study end (%)	8.08 (7.33; 9.09)	8.12 (7.33; 9.19)	8.04 (7.33; 8.99)	7.42 (6.87; 7.98)	8.94 (8.18; 9.92)

spurt might be directly associated with insufficient metabolic control. We therefore compared timing and degree of peripubertal growth velocity of our patients in relation to metabolic control with German reference data [10].

2. Methods

DPV (Diabetes Patienten Verlaufsdaten) is a diabetes registry for quality management and research that started in 1995. Approximately 325 paediatric diabetes centres in Germany and Austria participate in DPV. The participating centres enter their routine care data into an electronic health record; anonymized data are analysed every six months.

The inclusion criteria for this study were a continuous recording of height and HbA1c at least every six months from the age of seven to 16 years in patients with T1DM.

Patients with celiac disease, TSH > 10 μU/ml, eating disorders, and glucocorticoid or growth hormone therapy were excluded. Also, patients with duration of diabetes less than three months and patients with a BMI below the 3rd or above the 97th percentile at the age of seven years were excluded. A different quality of metabolic control during the first year of disease might influence growth and weight and may therefore not be compared to those who have suffered from type 1 diabetes for a longer period of time. We therefore added an analysis, comparing whether height velocity in patients with duration of 3–12 months differs from those with a duration exceeding 12 months and found no significant difference in height velocity between the groups.

In the DPV database, 9920 patients had diabetes onset before 7.5 years of age and were older than 15.5 years at the time of analysis. Applying all exclusion criteria, 1294 patients with a complete longitudinal dataset could be analysed (male $n = 664$, female $n = 630$). Clinical characteristics of these patients are depicted in Table 1.

HbA1c levels were determined using the methodology established at each centre. To adjust for differences among laboratories, the HbA1c values were mathematically standardized to the DCCT (Diabetes Control and Complications Trial) with a reference range of 4.05% to 6.05% [11] using the multiple-of-the-mean method.

To quantify the deterioration of HbA1c, we calculated the change of HbA1c in individual patients between two consecutive time points for every year (Δ HbA1c = (mean HbA1c age $(n+1)$) − (mean HbA1c age (n)). We used SAS version 9.3 for statistical analysis. p values were based on a general linear model. We compared the growth velocity data of our patients with data from a healthy control group surveyed by Brandt and Reinken [10] and used t-tests to assess for statistical significance.

Although there are newer reference data in German children available, we decided to use the reference data from Brandt and Reinken, since these in contrast to the more recent growth data had been collected longitudinally. Because body mass index (BMI) is not normally distributed, we used the LMS method to calculate SDS-BMI as a measure for the degree of overweight. The LMS method was chosen as it summarizes the data in terms of three smooth age-specific curves called lambda (L), mu (M), and sigma (S) based on German population-specific data [12]. The M and S curves, respectively, correspond to the median and coefficients of variation (CV) of BMI for German children at each age and gender, whereas L allows for the substantial age-dependent skewness in the distribution of BMI [11, 13]. The assumption underlying the LMS method is that after Box-Cox power transformation, the BMI data at each age are normally distributed [11].

3. Results

3.1. Metabolic Control. Mean HbA1c levels increased continuously from 7.3% (56.3 mmol/mol) at the age of seven years to 8.4% (68.3 mmol/mol) at the age of 16 years (Figure 1 and Table 2). Peak HbA1c in girls (9.37 [9.25; 9.50]) was significantly higher than peak HbA1c in boys (9.17 [9.05; 9.29]) (delta 0.20 [0.03; 0.37], $p = 0.02$). From 10 years onwards, mean HbA1c was always lower in boys as compared to girls except for a period of 1.5 years between 13.5 and 15 years of age.

The highest HbA1c increase in boys (increment to preceding measurement + 0.4, $p = 0.027$) occurred between

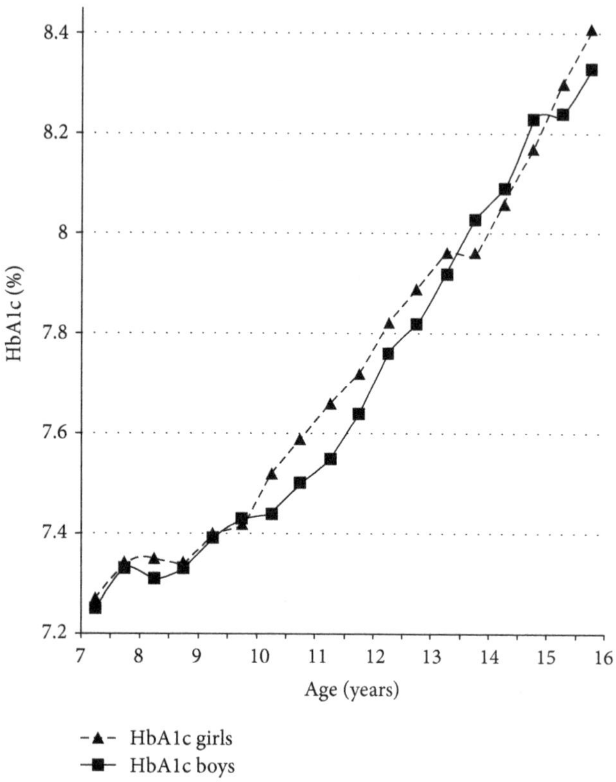

FIGURE 1: Gender-specific course of HbA1c concentration before and during puberty.

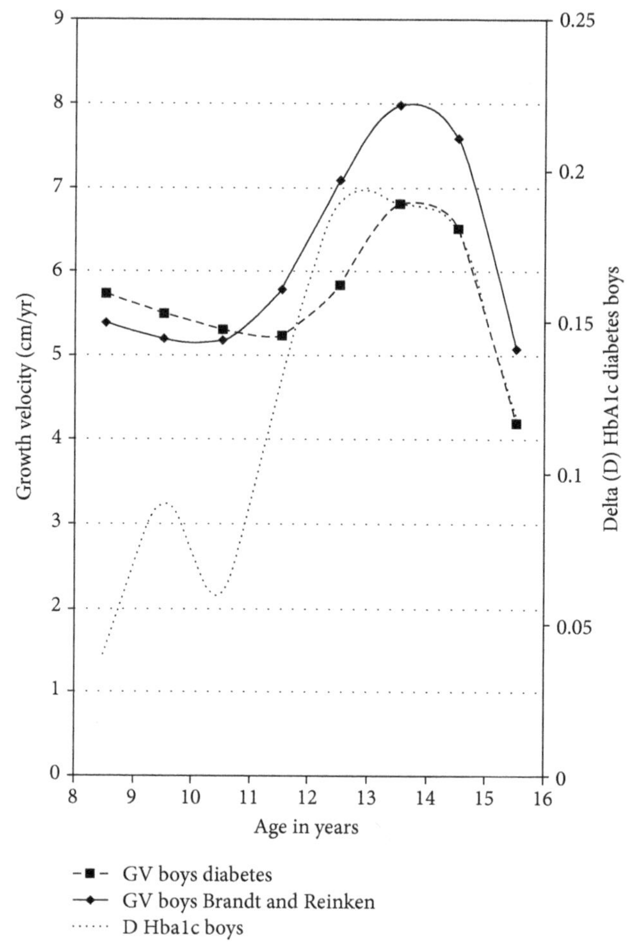

FIGURE 2: Growth velocity and delta HbA1c in boys with T1DM.

TABLE 2: Gender-specific HbA1c development in patients with T1DM before and during puberty. Change in HbA1c (%) was calculated by the difference of the HbA1c concentration between the actual and the preceding year.

Age (years)	Δ HbA1c boys	Δ HbA1c girls	p value (Δ HbA1c boys versus girls)
8-9	0.04	0.05	0.05
9-10	0.09	0.07	0.63
10-11	0.06	**0.14**	**0.012**
11-12	0.13	0.14	0.065
12-13	0.19	0.16	0.023
13-14	0.19	0.11	0.31
14-15	0.18	0.15	0.23
15-16	0.12	**0.24**	**0.018**

12 and 14 years, which covered the time of usual maximum growth spurt at the age of 13 to 14 years.

Girls exhibited their maximum growth spurt on average between 11 and 12 years of age. In girls, we found a significantly higher HbA1c increase between 10 and 11 years (increment to preceding measurement + 0.14, $p = 0.012$) and between 15 and 16 years (increment to preceding measurement + 0.2, $p = 0.018$) (Table 2). Thus, in girls, HbA1c increase was not strictly related to the time of maximal growth spurt (Figures 2 and 3).

3.2. Growth Velocity. We compared growth velocities of diabetes patients with growth velocity data from a healthy control group published by Brandt and Reinken [10]. We started to analyse and to compare growth velocity of our diabetes patients between the ages of eight and nine years with the data published by Brandt and Reinken.

This time interval from the start of the observation period was chosen to make sure that all patients were most likely to have finished remission and had made enough experience with diabetes management to exclude a respective influence on the quality of diabetes control.

Timing of pubertal growth spurt in girls and boys with T1DM did not differ from the healthy control population. However, in boys with T1DM, median growth velocity at the time of maximal growth spurt was significantly reduced by 1.2 cm compared to the data of Brandt and Reinken ($p < 0.001$; Figure 4). In girls, we found no difference in median maximum growth velocity ($p = 0.5$), but growth velocity declined more rapidly in diabetic girls after reaching pubertal peak height velocity compared to the reference population, as visualized in Figure 5. To compare patients who had adequate to those who had inadequate metabolic control, the respective groups were stratified by HbA1c. The group with good metabolic control was defined by a long-term mean HbA1c < 7.5% ($n = 647$, female $n = 308$,

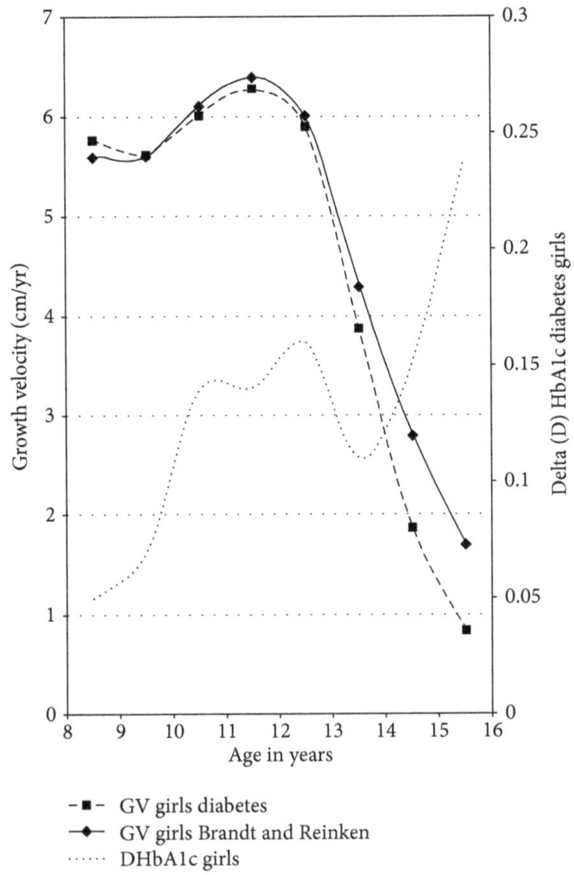

FIGURE 3: Growth velocity and delta HbA1c in girls with T1DM.

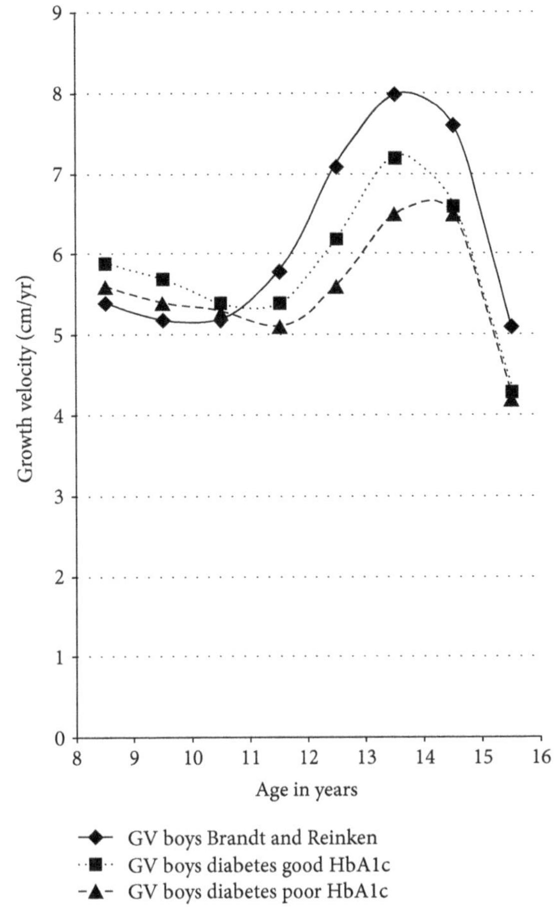

FIGURE 4: Growth velocity before and during puberty in boys with T1DM versus reference population.

male $n = 340$), and the group with poor metabolic control had a mean HbA1c equal or higher than 7.5% over all the years of documentation ($n = 647$, female $n = 323$, male $n = 324$).

The classification into two groups (good metabolic control and poor metabolic control) was based on medium HbA1c throughout all observation years, including six-month intervals. The median HbA1c of 7592 was chosen to divide our patients' group into two equally sized groups.

Compared to healthy children, growth spurt was impaired in both groups, but the impairment was more pronounced in patients with poor metabolic control (Figures 4 and 5).

To have a closer view on those with poor metabolic control, we subdivided this group into two parts: one part with poor metabolic control (HbA1c > 7.5%) ($n = 537$) and the other part with very poor metabolic control with a mean HbA1c > 9% ($n = 110$). As expected, the worst growth velocity was seen in those with a mean HbA1c > 9% (Table 3).

3.3. Height SDS. At the start of the age of seven years, diabetic girls and boys had reached a height SDS of +0.17 (interquartile range −0.45 to +0.85) compared to German reference data [12]. For both boys and girls with T1DM, height SDS during the observation period differed significantly from the reference population ($p < 0.0001$, resp.). However, at the end of this study at the age of 16 years, height SDS of both boys and girls was no longer significantly different from reference data (height SDS in girls + 0.04, interquartile range −0.65 to +0.69, n.s; height SDS in boys − 0.02, interquartile range −0.64 to 0.62, n.s.).

3.4. BMI-SDS. During the whole period from seven to 16 years of age, BMI-SDS of our patients was higher than the mean BMI-SDS of German reference data [13]. BMI-SDS declined from the age of seven until the age of 11.5 years but increased continuously thereafter (Figure 6). Girls with T1DM had a higher absolute mean BMI-SDS than boys with T1DM. This difference became increasingly obvious after the age of ten years.

By the age of 16 years, the mean BMI-SDS of girls was +0.61 (interquartile range + 0.12 to 1.06), and BMI-SDS of boys was + 0.18 (interquartile range −0.40 to +0.68). The median BMI (50th percentile) of 16-year-old girls in our cohort with T1DM was 23.4 kg/m^2 and corresponded to a BMI between the 75th and 90th percentile (exactly corresponding to the 81st percentile) of German reference data [12]. In 16-year-old boys, the median BMI of 21.5 kg/m^2 corresponded to a BMI between the 50th and 75th percentile (exactly corresponding to the 64th percentile) of reference data. For both boys and girls with T1DM, BMI-SDS differed significantly from the reference population

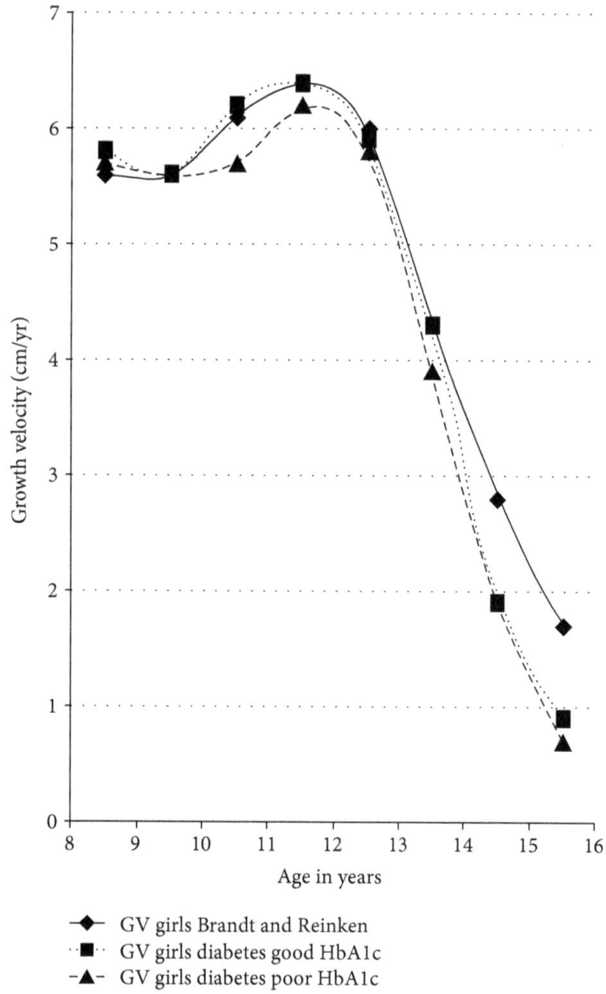

FIGURE 5: Growth velocity before and during puberty in girls with T1DM versus reference population.

TABLE 3: Growth velocity data of the whole dataset divided into good metabolic control (HbA1c < 7.5%), poor metabolic control (HbA1c > 7.5), and very poor metabolic control (HbA1c > 9%).

	Good metabolic control (HbA1c < 7.5%)	Poor metabolic control (HbA1c > 7.5%)	Very poor metabolic control (HbA1c > 9%)
n	647	537	110
Mean	5.38 (3.77; 7.02)	5.24 (3.63; 6.9)	4.86 (3.26; 6.46)

($p < 0.0001$, resp.) throughout the study period ($p < 0.0001$, resp.) and at the end of this study at an age of 16 years ($p < 0.0001$, resp.).

Interestingly, girls and boys with a satisfactory metabolic control exhibited a lower BMI-SDS than those with a mean HbA1c > 7.5% over the observation period. 16-year-old girls with adequate metabolic control had a BMI-SDS of +0.5 (interquartile range −0.05 to 1.0) versus +0.67 (interquartile range 0.25 to 1.13) in girls with poor metabolic control. In 16-year-old boys, the BMI-SDS was +0.15 (interquartile range −0.43 to 0.64) in those with good metabolic control versus +0.24 (interquartile range −0.37 to 0.69) in those with poor metabolic control.

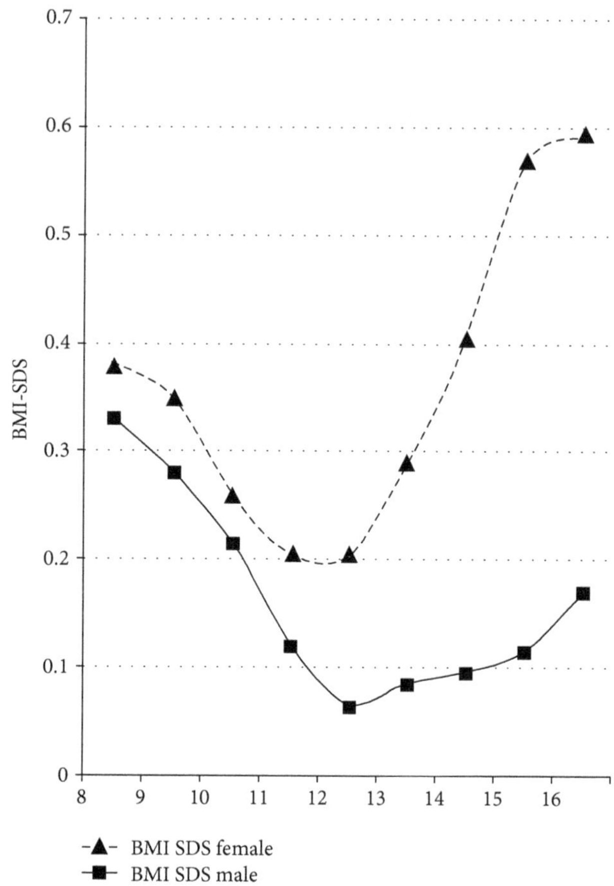

FIGURE 6: Gender-specific course of BMI-SDS before and during puberty.

3.5. Self-Monitoring of Blood Glucose (SMBG). Documented blood glucose self-monitoring frequency was not significantly different between girls and boys. The reported frequency of all patients, independent of treatment regimes, increased from the age of seven (mean 4.97 measurements per day) to 12 (mean 5.43 measurements per day) and declined afterwards. At 16 years of age, the reported frequency was not different from that with seven years of age. The mean SMBG over the whole period of time was 5.2 measurements a day. Girls and boys with a good mean HbA1c had a higher SMBG (arithmetical mean good HbA1c versus poor HbA1c: 5.5 versus 4.95 SMBG) than those with an inadequate metabolic control. In the course of the data collection and passing time, the percentage of patients using an insulin pump treatment increased from 1% to 36%.

Those patients who were using an insulin pump exhibited a higher frequency of SMBG in all age groups compared to patients using ICT. In both groups (ICT and CSII), the SMBG frequency declined with age. At the age of seven years, the mean SMBG was 4.97 for ICT versus 6.52 SMBG with insulin pump treatment. At the age of sixteen years, SMBG was 4.77 (ICT) versus 5.36 (CSII). Taken together, SMBG frequency in this cohort was influenced by age, time period, and mode of insulin treatment.

4. Discussion

Adherence to diabetes therapy and consecutive metabolic control in adolescent type 1 diabetes is challenging. Furthermore, diabetes control in puberty is modulated by a change in synthesis and secretion of several hormones, including growth hormone, which associate with changes in insulin sensitivity. In this longitudinal study, we found significant gender differences regarding metabolic control during puberty and marked differences with regard to gender-specific growth patterns.

Pubertal growth is characterized by the so-called pubertal growth spurt with a puberty-related increase of growth velocity. Change of growth velocity is a reliable sign of puberty [14]. In our study, we found that timing of pubertal growth spurt in girls and boys with T1DM did not differ from the healthy control described by Brandt and Reinken. However, mean growth velocity in diabetic boys at the time of maximal growth spurt was significantly reduced by 1.2 cm/year compared to that in healthy boys. In girls, we found no difference in median maximal growth velocity, which might be due to the relatively flat female pubertal growth spurt in comparison to the more pronounced male pubertal growth spurt. However, in girls with T1DM, growth velocity declined significantly faster after reaching peak growth velocity than in the reference population.

The reduced growth velocity in puberty can explain the loss of height during the course of diabetes [5]. Boys seem to lose height at the time of maximum growth spurt, whereas girls seem to lose height because of a more rapid decline in growth velocity afterwards. Nevertheless, it is rather relieving that height at the age of 16 years seems to be at exactly the same level like background population height, even though the height at the age of seven years lies above average (SDS +0.17). Whether the taller height at the age of seven reflects differences in the growth pattern of diabetic subjects due to altered nutrient intake and metabolic control remains a subject of speculation.

Several studies with small patient numbers tried to analyse growth data in patients with T1DM. Salerno et al. [6] followed 62 subjects with T1DM from the onset of the disease until final height. At diagnosis, height was above the genetic target height, but in the following years, they saw, similar to our results, a reduced height gain. The authors were not able to explain these findings, as it seemed to be independent of the duration of T1DM or of metabolic control. Ahmed et al. [15] examined 46 children with T1DM. Height was measured every three months, and bone age was assessed annually. In addition, HbA1c, IGF-I, and C-peptide were analysed. Similar to our study, the timing of peak height velocity was in the normal range in both sexes. However, in contrast to our study, maximum growth spurt was reduced in girls, but not in boys. In their study, bone age of girls with T1DM was advanced at the onset of puberty, potentially explaining the different findings. In a cohort of 72 Sudanese diabetic children who were treated with a conventional insulin regime using purified bovine insulin, growth velocity between diagnosis and final height was slow with a significant reduction in pubertal growth spurt [16]. The metabolic control of this cohort was rather poor with a mean HbA1c level of 9.8%. As expected, adolescents with poor metabolic control showed a more impaired growth velocity compared to patients with a satisfactory mean HbA1c over the whole period of time.

In accordance with others, we found an increase in mean HbA1c levels during puberty, which were clearly above target HbA1c levels recommended in current guidelines [7, 8, 17, 18].

In contrast to most other studies, concerning growth in diabetes, metabolic control in our collective was still quite good [16].

For nearly the whole period of puberty from ten to 16 years of age, boys had a lower mean HbA1c concentration than girls. This is in accordance with the majority of other studies demonstrating a sex difference with worse metabolic control in females [4, 19–22]. Only a few studies were not able to find differences in metabolic control between men and women [7, 15]. Indeed, for a short interval of 1.5 years, our data showed a higher mean HbA1c concentration in boys compared to diabetic girls. Interestingly, this covered the period of maximum male pubertal growth spurt. Puberty and especially pubertal growth spurt are triggered by an interaction of gonadotropic (GnRH-LH/FSH-sex steroid) and somatotropic (GH-IGF-1) hormone axes [23]. Estrogens lead to an increase in the amplitude of pulsatile GH secretion; GH opposes insulin effects on glucose metabolism with GH overexposure typically resulting in impaired glucose homeostatic control. Androgens play a major role in the dramatic change in linear growth during puberty [24]. It is a well-known phenomenon that the increase of growth velocity is more pronounced in boys than in girls; this may be a consequence of higher GH amplitude in males compared to females. Furthermore, this increase in GH secretion might be responsible for a more pronounced dawn phenomenon in boys and therefore might underlie a deterioration of metabolic control around the maximum growth spurt. In contrast to boys, in our study, the highest mean HbA1c increase in girls was not associated with pubertal growth spurt but took place after the main hormonal changes characterizing female puberty. Hormonal differences [4] and different coping with a chronic disease may therefore play a role in the observed gender differences in glucose control during puberty [22]. Other causative factors for higher mean HbA1c concentration in females could be the higher prevalence of eating disorders and insulin purging, which might be of higher importance regarding growth as compared to a temporary impaired metabolic control [25–27].

Hoey and the Hvidoere study group could show that the quality of life (QoL) plays an important role in achieving a good metabolic control and that this score is typically worse in girls [28].

In addition, worse metabolic control in females could be modulated by the gender difference in weight development. The girls included in our cohort showed a significantly higher mean BMI-SDS than boys, especially at the age of

15-16 years, with a higher risk to become obese [13]. Higher BMI-SDS in adolescents with T1DM was described earlier [7, 29] and could have a negative influence on insulin sensitivity. This is supported by another study demonstrating greater insulin resistance in girls than boys during puberty [30].

In addition, hormonal changes and increasing insulin resistance during puberty [25, 31], treatment adherence, and family dynamics significantly influence metabolic control and HbA1c [28, 32]. A previous analysis of DPV data from 1995–2006 showed that self-monitoring of blood glucose (SMBG) declined with age and was lowest in children aged > 12 years. Additional SMBG up to five measurements per day improved metabolic control (HbA1c) especially in adolescents [33]. Our data underline that a higher frequency of SMBG is associated with a better HbA1c. Still, the differences were small and not statistically significant. Since DPV uses patient-reported SMBG and relies on the correctness of the patients' report, we cannot exclude that patients with worse metabolic control incorrectly answered the SMBG frequency.

Our study has several limitations: (a) target height of most patients was not available since this is not part of the routine data collection. (b) Documentation of Tanner stages was available only in 13% and was thus not included in our analysis. (c) Due to strict requirement of a sufficient auxological dataset in DPV, a large number of patients documented in DPV were not suitable and had to be excluded. However, patients that had to be excluded due to lack of auxological data did not differ regarding diabetes duration, therapy, or diabetes control. Still, the patient number of our study still remains significantly larger than that of all previous reports. (d) Since our population had its diabetes manifestation at the age of seven or younger, it is a specific group of diabetes patients. Growth patterns of patients who were older at the onset of the disease may be different. (e) In this study, we used relatively old reference data, since these in contrast to the more recent growth data had been collected longitudinally. We thus cannot exclude that this might have an impact on the interpretation of height data at the age sixteen years, although in Germany in recent decades there has been only a minor secular trend in height.

In conclusion, we found only a minor albeit significant affection of the growth pattern in diabetic subjects compared to the reference population. Furthermore, we detected that gender-discordant metabolic impairment during puberty, which in males, but not in females, correlated with peak growth velocity. The discrepancy that growth velocity in boys was more impaired than in girls even though girls' metabolic control was even worse over the whole period of time needs further investigations.

Thus, the care of patients with T1DM during puberty requires an enormous effort from the patient, the family, and the health care team, not only to deal with the psychological challenges of a chronic disease during the difficult period of puberty but also to improve the puberty-related risks for a poor metabolic control, reduced growth, and delayed pubertal development, although the effects on growth seem to be small.

Conflicts of Interest

The authors declare that they have no conflicts of interest.

References

[1] T. Rohrer, E. Stierkorb, S. Heger et al., "Delayed pubertal onset and development in German children and adolescents with type 1 diabetes: cross-sectional analysis of recent data from the DPV diabetes documentation and quality management system," *European Journal of Endocrinology*, vol. 151, pp. 647–653, 2007.

[2] T. Rohrer, E. Stierkorb, M. Grabert et al., "Delayed menarche in young German women with type 1 diabetes mellitus: recent results from the DPV diabetes documentation and quality management system," *European Journal of Pediatrics*, vol. 16, pp. 793–799, 2008.

[3] K. K. Danielson, M. Palta, C. Allen, and D. J. D'Alessio, "The association of increased total glycosylated hemoglobin levels with delayed age at menarche in young women with type 1 diabetes," *The Journal of Clinical Endocrinology and Metabolism*, vol. 90, no. 12, pp. 6466–6471, 2005.

[4] E. Codner and F. Cassorla, "Puberty and ovarian function in girls with type 1 diabetes mellitus," *Hormone Research*, vol. 71, no. 1, pp. 12–21, 2009.

[5] W. Bonfig, T. Kapellen, A. Dost et al., "Growth in children and adolescents with type 1 diabetes," *The Journal of Pediatrics*, vol. 160, no. 6, pp. 900–903, 2012.

[6] M. Salerno, A. Argenziano, S. Di Maio et al., "Pubertal growth, sexual maturation, and final height in children with IDDM: effects of age at onset and metabolic control," *Diabetes Care*, vol. 20, no. 5, pp. 721–724, 1997.

[7] M. O'Hagan, J. N. Harvey, and for the Brecon Group, "Glycemic control in children with type 1 diabetes in wales: influence of the pediatric diabetes specialist nurse," *Diabetes Care*, vol. 33, no. 8, pp. 1724–1726, 2010.

[8] R. W. Holl, P. G. Swift, H. B. Mortensen et al., "Insulin injection regimens and metabolic control in an international survey of adolescents with type 1 diabetes over 3 years: results from the Hvidore study group," *European Journal of Pediatrics*, vol. 162, no. 1, pp. 22–29, 2003.

[9] J. Hamilton and D. Daneman, "Deteriorating diabetes control during adolescence: physiological or psychosocial?," *Journal of Pediatric Endocrinology and Metabolism*, vol. 15, no. 2, pp. 115–126, 2002.

[10] I. Brandt and L. Reinken, "The growth rate of healthy children in the first 16 years: Bonn-Dortmund longitudinal developmental study," *Klinische Pädiatrie*, vol. 200, no. 6, pp. 451–456, 1988.

[11] T. J. Cole, "The LMS method for constructing normalized growth standards," *European Journal of Clinical Nutrition*, vol. 44, no. 1, pp. 45–60, 1990.

[12] H. Stolzenberg, H. Khal, and K. E. Bergmann, "Body measurements of children and adolescents in Germany. Results of the German health interview and examination survey for children and adolescents (KiGGS)," *Bundesgesundheitsblatt - Gesundheitsforschung - Gesundheitsschutz*, vol. 50, no. 5-6, pp. 659–669, 2007.

[13] A. Schaffrath Rosario, B. M. Kurth, H. Stolzenberg, U. Ellert, and H. Neuhauser, "Body mass index percentiles for children and adolescents in Germany based on a nationally

representative sample (KiGGS 2003–2006)," *European Journal of Clinical Nutrition*, vol. 64, no. 4, pp. 341–349, 2010.

[14] L. Aksglaede, L. W. Olsen, T. Sorensen, and A. Juul, "Forty years trends in timing of pubertal growth spurt in 157,000 Danish school children," *PLoS One*, vol. 3, no. 7, article e2728, 2008.

[15] M. L. Ahmed, M. H. Connors, N. M. Drayer, J. S. Jones, and D. B. Dunger, "Pubertal growth in ID DM is determined by HbA1c levels, sex, and bone age," *Diabetes Care*, vol. 21, no. 5, pp. 831–835, 1998.

[16] A. Elamin, O. Hussein, and T. Tuvemo, "Growth, puberty, and final height in children with type 1 diabetes," *Journal of Diabetes and its Complications*, vol. 20, no. 4, pp. 252–256, 2006.

[17] The Diabetes Control and Complications Trial Research Group, "The effect of intensive treatment of diabetes on the development and progression of long-term complications in insulin-dependent diabetes mellitus," *The New England Journal of Medicine*, vol. 329, no. 14, pp. 977–986, 1993.

[18] K. K. Hood, C. M. Peterson, J. M. Rohan, and D. Drotar, "Association between adherence and glycemic control in pediatric type 1 diabetes: a meta-analysis," *Pediatrics*, vol. 124, no. 6, pp. 1171–1179, 2009.

[19] E. M. Gerstl, W. Rabl, J. Rosenbauer et al., "Metabolic control as reflected by HbA1c in children, adolescents and young adults with type-1 diabetes mellitus: combined longitudinal analysis including 27,035 patients from 207 centers in Germany and Austria during the last decade," *European Journal of Pediatrics*, vol. 167, no. 4, pp. 447–453, 2008.

[20] A. Setoodeh, F. Mostafavi, A. Rabbani, and T. Hedayat, "Female sex as a risk factor for glycemic control and complications in Iranian patients with type one diabetes mellitus," *Iranian Journal of Pediatrics*, vol. 21, no. 3, pp. 373–378, 2011.

[21] T. Danne, H. B. Mortensen, P. Hougaard et al., "Persistent differences among centers over 3 years in glycemic control and hypoglycemia in a study of 3,805 children and adolescents with type 1 diabetes from the Hvidore study group," *Diabetes Care*, vol. 24, no. 8, pp. 1342–1347, 2001.

[22] K. S. Bryden, R. C. Peveler, A. Stein, A. Neil, R. A. Mayou, and D. B. Dunger, "Clinical and psychological course of diabetes from adolescence to young adulthood: a longitudinal cohort study," *Diabetes Care*, vol. 24, no. 9, pp. 1536–1540, 2001.

[23] A. D. Rogol, "Gender and hormonal regulation of growth," *Journal of Pediatric Endocrinology and Metabolism*, vol. 17, Supplement 4, pp. 1259–1265, 2004.

[24] E. J. Richmond and A. D. Rogol, "Male pubertal development and the role of androgen therapy," *Nature Clinical Practice Endocrinology & Metabolism*, vol. 3, no. 4, pp. 338–344, 2007.

[25] S. T. Philippi, M. G. Cardoso, P. Koritar, and M. Alvarenga, "Risk behaviors for eating disorder in adolescents and adults with type 1 diabetes," *Revista Brasileira de Psiquiatria*, vol. 35, no. 2, pp. 150–156, 2013.

[26] D. Neumark-Sztainer, J. Patterson, A. Mellin et al., "Weight control practices and disordered eating behaviors among adolescent females and males with type 1 diabetes: associations with sociodemographics, weight concerns, familial factors, and metabolic outcomes," *Diabetes Care*, vol. 25, no. 8, pp. 1289–1296, 2002.

[27] N. Scheuing, B. Bartus, G. Berger et al., "Clinical characteristics and outcome of 467 patients with a clinically recognized eating disorder identified among 52,215 patients with type 1 diabetes mellitus: a multicenter German/Austrian study," *Diabetes Care*, vol. 37, no. 6, pp. 1581–1589, 2014.

[28] H. Hoey and on behalf of the Hvidoere Study Group on Childhood Diabetes, "Psychosocial factors are associated with metabolic control in adolescents: research from the Hvidoere study group in childhood diabetes," *Pediatric Diabetes*, vol. 10, Supplement 13, pp. 9–14, 2009.

[29] R. W. Holl, M. Grabert, W. Sorgo, E. Heinze, and K. M. Debatin, "Contributions of age, gender and insulin administration to weight gain in subjects with IDDM," *Diabetologia*, vol. 41, no. 5, pp. 542–547, 1998.

[30] A. Szadkowska, I. Pietrzak, B. Mianowska et al., "Insulin sensitivity in type 1 diabetic children and adolescents," *Diabetic Medicine*, vol. 25, no. 3, pp. 282–288, 2008.

[31] J. Raab, F. Haupt, O. Kondonouri et al., "Continuous rise of insulin resistance before and after the onset of puberty in children at increased risk for type 1 diabetes – a cross-sectional analysis," *Diabetes/Metabolism Research and Reviews*, vol. 29, no. 8, pp. 631–635, 2013.

[32] J. M. Rausch, K. K. Hood, A. Delamater et al., "Changes in treatment adherence and glycemic control during the transition to adolescence in type 1 diabetes," *Diabetes Care*, vol. 35, no. 6, pp. 1219–1224, 2012.

[33] R. Ziegler, B. Heidtmann, D. Hilgrad et al., "Frequency of SMBG correlates with HbA1c and acute complications in children and adolescents with type 1 diabetes," *Pediatric Diabetes*, vol. 12, no. 1, pp. 11–17, 2011.

Permissions

All chapters in this book were first published in JDR, by Hindawi Publishing Corporation; hereby published with permission under the Creative Commons Attribution License or equivalent. Every chapter published in this book has been scrutinized by our experts. Their significance has been extensively debated. The topics covered herein carry significant findings which will fuel the growth of the discipline. They may even be implemented as practical applications or may be referred to as a beginning point for another development.

The contributors of this book come from diverse backgrounds, making this book a truly international effort. This book will bring forth new frontiers with its revolutionizing research information and detailed analysis of the nascent developments around the world.

We would like to thank all the contributing authors for lending their expertise to make the book truly unique. They have played a crucial role in the development of this book. Without their invaluable contributions this book wouldn't have been possible. They have made vital efforts to compile up to date information on the varied aspects of this subject to make this book a valuable addition to the collection of many professionals and students.

This book was conceptualized with the vision of imparting up-to-date information and advanced data in this field. To ensure the same, a matchless editorial board was set up. Every individual on the board went through rigorous rounds of assessment to prove their worth. After which they invested a large part of their time researching and compiling the most relevant data for our readers.

The editorial board has been involved in producing this book since its inception. They have spent rigorous hours researching and exploring the diverse topics which have resulted in the successful publishing of this book. They have passed on their knowledge of decades through this book. To expedite this challenging task, the publisher supported the team at every step. A small team of assistant editors was also appointed to further simplify the editing procedure and attain best results for the readers.

Apart from the editorial board, the designing team has also invested a significant amount of their time in understanding the subject and creating the most relevant covers. They scrutinized every image to scout for the most suitable representation of the subject and create an appropriate cover for the book.

The publishing team has been an ardent support to the editorial, designing and production team. Their endless efforts to recruit the best for this project, has resulted in the accomplishment of this book. They are a veteran in the field of academics and their pool of knowledge is as vast as their experience in printing. Their expertise and guidance has proved useful at every step. Their uncompromising quality standards have made this book an exceptional effort. Their encouragement from time to time has been an inspiration for everyone.

The publisher and the editorial board hope that this book will prove to be a valuable piece of knowledge for researchers, students, practitioners and scholars across the globe.

List of Contributors

Byung-Seop Shin, Jong-Hwan Lee, Dae Kyun Ryu, Sojin Kim and Young Hee Shin
Department of Anesthesiology and Pain Medicine, Samsung Medical Center, Sungkyunkwan University School of Medicine, Seoul, Republic of Korea

Jeong Jin Min
Department of Anesthesiology and Pain Medicine, Samsung Medical Center, Sungkyunkwan University School of Medicine, Seoul, Republic of Korea
Department of Anesthesiology and Pain Medicine, Seoul National University Hospital, Seoul National University College of Medicine, Seoul, Republic of Korea

Yunseok Jeon
Department of Anesthesiology and Pain Medicine, Seoul National University Hospital, Seoul National University College of Medicine, Seoul, Republic of Korea

Nina Nielens, Olivier Pollé and Philippe A. Lysy
Pediatric Endocrinology Unit, Cliniques Universitaires Saint Luc, Av. Hippocrate 10, 1200 Brussels, Belgium

Annie Robert
Pôle Epidémiologie et Biostatistique, Institut de Recherche Expérimentale et Clinique, Université Catholique de Louvain, Av. Hippocrate 10, 1200 Brussels, Belgium
Ignacio Rodríguez-Rodríguez and Miguel-Ángel Zamora-Izquierdo
Universidad de Murcia, Spain

José-Víctor Rodríguez
Universidad Politécnica de Cartagena, Spain

Qixian Wang, Min Long, Hua Qu, Rufei Shen, Rui Zhang, Jing Xu, Xin Xiong, Hui Wang and Hongting Zheng
Department of Endocrinology, Xinqiao Hospital, Third Military Medical University, Chongqing 400037, China

Katerina Stechova and Pavlina Pithova
Department of Internal Medicine, 2nd Medical Faculty, Charles University and University Hospital Motol, Prague, Czech Republic

Jana Sklenarova-Labikova
Department of Paediatrics, 2nd Medical Faculty, Charles University and University Hospital Motol, Prague, Czech Republic

Tereza Kratzerova
Department of Physiology, 2nd Medical Faculty, Charles University, Prague, Czech Republic

Dominik Filipp
Laboratory of Immunobiology, Institute of Molecular Genetics of the ASCR, Prague, Czech Republic

Masahito Katahira
Aichi Prefectural University School of Nursing and Health, Nagoya 463-8502, Japan
Department of Endocrinology and Diabetes, Ichinomiya Municipal Hospital, Ichinomiya 491 8558, Japan
Department of Endocrinology and Diabetes, Ichinomiya Municipal Hospital, Ichinomiya 491 8558, Japan

Hidetada Ogata, Takahiro Ito, Tsutomu Miwata, Megumi Goto and Hiromi Takashima
Department of Endocrinology and Diabetes, Ichinomiya Municipal Hospital, Ichinomiya 491 8558, Japan

Shizuka Nakamura
Department of Endocrinology and Diabetes, Ichinomiya Municipal Hospital, Ichinomiya 491 8558, Japan
Department of General Internal Medicine, Matsunami General Hospital, Gifu 501-6062, Japan

Dan Yan, Qiqi Zhu, Jun Li and Qingquan Lian
Department of Anesthesiology, The Second Affiliated Hospital and Yuying Children's Hospital, Wenzhou Medical University, Wenzhou, China

Xiang Xie
Department of Anesthesiology, The Second Affiliated Hospital and Yuying Children's Hospital, Wenzhou Medical University, Wenzhou, China
Department of Anesthesiology, The University of Hong Kong, Pok Fu Lam, Hong Kong

Haobo Li, Chi Wai Cheung, Michael G. Irwin and Zhengyuan Xia
Department of Anesthesiology, The University of Hong Kong, Pok Fu Lam, Hong Kong

Yong-ping Fang
Department of General Surgery, Huizhou First Hospital, Huizhou, Guangdong, China

Joanna Gołębiewska, Andrzej Olechowski, Agnieszka Czeszyk-Piotrowicz and Wojciech Hautz
Department of Ophthalmology, The Children's Memorial Health Institute, Aleja Dzieci Polskich 20, Warsaw, Poland

Marta Wysocka-Mincewicz, Marta Baszyńska-Wilk and Artur Groszek
Department of Diabetology and Endocrinology, The Children's Memorial Health Institute, Aleja Dzieci Polskich 20, Warsaw, Poland

Mieczysław Szalecki
Department of Diabetology and Endocrinology, The Children's Memorial Health Institute, Aleja Dzieci Polskich 20, Warsaw, Poland
Department of Medicine and Health Sciences, UJK, Kielce, Poland

Tereza Vitvarová and David Neumann
Department of Pediatrics, University Hospital Hradec Kralove, Faculty of Medicine in Hradec Kralove, Charles University, Hradec Kralove, Czech Republic
Radka Šimáková
Philosophy Faculty, Palacky University Olomouc, Olomouc, Czech Republic

Jan Kremláček
Department of Pathological Physiology, Faculty of Medicine in Hradec Kralove, Charles University, Hradec Kralove, Czech Republic

Eleanor Race Mackey, Marni Jacobs and Randi Streisand
Children's National Health System, Psychology, Washington, DC, USA
University of Toronto, Toronto, Ontario, Canada

Lyndsay O'Brecht
University of Toronto, Toronto, Ontario, Canada

Clarissa S. Holmes
Virginia Commonwealth University, Pediatrics, Richmond, VA, USA
Georgetown University, Psychiatry, Washington, DC, USA

Chenyue Qian, Aiming Shi and Jie Pan
Department of Pharmacy, The Second Affiliated Hospital of Soochow University, Suzhou 215004, China

Heming Guo, Xiaohong Chen, Sicheng Li and Chen Fang
Department of Endocrinology, The Second Affiliated Hospital of Soochow University, Suzhou 215004, China

Xin Wang
Department of Endocrinology, Jiangsu Province Hospital of TCM, 155 Hanzhonglu, Jiangsu Nanjing 210029, China

Elzbieta Wierzbicka
Department of Human Nutrition, Warsaw University of Life Sciences (SGGW), Warsaw, Poland

Anna Swiercz
Department of Endocrinology and Diabetology, The Children's Memorial Health Institute, Warsaw, Poland

Pawel Pludowski and Maciej Jaworski
Department of Biochemistry, Radioimmunology and Experimental Medicine, The Children's Memorial Health Institute, Warsaw, Poland

Mieczyslaw Szalecki
Department of Endocrinology and Diabetology, The Children's Memorial Health Institute, Warsaw, Poland
Faculty of Medicine and Health Sciences, Jan Kochanowski University, Kielce, Poland

Ewa Rusak
Department of Pediatrics and Children's Diabetology, Medical University of Silesia, 40-752 Katowice, Poland

Anna Rotarska-Mizera and Joanna Polanska
Data Mining Division, Faculty of Automatic Control, Electronics and Computer Science, Silesian University of Technology, 44-100 Gliwice, Poland

Piotr Adamczyk and Bogdan Mazur
Department of Pediatrics, School of Medicine with the Division of Dentistry in Zabrze, Medical University of Silesia, 40-752 Katowice, Poland

Agata Chobot
Department of Pediatric Gastroenterology and Hepatology, Clinical Hospital No. 1, 41-800 Zabrze, Poland

Syed Wasif Gillani, Hisham A. Zaghloul and Mohi Iqbal Mohammad Abdul
College of Pharmacy, Taibah University, Al Madinah Al Munawarah, Saudi Arabia

Irfan Altaf Ansari
Department of Pathology, College of Medicine, Taibah University, Al Madinah Al Munawarah, Saudi Arabia

Syed Azhar Syed Sulaiman and Hassaan Anwar Rathore
School of Pharmaceutical Sciences, Universiti Sains Malaysia (USM), Penang, Malaysia

Mirza R. Baig
Dubai Pharmacy College, Dubai, UAE

M. Matta, C. Laporte, I. Berdugo and H. Hanaire
Service de Diabétologie et maladies métaboliques, CHU de Toulouse, 1 avenue Jean Poulhès, 31059 Toulouse Cedex 9, France

A. Pavy-Le Traon and N. Nasr
Service de Neurologie, Hôpital Pierre-Paul Riquet, Place du Docteur Baylac-TSA 40031, 31059 Toulouse Cedex 9, France
Institut des Maladies Métaboliques et Cardiovasculaires, INSERM, Université de Toulouse, 1 avenue Jean Poulhès, BP 84225, 31432 Toulouse Cedex 4, France

J. M. Senard
Institut des Maladies Métaboliques et Cardiovasculaires, INSERM, Université de Toulouse, 1 avenue Jean Poulhès, BP 84225, 31432 Toulouse Cedex 4, France
Service de Pharmacologie Clinique, Faculté de Médecine, CHU de Toulouse, 37 allées Jules Guesde, 31000 Toulouse, France

S. Perez-Lloret
Institute of Cardiology Research, University of Buenos Aires, National Research Council (CONICET-ININCA), Buenos Aires, Argentina

Datis Kharrazian
Harvard Medical School, Boston, MA, USA
TRANSCEND Research, Department of Neurology, Massachusetts General Hospital, Charlestown, Boston, MA 02129, USA
Department of Preventive Medicine, Loma Linda University School of Medicine, Loma Linda, CA, USA

Martha Herbert
Harvard Medical School, Boston, MA, USA
TRANSCEND Research, Department of Neurology, Massachusetts General Hospital, Charlestown, Boston, MA 02129, USA

Aristo Vojdani
Department of Preventive Medicine, Loma Linda University School of Medicine, Loma Linda, CA, USA
Immunosciences Laboratory, Inc., Los Angeles, CA, USA

Jiayin Zheng, Song Han, Yanlin Luo, Xiuli Sun, Ning Zhu, Li Zhao and Junfa Li
Department of Neurobiology and Center of Stroke, Beijing Institute for Brain Disorders, Capital Medical University, Beijing 100069, China

Yue Wang
Department of Neurology, Beijing Chaoyang Hospital, Capital Medical University, Beijing, China

Beatriz Tavira, Hugo Barcenilla and Rosaura Casas
Division of Pediatrics, Department of Clinical and Experimental Medicine, Faculty of Medicine and Health Sciences, Linköping University, Linköping, Sweden

Jeannette Wahlberg
Department of Endocrinology and Department of Medical and Health Sciences and Department of Clinical and Experimental Medicine, Linköping University, Linköping, Sweden

Peter Achenbach
Institute of Diabetes Research, Helmholtz Zentrum München and Forschergruppe Diabetes, Klinikum Rechts der Isar, Technische Universität München, München, Germany

Johnny Ludvigsson
Division of Pediatrics, Department of Clinical and Experimental Medicine, Faculty of Medicine and Health Sciences, Linköping University, Linköping, Sweden
Crown Princess Victoria Children's Hospital, Region Östergötland, Linköping, Sweden

Murat Karaoglan
Division of Pediatric Endocrinology, Gaziantep University Faculty of Medicine, Gaziantep, Turkey

Fahriye Eksi
Department of Medical Microbiology, Gaziantep University Faculty of Medicine, Gaziantep, Turkey

Matthew W. McDonald, Michelle S. Dotzert, Mao Jiang, Michael R. Murray and C. W. James Melling
Exercise Biochemistry Laboratory, School of Kinesiology, Western University, London, ON, Canada

Earl G. Noble
Exercise Biochemistry Laboratory, School of Kinesiology, Western University, London, ON, Canada
Lawson Health Research Institute, London, ON, Canada

John E. Bylander
Department of Environmental Sciences, Pennsylvania State University, Harrisburg, Middletown, PA 17057, USA

Faihaa Ahmed, Sabena M. Conley, Jean-Marie Mwiza and Elimelda Moige Ongeri
Department of Biology, North Carolina A&T State University, Greensboro, NC 27411, USA

Elizabeth Duarte Gómez and Miriam Castrati Nostas
Centro Vivir con Diabetes, Av. Simón López, No. 375, Cochabamba, Bolivia

Gabriel Andrew Gregory
International Diabetes Federation Life for a Child Program, Glebe, NSW 2037, Australia
NHMRC Clinical Trials Centre, University of Sydney, Sydney, NSW 2006, Australia

Graham David Ogle
International Diabetes Federation Life for a Child Program, Glebe, NSW 2037, Australia
NHMRC Clinical Trials Centre, University of Sydney, Sydney, NSW 2006, Australia
Diabetes NSW, Glebe, NSW 2037, Australia

Alicia Josephine Jenkins
NHMRC Clinical Trials Centre, University of Sydney, Sydney, NSW 2006, Australia

Angela Christine Middlehurst
International Diabetes Federation Life for a Child Program, Glebe, NSW 2037, Australia
Diabetes NSW, Glebe, NSW 2037, Australia

Fabiana Picconi, Laura Chioma and Simona Frontoni
Unit of Endocrinology, Diabetes and Metabolism, S. Giovanni Calibita Fatebenefratelli Hospital, Department of Systems Medicine, University of Rome Tor Vergata, Rome, Italy

Giorgia Mataluni and Girolama Alessandra Marfia
Unit of Disimmune Neuropathies, Department of Systems Medicine, University of Rome Tor Vergata, Rome, Italy

Lucia Ziccardi, Mariacristina Parravano and Antonio Di Renzo
IRCCS-G.B. Bietti Foundation, Rome, Italy

Dorina Ylli
Division of Endocrinology MedStar Washington Hospital Center, MedStar Health Research Institute, Washington, DC, USA

Patrizio Pasqualetti
Fatebenefratelli Foundation for Health Research and Education, AFaR Division, Rome, Italy

Valeria Studer
Unit of Disimmune Neuropathies, Department of Systems Medicine, University of Rome Tor Vergata, Rome, Italy
Neuroimmunology and Neuromuscolar Diseases Unit, Foundation IRCCS Neurological Institute Carlo Besta, Milan, Italy

M. Plamper, B. Gohlke and J. Woelfle
Pediatric Endocrinology Division, Children's Hospital, University of Bonn, Bonn, Germany

K. Konrad
Department of Pediatrics and Adolescent Medicine, University of Cologne, Cologne, Germany
Department of Pediatric and Adolescent Medicine, Elisabeth Hospital Essen, Essen, Germany

T. Rohrer
Department of Pediatrics, University of Saarland, Homburg, Germany

S. Hofer
Department of Pediatrics, University of Innsbruck, Innsbruck, Austria

W. Bonfig
Department of Pediatrics, Technical University Munich, Munich, Germany
Department of Pediatrics, Klinikum Wels-Grieskirchen, Wels, Austria

K. Fink and R. W. Holl
Institute for Epidemiology and Medical Biometry, ZIBMT University of Ulm and German Center for Diabetes Research (DZD), Neuherberg, München, Germany

Index

www.ingramcontent.com/pod-product-compliance
Lightning Source LLC
LaVergne TN
LVHW060536210926
848485LV00005B/1212